GW00722680

REGIONAL OPIOID ANALGESIA

DEVELOPMENTS IN CRITICAL CARE MEDICINE AND ANESTHESIOLOGY

Volume 20

Regional Opioid Analgesia

Physiopharmacological Basis, Drugs, Equipment and Clinical Application

by

J. DE CASTRO, M.D.
Department of Anaesthesiology, Université Libre de Bruxelles,
Hôpital St. Pierre, Bruxelles, Belgium

J. MEYNADIER, M.D.
Department of Anaesthesiology and Intensive Care,
Centre Oscar Lambret, Lille, France

M. ZENZ, M.D.
University Clinic for Anaesthesiology, Critical Care and Pain Management,
Bergmannsheil Bochum, Germany

Preface by
E.K. ZSIGMOND, M.D.
Chicago

Introduction by
T.L. YAKSH, Ph.D.
San Diego

Kluwer Academic Publishers
DORDRECHT / BOSTON / LONDON

Library of Congress Cataloging-in-Publication Data

Castro, J. de.
Regional opioid analgesia: physiopharmacological basis, drugs, equipment, and clinical application/ J. de Castro, J. Meynadier, M. Zenz.
     p.   cm.   -- (Developments in critical care medicine and anaesthesiology)
Includes index
ISBN 0-7923-0162-5 (U.S.)
1. Opioids -- Therapeutic use. 2. Conduction anaesthesia. 3. Analgesia. I. Meynadier, J. (Jacques)
II. Zenz. M. (Michael) III. Title. IV. Series.
[DNLM: 1. Analgesics -- therapeutic use. 2. Analgesics, Addictive -- therapeutic use. 3. Endorphins
-- therapeutic use 4. Pain -- drug therapy. QV 89 C355r]
RD86.064C37 1989
617.9'6 -- dc20
DNLM/DLC
for Library of Congress   89-2557

ISBN-13: 978-94-010-7543-5   e-ISBN-13: 978-94-009-2321-8
DOI: 10.1007/978-94-009-2321-8

Published by Kluwer Academic Publishers,
P.O. Box 17, 3300 AA Dordrecht, The Netherlands

Kluwer Academic Publishers incorporates
the publishing programmes of
D. Reidel, Martinus Nijhoff, Dr. W. Junk and MTP Press.

Sold and distributed in the U.S.A. and Canada
by Kluwer Academic Publishers,
101 Philip Drive, Norwell, MA 02061, U.S.A.

In all other countries, sold and distributed
by Kluwer Academic Publishers Group,
P.O. Box 322, 3300 AH Dordrecht, The Netherlands.

Printed on acid-free paper

In Memoriam

Joris de Castro
* 9 November 1918 – † 8 October 1990

Acknowledgements

We acknowledge with gratitude the valuable discussion we had with Prof. Ph. Bromage concerning the first version of our manuscript, and thank him most sincerely for his helpful criticisms stemming from that discussion.

We are also extremely grateful to Mrs. E. Weihs who didn't give up while preparing some 10 versions of the tables, figures and bibliography.

Our special thanks go to all our patients from whom we have learned most of our knowledge of regional opioid analgesia.

Preface

by E.K. ZSIGMOND, M.D.
Department of Anesthesiology
University of Illinois
Chicago
U.S.A.

It is, indeed, a distinct honor and privilege to be invited by the authors to write a preface to this monumental monograph, Regional Opioid Analgesia.

Regional Opioid Analgesia is a colossal undertaking by Drs. De Castro, Meynadier and Zenz shortly after the introduction of this revolutionary approach to pain relief which opened a new epoch in analgesiology. This is, indeed, the first authentic and comprehensive textbook encompassing the current knowledge on this novel approach to pain relief. We are indebted to the authors for introducing the new opioids to regional analgesia with the scientists, who developed the potent short and ultrashort acting opioids with high therapeutic indices, which many researchers dreamt about but never before materialized. The side effect liabilities of these new opioids are minute as compared to morphine and meperidine.

Regional Opioid Analgesia could not have been more authentically written than by Drs. De Castro,Zenz and Meynadier,who have conducted daily clinical investigations on all known opioids for regional analgesia as well as for neurolept analgesia. Therein lies the great value of this monograph: it is the most authentic work on this topic.

It was my good fortune to have met Dr. De Castro more than a quarter of a century ago. He gave me inspiration for hundreds of clinical investigations which benefited thousands of patients. From my personal acquaintance and visits with Dr. De Castro, I learned a great deal about his exceptional skills as a teacher. The text, tables and artistic figures of his own design unveil his genius as a didacta; an artist as well as a computer expert. Much of the educational material was organized and designed by the aid of his own computer in such a lucid way that the reader immediately grasps the essential correlations. Even clinicians not well versed in research can easily comprehend the basics of clinical pharmacology and pharmacokinetics of opioids, equipments and clinical applications. The monograph superbly fulfils its mission expressed in its subtitle.

Regional Opioid Analgesia ought to find its place on the shelves of all anaesthesia and hospital libraries, since it is not only the most up-to-date reference source for researchers and academicians but also is published at a time of great need for such a book. No doubt, clinicians who practice regional opioid analgesia will consult this monograph daily. The lucid and systematic presentation of the most extensive research information available on regional opioid analgesia will make this book the best reference book for clinicians of all disciplines for many years to come.

Table of contents

PART I: ANATOMICAL, PHARMACOLOGICAL, PHYSIOLOGICAL
AND TECHNICAL BASIS OF SPINAL REGIONAL OPIOID
ADMINISTRATION

The book under eight headings

1. Four new routes for the delivery of opioids as close as possible to their receptor sites producing maximal analgesic effects and using minimal drug amounts:
- epidural route (ED)
- intrathecal route (IT)
- intracerebroventricular route (IC)
- perineural route (PN).

2. Nearly all pure opioids agonists and agonist-antagonists can be administered by these four routes.
- However the opioid solutions must be:
  . preservative free
  . with a pH near to 7.4
  . in low volume.
- Lipophilic opioids (e.g. fentanyl and sufentanil) have real advantages compared to hydrophilic products (e.g. morphine).

3. Four major indications:
- Severe acute pain
  . postoperative pain
  . post-traumatic pain
  . delivery pain.
- Severe chronic pain
  . cancer pain.

4. Four potential side effects:
- respiratory depression
- urinary retention
- pruritus
- nausea, vomiting.
  Reduction of side effects is possible if several technical measures are taken.
  Treatment of side effects with naloxone is effective.

5. Three techniques of administration can be applied:
- repeated bolus
- continuous infusion
- continuous + on-demand administration (the most effective).

6. Chronic pain treatment may require a special equipment of progressive complexity:
- percutaneous catheter
- implanted tunnelled catheter
- implanted injection port
- infusion pump, portable or implanted.

7. A major problem with acute treatment is respiratory depression. It can be prevented by proper indication and adequate technique.

8. A major problem with chronic treatment is tolerance.
It can, however, be delayed by adequate measures.

Abbreviations frequently used in text, tables and figures

Routes of administration		Administered drugs		Goal analgesia	Combined Logo
		Opioid	Local anaesthetic		
epidural	ED ED	O 	 L	A A	EDOA EDLA
intrathecal	IT IT	O 	 L	A A	ITOA ITLA
spinal *	SP SP	O 	 L	A A	SPOA SPLA
intracerebro-ventricular	IC	O		A	ICOA
perineural	PN PN	O 	 L	A A	PNOA PNLA
regional	RG RG	O 	 L	A A	RGOA RGLA
intravenous	IV IV	O 	 L	A A	IVOA IVLA
intramuscular	IM	O		A	IMOA
parenteral	PE	O		A	PEOA
peroral	PO	O		A	POOA
sublingual	SL	O		A	SLOA
subcutaneous	SC	O		A	SCOA

* ED and/or IT = spinal

Introduction

by T.L. YAKSH, PH.D.
Department of Anesthesiology
University of California
San Diego
U.S.A.

The analgesic actions of systemic opioids are well known and their benefits to those in pain are a blessing. The delivery of these agents into the spinal space has resulted in a clinical tool which, its limiting side effects notwithstanding, provides a powerful and selective analgesia. The significance of this use is three-fold. First, spinal opioids practically add an important tool to the therapeutic armamentarium. Second, aside from clinical utility, these analgesic effects are of conceptual significance for they indicate the principle that *specific* facets of spinal cord function can be modified by the local use of receptor selective agents. As such, it is a practical recognition of the pharmacological complexity of the spinal dorsal horn. Thirdly, the historical development and rapid application of spinal opioids provide emphatic support for the premise that:

a fundamental appreciation of the mechanisms by which the nervous system processes sensory information represents the principle route by which rational advances in pain therapy will occur.

In these introductory comments for a scholarly compendium on the clinical use of spinal opioids, I would like to establish a perspective which emphasizes the implications of the above statement.

The physical energy of stimuli, continuously impacting on the inner and outer body surface, is transduced by modality specific nerve terminals into activity in the associated axon. Entering the spinal gray, these afferents make synaptic contact with the dendrites and cell bodies of second order neurons. In the most naive sense, this spinal system could be (and was) thought to serve only a repeater function, with each element faithfully mirroring a certain element of the stimulus environment. However, as in Alice in Wonderland, things are not as they seem. Examination of the afferent input, which excites a dorsal projection neuron, reveals that the most frequent occurrence is a high degree of modality and spatial convergence. Thus, the wide dynamic range neuron in the dorsal horn can be shown to receive excitatory input from AB/A-δ- and C-fibers; from visceral and cutaneous organs (i.e. cardiac sympathetic afferents and cutaneous afferents from the T-4 dermatome); and drive from afferents arising from distant dermatomes (Forman and Ohata 1980). Indeed, dorsal horn neurons have been shown to have whole body receptive fields, these distant inputs arising from long spino-bulbo-spinal excitatory loops (Giesler et al. 1981). In short, the organization of the dorsal horn is not a hard wired set of connections, mirroring the sensory environment, but a very plastic and potentially mutable substrate. The ability to modify the input/output of these convergent nets of dorsal horn neurons provides processing capabilities which far exceeds that possible with the same number of elements hard wired into an array.

However, to make use of this plasticity and to establish the characteristics of the dorsal horn neuronal net, the nervous system must have control over the several elements. This is clearly the case. There is an evolving appreciation by workers in the field that primary afferent input results in the activation of a complex integrative substrate in the dorsal horn which serves to organize, or encode, the information which is to be projected to supraspinal centres. Thus, with increasingly sophisticated physiological preparations, excitatory inputs arising from different classes of afferents have been routinely shown to be subject to powerful and selective facilitations and inhibitions by systems which are pre- and post-synaptic to the primary afferents (Cervero and Iggo 1980). How these influences interact to prepare the message is only poorly understood; yet, it is certain that this modulation in the spinal dorsal horn is mediated by specific intrinsic and bulbospinal systems.

Although the physiological effects noted above appear subtle, our developing sophistication with regard to the pharmacology and biochemistry of the spinal dorsal horn has clearly revealed that it rivals in complexity any region of the brain. Identification of populations of dorsal root ganglion cells and dorsal horn neurons containing one or more of some 10 peptides (Cameron et al. 1988), the demonstration of postsynaptic actions (Gamse an Saria 1986), and the observation of discretely distributed ligand binding sites associated with different subpopulations of neurons and dendrites (Seybold et al. 1986) clearly bodes for an incredible sophistication in the organization of the encoding circuitry. Current evidence, for example, suggests the location of certain small neuropeptides such as substance P, somatostatin and calcitonin gene-related peptide (CGRP) in small high threshold primary afferents (Inagaki and Kito 1986). While these may be released by "painful" stimuli, their role is clearly more complex as the terminals from which peptides are released frequently show multiple populations of synaptic vesicles, suggesting that the coding of the postsynaptic event in the second order neuron depends not upon a single transmitter, but upon the mix of two or more.

From a practical standpoint, the first application of knowledge viz a viz the spinal encoding of sensory information was a simple recognition of the role of the spinal cord as a pathway through which sensory information must pass and hence the utility of agents which could reversibly block all processing, i.e. local anaesthetics. The sophistication of the dorsal horn systems, along with its complex pharmacology, however suggests that the nature of the encoded message may be subtly sensitive to changes in local receptor activity. Thus, early studies emphasized the inhibitory association of opioid receptors with activity evoked by small (C-fiber: high threshold), but not large (AB: low threshold) afferents (Yaksh and Rudy 1978). The development of simple animal models for spinal administration permitted the direct assessment of the role played by these local receptor systems in modulating the behavioural reponse of the intact and unanaesthetized animal and the lack of drug toxicity. Such studies revealed that activation of the respective receptor systems could indeed alter *selectively* the response of the animal to a noxious stimulus, leaving the response to tactile/joint position and autonomic reflex function unchanged (Yaksh 1981). The relevance of spinal opioids to clinical pain has since expanded rapidly over the last 13 years, forming the focus and substance of the present book.

This application of spinal morphine for pain, arising from fundamental studies on spinal cord physiology and pharmacology, is a simple and practical manifestation of the subtle control which may be exerted by specific intrinsic systems over delimited aspects of spinal cord sensory processing. As important is the clinical utility of spinal opioids, it is, however, my opinion that the important outcome of this experience is conceptual: 1) spinal substrates are subject to specific pharmacologic manipulation; and 2) agents administered spinally exert their effects in the absence of an interaction with other supraspinal or peripheral systems which employ the receptor. Given these concepts, the impetus of current research into the complex anatomy, physiology and pharmacology of the spinal cord suggests prominent clinical advances involving the spinal use of receptor selective agents. Three major areas appear even now to herald the future.

First, other modulatory systems have been identified which can modify the dorsal horn response evoked by high threshold primary afferents. For example, adrenergic agonists and the functional effects on spinal pain encoding of the spinal alpha-2-receptor has led to the appreciation of the analgesic efficacy of spinally administered alpha-2-agonists (Yaksh 1985). Other modulatory systems have also been identified (Yaksh and Stevens 1988). Chapter 7 in this book details the even now rapidly developing literature in which alternate modulatory receptor systems may be employed to modify the spinal processing of somatic pain in man.

Second, while the emphasis on modulation has focused on the role it may play in modifying nociceptive input, it is clear from the above comments, that these systems are directed at all aspects of spinal sensory coding. Moreover, it appears that under normal circumstances, these modulatory receptor systems in the dorsal horn neuronal net are activated as part of the intrinsic coding of the sensory stimulus. Thus, it has been shown that high intensity afferent stimuli will activate bulbospinal and intrinsic systems which release noradrenaline and enkephalins, respectively (Tyce and Yaksh 1981; Yaksh and Elde 1981). We may pose the question as to what occurs when these spinal modulatory systems are antagonized? Surprisingly with many of the receptors associated with nociceptive modulation (e.g. opioid and alpha adrenergic), relatively little happens. In contrast, following the loss of other systems, such as those for GABA and glycine, a very prominent allodynea is observed, i.e. a light tactile stimulus, activating only low threshold afferents, is perceived as highly noxious (Yaksh 1989). This gives rise to the perhaps unexpected conclusion that input from high threshold afferents are exposed to little tonic control, while the input from low threshold afferent systems (e.g. light tactile) is under a powerful and pervasive spinal modulation, the loss of which converts the message evoked from an innoxious one to one with a decidedly noxious content. Given the changes in dorsal horn morphology and neurochemistry which occur following peripheral nerve lesions (Sugimoto et al. 1987), it might be speculated that changes in the functional modulatory state of the dorsal horn will occur and lead to a condition, such as neurogenic pain, where the normal message evoked by a low threshold afferent may become "miscoded" as a noxious event. It is generally conceded that such pain in man is relatively refractory to opioids. Given our understanding of the association of opioid receptors with small and not large (low threshold) primary afferents, such relative insensitivity might be anticipated. We must then consider that other pharmacological systems which modulate, for example, low threshold afferent input, may alter the pain of a neurogenic origin. In view of the complexity of the dorsal horn, I anticipate that a wide variety of pain syndromes will be found to result from various encoding dysfunctions which will be traced to specific spinal transmitter/receptor deficits. Because of the ubiquity throughout the neuraxis of many neurotransmitter receptor systems (e.g. GABA and glycine), such local deficits may be usefully addressed only by an interaction with the local *spinal* receptor system.

Thirdly, a variety of spinal receptor systems modulate functions which are responsible for motor and autonomic outflow. Though not discussed, the spinal substrates for these systems are every bit as pharmacologically complex as those systems within the dorsal horn. The inhibition of the micturition reflex by spinal opioids indicates the association of opioid receptors with spinal parasympathetic systems. In spinal injured patients, somatomotor spasticity and external sphincter spasticity can be diminished by the spinal administration of GABA and opioid agonists (Müller 1980). In this manner, one can obtain spinal drug levels which might be unachievable by systemic administration because of unacceptable side effects. These physiolgical effects reflect the association of opioid and GABAergic receptors on spinal motor neuron and interneuronal systems.

In short, though the clinical use of spinally administered drugs has found significant benefit for the use of opioids in controlling somatic pain, the pharmacological complexity of the spinal cord and the association of specific receptor systems with different spinal substrates suggests that in the future, spinally administered, receptor-selective agents may be administered for the functional control of systems far removed from those mediating the encodement of high threshold C-fiber input.

Finally, from my perspective, simple inspection of the information base outlined in this book emphasizes the value of basic animal studies in their ability to define and characterize the pharmacology, physiology and toxicology of drugs administered into the privileged space adjacent to the spinal cord. It is my belief that the safe spinal use of currently available drugs and the ethical application in man of the novel agents suggested by the animal studies require such fundamental investigations. The continued safety of the spinal approach, however, depends not only upon the hard won insights garnered from the animal studies but on the understanding and considered application by each clinician of the principles which govern the effects of the drugs he uses and the peculiarities of the routes by which he administers them. This book by Professors DeCastro, Meynadier and Zenz provides a thoughtful compendium of information relevant to the use of spinally administered drugs in general and the opioids in particular and will provide the clinician and basic scientist alike with much food for thought. My congratulations to them for a job very well done.

To conclude, while reading this volume, I was struck by the intellectual distance that this therapeutic concept has come since 1975. Details of drug dosing, kinetics of distribution, therapeutic indications and so forth have been provided by so many. Still, on this day, as I write this text, I am further struck by how far we have yet to go and how we must constantly be prepared intellectually for the unexpected. As the character in Kurt Vonnegut's novel "Cat's Cradle" said: "Strange travel invitations are dancing lessons from God".

6

References

Cameron, A.A., Leah, J.D. and Snow, P.J. The coexistence of neuropeptides in feline sensory neurons. Neuroscience 27:969-980, 1988.

Cervero, F. and Iggo, A. The substantia gelatinosa of the spinal cord: a critical review. Brain 103:717-772, 1980.

Foreman, R.D. and Ohata, C.A. Effects of coronary artery occlusion of thoracic spinal neurons receiving viscerosomatic inputs. Am. J. Physiol. 238:H667-H679, 1980.

Gamse, R. and Saria A. Nociceptive behavior after intrathecal injections of substance P, neurokinin A and calcitonin gene-related peptide in mice. Neurosci. Lett. 70:143-147, 1986.

Giesler, G.J., Yezierski, R.P., Gerhart, K.D. and Willis, W.D. Spinothalamic tract neurons that project to medial and/or lateral thalamic nuclei: evidence for a physiologically novel population of spinal cord neurons. J. Neurophysiol. 46:1285-1308, 1981.

Inagaki, S. and Kito, S. Peptides in the peripheral nervous systems. Progress in Brain Research 66:269-316, 1986.

Müller, H., Zierski, J. and Penn, R.D. (eds). Local-spinal Therapy of Spasticity, Springer-Verlag Berlin Heidelberg, 1988.

Seybold, V.S. Neurotransmitter Receptor sites in the spinal cord. In: Spinal Afferent Processing, Yaksh, T.L. (Ed.), Plenum Press, 1986, pp. 117-139.

Sugimoto, T., Takemura, M., Sakai, A. and Ishimaru, M. Rapid transneuronal destruction following peripheral nerve transection in the medullary dorsal horn is enhanced by strychnine, picrotoxin and bicuculline. Pain 30:385, 1987.

Tyce, G.M. and Yaksh, T.L. Monoamine release from cat spinal cord by somatic stimuli: an intrinsic modulatory system. J. Physiol. (Lond.) 314:513-529, 1981.

Yaksh, T.L. and Elde, R.P. Factors governing release of methionine enkephalin-like immunoreactivity from mesencephalon and spinal cord of the cat in vivo. J. Neurophysiology 46:1056-1075, 1981.

Yaksh, T.L. and Rudy, T.A. Narcotic analgesics: CNS sites and mechanisms of action as revealed by intracerebral injection techniques. Pain 4:299-359, 1978.

Yaksh, T.L. and Stevens, C.W. Properties of the modulation of spinal nociceptive transmission by receptor-selective agents. In: Proceedings of the Vth World Congress on Pain, Dubner, R., Gebhart, G.F. and Bond, M.R. (Eds.), Elsevier Science Publishers BV, 1988, pp. 417-435.

Yaksh, T.L. Spinal opiate analgesia: characteristics and principles of action. Pain 11:293-346, 1981.

Yaksh, T.L. Pharmacology of spinal adrenergic systems which modulate spinal nociceptive processing. Pharmacol Biochem Behav 22:845-858, 1985.

Yaksh, T.L. Behavioral and autonomic correlates of the tactile evoked allodynia produced by spinal glycine inhibition: effects of modulatory receptor systems and excitatory amino acid antagonists. Pain 37:111-123, 1989.

Part I

Anatomical, pharmacological, physiological and technical basis of spinal regional opioid administration

1. Developments, advantages and drawbacks of regional opioid analgesia

Centuries ago as well as today, opioids have been and still are the cornerstone of severe pain treatment. High specificity of the compounds and possibility of administration by all the classical medication routes provide an explanation for their success (Fig.1a).

Since 10 years the general administration routes of these substances have been extended in an important way by the use of regional routes (spinal, perineural, intracerebroventricular), giving way to brand new treatment techniques which can be called: "Regional opioid analgesia".

Overenthusiasm or understatement was the normal evolution of this important discovery. Today however, we have a sufficient extended background to make the point. Regional opioid analgesia already plays a substantial part in our actual therapeutic armamentarium, as it provides many successful application possibilities if the right indications with the right drugs and the right techniques are applied (Fig. 1b).

1979 is the year of a revolutionary new method, the spinal administration of opioids, intrathecally (Wang et al. 1979) and epidurally (Bahar et al. 1979). But actually, only few colleagues realized that the first year of spinal opioid application in man was 1977. In that year Wang reported on investigations in rats and mentioned, in the last paragraph of his publication, the first preliminary results in man, which were encouraging (Fig. 2).

The Mayo Clinic has been one of the main centres for the development of this important new method. Over there, in 1976, Yaksh and Rudy demonstrated in animals that segmental analgesia could be induced by intrathecal spinal administration of opioids. At the same clinic, one year later, Wang applied this finding successfully to relieve cancer pain in man. This new approach to opioid therapy rapidly gained in popularity and numerous enthusiastic reports followed in quick succession. Surprisingly it took more than two years from the publication of the basic experiments of Yaksh and Rudy and the first preliminary mention of Wang until suddenly in late 1979 and early 1980 the medical world became aware of this new method. Seldom has a "revolution", as it has been called, been hidden for such a long time.

Several historical steps and seminal laboratory discoveries preceded and paved the way for the revolution in neuroxial pharmacology and therapy that

12

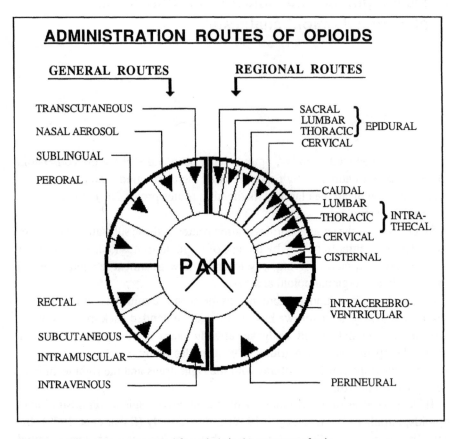

Fig. 1a. Administration routes used for opiods in the treatment of pain.

followed the first tentative clinical reports of intraspinal opioids as follows:

- Intrathecal administration of morphine combined with a local anaesthetic (eucaine) was already reported in 1901 by Kitagawa as providing long lasting pain relief. However, this technique was not used again until 75 years later (Matsuki 1983).
- Until 1972 the assumption prevailed that opioids produced analgesia by predominantly blocking the pain signals in the brain as well as by disrupting the affective pain component. The spinal cord was only considered as a place of neurotransmission between peripheral stimuli and brain.
- 1972 Jurna: observation in rats by section of the spinal cord at thoracic level: intraperitoneal morphine injection still produces an inhibition of the escape reflex in the hot plate test.

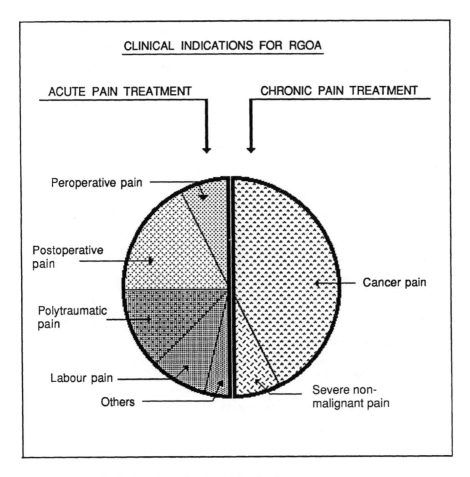

Fig. 1b. Potential indications for regional opioid analgesia.

- 1973 Pert and Snyder, Simon et al.: opioid receptor localization in the brain and in the spinal cord.
- 1974 Besson et al.: effects of opioids on the posterior horn of the spinal cord cells.
- 1974 Calvillo et al., Kitahata et al.: discovery that opioids were also capable of blocking pain pathways at the level of the spinal cord in the Rexed's laminae I, II and V.
- 1975 Terenius and Wahlström: identification of endorphins in the human CSF.
- 1976 Guillemin et al.: identification of pituitary endorphins.
- 1976 Yaksh and Rudy: demonstration of analgesia mediated by a direct spinal action of opioids.

Regional Anesthesia
Vol. 2, No. 3
3-4, 1977

Analgesic Effect of Intrathecally Administered Morphine

Josef K. Wang, MD

Dr. Wang is assistant professor of anesthesiology, Mayo Medical School, and a consultant to the department of anesthesiology, Mayo Clinic and Mayo Foundation, Rochester, Minn.

The author wishes to thank Dr. Frederick W. L. Kerr for his valuable scientific advice.

Abstract: *Morphine sulfate, a narcotic analgesic, possesses the undesirable side effects of central depression, tolerance, and dependency. Opiate receptors have been found in the brain and the spinal cord. Intrathecally applied opiates produce potent analgesia that can be antagonized by naloxone. The time-response study with tail-flick response after intrathecal injections of a small dosage of morphine (25 μg) demonstrated a long-lasting analgesia. Intrathecal injections of morphine or opiate-like peptides may become a predictable modality of pain relief without attendant loss of other neurologic function.*

(last paragraph)

A clinical trial with intrathecal administration of morphine for intractable pain of inoperable cancer is being conducted at the Mayo Clinic. The preliminary results are very encouraging. This modality of pain control may be effective for pain syndromes, without the attendant loss of other neurologic function. More studies are needed to establish its practical application.

THE LANCET, MARCH 10, 1979

Preliminary Communication

EPIDURAL MORPHINE IN TREATMENT OF PAIN

M. BEHAR   F. MAGORA
D. OLSHWANG   J. T. DAVIDSON

Hebrew University-Hadassah Medical School, and Hadassah University Hospital, Jerusalem, Israel

Summary   Epidural injections of 2 mg morphine were given to 10 patients with severe acute or chronic pain. All cases had considerable amelioration of pain, which commenced within 2–3 min, reached a peak in 10–15 min, and was effective for 6–24 h. It is suggested that the morphine reached the subarachnoid space and produced its effect by direct action on the specific opiate receptors in the substantia gelatinosa of the posterior-horn cells of the spinal cord.

THE LANCET, APRIL 18, 1981

M. BAHAR

Fig. 2. Partial reproduction of the first clinical reports about the spinal use of opioids in man:
a) Wang (1977) for the intrathecal route.
b) Bahar et al. (1979) for the epidural route.
(Bahar and Behar cited in the Lancet are the same person, difficulty with Hebrew vowels led to an error in translation, and Bahar is the correct spelling)

- 1977 Wang: first preliminary report on spinal opioid analgesia in man (Fig. 2).
- 1979 Bahar et al.: first report on epidural morphine analgesia in man (Fig. 2).
- 1979 Wang et al.: first report on intrathecal morphine analgesia in man.
- 1980 Freye and Arndt (b): intracerebroventricular injection of fentanyl in animals.
- 1982 Leavens et al., Roquefeuil et al.: intracerebroventricular injection of morphine in man.

To conclude about all these important investigations, it can be stated that opioids act not only by binding to certain brain receptors but also act more peripherally from the brain at opioid receptors, e.g. in the spinal cord. Consequently, by injection of the opioids near the receptor sites it is possible to decrease the amount of drugs needed to induce analgesia. Furthermore, this regional technique limits more segmentally the effects on extension and intensity of analgesia. It is a fact that the discovery of selective mechanisms for pain inhibition at the spinal cord level opened up a new area for acute and chronic pain management (Cousins and Mather 1984 b).

Definition

Regional opioid analgesia can be defined as the introduction of opioids in the epidural, caudal, intrathecal (subarachnoidal), intracisternal, intracerebroventricular or perineural space for the management of acute or chronic pain. The name of spinal opioid analgesia is used if the technique is limited to the application of opioids on the spinal part of the CNS.

Actually the word analgesia is incorrect for the effect of spinal opioids. The action is limited to a decrease or partial suppression of pain or hypalgesia. Spinal opioids do not cause a complete absence of pain like local anaesthetics. Typical localized surgical pain stimuli are felt unchanged, the needle prick is not modulated, but the dull and less localized second pain is suppressed. It can be postulated that the slow pain afferents (C-fibres-paleospinothalamic pathway) are well inhibited, whereas the fast myelinated pain afferents (A-δ-fibres, neo-spinohypothalamic pathway) are not modulated. The spinal opioid analgesia is selective, leaving some sensory function (touch, proprioception), motor and sympathetic function uneffected (Jurna 1983).

In the concept of "selective spinal opioid analgesia" suggested by Cousins et al. (1979 b), selectivity is only to be applied on the spinal action on the nociceptive fibres at the spinal level (in contrast to the action on the local anaesthetics). Segmentation of effects is initially limited to area surrounding to the injection level but does not exclude the cephalidad migration of opioids following spinal administration.

Despite this fact, we follow the common use of the literature and call the method spinal opioid analgesia.

Advantages compared to parenteral opioids

By using the spinal route, distances for the opioid to reach the specific spinal receptors are shorter, waste is decreased so that more intense and longer analgesia with lower doses and less side effects are obtained (Kitahata and Collins 1984 a). Moreover, the analgesia is predominantly segmentally confined to the site of injection.

Advantages compared to local anaesthesia

The major advantage of spinal opioids compared to spinal anaesthesia with local anaesthetics is the absence of a pronounced sympathetic block, postural hypotension and motor block, potentially allowing the patient to walk easily. Cardiovascular collapse or convulsions, which are the major complications of local anaesthetic blocks, are avoided (Tab. 1, 2, 3).

Table 1. Spinal opioid analgesia: potential advantages.

- **Pure antinociception?**

- **Selective analgesia without:**

    - Sensory block
    - Motor block
    - Sympathetic block

- **With small doses effects are:**

    - More intense
    - Longer lasting
    - Fewer side effects

- **Increased efficacy by reduced:**

    - Protein binding
    - First pass effects
    - Liver enzyme induction

Table 2. Comparison of the effects of opioids and local anaesthetics administered by spinal routes.

Effects	Opioids	Local anaesthetics
Sympathetic block **Motor block** **Sensory block** **Segmental block**	no no mainly pain yes (potentially rostral spread)	yes slight - complete all qualities (pain, touch, temp.) yes
Vascular uptake •dose dependent •reduced by epinephrine **Duration**	yes yes short - long	yes yes short

Side effects
•hypotension
•respiratory depression
  ••central
  ••peripheral
•urinary retention
•constipation
•pruritus
•nausea, vomiting
	no
	
	yes (dose-dependent)
	no
	yes
	yes
	yes
	yes
		yes
		
		no
		yes if high level
		yes
		no
		no
		no

Tachyphylaxis	yes	yes
Dependence	yes	no

Note: pethidine seems to be an exception, when it is administrated via an intrathecal route at doses of 1 mg/kg bw, it produces, just like local anaesthetics, a sympathetic and a motor block.

Table 3. Potential discreet signs of motor and/or sympathetic block observed after spinal opioids.

- Dysuria
- Ejaculation difficulties
- Urinary retention
- Constipation
- Miosis
- Redness of the face
- Temperature increase in the extremities
- Nausea and vomiting
- Muscle weakness

18

Drawbacks

In spite of initial dreams, spinal opioids have failed to solve the main problem to have only a good effect without any side effect. Discreet signs of desequilibrium in the motor or sympathetic system may become apparent (Tab. 3). Urinary retention, nausea, vomiting, itching are certainly no life-threatening complications. But still the problem of respiratory depression remains, making the therapeutic window between pain relief and danger alarmingly narrow (Bromage 1985). "Vigilance is still the price that must be paid for safe analgesia" (Bromage et al. 1983 b). We have to recognize that even "safe" analgesia is not at all always safe for the patient (see Chapter 6).

There is no available opioid free from these dangers, but there are drugs less likely to induce central side effects. There is no analgesic method without any danger but there are certain methods which are less dangerous. And there are no clinical settings where respiratory depression has never been reported; but there are clinical settings which are more or less likely to induce these complications.

2. Anatomy and physiology

2.1 Nociception and nociceptive pathways

Pain is induced when a tissue damage liberates algogenic substances like bradykinin, histamine, hydroxytryptamine or H^+-ions. Moreover phospholipase is activated, which contributes to the formation of prostaglandins. Those prostaglandins do not activate nociceptive nerve endings but increase their susceptibility to algogenic substances (Ferreira 1980). The endogenous pain substances electrically activate peripheral nerve endings, the nociceptors. The same electrical activation can be performed by direct mechanical, thermal or chemical stimulation of nerves or nerve endings. According to the used stimuli we can distinguish between nociceptors, mechanoreceptors, thermoreceptors and polymodal receptors. Nociceptors are distributed over the whole body from the skin surface to the viscera (Fig. 3, 4, 5, 6).

The afferents of *nociceptors* are A-δ- or C-fibres. Both fibre groups also conduct the modulation of other parameters like, e.g., temperature. Pain is commonly divided in two components and related to the two different fibres. The well localized sharp pain is being conducted as the first impression via A-δ-fibres. With a slight latency of about one second the dull pain is transmitted by C-fibres.

The A-δ-fibres that are myelinated conduct with a greater velocity than the unmyelinated C-fibres. A peripheral nerve contains up to 50 % of afferent fibres. Those primary afferents converge into the dorsal root as they enter the dorsal horn of the grey matter of the spinal cord.

Nociceptive and non-nociceptive stimuli are transmitted to two different neurons within the dorsal horn: "class 2"-neurons, afferents from mechanoreceptors (A-β-fibres) and "class 3"-neurons, nociceptive afferents from C- and A-δ-fibres. The dorsal horn neurons are the connecting link between transmission, afferent answers (sympathetic, motor), and inhibitory interneurons. The dorsal horn is the central switch-board of the spinal cord. Here all the different pathways with different transmitters are connected (Fig. 4).

The grey matter of the spinal cord is subdivided into laminae described by Rexed (1952). However, it has to be realized that a clear distinction between the different laminae is difficult to make, because they do not have clear cut edges and the dendrites range into different neighbouring laminae (Fig. 3, 4).

20

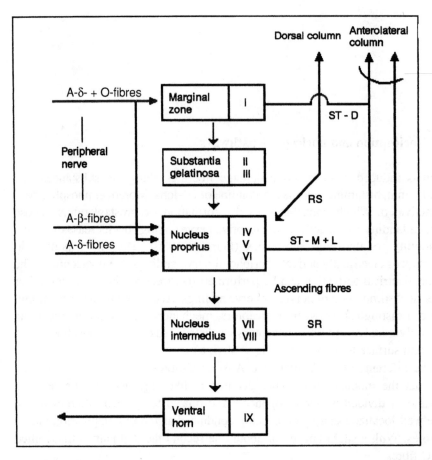

Fig. 3. Schematic representation of the stratification of the laminae (I to IX) of the spinal cord and the transmission of pain stimuli.
- Lamina I and Laminae II and III (substantia gelatinosa) in the dorsal horn receive afferent A-δ and C- fibres and carry pain.
- Laminae IV and V and VI (nucleus proprius) receive afferent A-δ fibres.
- Ascending fibres pass up the median and lateral spinothalamic tracts (ST-M and L), the spinoreticular tract (SR) and the dorsal spinothalamic tract (ST-D).
- There is a descending inhibitory reticulospinal input (RS) to lamina IV.
(Adapted from Budd 1982 and Bullingham in Smith and Covino 1985.)

Lamina I forms the marginal layer. It receives terminals of nociceptive afferents. Lamina I contains cells responding only to noxious stimuli. *Laminae II
and III* constitute the *substantia gelatinosa*, the central area for the action of
spinal opioids. Both layers form an area where integration and modulation of
noxious impulses occur. Nociceptive information conducted over C- and A-δ-

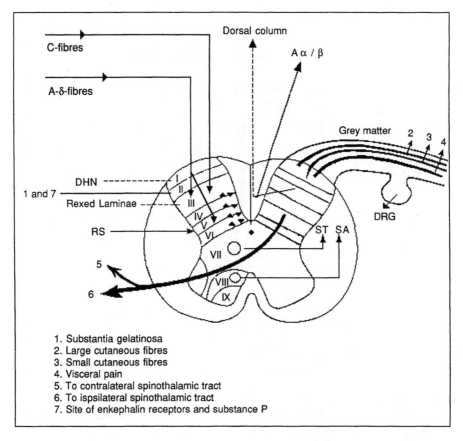

Fig. 4. Detailed diagram of the dorsal root ganglion (DRG) and the dorsal horn neuron (DHN) with the various laminae where synaptic connections occur.
- A-δ-fibres and C-fibres synapse with cells in the dorsal horn, which are divided into 9 laminae.
- Laminae II, III: substantia gelatinosa, carry pain.
- Laminae IV-V-VI: nucleus proprius, receive A-δ-fibres.
- Ascending fibres pass up the spinothalamatic (ST) and spinoreticular (SR) system.
- RS is a descending reticulospinal input to lamina V.
(Adapted from Budd 1982, Bullingham in Smith and Covino 1985)

fibres arrives at the substantia gelatinosa via synaptic connections from lamina I. *Lamina IV* is the terminal for light mechanical stimuli. *Lamina V* is involved in pain transmission while the cells are responding to mechanical, thermal and chemical stimuli. The ventral boundary of the dorsal horn is made up by *lamina VI*.

The cells in this lamina are responding to cutaneous afferents and muscle afferents. *Laminae VII* and *VIII* make up the ventral horn and continue with the

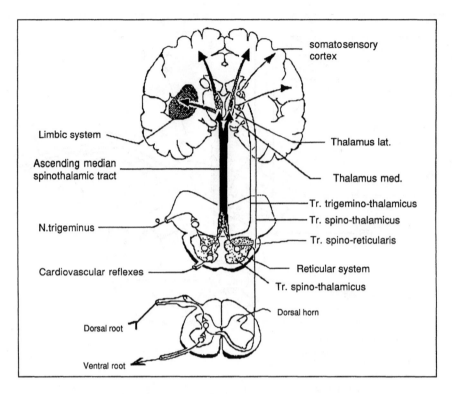

Fig. 5. Schematic representation of the central transmission of pain stimuli.
Nociceptive stimuli enter into the CNS via dorsal horn roots and N. trigeminus for integration.
Ascending pain stimuli travel via 2 systems:

a) Medial system: Reticular system
                         Central thalamic nuclei
                         Reticular ascending system
                         Activating system
                         Limbic system

b) Lateral system: Thalamic somatosensor nuclei
                         Tr. spinothalamicus
                         Tr. trigemino-thalamicus
                         Somatosensor nuclei
                         Lateral thalamus
                         Somatosensor cortex

(Adapted from Zimmermann and Handwerker 1984)

spinoreticular tract. Laminae I, IV, V, VI are sources for ascending pathways, whereas laminae II and III are mainly inhibiting interneurons.

Pain information is conducted mainly via the anterolateral column of the contralateral side. This column contains the spinothalamic tract, the most important

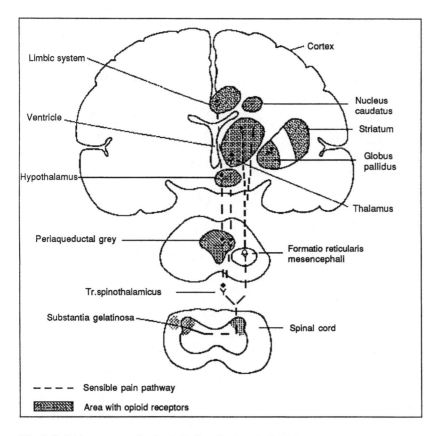

Fig. 6. Opioid receptor and enkephalin localizations in the CSF. High opioid receptor density is found: - longitudinally along the dorsal horn
- in its rostral extension into the trigeminal nucleus of the brain stem
- in the locus coeruleus
- in the periaqueductal grey
- in the midline raphe nuclei
- in the amygdala.
Pain pathways travel through the zones with high opioid receptor density.
(Adapted from Covino and Scott 1985)

pathway for signalling noxious stimuli in man. A subdivision is made between the paleospinothalamic pathway for transmission of dull pain and the neospinothalamic pathway for coding of sharp pain. The spinothalamic tract is mainly transmitting stimuli to the thalamus, from where the information is sent to the limbic system (for emotional and affect-coding of noxious stimuli) and to the hypothalamus (for control of vegetative function) (Fig. 6, 7).

24

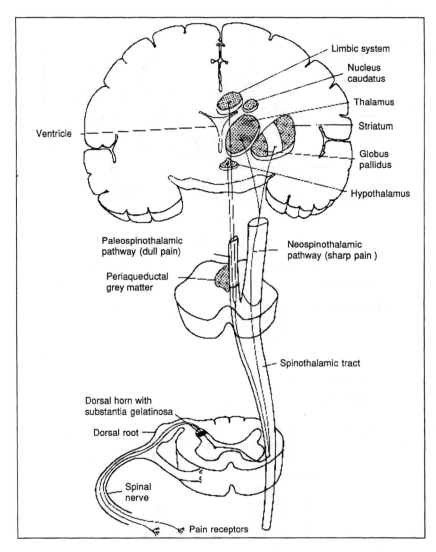

Fig. 7. Schematic representation of the pain pathways.
(Adapted from Covino and Scott 1985)

The other tract, the spinoreticular tract, is included as well in pain transmission as in inhibitory control of nociceptive input. The spinoreticular tract connects spinal cord and reticular formation. From there, connections are made to the periaqueductal grey and the raphe magnus, centres for vegetative, sleep and vigilance controls. From the periaqueductal grey matter, the raphe magnus and from the reticular formation, the descending inhibitory mechanisms are controlled. As will be seen later all these centres are involved in opioid analgesia because they contain a great proportion of opioid receptors.

Pain is realized in the cortex where all information with all the emotional and vegetative side information from the brain nuclei converges. There is no pain perception in the cortex without this modifying information aside.

2.2 Anatomy of opioid receptors

Opioid receptors are the specific binding sites for exogenous or endogenous opioid substances. Since 1973 their localization has been investigated, when Pert, as a student of Snyder, and Simon et al. demonstrated opioid receptors in brain and spinal cord (Fig. 8, 9, 10, Tab. 4).

On the basis of the anatomical correlates of pain pathways it is obvious that opioid receptors are mainly distributed in the neighbourhood of those spinal cord and brain areas involved in pain transmission.

After initial in vitro studies, opioid receptors have been visualized thanks to in vivo labelling and following autoradiography (Pert and Snyder 1973, 1976). The

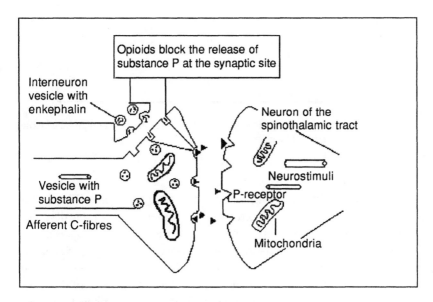

Fig. 8. Transmission of the pain impulses at the first relay in the dorsal horn of the spinal cord. Exogenous, as well as endogenous opioids (endorphins, enkephalin) are able to block the release of transmitter substance P.
(Adapted from Freye 1987)

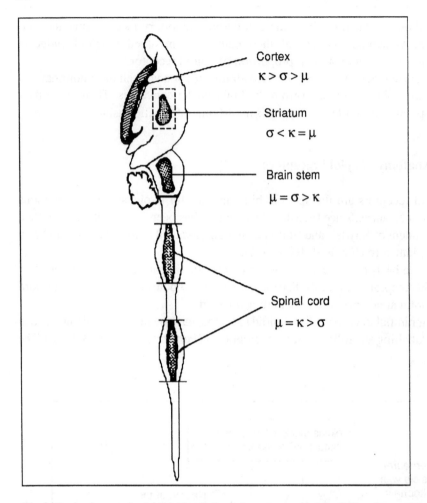

Fig. 9. Predominance of opioid binding in the various structures of the CNS as they are identified by means of displacing prototype ligands.
(Adapted from Freye 1987)

studies show a wide range of densities in various brain regions. Whereas the cerebral cortex contains only a limited autoradiographic receptor density, other areas are presenting a high density. Among these we can find: area striata, habenula, amygdala, reticular formation, midbrain-pons, thalamus, periaqueductal and periventricular grey matter. The marked difference of grain distribution outlines the specific opioid receptor sites. It is not a consequence of diffusion.

Within the spinal cord, the autoradiographic density is limited to a sharp, narrow band corresponding to lamina I and lamina II (substantia gelatinosa). The density in the substantia gelatinosa is 5- to 10-fold higher than in other areas of the grey or white matter of the spinal cord (Atweh and Kuhar 1977). Further-

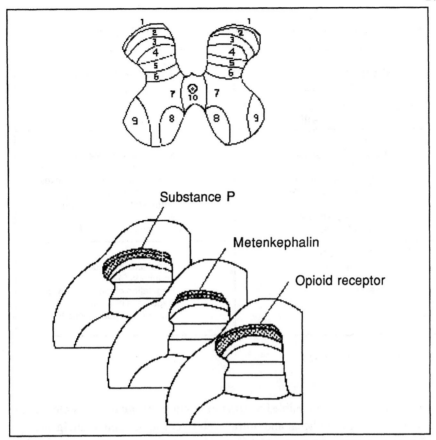

Fig. 10. Dorsal quadrant of the cord with the dorsal horn and the substantia gelatinosa. Localization of substance P, metenkephalin and opioid receptors in the cord. (Adapted from Besson et al. 1978)

more, the highest concentration of substance P and metenkephalin are found in laminae I and II. This fact demonstrates the close interrelationship between the different pain-mediating and modulating systems.

Anatomically it is essential to realize that the opioid receptors are mainly distributed over areas close to the subarachnoid space. In this way, exogenous opioids can easily reach areas with a high content of opioid receptors. Laminae I and II of the dorsal horn are the nearest laminae to the dorsal edge of the spinal cord and the closest to communication with CSF. The periaqueductal and periventricular grey matter are located close to the third and fourth ventricles, which is again close communication with the drugs contained in the CSF.

On the other hand, it has to be realized that the map of the distribution of opioid receptors strikingly parallels the paleospinothalamic pathway (dull pain). The other high density area lies in parts of the limbic system, which is involved in the emotional control of pain.

Table 4. Localization and possible functions of opioid receptors in the mammalian brain.

Localization	Possible function
SPINAL CORD - Laminae I - II - III	- Spinal analgesia

BRAINSTEM
  - Periaquaeductal grey
  - Area postrema
  - Vagal nuclei (nucleus tractus
    solitarius, n. commissuralis,
    n. ambiguus)
  - Medial and lateral optic nuclei
  - Locus coeruleus
	- Supraspinal analgesia
	- Nausea and vomiting
	- Regulation of visceral reflexes
	  (respiratory depression,
	  orthostatic hypotension)
	- Miosis
	- Euphoria

PROENCEPHALON
  - Limbic system
 	
  - Basal nuclei
  - Median eminence
	- Regulation of mood
	  (euphoria ?)
	- Regulation of motor behaviour
	- Regulation of neuro-
	  endocrinological function

(Adapted from Snyder 1977)

Opioid receptors responsible for pain modulation are situated very close to the injection sites of intrathecal and intracerebroventricular opioid analgesia.

But, opioid receptors responsible for side effects — respiratory depression, nausea, vomiting — are also distributed in the same close vicinity of the CSF space, e.g. in the area postrema on the ground of the IV ventricle. The anatomical origin of wanted and unwanted effects of the opioids shows a narrow neighbourhood.

2.3 Anatomy of the epidural and the intrathecal spinal space

The very high density of receptors in the substantia gelatinosa (Laminae II, III) opened the way for a topical rather than a systemic application of opioid substances. The great (theoretical) advantage of this method is the close vicinity of the injection site and the specific receptors for the injected drugs. It represents the only clinical method in pain therapy where the injected agonist can be brought into the immediate area of his receptor.

It is the aim of regional opioid techniques to place the drug as near as possible to his specific receptor by direct administration into:
- the spinal canal
  . epidural (ED) space

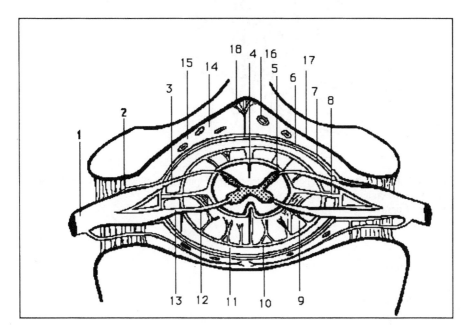

Fig. 11. Cross section of the spinal cord, membranes and nerve roots.

1. N. spinalis	10. Arachnoidea spinalis
2. Ganglion spinale	11. Cavum subdurale
3. Radix dorsalis	12. Radix ventralis
4. Septum medianum spinalis	13. Nerve root
5. Pia mater	14. Postepidural space
6. Dura mater spinalis	15. Epidural fat
7. Internal membrane of the dura mater or arachnoid mater	16. Epidural veins
	17. Ligamentum flavum
8. Ligamentum denticulatum	18. Plica mediana dorsalis
9. Cavum subarachnoidale	

(Adapted from Covino and Scott 1985)

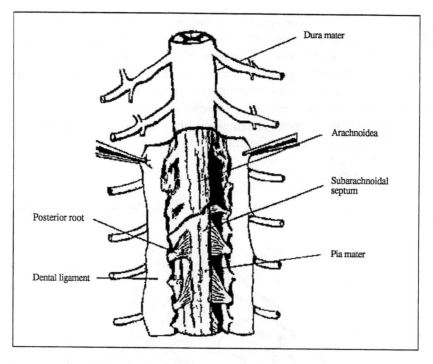

Fig. 12. Spinal membranes and nerve roots segment of spinal cord viewed from behind, with portions of the dura mater and arachnoid removed.
(Adapted from Netter 1977)

. intrathecal (IT) space
. intracisternal space
- the intracerebroventricular space (IC).
The *spinal canal* contains the spinal cord and its three coverings:
- the dura mater
- the arachnoid mater
- the pia mater (Fig. 11, 12).

The *dura mater* forms a loose sheath around the spinal cord. The dura mater consists of white collagen fibres with an admixture of elastic fibres (Williams and Warwick 1980). It does not represent a complete barrier to the movement of opioids between the epidural and the subarachnoidal space. The facility and depth of penetration of opioids into the spinal cord appear to be related to the physiochemical properties of the employed opioid (Covino and Scott 1985). These will be discussed in detail later.

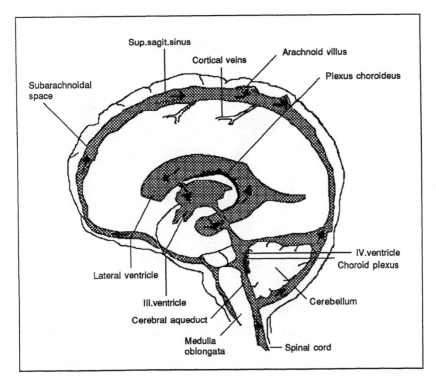

Fig. 13. Schematic representation of the CSF circulation in the brain.
(Adapted from Allinson 1978)

The *arachnoid mater* is the internal layer of the dura, a thin membrane lying close to the dura mater but easily separated from it.

The *pia mater* surrounds the surface of the entire CNS and is closely attached to the spinal cord and the spinal nerves. It is a vascular membrane containing collagen, elastin and reticulin fibres. The pia mater supplies the brain and the spinal cord with blood vessels and makes up the fibrous part of the plexus choroideus in the brain ventricles.

The meninges create two separate spaces which can be used for two different clinical methods:

- the epidural space (ED)
- the subarachnoidal space usually named intrathecal (IT) space.

The *epidural space* is the part of the spinal canal outside the dura mater, enclosed by the connective tissues covering the vertebra and the ligamentum flavum. It contains fat and blood vessels. It can be considered as a closed com-

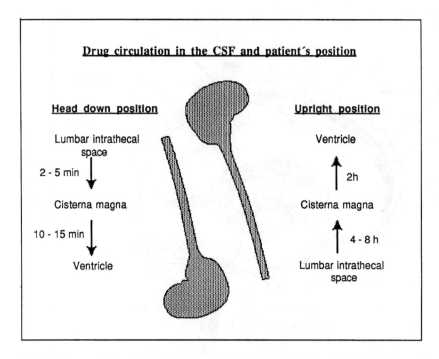

Fig. 14. Changes in the circulation times in the CSF in relationship with the patient's position after intrathecal injection.
(Adapted from Allinson 1978)

partment internally limited by the dura and by the connective tissue lining externally the spinal canal (Williams and Warwick 1980). Fluids injected into the epidural space can spread up to the base of the skull or down to the sacral hiatus.

The epidural space measured by X-Rays shows the following anatomy (Reynolds et al. 1985):

- ventral epidural space 1 mm
- lateral epidural space 2 mm with a sawtooth shape to the dorsal epidural space
- dorsal epidural space 1.1-2.9 mm at the rostral laminae and 3.8-6.5 mm at the caudal laminae.

The *subarachnoid space* is the interval between the arachnoid and pia mater. It contains the cerebrospinal fluid (CSF).

The space between the arachnoidea and the dura mater is the *subdural space* which is not only a potential space containing lymph, but the subdural space may be accidentally and rarely injected with opioids (Hartrick et al. 1985) or local anaesthetics (Stevens and Stanton-Hicks 1985), e.g. when a catheter migrates into that space. This presents an enormous danger because the spreading of the injected solution is unpredictable and reaches the brain in most cases.

The *spinal root sleeves* exhibit arachnoid protrusions, when entering the dura mater. They are important for the penetration of drugs epidurally administered into the CSF and also for the drainage of the CSF.

The *CSF* is produced by the plexus choroideus of the third and fourth ventricles. The volume produced per hour is about 15-30 ml, which contributes to a daily production amount of 150-200 ml CSF (Fig. 13, 14). The same volume, which is produced, has to be absorbed. Absorption is performed by protrusions of the arachnoidea, by the arachnoid villi, by the capillaries of the pia mater and by the ependyma of the brain ventricles. The CSF fills the cavum subarachnoidale, the space between the pia mater and arachnoidea. This space extends approximately from the brain ventricles to the level of the third sacral vertebra, whereas the spinal cord terminates at the level of the first lumbar vertebra. For clinical practice, the physical properties of the CSF have importance, above all the pH, the specific gravity, and the protein content.

3. Micropharmacology of antinociceptive substances in the spinal cord

Opioid receptors are distributed through the entire body primarily not to act with injected morphine but to act with endogenous substances which have nociceptive stimuli modulating activity. Those endogenous drugs belong to the group of about 30 neuropeptides, whose members are, among others, endorphins and substance P.

3.1 Endorphins

"Endorphins" or "endogenous morphines" represent all endogenous substances with an opioid-like action. The common chemical structure of endorphins is a peptide structure (opioid peptides). The endorphins are the natural ligands of the opioid receptors. They induce the same characteristic opioid actions like the exogenous opioids (Guillemin et al. 1976).

The family of opioid peptides derives from 3 precursors which are pro-opiomelanocortin, pro-enkephalin and pro-enkephalin B. Each precursor and each endorphin consist of a sequence of 5 amino acids Tyr-Gly-Gly-Phe-x (x=Leu or Met) at least. This sequence seems essential for opioid receptor affinity. Thus each endorphin consists of either metenkephalin or leuenkephalin plus a sequence of other amino acids. Most of them are quite unstable substances and are quickly split by peptidases (Tab. 5, 6, 7 a b).

Endorphins are distributed in brain centres with opioid receptors, in the brain stem and in the spinal cord. High concentrations are identified in the caudate nucleus, the substantia nigra, periaqueductal and periventricular grey matter, area postrema, hypothalamus, amygdala (Tab. 4).

All groups of opioid-like neuropeptides are especially concentrated in the substantia gelatinosa of the dorsal horn (Hoekfelt et al. 1982; Duggan 1985). Metenkephalin is particularly released by descending axons in the substantia gelatinosa of the spinal cord where modulating pathways terminate as a response to afferent painful inputs to rostral brain centres (Jurna 1983).

Again, it is essential to realize the anatomical parallelism, between opioid receptor sites, distribution of endorphins and the vicinity to the CSF space, the potential depot of exogenous spinal opioids.

Opioid-like peptides act as transmitters and modulators of nervous information or as neurohormones (Jaffe and Martin WR 1985). The opioid-like peptides bind to opioid receptors of postsynaptic interneurons and prevent the reception and liberation of substance P, a predominantly excitatory protein (neurotransmitter of primary sensory fibres) necessary for the transmission of noxious information released by A-δ- and C-fibre afferents.

Endorphins stimulate descending inhibitory pathways from the brainstem that project to the dorsal horn. The spontaneous activity of opioidergic neurons leads to postsynaptic inhibition of the spinofugally projecting neurons (Cervero 1986).

The endorphins can combine with the opioid receptors at different levels and in various quantities depending on the painful stimuli. In this way they realize a fairly significant analgesia. However, as a consequence of their small meta-

Table 5. Endogenous opioid precursors and peptide families.

Peptide precursor	Peptide families	Peptides
1. Proenkephalins (proenkephalin A or PEA)	Enkephalin	Met-enkephalin Leu-enkephalin Met-E-Arg-Phe Met-E-Arg-Gly-Leu Peptide E Metorphamid
2. Pro-opiomelanocortin (POMC)	Endorphins	α - MSH β - MSH γ - MSH ACTH α - LPH β - LPH Met-enkephalin β - endorphin
3 Pro-dynorphin (proenkephalin B or PEB)	Dynorphins	Leu-enkephalin Dynorphin A Dynorphin B α - neo endorphin β - neo endorphin
4. Other peptides with opioid activity		β - caseomorphin Anodinin Kiotorphin etc.

MSH = melanostimulating hormone
LPH = lipotrophin hormone
(Adapted from Jaffe and Martin 1985; Millan 1986; Puig Riera de Coneas 1986)

Table 6. Anatomical distribution of opioid peptides and receptors in the CNS and outside.

1. Enkephalins	- primarily in interneurons with short axons
	- in a few long fibre tracts
	- substantia gelatinosa of the dorsal horn
	- nerve plexus
	- exocrine glands of stomach and intestine
2. Endorphins	- pancreatic islet cells
	- pituitary
	- arcuate nucleus
	- limbic and brainstem areas
	- nucleus tractus solitarii
	- nerve plexus
	- substantia gelatinosa of the dorsal horn
3. Dynorphins	- laminae I, II of the spinal cord
	- spinal trigeminal nucleus
	- periaqueductal grey
	- hippocampus
	- locus ceruleus
	- cerebral cortex
	- median eminence

(Adapted from Duggan 1985; Jaffe and Martin 1985; Hoekfelt et al. 1982)

bolic stability, the clinical evidence for a real analgesic action is limited. Injected intracerebroventricularly or intrathecally (Oyama et al. 1980 b) β-endorphin, which is one of the more stable substances, has a pronounced antinociceptive action.

D-ala-D-leu-enkephalin or DADL is an opioid peptide located in the dorsal horn of the spinal cord, acting on the δ-opioid receptors (Atchison et al. 1984; Onofrio and Yaksh 1983). It requires approximately the five-fold amount of naloxone to antagonize its antinociceptive effects in comparison to morphine (Yaksh et al. 1986 a).

Focal electrical stimulation of brain areas with high concentration of endorphins induces naloxone-reversible analgesia (Akil et al. 1976; Besson et al. 1978).

The life of the endogenous endorphins is very short. Metenkephalin has a plasma half-life time in the millisecond range. Therefore a continuous secretion of these substances is necessary and in cases of chronic pain this secretion may become exhausted. Moreover, in clinical conditions, we note that such secretion is mostly insufficient to suppress the severe pain periods, even if they are short.

Therefore the search for substitution of these endorphins by more stable exogenous opioids seems logical. One can freely accept that the injection of an

Table 7a. Endogenous substances acting in animals as spinal modulators of nociceptive stimuli with exogenous agonists and antagonists.

Endogenous modulating systems and receptors		Type of nociceptive modulation in animals: ↗0↘	Exogenous substances	
			agonists	antagonists
1. Opioid peptide system 1.1. Opioid neuropeptides				
?	μ	↘	Morphine	Naloxone
?	μ1	↘	Meptazinol	Naloxone
Enkephalins	δ	↘	DADL	Naloxone
Endorphins	ε	↘	β- endorphin	Naloxone
Dynorphins	κ	↘	Spiradoline	Naloxone
			Buprenorphine e.g.	Naloxone
?	δ	↘	SKF-10 047	Naloxone
1.2. Aminopeptidases		↗		Thiorphan Bestatin Ketalorphan
2. Non opioid neuropeptides				
Calcitonin		↘	Calcitonin	
Calcitonin gene rel. pept.		↘		
Cholecystokinin		↗	Proglumide, Xylamide	
Glycine		↘		
Neurotensin		↘	Neurotensin	
Somatostatin		↘	Somatostatin	
Substance P		↗ or ↘		
Thyrotropin rel. Hormon		↘		
Vasopressine		↘	ADH	

↘ = decrease   ↗ = increase

Adapted from: Bates et al. 1983; Dalmas et al. 1987, 1988; de la Beaume et al. 1983; Goldstein 1976; Hylden and Wilcox 1983; Kuraishi et al. 1985; Reny Palasse and Rips 1987; Roques et al. 1984; Spampinato et al. 1984; Sawynok et al. 1984; Thurston et al. 1987; Watkins et al. 1985 a, b; Yaksh 1983 a, Yaksh 1988 a; Yaksh et al. 1988 b; Yaksh and Stevens 1988 c; Yamamoto et al. 1982.

opioid directly in the vicinity of the receptors (for instance the receptors of the spinal cord) can produce a more selective analgesia with a smaller quantity of the analgesic drug, producing pain suppression of longer duration than that obtained by parenteral routes.

3.2 Multiple opioid receptors

Not all of the effects of different opioids can be explained on the basis of interaction with a single opioid receptor. The pioneering studies of Martin WR et al. (1976) in the spinal dog led to a conception of multiple opioid receptors.

Table 7b. Endogenous substances acting in animals as spinal modulators of nociceptive stimuli with exogenous agonists and antagonists. (cont'd)

Endogenous modulating systems and receptors	Type of nociceptive modulation in animals: ➚ 0 ➘	Exogenous substances	
		agonists	antagonists
3. Neuroamines 3.1. Noradrenergic system			
α 1	➘	Methoxamine	Prazocin
α 2	➘	Guamfucine, Clonidine, ST-91 Medetomidine	Yohimbine
β	0	Isoproterenol	Propranolol
3.2. Serotoninergic system	➘	5 HT	Ketanserine
3.3. Gaba-ergic system			
Gaba A	0	Muscinol	Bicuculine
Gaba B	➘	Baclofen, Midazolam, Aminooxyacetic acid	Strychnine Flumazenil
3.4. Adenosine system			
A 1	➘	L-N6-phenylisopropyl-adenosine	8-phenyl-theophyline
A 2	➘	5-N-ethylisopropyl-adenosine	8-phenyl-theophyline
3.5. Cholinergic system			
Muscarine	➘	Carbachol, Oxotremorine	Atropine
Nicotine	0	Nicotine	Tubocurare

➘ = decrease   ➚ = increase   0 = ineffective

Adapted from: Dalmas et al. 1988; Germain et al. 1987; Glynn et al. 1987 b; Goodchild et al. 1987; Hartvig et al. 1987; Henry 1982; Kitahata 1989; Ossipov et al. 1989; Post and Freeman 1984; Post et al. 1987 b; Whitwam et al. 1982; Wilson and Yaksh 1978; Yaksh 1988 a; Yaksh et al. 1988 b.

Three different drugs elicited three distinct opioid syndromes. The hypothesis of Martin WR et al. was that different syndromes result from actions upon different receptors. Named after their prototype agonists they were called μ (m)-morphine, κ (k)-ketocyclazocine and σ (s)- SKF 10 047. The effects of all three drugs could be antagonized by the pure antagonist naltrexone indicating that the three used drugs were agonists.

The existence of at least 8 types of opioid receptors has been suggested but, reasonable evidence for five major categories of receptors exist; μ- κ-, δ-, ε-, and σ-receptors (Martin WR et al. 1976; Martin WR 1979; Herz 1984). Upon each receptor a given substance may act as an agonist, a partial agonist or an antagonist (Jaffe and Martin 1985), (Tab. 8, 9, 10).

The *opioid receptor* system includes:
- μ-receptors, activated by μ-agonists, such as morphine and β-endorphin, fentanyl, sufentanil etc. The identity of the natural ligand is uncertain but it has

Table 8. Opioid receptors, typical effects and ligands.

Receptor type	Endogenous ligand typical neuropeptide	Exogenous ligand typical alcaloid	Typical preferential effects
μ	?	- morphine - fentanyl	- analgesia - resp. depression - euphoria - physical dependence - bradycardia - antidiuresis - depression of T° regulation - miosis
δ	leucine enkephaline (DADL)	- enkephalins	(analgesia)
κ	dynorphin	- bremazocine - ketazocin	- spinal analgesia - sedation, dysphoria - miosis - diuresis - no resp. depression - no morphine-like physical dependence
ε	β - endorphin	–	- analgesia

σ	–	- SKF-10 047
		- N-allylnor-metazocine
		- phencyclidine
			- dysphoria
			- resp. stimulation
			  • tachypnea
			- vasomotor stimul.
			  • tachycardia
			  • hypertonia
			- mydriasis
			- no analgesia

The σ-receptor is not a real opioid receptor, but the dysphoric effects produced by binding to this receptor are antagonized by naloxone (Basbaum 1986).
The opioid receptors in the substantia gelatinosa are: $\kappa = 50\%$, $\mu = 40\%$, $\delta = 5\text{-}10\%$ (Andersen 1986 b)
(Adapted from Dudziak 1986; Goodman-Gilman 1985; Herz 1986 a; Martin et al. 1976)

high affinity for morphine-like compounds
 - μ_1-receptors activated by meptazinol
 - δ-receptors, activated by δ-agonists, such as DADL; the natural ligand is methionin-enkephalin
 - κ-receptors, the natural ligand is dynorphin agonists (spiradoline, nalbuphine, butorphanol)

Table 9. Functional correlates of opioid receptor types.

FUNCTIONS	RECEPTORS				
	μ	κ	σ	δ	ε
- Analgesia: • cerebral level	+	−	−	−	+
• spinal level	+	+	+	−	−
- Vigilance:	−	↓	−	↑	−
- Respiratory function:	↓	−	−	↑	−
- Heart rate:	↓			↑	−
- Cardiovascular tonus:	−	↓	↓	−	−
- Endocrine system:	+	−	+	−	−
- Diuresis:	↓	↑	−	−	−
- Constipation:	+	−	−	−	−
- Euphoria:	+	−	−	−	−
- Dysphoria:	−	+	+	+	−
- Alterations in affective behaviour:	−	−	+	+	−
- Pupil diameter:	↓	↓	−	↑	−
- Nausea:	+	−	−	+	−
- Muscle rigidity:	↑	↓		↑	−
- Dependence:	+	±	−	−	−

- = no effect, + = effect, ↑ = increase, ↓ = decrease
(Adapted from Herz 1986 a; Jaffe and Martin WR 1985)

- ε-receptors, the natural ligand is β-endorphin
- σ-receptors: no natural ligand found, agonist (SKF-10 047)
All the receptors are inactivated by naloxone.
Pharmacological effects of opioid drugs and peptides are related to interactions with a particular constellation of receptors (Tab. 9).
There are distinct differences between cerebral and spinal pain modulating

Table 10. Classification of opioid drugs according to their receptor affinity.

Drugs	Receptor types			
	μ	κ	σ	δ
1 - PURE AGONISTS				
- morphine	HA	LA	LA	-
- DADL	CA	-	-	HA
2 - PURE ANTAGONISTS				
- naloxone	CA	CA	CA	CA
- naltrexone	CA	CA	CA	CA
3- MIXED AGONIST-ANTAGONISTS				
- nalorphine	CA	PA	HA	-
- pentazocine	CA	HA	HA	-
- nalbuphine	CA/PA	PA	LA	-
- butorphanol	CA/PA	PA	LA	-
- SKF - 10 047	?	CA	HA	-
4 - PARTIAL AGONIST-ANTAGONISTS				
- buprenorphine	PA/CA	HA	LA	-

LA = low agonist affinity
HA = high agonist affinity
PA = partial agonist affinity
CA = competitive antagonist affinity
 – = no affinity
(Adapted from Jasinski 1984; Martin WR 1983)

systems as regards the involvement of opioid receptors and respective ligands. At the supraspinal level, β-endorphins and μ-receptors seem to play a key role in pain control. κ-receptor ligands do not affect pain modulation at the midbrain level, but at the level of the spinal cord.

At the spinal level, μ-, δ-, and κ-receptor ligands are effective modulators of nociceptive transmission. But there are some differences in the relative efficiency of the various ligands against different pain stimuli pointing to receptor selectivity in antinociception.

Schmauss and Yaksh (1985 a) have shown that visceral pain is more responsive to κ -agonists than δ-agonists and that the reverse holds for cutaneous electrical stimulation. This has led to the speculation that spinal κ-agonists might be used for one type of pain while the δ-agonists would best be reserved for a different group of pain problems (Coombs 1986 a).

The role of different types of opioid receptors and their respective ligands has also encouraged the search for new opioid analgesics producing less respiratory depression and reduced dependence liability (Herz 1986 a). Thus U-5O.488 H is a selective κ-agonist opioid with an analgesic potency of approximately 1/13 of morphine. The substance provides epidural analgesia in rats and does not interact with any subtypes of opioid receptors that mediate respiratory depression. It is proposed for clinical investigation by Castillo et al. (1986 a).

3.3 Opioid agonists, opioid antagonists

3.3.1 AGONISTS

Substances act as agonists primarily at μ- and κ-receptors. The classical μ-agonist is morphine.

3.3.2 ANTAGONISTS

Opioid antagonists (Tab. 10) can be grouped into three classes (Jasinski 1979):

- pure antagonists
- mixed agonist-antagonists
- partial agonist-antagonists.

3.3.2.1 Pure antagonists

Pure antagonists are compounds that produce competitive antagonism without producing agonistic effects (e.g. naloxone).

3.3.2.2 Mixed agonist-antagonists

Mixed agonist-antagonists are compounds that produce agonistic or partial agonistic effects at κ- and σ-receptors and competitive antagonism at the μ-receptors that resembles nalorphine and cyclazocine (e.g. pentazocine).

In this way, pentazocine acts as an antagonist at the μ-receptor and as an agonist at the κ- and σ-receptor. The agonistic action at the σ-receptor is responsible for the hallucinogenic and dysphoric effects of pentazocine and butorphanol.

3.3.2.3 Partial agonist-antagonists

Partial agonist-antagonist are compounds that can partially antagonize strong agonists at one receptor and that resemble those of morphine (Jasinski 1978; Martin WR 1979; Houdé 1979) .

Partial agonist-antagonists have both an agonistic and antagonistic effect on the same receptor. When given alone they induce agonistic activity. When partial agonists are administered after pure agonists they have antagonistic activity. The partial agonists have a bell-shaped dose-response curve. In low and median doses their agonistic effect is increasing by dose increments. With further increments there is a plateau with no increasing effect and additionally increasing the dose, there might even appear antagonistic effects at the same receptor. A representative of this group is *buprenorphine*.

The antinociceptive effects of opioid antagonists differ from those of opioid agonists by the following properties:

1. Analgesia is limited by a plateau (ceiling effect) and a bell-shaped dose-response curve. The margin between effective doses and the dose producing ceiling effect responses is narrow. Increasing the dose leads to a diminished response and relative high doses produce excitation and the reversal of the depressive effects.

   Pure agonists also produce ceiling effects. However the dose margin between effective doses and plateau effects or excitation is very large.

2. Antagonistic effects are only seen if the antagonist is administered after an agonist.

3. Opioid antagonists produce tolerance and addiction (exactly like all opioids) but tolerance develops slower and dependence seems to be easier to treat with these compounds (De Castro and Kubicki 1980 b). The continued development of opioid selective agonists will provide the opportunity to alternate among receptor selective opioids and allows recovery of function of the receptor while activation of another receptor produces analgesia. This innovation may improve chronic pain management with spinal opioids (Inturrisi 1987). Possibly the ideal opioid would be a pure agonist at the κ-receptor. Such a drug would induce analgesia and sedation without respiratory depression. Furthermore it is suspected that κ-agonists have less dependence liability than e.g. morphine. But up to now no pure κ-agonist has been introduced into clinical practice.

3.4 Endogenous non-opioid neuropeptides and neuroamines

According to the investigations of Yaksh and Reddy (1981), Onofrio and Yaksh (1983 a), Yaksh et al. (1988 a) and to an overview of Dalmas et al. (1988), at least

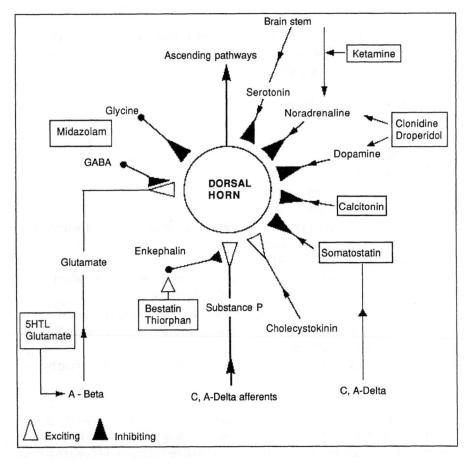

Fig. 15. The influence of several neurotransmitters on the modulation of the neuronal activity in the dorsal horn. A hypothetical dorsal horn neuron and excitatory and inhibitory pathways with known neurotransmitters; modulators of the nociceptive neurotransmission. Note that the descending inhibitory system contains both serotonin and noradrenalin. Beside these compounds acetylcholine, angiotensin II, dynorphin, glycine neurotensin and oxytocin seem to play a role in pain inhibition. (Adapted from Zimmermann and Handwerker 1984; Andersen 1986 a)

eight separate receptor systems are identified in the interneurons of the dorsal horn (Fig. 15, Tab. 7). They are able to modify the transmission of nociception.

It is suggested that peptidergic together with monoaminergic mechanisms are involved in the modulation of nociceptive information at the first stage of integration in the dorsal horn of the spinal cord (Zieglgaensberger and Butor 1985). It is now accepted that among others, the following systems can modulate the physiological response to painful stimuli:

1. The opioid peptide system with six distinct classes of spinal opioid receptors: μ_1, μ_2, δ, κ, σ, ε (see 3.2.).
2. Numerous non-opioid peptides
   - calcitonin
   - calcitonin gene related peptid
   - cholecystokinin
   - neurotensin
   - somatostatin
   - substance P
   - thyrotropin releasing hormon
   - vasopressine (ADH).
3. A noradrenergic system with the α_2-adrenergic receptor system activated by clonidine and D-medetomidine.
4. A serotoninergic system, 5HT.
5. AGABA ergic system linked to spinal nociceptive processing and activated by baclofen, amino-oxyacetic acid and midazolam.
6. An adenosine system with α_1-α_2-receptor activated by L-N6 phenylisopropyl adenosine and 5 N-ethylcarboxamide adenosine, antagonized by 8-phenyltheophylline or caffeine.
7. A cholinergic system with muscarine and nicotine receptors activated by carbachol (antagonist: bicuilline) and oxotremorine.

These modulators are other classes of agents that have shown to alter the pain behaviour. However, absence of adequate structure activity or effects on the motor system make the interpretation of their analgesic effects difficult to access (Yaksh 1987 a; Yaksh et al.1988 a).

The systems are independent, complementary and additive in the pain stimuli modulating processes of the dorsal horn. They develop tolerance and tachyphylaxis but cross-tolerance between the systems is not observed.

Activation of the non-opioid receptors produces only partial inhibition of the nociceptive stimulation. Synergistic interactions are observed, e.g., between α_2 and μ-agonists.

All these spinal modulators of pain stimuli are located in the axon synapses and the outer side of the nerve cell membranes. They produce in the internal cell structure changes in the energy supply systems cAMP and gAMP and in the ion flux with the end result of hypo- or hyperalgia. The spinal administration of receptor selective agents other than the opioid alcaloids, may possess advantages in acute or chronic pain therapy or both.

The most representative modulating systems will be discussed further in Sections 3.4.1. and 3.4.2.

3.4.1 Substance P

Substance P is a neuropeptid with 11 amino acids with the following sequence:

Arg-Pro-Lys-Pro-Gln-Gln-Phe-Phe-Gly-Leu-Met-NH$_2$

It is widely distributed in the central and peripheral nervous system. Substance P is produced in the spinal ganglion cells and by axonal transport transmitted to nerve endings peripherally and centrally.

Substance P generally acts excitatory as a neurotransmitter of nociceptive sensory afferents. But substance P not only reduces the pain threshold, it also has been reported to be responsible for analgesia. The dose-response curve is bell-shaped with increase of doses leading to no further activity or even hyperalgesia. Another explanation is the fact that also sensory neurons can be also activated (hyperalgesia) as descending control systems (analgesia) (Frederickson et al. 1978; Malick and Goldstein 1978). Substance P injected intrathecally antagonizes both the spinal antinociceptive effect of morphine and of noradrenaline (Sawynok et al. 1984).

The action of opioids and substance P are antagonistic. It is suggested that endorphins presynaptically inhibit the release of substance P, and postsynaptically decrease the action of substance P by substituting it at the receptor.

3.4.2 Other peptides and amines

Descending pathways from the higher centers of the CNS can modify noxious inputs to the sensory functions of the dorsal horn at the spinal level. The pharmacology of these descending systems is extraordinary complex. There exist descending inhibitory tracts from the formatio reticularis to the dorsal horn which are activated by 5-HT, *noradrenaline* and *adrenaline*, endogenous opioids and various other putative substances, as revealed by recent immunocytochemical techniques (Besson 1988). Intrathecal administration of noradrenaline and various other α_1-agonists (e.g. methoxamine) and α_2-agonists (e.g.ST91 and clonidine) produced a dose-dependent antinociception in rats (Reddy et al. 1980). These effects were clearly due to an action on spinal receptors.

Clonidine

Clonidine, produced a dose-dependent, long lasting elevation in the shock titration threshold after intrathecal injection. The action could be antagonized by yohimbine and phentolamine, but not by naloxone. Selectively activating α-adrenergic receptor systems lead to powerful analgesia (Yaksh and Reddy 1981; Kitahata 1989; Murata et al. 1989; Ossipov et al. 1989).

β-agonists like isoproterenol have antinociceptive effects as well (Yaksh et al. 1988 a b).

Somatostatin

Somatostatin, a peptide of 14 amino acids mainly involved in inhibitory growth hormone release, is widely distributed in the CNS.
 Somatostatin is an inhibitor of:

- synthesis of cyclic AMP (in some cell types)
- liberation of histamine
- secretion of pepsin, cholecyctokinin, pancreozynin, gastrin and pentagastrin, secretin, glucagon, insulin, renin, TSH, GH, ACTH (Barros D'Sa et al. 1975; Fehm et al. 1976; Konturek et al. 1976 and Lucke et al. 1975).

In the spinal cord, somatostatin is found in laminae II and III (substantia gelatinosa) of the dorsal horn. The substance plays a modulating role in the transmission of nociceptive stimuli.

3.5 Other exogenous substances with spinal anti-nociceptive action

Anti-enkephalinases

Thiorphan, bestatin and ketalorphan are enkephalinase antagonists. Enkephalinases are enzymes involved in the catabolism of endorphins. Enkephalinase antagonists are able to increase the analgesic effect of endogenous opioids (Roques et al. 1984).

Ketamine

Spinal analgesia with ketamine is reported in animals by Kawana et al. (1987); Whizar Lugo and Cortex Gomez (1987).

Baclofen

A derivate of gamma-aminobutyric acid (GABA) reduces nociceptive reflexes after its administration (Wilson and Yaksh 1978). Additionally, baclofen produces a dose-dependent muscle relaxation. The effects can not be antagonized by naloxone, and there is no cross-tolerance to opioids (Levy et al. 1977).

The substances discussed in sections 3.4 and 3.5 are still under animal investigation in order to discover spinal analgesics for alternative or associated use with opioids. Some among them have reached a clinical investigation phase. They are further discussed in Section 7.4.

Conclusions

Pain impulses travel from the periphery in different pathways. Upon entering the CNS, the impulses undergo modulation in the dorsal horn of the spinal cord.

This modulation is a complex process. Many neurotransmitters participate in the processing of pain impulses and play a role in whether or not a pain stimulus will ultimately produce the sensation of pain.

Obviously, applying either these neurotransmitters or their analogues to the spinal cord or brain can also affect the transmission of pain within the CNS. It is this realization that forms the physiopharmacological basis for the application of opioids within the spinal canal to produce analgesia (Naulty 1986 a).

4. Pharmacokinetics of opioids

All the opioids have a common chemical structure (Fig. 16):

- a basic amino group of different length
- an aromatic moiety
- a basophilic centre.

Those common features appear to constitute the fundamental structural requirements for opioids (Casy 1971). However, pharmacokinetic factors display striking differences: e.g. molecular weight, lipid solubility, protein binding, ionization, influence the action of opioids, increase or decrease the transport across membranes, the receptor binding affinity, the diffusion into the CNS, the analgesic action, etc. (Tab. 11, 12).

The pharmacokinetic study of opioids provides an important step towards our understanding of their mode of action and consequently their proper application. Indeed, analgesia, safety, efficacy, onset and duration of action, clearance from the blood and the CSF, distribution into the tissues and safety of spinal opioids is determined by the physicochemical properties of each particular drug.

Comparative data on the physicochemical properties of the eight most used opioids (morphine, alfentanil, buprenorphine, fentanyl, methadone, pethidine sufentanil) are given in Tab. 13. However, the presented data are to be interpreted with great caution for several reasons:

1. Pharmacokinetic data for opioids are obtained by drug dosages in blood plasma or CSF by radioimmuno- or gas-chromatographic assay methods. Radioimmuno-assay methods codetermine the opioid and its metabolites, e.g. glucoronide and cross-reactions with metabolites may provide problems of non-specificity in the dosage. Gas chromatographic assay methods allow purification of the sample by selective extraction and so they are more specific. However, in the context of clinical studies, many methods are not sensitive enough.
2. Values of clinical interest are mainly those which are related to the conditions existing in the human body, that is 37°C and a pH of 7.4. But most values are not obtained under such conditions.
3. All the pharmacokinetic values are pH and temperature dependent (Kaufman et al. 1975), they will change during particular physiological or pathological situations. They may also be modified by drug associations.

COMMON STRUCTURE OF DIFFERENT OPIOIDS
USED FOR RGOA

$$-\overset{\displaystyle |}{\underset{\displaystyle |}{C}}-C-C-N-$$

<u>4 - PHENYLPIPERIDINES</u>

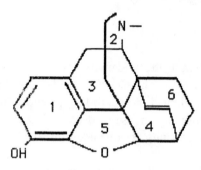

1 RING :   PRODINES

2 RINGS : PETHIDINES

3 RINGS : BENZOMORPHANS

4 RINGS : MORPHINANS

5 RINGS : MORPHINES

6 RINGS : ORIPAVINES

<u>PHENYLPERIDINES</u>

Fig. 16. The common "analgesiphoric" structure of opioids is represented by the sequential structure of a quaternary carbon atom, a C-C bridge and a nitrogen atom.
The most used substances are anilinopiperidine or phenylpiperdine derivatives.

Table 11. Physicochemical factors affecting the penetration of opioids into the CSF.

Penetration of opioids into the CSF

I - Direct relationship:
- Free fraction in plasma at pH 7.4 (unbound to protein)
- Un-ionized base at plasma pH 7.4
- Lipid solubility at plasma pH 7.4

II - Inverse relationship
- Molecular weight
- Plasma protein binding at plasma pH 7.4
- Ionization constant, pKa at plasma pH 7.4

Table 12. Drug properties contributing to high efficacy and long action of spinal opioids.

• High lipid solubility • High specific receptor affinity • Low protein binding • Low ionization	**High efficacy**
• High molecular weight • Low lipid solubility (low BBB crossing capacity) • Stability of receptor binding	**Long acting**

BBB = blood brain barrier

4. Patients in pain are submitted to a great inter-individual variability in nociceptive stimuli modulation, in opioid receptor sensibility, and in placebo
   effects. As a consequence, in the clinic, the three most important opioid
   parameters (onset, peak effect, and duration of analgesia) can only be
   evaluated very approximately.
5. The data presented in Tab. 13 are adapted from different sources and different authors and thus merely obtained under different experimental conditions. That is the principal reason why data may differ from author to author.
   Therefore, they are to be considered as indicative rather than absolute values.

Table 13. Comparative pharmacokinetic data of eight opioids used in spinal analgesia.

	Units	Morphine	Methadone	Pethidine	Alfentanil	Fentanyl	Sufentanil	Lofentanil	Buprenorphine
Molecular weight	Dalton	285	309	297	416	336	387	409	468
Lipid solubility	Log P	0	2.06	1.33	2.11	2.98	3.24	3.16	3.96
Ionisation constant	pka	8.15 - 9.55	9.30	8.50	6.50	8.43	8.01	7.82	8.40
Un-ionized fraction	%	24	1	5	89	9	20	27	
Protein binding	%	35	92	65	88	79	91	93.5	96
Tot.dist. volume	l/kg	3.0	2 - 12	2 - 8	0.86	4.0	2.9	3.0	2.5
Plasma t 1/2 β	min	177	1080	192	94	219	164	320	120 - 290
Clearance	ml/kg/min	14.7	1.8	12	6.4	13	12.7	10	13 - 18
Rel.pot. CNS entry		1	12	Ø	10	155	133	299	Ø
Specific receptor binding	%	Ø	Ø	Ø	50	75	90	Ø	Ø

Ø = no information available
NB: all data are approximations as there is some variation in published values

4.1 Molecular weight [dalton]

The molecular weight of an opioid base is an important factor for the permeability through the dura mater (Fig. 17). There is an inverse ratio of dura permeability and molecular weight. Opioids with low molecular weight have a high permeability through the dura mater (Moore et al. 1982). The permeability of the lumbar dura mater is 9 times greater for morphine (mw: 285) than for buprenorphine (mw: 468). But as also other factors determine the whole amount of drug transported, the total dose of epidural morphine or buprenorphine transferred across the dura is 20 % and 0.17 %, respectively (Moore et al. 1982). The molecular weight of morphine and pethidine (mw: 247) is comparable to that of local anaesthetics. Both opioids and the local anaesthetics have a similar permeability at the dura mater.

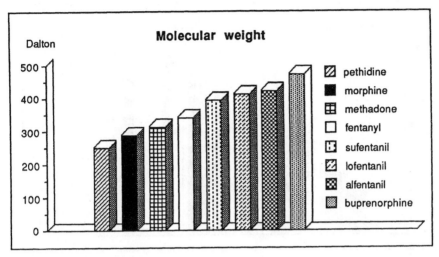

Fig. 17. Molecular weight: schematic representaion for 8 opioids.
The molecular weight is the sum of the atomic weights of all the atoms in the opioid base molecule
(Adapted from Cousins and Bridenbaugh (1986)).

4.2 Lipid solubility, hydrosolubility

Lipid or hydrosolubility (Fig. 18, 19, Tab. 14, 15, 16, 17) is measured by an experimentally determined constant: the partition coefficient (P), which measures at a given temperature and pH the ratio of the drug in the hydrophobic phase (e.g. octanol) [Co] to the neutral drug in the hydrophilic phase (water) [Cw].
P=Co/Cw.

Measurements of P are done at 21-23°C and at pH providing an un-ionized form of the compound. For practical reasons P can be expressed as log P.

Lipid solubility is one of the most important pharmacokinetic parameters for the action of opioids. The more lipid soluble the opioid, the more rapid will be the absorption from the epidural space into the blood flow and into CSF (Gourlay et al. 1985) .

Lipid solubility allows the rapid access across the blood/brain barrier into the CNS. The compounds with high lipid solubility and consequently low hydrosolubility such as buprenorphine, sufentanil, lofentanil or fentanyl diffuse easier across biological lipophilic membranes than compounds with low lipid solubility such as morphine, dihydromorphine, hydromorphone, ketobemidone (Herz et al. 1970). High hydrosolubility is also responsible for a slow reabsorption from the CSF back to the systemic circulation. Consequently, the most hydrophilic substance morphine has the longest duration of action after epidural or intrathecal administration.

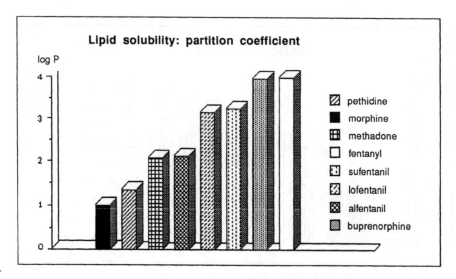

Fig. 18. Lipid solubility coefficient: schematic representation for 8 opioids.
- Lipid solubility is traduced by the partition coefficient P
- Log P: the logarithmic expression of P, the logarithm is chosen for reason of easy reading of the values.
- P n-octanol-water: measured in experimental conditions at room T° (21-23°C) and pH providing the un-ionized form of the compound.
- Theoretical P: the interesting values for the clinic are those existing at T°37°C and pH.7.4. Such values can be only obtained by estimation.
- Pi+Pu: theoretical partition coefficients estimated for physiological conditions of body T° and of pH 7.4.
(Adapted from Cousins 1987 b; Hug and Chaffman 1984 a; Mather 1983 a, b)

There is also a correlation between lipid solubility and analgesic activity after the intravenous and spinal administration. Lipophilic drugs like fentanyl are much more potent than hydrophilic ones when given intravenously. For intrathecal opioids there is a significant inverse correlation so that the most lipid soluble drugs were the least potent (Mc Quay et al. 1989). This in part is due to the fact that lipophilic substances have better penetration capabilities to lipophilic membranes and tissues. Bullingham et al. (1982) calculated theoretical values for the distribution of opioids between the CSF and the spinal cord. He concluded that the percentage of the initial intrathecal dose taken up into the spinal cord is directly related to lipid solubility. The uptake is more than 95 % for high lipophilic compounds such as fentanyl and only 4 % for morphine.

Due to rapid penetration and rapid reabsorption lipophilic opioids remain only a limited time within the CSF.

The lipophilic opioids also rapidly diffuse into the lipid rich areas of the spinal cord thereby effectively reducing the amount that is available for cephalidad

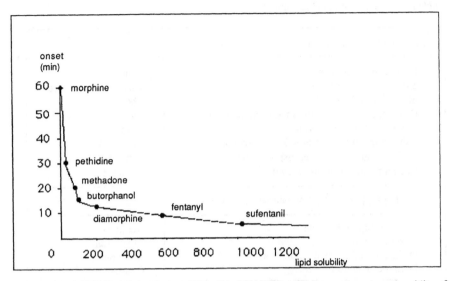

Fig. 19. Relationship between lipid solubility, blood/brain barrier penetration rate and rapidity of onset for spinal opioids.

Low lipid solubility and limited rate of blood/brain barrier penetration results in slow onset and dissipation of opioids effects. Low blood/brain barrier solubility results in a very rapid onset of opioid effects.

(Adapted from Naulty 1986; Stanski 1987)

Table 14. Classification of opioids by their lipophilic properties.

Low lipophilic properties	morphine nicomorphine hydromorphone
Medium lipophilic properties	diamorphine pethidine methadone
High lipophilic properties	alfentanil phenoperidine fentanyl lofentanil sufentanil buprenorphine

Table 15. Properties of lipophilic opioids.

1 - Lipophilic opioids administered epidurally	
- Deposit in fat tissues	Increased
- Systemic reabsorption	Faster and increased
- Stay in extradural space	Shorter
- Direct transit through dura mater to the medulla	Easier but lower
- Blood-brain-barrier crossing	Easier
- Indirect transport (systemic) to the medulla	Increased
- Diffusion along the cerebrospinal axis	Increased
- Concentration at receptor level	Reduced
2 - Lipophilic opioids administered intrathecally	
- Relationship IT/IV dose	Reduced
- Onset of action	More rapid
- Diffusion in the blood circulation	More rapid
- Duration of action	Shorter
Hydrophilic opioids have the opposite properties	

(Adapted from Herz 1986b; Moore et al. 1982; Phillips et al. 1984; Watson et al. 1984)

migration via the CSF flow (Gourlay et al. 1985).

Analgesia is more segmental with lipophilic drugs, and the risk of transport within the CSF to brain centres is lesser. On the other hand, hydrophilic opioids e.g. morphine remain for a long time within the CSF so that they are exposed to the slow CSF circulation, diffuse in rostral direction, and can induce delayed respiratory depression. These mechanisms were strongly established by two studies of Bromage and co-workers (Bromage et al. 1980 b, 1982 b). The first study with the slightly lipophilic hydromorphone demonstrated analgesia with segmental limits. Respiratory response to CO_2 was less affected by epidural than by intravenous injection. Dramatic differences with a similar protocol were obtained when the hydrosoluble morphine was administered. The CO_2-response curves were markedly depressed for more than 12 hours. And analgesia was no longer limited segmentally, rostral spread was evident, reaching even the trigeminal area within 7 hours. These data demonstrate the striking differences between hydro- and liposoluble opioids. The data clearly favour lipophilic opioids for spinal administration.

Table 16. Relationship between lipid solubility and analgesic potency of opioids.

	Absolute P n: octanol-H_2O	Medium effective dose mg/70 kg bw	
		IV route	ED route
Morphine	1.42	10	2
Pethidine	38.80	100	25
Methadone	116	10	5
Alfentanil	131	0.5	0.5
Fentanyl	813	0.1	0.1
Lofentanil	1450	0.02	0.02
Sufentanil	1778	0.005	0.005
Burprenorphine	Ø	0.3	0.3

Table 17. Relationship between lipid solubility of different opioids and the onset and duration of their analgesic effect following use of ED route.

	Partition coefficient, ratio to M=1	ED dose (mg)	Onset (min)	Duration (h)
Weak lipid solubility Morphine	1	2	20-35	8-22
Medium lipid solubility Pethidine Methadone	28 82	50 5	15-20 12-17	7-10 7-9
High lipid solubility Alfentanil Fentanyl Lofentanil Sufentanil Burprenorphine	89 676 1265 1241 670	0.5 0.1 0.005 0.05 0.03	5 4-6 20-30 5-10 5-10	1.5 2-3 5-10 2-10 4-10

M = morphine
(Adapted from Smith and Covino 1985; Hug 1984 b)

4.3 Ionization

The ionized (H^+, A^-) and the un-ionized (HA) forms of a substance exist in equilibrium in a solution as:

$$H^+ + A^- \rightleftharpoons HA$$

The Henderson-Hasselbach equation is a formula used to calculate the pH of blood from the ratio of plasma-combined CO_2 to free CO_2 (CO_2 in simple solution):

$$pH = pKa + \log \left(\frac{[HCO_3^-]}{[H_2CO_3]} \right)$$

The ionization is related to the pH. The pKa, the negative log of the apparent ionization constant, represents the pH at which the ionized and un-ionized forms of the compound are equal. Strong acids are characterized by small values of pKa and vice versa. The pKa of most opioids can vary from 7.9 to 9.4. So, they are weak bases. That means most opioids are at physiologic pH (7.3 in the CSF) predominantly ionized and have difficulties in crossing biological membranes. By increasing the pH the proportion of the un-ionized opioid form is increased and absorption will be improved (Payne 1987 b). Alfentanil with a pKa of 6.5 at 25 ° C represents an exception. This substance has already at pH 7.4 an un-ionized fraction of 89%. Alfentanil is the only opioid where the un-ionized form predominates at physiological pH. So, alfentanil, in respect of ionization, is a drug with a fast permeability through biological membranes and limited binding properties at the receptor (Fig. 20 a, b).

The un-ionized moiety of opioids is lipid soluble and kinetically mobile across lipid membranes and into lipid stores. However, it is pharmacologically inactive.

The charged, ionized moiety is pharmacologically active but kinetically immobile.

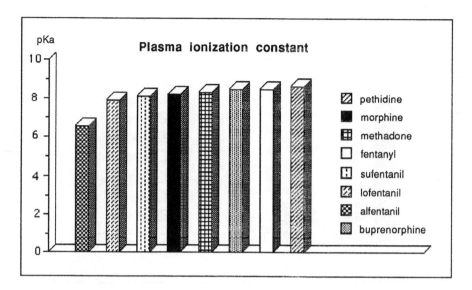

Fig. 20a. Schematic representation of the plasma ionization constant for 8 opioids.
- pKa: ionization constant, the pH of a compound at which the un-ionized and ionized concentration are equal.
(Adapted from Cousins and Mather 1984 b; Hug and Chaffman 1984 a; Hug 1984 b; Kaufman et al. 1975; Mather 1987; Stanski 1987)

For some opioids two pKa-values are determined. This is due to the fact that the amine group and the phenolic group have different ionizations. For example, the tertiary amine of morphine has a pKa of 7.9, and the phenol group one of 9.6. (Dahlström et al. 1986 b) Ionization depends also on the temperature at which the measurements are performed. So, the literature quotes a wide variation in pKa-values depending on the fact of whether the investigation is performed at body temperature of 37°C or at room temperature of 20°C (Kaufman et al. 1975). However, it can be anticipated that in all opioids tissue buffering ensures a rapid equilibrium in fluids like CSF or blood.

4.4 Protein binding

In blood and other fluids, drugs are bound to proteins in a reversible way.

Thereby, a drug is always present in two forms in body fluids, bound and unbound. Only the free compound of the drug crosses biological membranes and is pharmacologically active for the specific effect (Fig. 21).

The protein content of the CSF is very low. So, protein binding in this compartment does not very much influence the fixation of a drug within the CSF.

62

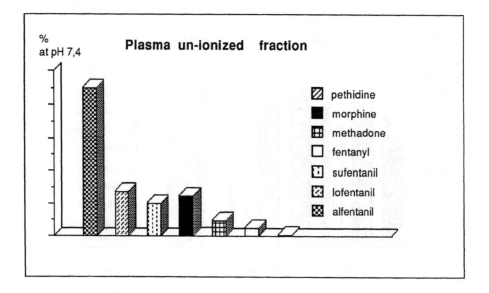

Fig. 20b. Schematic representation of the plasma un-ionized fraction for 7 opioids.
- Un-ionized fraction: % drug un-ionized in plasma
- Ionized fraction: % drug ionized in plasma
- Most opioids at pH 7.4 are ionized in excess compared to the un-ionized part (73-99% compared to 1-27%)
- Alfentanil is an exception at pH 7.4: ionized part is lower than 11%, the un-ionized part 81%
- Alfentanil has also compared to other compounds of the fentanyl family a lower lipid solubility of the free base (log P = 2.11 compared to 3.16-3.98)
- These two properties provide particular distribution and binding characteristics for alfentanil. (Adapted from Cousins and Mather 1984 b; Hug and Chaffman 1984a; Hug 1984 b; Kaufman et al. 1975; Mather 1987; Stanski 1987)

In contrast, after a systemic injection of the same substance binding to plasma proteins may play a very important role during its systemic circulation.

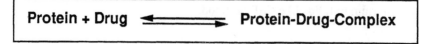

The very low protein content of the CSF presents another characteristic: its spread is not homogenous since a gradual decrease is observed from the lumbo-sacral area to the cerebral ventricle. Consequently, the higher the point of injection of the opioid on the vertebral column, the lesser the role of protein binding. It follows that after administration of the opioid at a high level, near the cerebrum, the potency of the opioid or of the local anaesthesic is greatest (Cousins and Mather 1984 b).

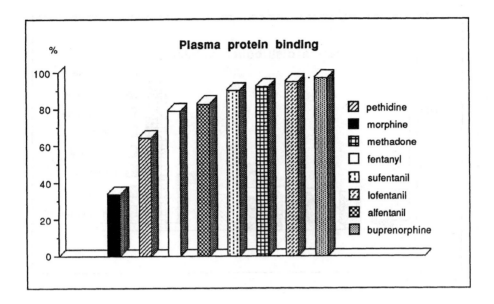

Fig. 21. Schematic representation of plasma protein binding for 8 opioids.
(Adapted from Bower and Hull 1982; Hug 1984 b; Mather 1987; Reitz et al. 1984; Stanski 1987)
- Plasma protein bound fraction: % drug bound to plasma (inactive part) protein at 50 ng/ml.
- Free plasmatic fraction: % drug not bound in the plasma (active part)

4.5 Distribution volume

The distribution volume is the relationship between the injected dose and the plasma concentration. Different distribution volumes can be distinguished (Fig. 22).

Initial distribution volume: ratio between the administered dose of a drug and the plasma concentration of the drug extrapolated at the time zero after the injection.

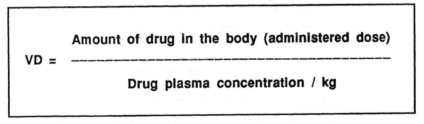

Apparent distribution volume: ratio between the amount of the drug in the tissues and its plasma concentration at the time of equilibrium between the two compartments.

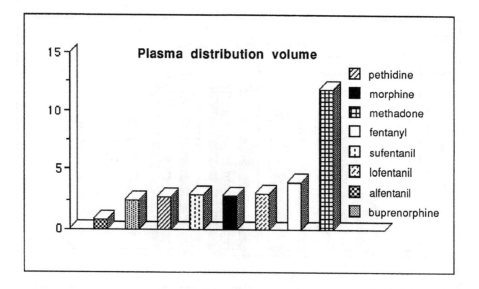

Fig. 22. Schematic representation of plasma distribution volume for 8 opioids.
- VD: apparent volume of distribution, terminal phase. The apparent volume into which a drug
  distributes in the body at equilibrium, in relation to the body weight.
  This is the ratio of drug/plasma concentration/kg
- VC: apparent volume of central compartment.
(Adapted from Bovill et al. 1982, 1984; McClain and Hug 1980; Mather 1987; Stanski 1987)

The difference between steady state and initial volume gives an indication of
the extent of tissue distribution of the drug as soon as equilibrium is reached,
or:

VD ss = apparent volume of distribution at steady state.

$$VD_{ss} = \frac{Qd\ eq}{Cp\ eq} = \frac{\text{Quantity of drug distributed through the whole body at equilibrium}}{\text{Concentration of drug in plasma at equilibrium}}$$

A high volume of distribution means that a greater proportion remains within
the tissue and a minor proportion in the plasma, from which it can be eliminated
by hepatic metabolism. For example the distribution volume of fentanyl is 12-
fold higher than that of alfentanil. Thus, the tissue localization of fentanyl is also

12-fold higher. Consequently, the risk of delayed respiratory depression is extremly higher for fentanyl than for alfentanil, because fentanyl may be redistributed from tissue depots. For spinal opioids the plasma distribution volume is not as important, because only a limited amount of the drug is resorbed to systemic circulation. In contrast to plasma volume of distribution the CSF compartment is less than 1/3000 compared to the central compartment. Consequently, even small amounts of opioid applied intrathecally will give rise to enormeous CSF concentrations and small CSF distribution volumes (Nordberg et al. 1984 a).

Several drug properties may influence the VD:

- protein binding (plasma, tissues)
- physiological properties (molecular weight, pH, pKa)
- affinity for particular tissues (e.g. lipids for high liposoluble drugs)
- membrane crossing ability.

Several physiological characteristics may modify the VD:

- age (great differences for neonates and elderly)
- pregnancy
- obesity
- hepatic or renal insufficiency
- infections
- heart disease
- thyroid hyperactivity.

4.6 Plasma half life times

The plasma half life time represents the time interval to reduce the plasma concentration of a given drug amount to its half value by resorption, distribution or elimination processes (Fig. 23).

The total half life of a substance is determined by different subgroups of half life times. T $1/2 \pi$ is the resorption half life time to shallow compartments, t $1/2 \alpha$ represents the distribution half life time to peripheral compartments, and the t $1/2 \beta$ represents the elimination half life time. Those times play an important role, when opioids are given parenterally, because most of the substance remains within the plasma due to the limited transport over the blood/brain barrier. The conditions are different for epidural or intrathecal administration of opioids. Here, receptor binding and lipid solubility determine the time-effect-curve. The terminal elimination half life of morphine in CSF is comparable to the morphine half life in plasma (Nordberg et al. 1983).

66

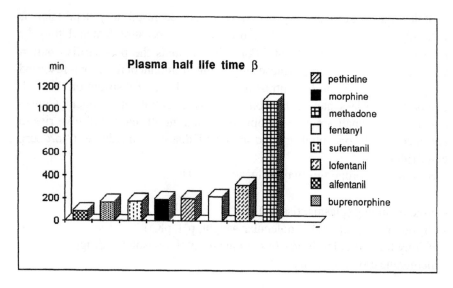

Fig. 23. Schematic representation of plasma elimination half-life time β.

$$-t\,1/2\,\beta \;=\; \frac{0.683 \times VD}{Cl}$$

(Adapted from Bovill et al. 1982,1984; McClain and Hug 1980; Mather 1987; Stanski 1987)

4.7 Clearance

The total body clearance includes all the elimination processes in a single expression:

$$Cl \;=\; K_\varepsilon \times VD$$

K_ε = the rate constant of elimination (hours or minutes).
$\qquad K_\varepsilon = 0.693/t\,1/2\,\beta$
VD = the volume of distribution (ml)
Cl = the expression of the extent to which a substance after distribution is removed from the body in unit of time (Fig. 24).
The plasma clearance is the extent, to which a substance after distribution is

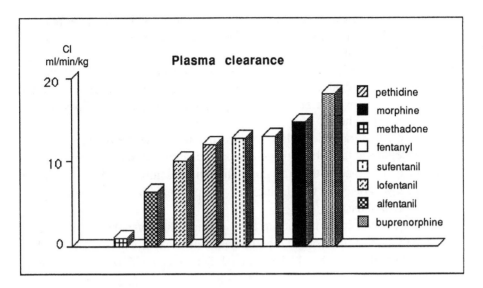

Fig. 24. Schematic representation of plasma clearance of 8 opioids.
- Plasma clearance (Cl): reflects removal of drug from plasma per unit time.
(Adapted from Bovill et al. 1982; Mather 1987; Stanski 1987)

cleared from the plasma by the kidneys, liver, intestine, lungs e.g., and is expressed by ml/kg/hour.

The CSF clearance is the rapidity of elimination of the substance from the CSF. Age, obesity, renal and hepatic insufficiency may be responsible for a reduced clearance and hence prolonged opioid effects. Special attention is to be given to alfentanil, which is the only opioid with a significantly lower distribution volume than most other opioids and a relative low clearance.

4.8 Permeability across biological membranes

The transport across biological membranes is determined by certain factors: vascularity of the tissue, ionization, protein binding, lipid solubility and volume of the solution (Fig. 25).

1. Small molecules diffuse easier than great ones. The size of a molecule depends on molecular weight, molecular shape and the binding of the molecule to proteins.
2. The un-ionized form of the drug diffuses easier.
3. Lipid soluble drugs diffuse easier than hydrosoluble drugs.

Administered intravenously only a small fraction of an opioid penetrates into the CNS. Only 0.1% of morphine reaches the CNS-receptor sites. That represents 0.01 mg of a dose of 10 mg morphine given intravenously (Stanley 1980). Surprisingly, the same is true for both the hydrophilic morphine and the lipophilic methadone (Payne et al. 1986). The method of intraspinal opioid administration has the advantage of bypassing the blood-phase before entering the CNS-tissues with the receptor sites.

However, epidural opioids have to pass the dura mater before reaching the opioid receptors at the substantia gelatinosa. As discussed in the above sections, some factors influence the transport. High lipid solubility, high un-ionized fraction, low molecular weight increase the permeability through biological membranes and tissues.

The dura mater itself has no uniform permeability over the whole length. Related to the thickness of the membrane the permeability is better in the thin lumbar dura than in the thicker cranial dura mater (Moore et al. 1982).

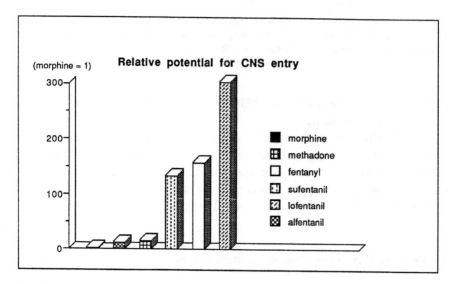

Fig. 25. Schematic representation of relative potential for CNS entry for 6 opioids.
- The dura permeability as measured in vitro by Moore (1982) indicates a linear relationship to the inverse of the square root of molecular weight.
- The permeability of the same opioid across the lumbar dura is usually significantly greater (± 30%) than that for the cranial dura which accords with the greater thickness of the cranial dura.
- Low molecular weight and slow absorption produce high dural transfer.
- The relative potential for entering the CNS: partition coefficient at pH 7.4 multiplied by the free fraction of drug in plasma and divided by the value for morphine (Hug 1984 b).
- The most important factors of diffusion into the CNS are the lipid to water partition coefficient and the degree of ionization (only an un-ionized drug penetrates into the brain).
- Epinephrine reduces the vascular resorption of opioids.
(Adapted from Hug and Chaffman 1984 a; Hug 1984 b; Moore et al. 1982)

Hyperthermia or inflammation increases the meaningful permeability (Allinson and Stach 1978). Concluding from the study of Moore et al. (1982) the dural transfer is increased by:

- low molecular weight (most important factor)
- high volumes
- slow vascular and tissue absorption rate
- molecular shape (extended shape)
- high injection pressure.

The role of lipid solubility itself is for dural transfer a minor one. Theoretically, the best transfer rates should be obtained for morphine or pethidine, the drugs with the smallest molecular weight. The calculated amount of morphine or buprenorphine crossing the dura is calculated by 20 % or 0.17 %, respectively (Moore et al. 1982). Perhaps the action of the dura mater is more or less a molecular sieve.

To reach the subarachnoid space there are secondary pathways beside the transport via the dura mater. The blood vessels around the dorsal nerve root give access to the CSF (Cousins and Mather 1984 b). This bypass is greater for the lipophilic drugs, which also enter easily into the systemic circulation. Another amount of the opioid can enter the CSF via the arachnoid granulations located at the entry zone of the nerve root sleeves.

An important clinical point is the fact that the transport across the dura mater is equal in both directions. That means all substances quickly entering the CSF (e.g. lipophilic ones) also leave the CSF as quickly. This represents the danger of all the hydrophilic opioids like morphine, which are crossing the dura quickly but which remain within the CSF for a long time free for transport to brain centres. This transport is responsible for side effects.

The problems of placental barrier crossing are governed by the same parameters as those described for the haemato/meningeal barrier. Therefore, if opioids are administered by the spinal route in obstetrics, the rules are the same for mother and child. But before crossing the placental barrier the substance has to be reabsorbed by the systemic circulation. Lipophilic opioids have our preference because the lipophilic placenta is binding those substances easier than hydrophilic opioids.

4.9 Diffusion of spinal opioids

The distribution of an opioid from the epidural space develops in different directions. Four main pathways give access to a network of secondary ones (Figs. 26 a b, 27).

A first fraction of the opioid crosses directly the relative barrier imposed by the dura mater and enters the CSF.

A second fraction of the injected opioid is reabsorbed by the systemic circulation and the extent of this reabsorption is very similar to that seen after an intramuscular injection (Chauvin et al. 1982 a, b). A small part of this fraction of the drug reaches the spinal and central opioid receptors by the normal blood circulation.

It should be noted that the plexus of the vena vertebralis interna has no valves and has indirect communication with the intracranial venous sinuses above, and the azygos system below. This would explain the fact that, in the presence of hypertension in the epidural space, the venous flow is mainly directed to the brain. In this situation, e.g. during a Valsalva manoeuvre, the substances injected into the epidural space can reach the rostral centres directly and rapidly.

A third fraction of the opioid is mixed with the passive rapid circulation flow of the intracranial CSF through dural root sleeves and via arachnoid villi (Cousins and Mather1984 b). This occurs mainly in cases of Valsalva or coughing.

A fourth fraction is temporarily inactive in the form of a depot absorbed in the fatty tissues near the injection area, from where it is either progressively reabsorbed by the parenteral route, or where it remains available for transdural spread into the CSF without being bound to the specific receptors. From the CSF it can migrate rostrally, moving in a slow and passive flow to reach, within 3 to 5 hours, the opioid receptors located in the brainstem.

Differences exist within this fraction between lipid soluble and hydrosoluble opioids. The lipophilic ones quickly bind to the lipid tissues (CNS), so that a minor proportion of them remains free within the CSF than is the case with the hydrophilic opioids.

In conclusion, at least 4 routes exist from the epidural space to the CSF (Fig. 26 a).

These different options governed by physical, physicochemical and biological variables explain the reported variability in both plasma and CSF levels after epidural opioid injections.

From the moment an opioid has entered the CSF it is submitted to the diffusion and circulation modalities of the subarachnoid space. Protein binding and metabolism of the opioid in the CSF can be dismissed.

The mechanism of bulk movement of spinal CSF in a cranial direction is unclear but changes in intra-abdominal and intrathoracic pressures and turbulences produced in the CSF by injection of solutions with volumes exceeding 10% of the spinal CSF volume (> 15 ml) are important factors (Payne 1987 a).

Normally, it takes several hours before the liquor circulation has brought a drug into the ventricle system. (DiChiro et al. 1976) (Fig.14). But also a fast

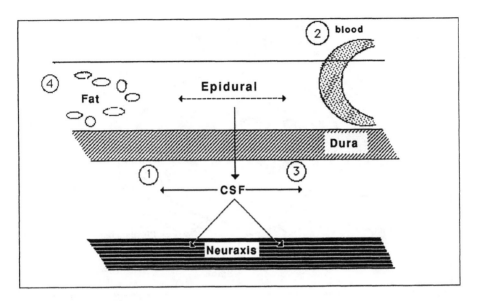

Fig. 26a. Diffusion pathways after EDOA (longitudinal view)
1. diffusion through the dura
2. vascular absorption
3. root sleeves and arachnoid villi
4. fat uptake
(Modified adaption from Bromage 1984 a)

movement is possible. A water soluble contrast medium spreads within 10 to 15 minutes to the lateral ventricle, when a head down position is held by the patient. (Allison and Stach 1978). Consequently, the same is true for morphine and other hydrophilic opioids. But we have to be aware that the dangerous CSF circulation is not the fast one, but much more dangerous is the slow one which exposes the patient to possible side effects after 12 hours at a time when we do not expect any danger. This danger is greater with the hydrophilic opioids, as mentioned above. The hydrophilic stubstances diffuse very slowly into the neuraxis and, consequently, the amount of drug exposed to CSF circulation is extremely higher than in liphophilic opioids.

Only the first point of the four uptake routes, direct transdural diffusion to the opioid receptors, contributes positively to the main object of the epidural opioid treatment, that is analgesia (Fig. 27). The three other ways represent possible bypasses to side effects and delayed respiratory depression. The latter point explains why, in intraspinal opioids, all the attention must be concentrated on modalities reducing the extensive spread of the opioid (Tab. 18, 19). An extensive spread of the opioid injected epidurally and consequently more intense

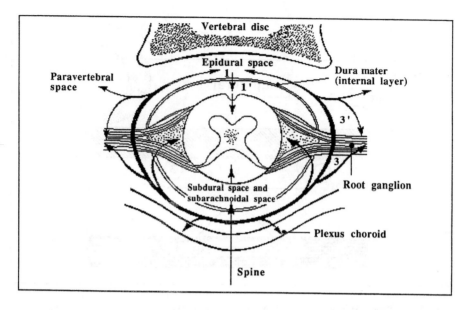

Fig. 26b. Diffusion pathways after EDOA (transversal view).
1 - diffusion through the dura to CSF
1'- diffusion from CSF to cord
2 - dural root sleeves to nerve root and cord
2'- dural root sleeves to spinal nerve
(Adapted from Lecron 1986)

depressive effects may occur in the following situations:

- epidural stop by hernial disk
- a cava obstruction and distended extradural veins
- aged arteriosclerotic or diabetic patients (extradural diffusion is increased in these patients)
- inadvertent dural puncture
- subdural injection by needle or catheter (Stevens and Stanton-Hicks 1985).

4.10 Specific receptor binding activity

Opioids have no effect in the CSF but in the spinal cord, which is lipid.Thus the more lipid soluble drugs will be taken up into the spinal cord more quickly than water soluble drugs (Glynn et al.1987 b).

The affinity of an opioid to bind with his specific receptor, the specificity and the strength of this binding and finally the time that the opioid occupies the receptor reflect the potency and the duration of analgesia (Tab. 20 a, b). The

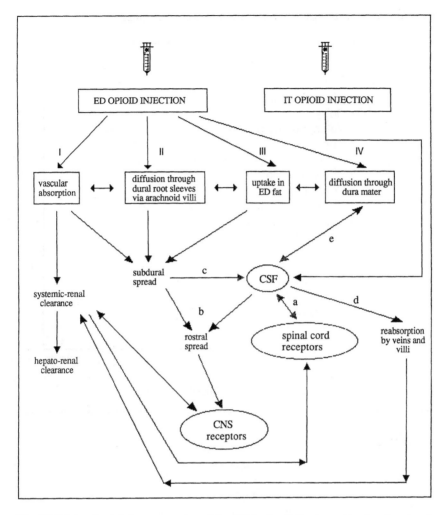

Fig. 27. Schematic global representation of the distribution following epidural or intrathecal administration.

binding assays of opioids to the opioid receptors can be evaluated by quantitative and qualitative parameters. Rapidity, strength, duration of binding or time before dissociation from receptors can be measured in vitro in cell membrane suspensions mixed with the radioactive ligand. Binding affinities correlate highly significantly with the analgesic potency measured in vivo (Tab. 20 b). Lipid solubility, ionization, molecular weight and other physicochemical properties have no or very little influence on receptor binding. Among the strong pure agonists lofentanil binds to the receptor over a long period of time. Fentanyl has a faster dissociation rate, and alfentanil has the most rapid dissociation from the receptor.

Table 18. Some parameters and technical modalities affecting the diffusion of spinal opioids.

---

1 - Technique

- ED or IT administration
- Dose
- Volume of the bolus
- Specific gravity
- With or without epinephrine
- Site of injection
- Position of the patient
- Speed of injection, turbulence

2 - Individual factors

- Epispinal vascularisation
- Obesity, age, epidural fat
- Permeability of the spinal dura mater
- Intraspinal pressure
- Intraabdominal and intrathoracic pressure

Table 19. Modalities to reduce intraspinal spread of opioids.

AVOID

- Hydrophilic opioids
- High volume
- Injection at high level
- Intrathecal injection
- Epinephrine (in combination with morphine)
- Forced injection
- Brisk movements and cough during injection

PREFER

- Lipophilic opioids (e.g. fentanyl and sufentanil)
- Reduced volume
- Dilution in small volume: 5 - 10 ml
- Slow injection

Table 20a. Comparative estimation of receptor interactions.

	Dissociation time (min) $t_{1/2}\alpha$ $t_{1/2}\beta$	% Specific binding	Kd nmol
Alfentanil	too rapid to be mesaured	50	0.25
Fentanyl	5 1.2	75	1
Sufentanil	125 25	90	0.13
No information on other opioids			

- The binding assays of opioids to the opioid receptors can be evaluated by quantitative and qualitative parameters.
  Rapidity, strength, duration of the binding with or the dissociation from the receptors can be measured in vitro on a cell membrane suspension mixed with a radioactive ligand.
- Specific binding % of receptors occupied.
- Dissociation times: speed of dissociation from the opioid receptors:
  . t 1/2 α = rapid dissociation time
  . t 1/2 β = slow dissociation time
- Kd: value of the binding equilibrium constant of the labelled ligand.
(Adapted from Leysen et al. 1980; Leysen and Gommeren 1983; Hug and Chaffman 1984 a; Hug 1984 b)

Stereospecificity is another factor since the opioid must be recognized by his specific receptor. The behaviour of opioids given by the spinal route is not different from that after their parenteral administration. Example: the dextrorotatory isomer of morphine is totally inactive, the active form of morphine is the natural levorotatory molecule.

Another example is the lability of met-enkephalin and leu-enkephalin. Both endorphins are degraded very quickly by peptidases. But, when changing their structure by introduction of D-amino-acids their stability is increased. The greater stability is due to a greater affinity to the specific opioid receptors.

For the stereospecific binding at the receptor ionization plays an important role, too. For the receptor only the ionized fraction of the substance is acceptable, whereas for transport to the receptor the un-ionized fraction is the active form.

4.11 Rediffusion

There appears to be very little metabolism of opioids either in the CSF or in the spinal cord and so the elimination of the drug from the cord will be done via the CSF and the bloodstream (Glynn et al. 1979).

Table 20b. In vitro receptor binding affinities.

Opioids	κ (nmol/l)
• Lofentanil	0.06
• Sufentanil	0.13
• Fentanyl	0.5
• Buprenorphine	1.13
• Naloxone	5.2
• Morphine	10 (approx.)
• Pethidine	10000 (approx.)

Receptor binding affinity of opioids measured in vitro, correlates with analgesic potency.
(If the needed opioid concentration is low the receptor binding affinity is high. Thus a low κ-value represents high receptor binding affinity.)
(Adapted from Leysen and Gommeren 1983; Boas and Villiger 1985)

Five clearance routes can be followed by the opioid (Fig. 27):

1. Migration to the opioid receptors located in the spinal cord in the vicinity of the injection level, where receptor binding produces the specific analgesic effect.
2. Dilution by new CSF.
3. Reabsorption by veins and villi (arachnoid, arachnoid villi, choroid plexus).
4. Rediffusion through the dura mater and other neural sleeves.
5. Rostral spread and migration to the higher centres in the CNS.

An important role in the clearance has the venous drainage of the spinal canal. Blood drains into a tortuous venous plexus within the pia mater, which contains six longitudinal vessels. These are connected with the internal vertebral plexus in the epidural space, which is drained via the intervertebral veins into the azygos and hemiazygos system.

Blood from the vertebrae drains into both the internal and external vertebral plexuses. To reach the external plexus the veins must traverse the intravertebral foramina.

The clearance of the opioid from the CSF can be increased by:

- disturbed CSF production
- bulk flow of CSF
- passive and active CSF circulation
- active transport: Valsalva
- changes in position, high pressure, temperature increase.

Recently, lipid solubility has been demonstrated as an important factor in CSF distribution and clearance (Payne et al. 1987 a). In adults, even the lipophilic substances methadone and naloxone were cleared from CSF during descent or ascent. In contrast, more hydrophilic opioids like morphine or hydromorphone are distributed caudal-rostral and rostral-caudal in CSF (Payne et al. 1987 a).

High lipid solubility facilitates diffusion and rediffusion. Changes in intraspinal pressure can modify rediffusion. In case of hypertension in the intrathecal space the villi are more developed and due to an increased contact surface the reabsorption of the opioid in the CSF, consequently, is also increased. In case of extrinsic or intrinsic compression of the CSF the diffusion of the opioid to the cerebrum is as well accelerated.

4.12 Physical characteristics of opioid solutions

4.12.1 VOLUME, DENSITY, SPECIFIC GRAVITY, BARICITY

The physical characteristics of opioid solutions are an important determinant of CSF drug distribution.

The volume is the space expressed in ml occupied by the solution in the epidural area. Studies relating the volume of the injected opioid solutions to the degree of spread have been conflicting. Many workers have found that volume bore little relationship to spread whereas others have reported that volume influenced spread and duration of analgesia. The smallest volume still compatible with plain activity is perhaps the right choice.

The density is the ratio of the concentration of the solution to its volume expressed as g per ml. The density of the injected solution plays a very important role with reference to intrathecal opioid injections. Using the latter technique it is essential to remember that the density of the cerebral spinal fluid is relatively constant between 1003 and 1012. With regard to epidural injection the density of the solution produces no changes in its effects. The double blind studies of

Bläss (1982) made quite clear that there was no difference in the efficacy produced by 2 mg epidural morphine dissolved in 5% glucose and the same quantity dissolved in saline 0.9%.

The specific gravity is the weight of a solution compared with that of distilled water.

The baricity of a solution injected into the CSF is defined as the ratio of:

$$\text{baricity} = \frac{\text{density of a solution (g/ml)}}{\text{density of CSF (1.003 g/ml at 37°C)}}$$

The baricity of the CSF is 1.00 by definition.

An *hyperbaric solution* is a solution producing, in ambiant air, a pressure greater than one atmosphere. Glucose 10% can be added by the operator to the opioid solution to produce hyperbaric solutions. These solutions may be used only for intrathecal procedures below the diaphragma.

Isobaric solutions are opioid solutions without addition of glucose.

The distribution of intrathecally administered hypobaric (<0.9990) or hyperbaric (>1.0015) solutions in the CSF is influenced by the position of the patient, whereas isobaric solutions are not.

4.12.2 CHANGES IN BODY TEMPERATURE

In the case of significant hyperthermia or inflammation there is an increase of the meningeal permeability (Allinson and Stach 1978).

4.12.3 CHANGES IN INTRASPINAL PRESSURE

Changes in intraspinal pressure can modify rediffusion. In the case of hypertension in the intrathecal space the villi are more developed and with an increased contact surface, the reabsorption of the opioid in the CSF, consequently, is also increased. But in the case of extrinsic or intrinsic compression of the CSF, the diffusion of the opioid to the cerebrum is accelerated as well.

On the other hand, in the case of hydrocephalus internus, the villi are less developed and evacuation and reabsorption of the opioids decrease.

4.13 Special pharmacokinetics of spinal opioids

Plasma concentrations

Opioids injected in the epidural space are rapidly absorbed into the general circulation. Absorption time profiles closely resemble those obtained after intravenous or intramuscular administration. Interindividual variations are pronounced.

(For morphine see: Chauvin et al. 1981 a, 1982 a, 1988; for alfentanil see: Chauvin et al. 1983; Levron et al. 1983; for sufentanil see: Camu et al. 1985.)

CSF concentrations

Studies on pharmacokinetics of opioids in the CSF after spinal administration are rather rare because repeated concentration dosages of the spinal fluid are to be performed. Morphine, pethidine, or alfentanil have been investigated by: Chauvin 1988; Chraemmer -Jørgensen et al. 1981; Cousins and Mather 1984 b; Glynn et al. 1981; Jayais et al. 1982; Levron et al. 1983; Max et al. 1985; Nordberg et al. 1983, 1984 a; Sjöström et al. 1987 a, b; Strube et al. 1984 a.

Despite very rapid vascular uptake, opioids penetrate into the CSF to such an extent that the concentrations in the lumbar CSF far exceed the corresponding plasma concentrations. For epidural morphine (2-6 mg) the CSF concentrations increase slowly and, after 30 min, may become 50 to 250 times higher than the corresponding plasma concentrations, maximal concentrations 100 ng/ml. They remain above 20 ng/ml as long as 20 hours after the injection (Nordberg et al. 1983). Half-life times are in the same range as values obtained after intravenous administration of morphine (Nordberg et al. 1984 c) and alfentanil (Levron et al. 1983). After intrathecal morphine 1.0 mg, peak concentrations are in the order of 60,000 to 70,000 ng/ml.

After epidural pethidine the diffusion in the CSF is more rapid. Peak concentrations are reached in 15 min. They are clearly lower than those seen after morphine. After 4 to 6 hours pethidine has completely disappeared from the CSF. Interindividual variations are always very high (Chauvin 1988).

4.14 Pharmacokinetic variability

The effect of a spinal opioid injection is the global result of several factors:

- direct effects on the spinal receptors
- indirect effects produced by the parenteral uptake

Table 21. Comparison of the duration of analgesia, obtained by some opioids administered in equi-analgesic doses by the epidural, the intrathecal, the intravenous and the intramuscular route.

Products	Dose	Onset	Duration		Dose	Duration	
		ED	ED	IT		IV	IM
	(mg/70 kg)	(min)	(h)	(h)	(mg/70 kg)	(h)	(h)
Short acting drugs							
Alfentanil	0.5	5	1 1/2		0.5 - 1	1/2	
Nicomorphine	2 - 5	20	3 1/2		10	2.5	
Medium acting drugs							
Sufentanil	0.05	5 - 10	6		0.02	1	-
Fentanyl	0.1	4 - 6	2 - 3		0.1	1	-
Methadone	5	10 - 12	7 - 9		10	4 - 6	4 - 6
Pethidine	25 - 50	5 - 20	7 - 10		100	2 - 4	2 - 4
Pentazocine	20	15	10		30 - 60	2 - 3	2 - 3
Butorphanol	0.5 - 2	15	6 - 10		4	3 - 4	4 - 5
Long acting drugs							
Hydromorphone	1	10 - 20	11 - 14		1 - 2	4 - 6	4 - 5
Diamorphine	5	5	12	22	10	3 - 4	4 - 5
Nalbuphine	10	15	13		10	3 - 4	3 - 5
Buprenorphine	0.15 - 0.3	10 - 20	4 - 10	10	0.15 - 0.3	6 - 8	6 - 10
Lofentanil	0.005	20 - 30	5 - 10		0.002	8 - 12	-
Morphine	2 - 5	20 - 35	8 - 22	25	10 - 20	4	4

(Adapted from Martindale 1982 for IV route; from Bromage et al. 1980a; Camu et al. 1985; Chauvin et al. 1983; Cousins and Mather 1984 b; De Castro and Lecron 1981 b; Dirksen 1980 b; Glynn et al. 1981; Jacobson et al. 1983; Kalia et al. 1983; Kitahata and Collins 1984 a; Lecron et al. 1980 b; Mok et al. 1984 b; Naulty et al. 1984; Zenz et al. 1981 d, 1982 a for the ED route; from Glynn 1987 a for the IT route and the IM route.)

- migration of the substance to the higher cerebral centres
- individual factors (age, illness).

The real importance of each modality is not to be foreseen because it depends on multiple pharmacokinetic, physicochemical and pharmacodynamic parameters, specific for each opioid and each patient (Lanz et al. 1986 b). Some parameters act additively some others in the opposite way. It is also evident that the effect is not the same for different ways of administration (Bromage et al. 1982 b).

The most important physicochemical parameters for several pure opioids are comparatively summarized in Tab. 13, 20, 21, 22 and Fig. 17 to 25. However, the data are collected from different sources and have not been obtained in identical experimental conditions. Therefore it is necessary to interpret them merely on an indicative basis. Lipid solubility, ionization and molecular weight seem to be the most important pharmacokinetic parameters of these substances.

It is also to be remembered that pharmacokinetic data are potentially affected by kidney and liver dysfunction, concomitant agents, type of surgery, severity

Table 22. Pharmacokinetic parameters of opioids for different routes of administration.

Dose: mg/70 kg bw			Plasma t 1/2 β (min)	Total VD * (l/kg bw)	Plasma clearance (ml/kg bw/min)
Morphine	IV	10	120 - 200	1.4 - 4.6	10 - 23
	ED	3	87 - 115		
	ED	0.05	162		
	ED	2	173		
	IT	0.5	170	8.8	2.81
	IT	0.25	310	10.8	3.45
Fentanyl	IV	0.1	80 - 420	2.1 - 6.4	10 - 22
	ED	0.1	240	7.58	
Alfentanil	IV	0.3	7 - 110	0.3 - 0.8	3 - 8
	ED	1.0	89.4	0.33	3.0
Sufentanil	IV	0.01	100 - 240	2 - 3.4	9 - 15
	ED	0.075	170	9.5	3.25
Pethidine	IV	100	100 - 360	2.4	8 - 18
	ED	30	90		

*VD = volume of distribution
(Adapted from Camu et al. 1985; Chauvin et al.1983; Gustafsson et al. 1984; Levron et al. 1983; Nordberg et al. 1983; Nordberg 1984 b; Shipton et al. 1984 b; Sjöström et al. 1987 a,b; Tamsen et al.1983).

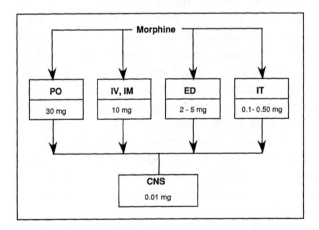

Fig. 28. Estimation of the necessary morphine (M) dose (70 kg bw) administered by peroral route (PO), intravenous (IV) or intramuscular (IM) route, epidural route (ED) or intrathecal (IT), in order to obtain a brain concentration of the opioid producing analgesia of the same depth but with important differences in rapidity of onset and duration of action. Note, it has been estimated that only 0.1% of the IV injected drug can reach the CNS.
(Adapted from Nordberg et al. 1983; Stanley 1980)

of pain, certain illnesses, obesity, age, race, sex, etc. (Kaiko et al. 1986).

Renal failure decreases the clearance of morphine (Moore et al. 1986).

Hepatic dysfunction may be accompanied by a lower clearance and an increased t 1/2 β than those seen in patients with a normal liver function (Ferrier et al. 1985; Levron et al. 1983; Shafer et al. 1986 a).

Obesity produces lower clearance and increased elimination half-life time (Bentley et al. 1983).

In geriatric patients clearance is reduced and elimination half-life time is increased but volume distribution remains unchanged (Helmers et al. 1984).

Children have, per kg body weight, a lower distribution volume than adults and present a lower fat deposit of the administered drugs. That is the reason why in children after repeated opioid injections, a lower accumulation trend of opioids may be expected. Also plasma elimination half-life time is shorter and clearance is increased. These two properties observed regularly in children may explain a more rapid recovery time with a need for more frequent opioid injections (Meistelman et al. 1987; Roure et al. 1987; Sale et al. 1986).

Onset, and even more duration of analgesia are two opioid parameters which can only be roughly evaluated in a clinical practice (Tab. 21). Nevertheless, it is evident that the duration of analgesia following epidural or intrathecal administration is, as with most opioids, consistently greater than that achieved from intravenous or intramuscular injection, thus providing good evidence for the dominant spinal effect of the analgesics given in this way (Glynn 1987 a).

This situation is not so clear cut for buprenorphine, lofentanil and methadone. Buprenorphine and lofentanil (two opioids hardly to antagonize, even by massive naloxone doses) are clearly different from the other substances. Their long duration of action is merely determined by their strong receptor binding affinity (Tab. 20 b). Absorption, distribution and excretion differences resulting from different administration routes play only a minor role in their activity profile. The epidural or intrathecal administration of such compounds does not necessarily result in longer lasting spinal analgesia than that observed after parenteral use of the same products. For the long lasting effects of methadone by all administration routes, the reported evaluations are very different. The racemic mixture of methadone (in which (-) methadone is 8-50 times more potent), the long plasma half-life time with large interindividual variations, and the multiple active metabolites, are important enough to explain the reported discrepancies.

It is above all essential to remember the enormous differences between intravenous and intraspinal opioid administration (Fig. 28, Tab. 21, 22). Facing the fact that only 0.1 % of the intravenous injected opioid reaches the CNS, the obtained CSF concentrations after spinal administration (epidural and intrathecal) are extremely high (Chauvin 1988; Cousins et al. 1979 a; Dahlström et al. 1986 b; Moulin et al. 1986 a; Nordberg 1984 b). Only for the epidural route the dura mater represents a relative barrier, which is very permeable. The further transport from the CSF to the CNS is determined above all by the lipid solubility. Highly liposoluble drugs are rapidly absorbed by the lipid tissues of the spinal cord. On the other hand, hydrophilic opioids remain within the CSF for many hours and their rostral transport seems inevitable (Bromage 1984 b). In this respect we can distinguish between high CSF clearance drugs (lipophilic) and low CSF clearance drugs (hydrophilic) (Moulin et al. 1986 a). By the way, the same is true for intravenous injections (Hartvig et al. 1986), the slightly lipophilic pethidine being cleared from the brain much faster than the hydrosoluble morphine.

Conclusions

Pharmacokinetics cannot determine all the factors influencing the clinical action of a drug. Certainly, the nature of pain, the indication for treatment and the patient himself play the most important roles.

Future knowledge will certainly give access to some deeper insights. Pharmacokinetics can be helpful. However, the real answer to the various aspects and problems related to spinal opioids must be given by the clinical practice and the individual response of the patient.

5. Pharmacodynamics of opioids

Nearly all effects of the opioids (analgesia, sedation, respiratory depression) result from an interaction with a specific opioid receptor. The desired interactions of spinal opioids are those with the spinal receptors. But rostral distribution and effect on brain receptors as a source of undesired actions can neither be completely prevented nor completely excluded.

Epidural or intrathecal opioids produce a significant elevation of the pain threshold. The effect is characterized by:

- dose dependency
- stereospecificity
- highly regular structure activity relationship
- dose-dependent antagonism by naloxone.

Spinal opioids at analgesic doses, unlike local anaesthetic agents, have neither effect on the response to light touch nor do they have any direct effects on the sympathetic nervous system or voluntary motor function. However, there is clear clinical evidence that spinal opioids do not act as pure antinociceptive substances and do not only selectively block pain transmission. Side effects always appear inherent with the analgesic effect of spinal opioids (Bromage et al. 1980 c; Bromage et al. 1982 b). The degree of those side effects certainly can be different with different methods, different drugs and different doses. Therefore, the main point for the clinical practice will be to evaluate very carefully the right patient, the right drug given in the right dose and using the right technique.

5.1 Analgesia

The intensity and duration of analgesia are related to the pharmacokinetic characteristics of the opioid. In view of a good analgesic action there is an obvious advantage for morphine (low lipid solubility = long lasting effects). But regarding the safety there is a clear disadvantage for morphine (low lipid solubility = rostral spread). So, the main point for deciding is not effectiveness of analgesia but security for the patient.

As mentioned earlier, the analgesia after epidural opioids is actually a hypalgesia, not fully comparable to that obtained with local anaesthetics. The special character of hypalgesia is documented only anecdotally (Zenz et al. 1981 b). It seems that the dull pain, corresponding to the paleo-spinothalamic pathway, is more affected by spinal opioids than the sharp pain. This would imply important consequences for the postoperative period. The diffuse wound pain is clearly diminished, whereas the sharp pain (peritoneal reactions) remains fairly unaffected. This is certainly an advantage for the early diagnosis of surgical complications which, in the case of regional blocks, are masked by the completeness of analgesia. Using different opioids, there are no proven differences in efficacy if equipotent doses of different compounds are used.

The use of the visual linear analogue scale (VAS) is the most practical method for evaluating pain and pain relief (Revill et al. 1976; Scott and Huskisson 1976)

5.1.1 RELATIONSHIP BETWEEN ADMINISTRATION ROUTE AND DOSE

One of the most outstanding advantages of spinal administration of opioids is the long duration of action in comparison to conventional analgesia provided by parenteral administration routes (Tab. 21, 22, Fig. 28).

Comparative studies were carried out with hydrophilic opioids given at approximately equianalgesic doses epidurally (morphine 5 mg) or intravenously (morphine 5-10 mg) (Bromage et al. 1982 b; Rutter et al. 1981; Torda and Pybus 1982). A duration of the analgesic action of, respectively, 18 and 11 hours for the epidural route and 3 hours for the intravenously route were found.

For lipid soluble opioids the differences between the duration of analgesia after epidural or intravenous administration are less important (Tab. 21).

The differences in bioavailability as a function of the administration route was studied after 10 mg of morphine was injected intravenously or intramuscularly. Only 0.1% or 0.01 mg penetrates into the central nervous system. To obtain the same concentration in the CNS only 5 mg of epidural or 0.25-0.5 mg of intrathecal morphine were needed (Nordberg et al. 1984 b).

This indicates that the relative potencies of morphine for the three routes of administration are as follows :

- intravenous or intramuscular   = 1
- epidural   = 2
- intrathecal   = 20-40 (Fig. 28)

Holland et al. (1981) and Reiz et al. (1981 a) failed to obtain similar results. They estimated that the effective intrathecal morphine dose may be only 5 to 10 times smaller than the effective intramuscular dose.

5.1.2 RELATIONSHIP BETWEEN DOSE AND DEPTH OF ANALGESIA

The direct relationship between dose and depth of analgesia is not as evident after epidural administration as after intravenous administration of opioids. An increase in dosage is not necessarily accompanied by a better result (Crawford 1981; McClure et al. 1980; Martin R et al. 1982). It has been demonstrated that 6 mg as well as 8 mg of morphine administered epidurally may produce an approximately identical acute effect (Pybus and Torda 1982). It becomes evident that a ceiling effect was rapidly obtained with spinal opioids and that an increase in dose was without any result as soon as a sufficient analgesia was reached. Five mg epidural morphine provided a significant improvement in postoperative analgesia compared to control groups. However, further increasing the dose to 10 mg morphine did not increase the analgesic effect but gave rise to respiratory depression 10 hours after drug administration (Allen et al. 1986).

An hyperalgesic response in a patient receiving high concentrations of intrathecal morphine was reported by Ali (1986). Yaksh et al. (1986 b) speculated that high concentrations of spinal opioids could exert an antagonism on the analgesic effect otherwise mediated by the action of the same morphine on spinal opioid receptors.

Individual variability in dose response is an important characteristic of spinal opioids.

On one hand, this variability is so high and on the other hand the dose/side effect relationship is so narrow (twice the normal dose), that in some situations titrated administration of spinal opioids against response is now recommended by many authors.

Successful use of spinal opioids in opioid-naive patients requires that the dose is carefully adjusted depending on the patient's response.

The use of a dose in an individual acute patient of twice that required for analgesia could lose all of the potential advantages (Cousins 1987 b).

5.1.3 RELATIONSHIP BETWEEN DOSE AND DURATION OF ANALGESIA

A direct relationship between dose and duration of analgesia can be observed after the epidural administration of opioids. For example 2 mg, 4 mg, 6 mg and 8 mg of morphine injected epidurally produced a duration of analgesia of 514, 543-718, 722-938, and 865 min, respectively (Nordberg et al. 1983; Pybus and Torda 1982).

As already pointed out, the longer duration of analgesia is the sole (and questionable) justification for the use of a higher dose than the minimal effective dose necessary for a sufficient analgesic effect.

88

However, it must be kept in mind that an increase in the desired effect is always accompanied by a proportional increase in side effects.

5.1.4 RELATIONSHIP BETWEEN LIPID SOLUBLE SUBSTANCES AND DURATION OF ANALGESIA

Although the duration of analgesia is quite variable with various opioids, most substances achieve a duration considerably in excess of that which may be obtained by a parenterally administered opioid or by the spinal administration of a local anaesthetic. The most hydrophilic products have the longest duration of action. The most lipid soluble opioids have the shortest duration of action. Nevertheless, exceptions to this rule exist, e.g. buprenorphine, notwithstanding its higher lipid solubility (but with a higher opioid receptor affinity), acts much longer than fentanyl (Tab. 21).

An affinity for the lipids influences not only the rate of uptake by neuronal tissue and hence latency of onset. However, the same is also true for the rate of rediffusion from the spinal cord and the subarachnoid space thereby determining the duration of action (Stanton-Hicks 1985).

Diamorphine (5 mg epidurally) although being a lipophilic substance also evokes an analgesia of relatively long duration. In this case, however, the long-lasting effect is produced by the active metabolites, the lipophylic acetyl-morphine and the hydrophylic morphine (Watson et al. 1984).

Further, there is a striking difference in the segmental distribution between different drugs. Lipophilic opioids tend to induce a clearly segmental analgesia, whereas the rostral spread with hydrosoluble opioids is quite unpredictable (Bromage et al. 1980 b, 1982 b).

5.1.5 RELATIONSHIP BETWEEN ANALGESIA AND PAIN AETIOLOGY

Intraspinal opioids may be ineffective or provide poor pain relief in the following clinical situations:

- pain caused by movements
- pain resulting of a fracture or a compression of large nerve trunks
- pain from deafferentation or from spinal cord compression
- psychosomatic pain.

5.2 Cardiovascular system and sympathetic nervous system

Heart frequency, blood pressure and cardiac output remain stable after spinal opioids (Child and Kaufman 1985; Bromage et al. 1980 b).

In contrast to intravenous morphine, which causes a significant decrease in cerebral and spinal cord blood flow in dogs, intrathecal morphine had no haemodynamic or circulatory side effects (Matsumiya and Dohi 1983).

One of the most striking differences between spinal opioids and local anaesthetics is their respective effect on the sympathetic function. Local anaesthetics block the sympathetic afferent fibres in relation to the segmental extent of the blockade. In contrast, little or no sign of sympathetic block occurs with epidural opioids apart from miosis, which is recognized, if the opioid spreads far enough rostrally, to involve the ependymal medullary nuclei. Peripheral vasodilatation is not apparent and the normal sympathetic response to a Valsalva manoeuvre is unaffected (Bromage et al. 1980 b). The psychogalvanic reflex remained uneffected after spinal opioids, but was abolished after local anaesthetics (Bromage et al. 1980 b). Plethysmographic recordings demonstrated the enormous increase of arterial blood flow in the blocked area after epidural bupivacaine. In contrast, epidural morphine did not change arterial blood flow or venous capacity (Zenz et al. 1981 g). Thus, vascular pooling and orthostatic hypotension are not likely to present a problem after intraspinal opioids (Bromage 1985).

5.3 Respiratory system

Respiratory depression is one of the most severe side effects in opioid therapy. Also epidural opioids are not free of this effect. There is a dose related depression of the CO_2-response curve after epidural morphine (Rawal and Wattwil 1984 a). The respiratory depression after morphine lasts for up to 24 hours (McCaughey and Graham 1982) and is a consequence of the rostral spread of the opioid (Bromage et al. 1982 b).

But again, marked differences exist between the different opioids. The respiratory depression seems less important after lipophilic opioids (Bromage et al. 1980 b, 1982 b) and some authors conclude that there is no danger of delayed depression after epidural fentanyl (Lam et al. 1983). In lipophilic opioids, the depression of the respiratory centre is greater after the intravenous than after the epidural administration (Bromage et al. 1980 b). Kappa-agonists are suggested to induce no danger of respiratory depression at all (Castillo et al. 1986 a, b).

A discreet clinical respiratory depression with transient bradypnea is present in the majority of cases treated. The biological changes typical for respiratory depression ($PaCO_2$ increase) are always evident. However, it is surprising that some patients tolerate more than 50 mg of morphine without any clinical sign of

90

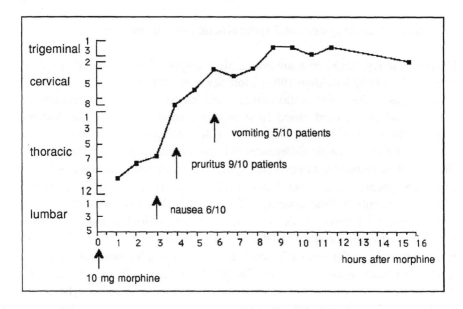

Fig. 29. Relationship between appearance of side effects and rostral spread of morphine.
(Adapted from Bromage et al. 1982 a)

respiratory depression (Greenberg et al. 1982; Woods and Cohen 1982; Zenz et al. 1985 a), whereas other patients get depressed after less than 10 mg of morphine (Crawford 1981 a; Nordberg et al. 1983). An important explanation might be the different degrees of pain.

As a theory, it can be advanced that in severe pain all opioid receptors are highly susceptible to opioids: pain opens the opioid (pain) receptors. In contrast, in painfree states or with only moderate pain the opioid receptors are fairly closed, so that most of the substance diffuse rostrally to the respiratory centres (Fig. 29, 30).

It has been demonstrated that respiratory depression is significantly more pronounced in volunteers than in patients suffering from pain (Rawal and Wattwil 1984 a). Thus, it can be explained, why opiate-naive pain patients tolerate extremely high doses of opioids without any sign of respiratory depression. Also, it has been demonstrated that the prophylactic administration of opioids in patients whose pain level is unknown increases the risk of respiratory depression (Gowan et al. 1988). Pain is a potent stimulator of respiratory drive (Hanks et al. 1981; Hanks 1984) or a potent stimulator of the opioid receptor's susceptibility.

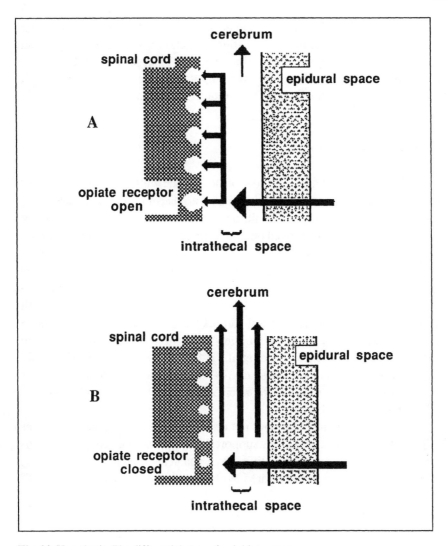

Fig. 30. Hypothesis: The differential state of opioid receptors.

A: In pain states the opioid receptors are open and susceptible to opioid substances so that not much of the opioid can diffuse rostrally

B: Without pain most of the opioid receptors are closed so that most of the opioid diffuses rostrally to the vital centres and induces respiratory depression.

(Zenz 1986 d)

5.4 Muscular system and gastrointestinal system

The muscular system and the gastrointestinal system are only moderately modified. Motor power and coordination are unaffected by epidural opioids. However, muscle tone and spasticity seem slightly diminished by spinal opioids

(Müller et al. 1985 c). The site of action is thought to be the polysynaptic reflex arc of the stretch reflex. However, intestinal muscles are also affected by spinal opioids in chronic therapy. Constipation may become a severe problem.

ED morphine produces delayed gastric emptying, ororectal transit and transit through the small intestine in healthy volunteers (Thorén et al. 1989).

5.5 Central nervous system

Even if deep analgesia with light sedation occurs, the motor system, the sensory system, and the neuroreflexes remain intact. Intrathecal opioids decrease spasticity in patients with CNS disease although they neither affect the neurotransmission of somatosensory evoked potentials nor decrease the monosynaptic H-reflex (a spinal motor reflex).

Local anaesthetics on the contrary completely abolish these reflexes (Chabal et al. 1988). A miosis is nearly always noticed. Miosis is assumed to be due to an action on the oculomotor nucleus. But evidence for this is not obtained in all species. Postoperatively, the epidural administration of low doses of morphine (2-3 mg) results in pain relief that parallels powerful depression of lower limb nociceptive flexion reflexes. Willer et al. (1985) demonstrated that 40-50 min after epidural morphine an increase of 87% of the reflex threshold appears as well as a 80-90% depression of the nociceptive responses when elicited by a constant level of stimulation.

Low dose epidural morphine does not effect non-nociceptive spinal reflexes (Willer et al. 1988). These findings support the hypothesis that epidural opioids used in low doses produce a selective spinal analgesia in man.

ED or IT morphine is associated with significant decrease in body $T°$ (Bernstein et al. 1988).

5.6 Endocrine and metabolic system

External stress, pain, bloodloss, trauma, and surgery result in significant endocrine and metabolic responses. A rise in secretion of most hormones is produced. Plasma concentrations of cortisol, ACTH, aldosterone (AD), plasma renine activity (PRA), prolactine (PL), antidiuretic hormone (ADH) and growth hormone (GH) are increased in a direct relationship with the intensity and duration of the aggression (Stoner and Hall 1979; Oyama 1980 c). In pregnant women beta endorphin shows a massive rise with the onset of labour (Budiamal et al. 1981). Plasma adrenaline, noradrenaline, glucose, glycerol, FFA and lactate concentration are increased by stress and pain.

These stress responses may be transiently blocked or even inhibited depending on:

- the technique of anaesthesia
- the depth of anaesthesia
- the anaesthetic substances used (Clark 1970; Kehlet 1982).

Volatile and gaseous anaesthetics are poor inhibitors of surgical stress responses (Arroyo et al. 1983). Local anaesthetics almost completely inhibit hormonal hyperactivity (Arroyo et al. 1982, 1983; Engquist et al. 1977; Ponz et al. 1982 a, b; Traynor and Hall 1981; Traynor et al. 1982). Opioids, if used in high intravenous doses, are potent inhibitors of cortisol, ACTH, GH and AD increase and poor inhibitors of PRA hyperactivity (Arroyo et al. 1983 a, b; Philbin and Coggins 1978; De Castro et al. 1982; Hall et al. 1978). Nevertheless, the administration of low opioid doses, itself without any pain or surgery, may produce an increase of several hormonal stress parameters (Goodman and Gilman's 1985).

The hormonal inhibition produced by spinal opioids was studied by Bonnet et al. (1982); Christensen et al. (1982 b); Downing et al. (1986); Haekanson et al. (1985); Hjortsø et al. (1985 a); Jørgensen et al. (1982); Korinek et al. (1982, 1985); Normandale et al. (1985); Rutberg et al. (1984); El Baz and Goldin (1987) with morphine, by Bormann et al. (1982 b, 1983 b, c) with fentanyl, and by Ponz et al. (1982 a) with fentanyl or buprenorphine in combination with etidocaine.

The endocrine response to pain in the postoperative period after abdominal surgery under epidural administration of morphine 4 mg or bupivacaine 0.5% was compared by Rutberg et al. (1984). In both groups, cortisol was increased immediately after surgery. Plasma epinephrine concentration was lower immediately after surgery only in the group which received a local anaesthetic. The plasma norepinephrine concentrations remained unchanged after local anaesthesia, while an increase occurred after epidural morphine. Similar results were obtained by Håkanson et al. (1985). The local anaesthetic group had significantly lower blood glycerol and lactate concentrations than the group with epidural morphine.

Thoracic epidural morphine differs from thoracic epidural local anaesthetics in being much less capable of suppressing the metabolic response (Håkanson et al. 1985; Normandale et al. 1985).

Following abdominal surgery, ADH was significantly increased even when an opioid was associated to a local anaesthetic (Korinek et al. 1985; Håkanson et al. 1985; Hjortsø et al. 1985 a).

Epidural morphine used in doses of 4-7 mg, notwithstanding the analgesic efficiency, did not block the endocrine stress response during the postoperative period (Jørgensen et al. 1982; Korinek et al. 1982, 1985).

Some results indicate that the protective effect of local anaesthetics or fentanyl are superior to those obtained with morphine. It is however, very difficult to make really comparable evaluations. After abdominal surgery, Bormann et al. (1983 b) investigated two series of patients : one series received epidural fentanyl (0.1-0.2 mg) and the other series received intravenous fentanyl in equipotent doses. In the epidural group the inhibition of the postoperative increase of ADH was significantly greater than that in the intravenous group. Comparable results were presented by El Baz and Goldin (1987). They found that after cardiac operations epidural morphine was able to suppress the stress response significantly more than intravenous morphine.

In experiments in cats, epidural fentanyl counteracted the inhibition of gastrointestinal mobility mediated by the autonomous nervous system (Lisander and Stenquist 1985). In clinical settings such a spinal effect may partially counteract a tendency to postoperative paralytic ileus.

The endocrine anti-stress protection of intrathecal opioids is generally greater than that obtained by the epidural route. The final results depend on the one hand on the doses used and on the other hand on the extent of the surgery. According to the study of Sebel et al. (1985) intrathecal morphine administered for cardiac surgery was totally insufficient to provide a satisfying protection against stress.

Intrathecal morphine (0.8 mg) had no effect upon the hyperglycemic response to cholecystectomy but attenuated the increase in serum cortisol concentration (Downing et al. 1986).

Conversely, Child and Kaufman (1985) observed that for abdominal surgery diamorphine used in intrathecal doses of 0.35 mg provided a better protection against stress reactions than fentanyl used in intravenous doses of 0.2-0.35 mg.

Comparing epidural local anaesthetics with epidural morphine the catecholamine responses and the nitrogen loss was more decreased by local anaesthetics. However, also epidural morphine had a nitrogen sparing effect due to an inhibition of the catecholamine response (Tsuji et al. 1987).

The results of all these studies suggest that the endocrine and metabolic response to surgery is predominantly released by neurogenic stimuli other than pain stimuli. So, opioid receptors and nociceptive pathways are only minimally involved in endocrine metabolic changes.

Conclusions

The pharmacodynamic properties of spinal opioids are the same as their well known effects observed after parenteral use.

However, by the spinal route the effects are generally slower in onset and longer lasting. The pharmacodynamic changes are less brisk because they have time for equilibration.

6. Side effects

6.1 Generalities

In its present form spinal opioid analgesia does not provide pure antinociception as anticipated and desired. A number of side effects involving respiratory, urinary, neuromuscular, gastro-intestinal and sexual functions may also occur. They demonstrate an occurrence in relationship to the segmental progression of analgesia and rostral spread of the opioid.

Side effects of epidural opioid analgesia can be divided in relatively frequent and in rare side effects.

- The most frequent among them are: respiratory depression (early or delayed), urinary retention, nausea and vomiting, dizziness, pruritus, drowsiness, hypothermia.
- The less frequent are: constipation (although important in chronic opioid therapy), oliguria, inability to ejaculate, headache, redness, agitation, dysphoria, miosis, muscle weakness, hallucinations, catatonia, abdominal spasm, diarrhea, shivering, hypotension, withdrawal syndrome in addicts. Accidental intravenous or intrathecal administration may produce overdose effects.

The side effects produced by the spinal opioids are very different in importance and frequency according to the context in which they are used: indications, type of opioid used, mode of administration, epidural or intrathecal route are very important factors for the development of side effects (Tab. 23 to 25).

The risk of delayed respiratory depression is most serious in the treatment of postoperative and post-traumatic pain and is nearly non-existent in chronic cancer pain treatment. On the other hand, tolerance is the most important problem in cancer patients and has only reduced importance in postoperative pain.

The most serious side effects observed (mostly at the beginning of the treatment) after the chronic administration of opioids by the epidural route are respiratory depression, either immediate or tardive, pruritus, urinary retention, nausea and vomiting, drowsiness, tolerance and physical dependence.

Tab. 26 summarizes the results of Reiz and Westberg (1980) concerning 1200

Table 23. Spinal opioids, relationship between side effects and indications.

Side effects		Indications (type of pain)			
		Post op.	Post traum.	Delivery	Cancer
Respiratory depression	immediate	+	+	+	(–)
	delayed	+ +	+ +	+ +	(–)
Urinary retention		+ +	+ +	+ + +	+
Pruritus		+	+	+ +	+
Nausea, vomiting		+	+	+	+
Drowsiness		+	+	(–)	(–)
Dysphoria, euphoria		+	+	(–)	(–)
Tolerance		–	(–)	–	+ +

Table 24. Spinal opioids, relationship between side effects and type of drug.

Side effects		Lipid solubility	
		Low Morphine	High Fentanyl, sufentanil etc.
Respiratoy depression	immediate	+	+
	delayed	+ +	(–)
Urinary retention		+ +	+
Pruritus		+	+
Nausea, vomiting		+ +	+
Drowsiness		+ +	+
Dysphoria, euphoria		+ +	(–)
Tolerance		+	+

cases with 2 mg of epidural morphine, and also the results of Gustafsson et al. (1982 d) in a multicentre study performed in Scandinavian hospitals. About 9000 patients following epidural morphine 2-4 mg, and 150 patients following intrathecal morphine at doses of 0.8-2 mg were investigated.

Tab. 26 also shows the results of Stenseth et al. (1985 a) obtained in 1085 patients during the postoperative period, after the use of epidural morphine 4-6 mg.

Respiratory depression is certainly not only a serious side effect seen after the

Table 25. Spinal opioids, relationship between side effects, mode of administration, route of administration.

Side effects		Mode of administration		Route of administration	
		Bolus	Continuous infusion	ED	IT
Respiratory depression	immediate	+	+	+	+
	delayed	+ +	+	+ +	+ + +
Urinary retention		+ +	+	+	+
Pruritus		+ +	+	+	+
Nausea, vomiting		+ +	+	+	+
Drowsiness		+ +	+	+	+
Dysphoria, euphoria		+ +	+	+	+
Tolerance		+ +	+	+ +	+
Technical problems		+	+ +	+ +	+
Danger of infection		+ +	+	+	+ +

Table 26. Clinical reports on side effects following the epidural and intrathecal administration of morphine.

	Reiz and Westberg (1980)	Gustafsson (1982)		Stenseth et al. (1985 a)	Meynadier Blond (1986 a)
- Technique	EDOA	EDOA	ITOA	EDOA	ITOA
- Number of cases	1200	9000	150	1085	126
- Type of pain	Postop.	Postop.	Postop.	Postop.	Cancer
- Morphine doses (mg/70 kg)	2	2	0.8 - 2	4 - 6	1.6 - 2.6
- Severe resp. depression (%)	0.1	0.9	9	0.9	0
- Nausea and vomiting (%)	17	34		34	44
- Severe pruritus (%)	15	25		11	29
- Urinary retention (%) *	2	10 - 25		42	9

*Patients without urinary catheter.

use of spinal morphine (Tab. 27), it may also appear after all the other spinal opioids. However it must be underlined that the severity and the delayed appearance of the phenomenon is without any doubt most pronounced after morphine (Doblar et al. 1981; Downing et al. 1984; Holland et al. 1982; Kafer et al. 1983;

98

Table 27. Spinal morphine: incidence of severe respiratory depression.

	ED morphine 4 mg / 70 kg	IT morphine 1 - 2 mg / 70 kg
• Early or delayed respiratory depression (%)	0.08	0.36

(Adapted from Rawal et al. 1986 a)

Knill et al. 1982; McCaughey and Graham 1982; McDonald 1980; Møller IW et al. 1982; Nielsen et al. 1981; Perez-Saad and Bures 1983; Petit et al. 1983a; Rawal et al. 1983 a, 1986 a; Rybro 1982).

The overall incidence in large retrospective studies have varied from 0.25% and 0.4% to 9%. The highest incidence occurred in investigations in which epidural morphine was administered until complete pain relief (Gustafsson et al. 1982 b; Stenseth et al. 1985 a).

Dose reduction, progress in experience, and selection of more lipophilic products will produce better results (Suzuki 1985). Most of the side effects seen after spinal opioid treatment are the same as those occurring after the parenteral use of opioids. However, their severity and frequency were less pronounced.

The side effects may occur at different periods after administration, indicating that they are induced by perturbances at different action sites (Bromage et al. 1982 a) (Fig. 29).

6.2 Side effects of epidural opioids

6.2.1 EARLY AND DELAYED RESPIRATORY DEPRESSION

6.2.1.1 Aetiology and characteristics

Delayed respiratory depression seen after spinal opioids is due to a cephalidad spread of the opioid in the CSF. Following diffusion of the substance from the intrathecal space to the ventricle system, they produce reactions with opioid receptors in the arcuate nucleus (Jørgensen et al. 1981).

It is well known that the parenteral use of an effective dose of an opioid is always accompanied by some degree of respiratory depression and, in many cases, this depression can only be highlighted by the rebreathing CO_2 stimulation test. The administration of opioids by the epidural route follows the same rule. The clinical observation alone is often misleading. The therapeutic margin between pain relief and respiratory depression is often alarmingly narrow, especially in the case of intrathecal opioids. Dose-response data suggest that the ratio between the spinal analgesic dose and the dose that causes severe respiratory depression in acute patients, is not much in excess of 2 (Cousins 1987 c).

Time course

Following the use of morphine, the respiratory depression generally appears 4-8 hours after an epidural injection (McCaughey and Graham 1982). In some cases the depression is still present 24 hours later (Morgan M 1982; Nielsen et al. 1981). This respiratory depression has the same severity and frequency as that seen after systemic injection of morphine (Gustafsson et al. 1982 d).

It is possible to observe two types of relatively severe respiratory depression:

- Firstly, the appearance of a brisk and rapid respiratory depression produced by overdose and massive systemic reabsorption of the product.
- Secondly, a more insidious and sometimes very delayed respiratory depression (5-12 hours after the epidural injection). The latter is most likely caused by rostral intrathecal spread of morphine from the lumbar region to the cerebroventricular structures (Glass 1984; Glass et al. 1985).

The vast range of susceptiblility to the respiratory depressant effects of epidural or intrathecal administered opioids must be underlined (Jyu and Lamb 1985).

Spinal opioids provide excellent analgesia. However, delayed respiratory depression continues to be a problem in a manner that is not entirely predictable. Risk factors are: inadvertent overdose, advanced age, coexisting administration of parenteral opioids, pre-existing disease, but the risk exists also in absence of any suspected risk factors (Etches et al. 1989).

Severity

It is also highly noteworthy that the frequency and the severity of respiratory depression is very different in opioid-naive patients, compared to those more or less accustomed to some form of opioid treatment. Severe respiratory depression is practically never seen in patients with severe chronic pain; they have already developed a relatively high degree of tolerance against opiates (Coombs et al. 1983 f; Glynn et al. 1979; Zenz et al. 1980). On the other hand, pain is a potent central nervous stimulant, so that even opioid-naive patients do not develop respiratory depression (Hanks et al 1981; Hanks 1984) (Fig. 30).

Very severe cases of respiratory depression are not frequent: 0.1% after epidural morphine and 0.4 % after intrathecal (Rawal et al. 1986 a), but a significant rise in $PaCO_2$ is frequent (Gerig and Kern 1982), (Tab. 27). Prolonged supervision of patients and special information for the nursing team about all the elements contributing to these side effects, to their prophylaxis and to their treatment are mandatory (Bennett and Adams 1983).

6.2.1.2 Monitoring

The nursing staff must be particularly well trained in the recognition of the early clinical signs of insidious respiratory depression:

- satisfied patient
- no respiratory distress
- superficial respiration
- decreased respiratory frequency
- somnolence
- cyanosis
- miosis
- end-tidal CO_2 and PCO_2 increased
- Sa O_2 and PO_2 decreased

Patients treated with spinal opioids after surgery or trauma must not be sent back to their wards unless a "roombound" nurse can check the patients for the first 24 hours after initiating the therapy (Andersen 1983).

A method presented by Busch and Stedman (1987) with an incidence of 95% of the patients being managed in private or semi-private rooms for postoperative epidural morphine is highly dangerous. Its conclusion that epidural morphine is an acceptable modality of pain relief for surgical patients in private rooms absolutely cannot be agreed with.

a) Clinical observation

Accurate observation of respiratory frequency and amplitude are still the most important methods. The inadequacy of the respiratory rate is the only indicator of respiratory depression to remember (Writer et al. 1986). The pattern of respiratory depression following epidural opioid administration is different from that following parenteral use. Frequency is often unchanged but minute ventilation decreases and respiratory depression is not always detected by the respiratory rate alarm (Brown et al. 1985; Knill et al. 1981; Rawal and Wattwil 1984 a).

Do not forget that a patient with opioid respiratory depression does not present any respiratory distress. He remains a satisfied patient, even feeling more satisfied than before, slipping progressively into a state of decreased vigilance with periods of "oubli respiratoire".The three most important elements in the appearance of clinically serious respiratory depression are:

- a low pain level
- a depressed vigilance (e.g. due to the action of sedatives)
- miosis

b) Electronic monitoring

Several electronic devices are at our disposal (commercial names and manufacturers: see Technical data, Chapter 20).

- Pupil measurement device

In man all opioid analgesics tend to cause pupillary constriction. Pure opioid overdosage characteristically induces pin-point pupils whereas in case of respiratory depression leading to hypoxia, mydriasis may develop.

Partial agonists produce firstly a plateau effect and in higher dose a biphasic effect on the pupillary diameter (Martin WR 1983).

The pupillary constriction is **dose-related** and is also closely related to the analgesic potency. Thus it can be used to monitor the depth of depression after effects or remorphinization of opioids.

The pupil measurement device is a portable pupil scan that can measure pupil diameters under widely variable **ambient** light conditions. It measures and displays the minimum pupil diameter produced by a light stimulus of programmable duration, the recovered diameter, 3 sec after stimulus, and the elapsed time from stimulus to minimum diameter. Activated by a finger switch on the manual optical unit, the measurement cycle and data capture are fully automatic. Memory capacity allows storage of up to 30 measurements for each series of 5 patients before reset. Stored data may be recalled to the display or printed. The optical unit weight is 400 g.

The correlation of the pupillary diameter with ventilatory CO_2 sensitivity and respiratory depression was studied during a period of 20 hours after administration of epidural opioids using the Essilor pupillometer and a modified Read rebreathing technique (Ravenborg et al. 1987). The pupillary response may be used as a practical indicator of respiratory depression (see: Chapter 20, Technical data).

- Respiration monitor

The Cardiff respiratory monitor is a relatively simple device which assesses abdominal and suprasternal movements. Two plastic foam sensors, one placed in the suprasternal notch and the other on the abdominal wall at the place of maximal excursion during quiet breathing are connected to a differential transducer. If there is no pressure change after 20 seconds between the capsules, this will cause the alarm to be activated (Harmer et al. 1985).

The Respi Rate is another non-invasive respiration monitor with apnea alarm.

However, current clinical practice has shown that routine use of a respiratory rate monitor provides frequent false alarms and often poor patient acceptance. Respiratory rate is not a reliable predictor of adequate ventilation when epidural opioids are used.

Pulse oximeters and end-tidal CO_2 monitors are also useful adjuncts in evaluating the patient's respiratory status.

- Pulse oximetry (SaO_2) (see Chapter 20)

Since hypoxemia is the most serious consequence of respiratory depression, it seems most sensible to monitor arterial oxygen saturation. Chubra-Smith et al. (1986) has shown that there exists a direct correlation between SaO_2 and PaO_2 during and after anaesthesia. The SaO_2 is consistently lower than the corresponding PaO_2 measurement, thus providing a continuous estimation of the minimum PaO_2 level throughout anaesthesia and recovery.

The use of a pulse oximeter as a monitor of patient oxygenation after epidural opioid analgesia is easy, practical, and well accepted by patients and ward nurses. It provides a valuable alarm in the presence of respiratory depression if the low alarm of the oximeter is set at an SaO_2 of 85% (Choi et al. 1986).

The pulse oximeter is becoming a widely accepted device because its simplicity and its ability to provide continuous, non-invasive data with regard to arterial oxygenation. It is undoubtedly a significant advance. It is however important to remember that there is no correlation between SaO_2 decrease and respiratory rate when patients are breathing room air or supplemental oxygen (Cheng and Stommel 1988).

- Transcutaneous PCO_2

PCO_2 values follow the trend of PaO_2. If perfusion in the heated skin is adequate, it can give an early warning of decreased oxygen delivery. Combined transcutaneous O_2CO_2 monitors increase the utility of these non-invasive sensors.

- End-tidal CO_2

The ET CO_2 monitor is also a useful adjunct in evaluating the patient's respiratory status. ET CO_2 is perhaps better than SaO_2 in following the respiratory rate (Cheng and Stommel 1988).

In conclusion, electronic monitoring devices are useful adjuncts in evaluating the patient's respiratory status, nevertheless we continue to rely above all on frequent nursing assessment of ventilation and sedation.

6.2.1.3 Factors increasing or reducing the risk of delayed respiratory depression

Increased risk factors

a) Patients:

- opioid-naive patients
- old age, debilitated patients
- chronic respiratory disease
- obesity
- Adams-Stokes attacks
- sleep apnea syndrome
- prophylactic spinal opioid administration

Lamarche et al. (1986) has drawn attention to the increased risk presented by patients with a sleep apnea syndrome (loud snoring, excessive daytime somnolence, upper airway abnormalities and apneic spells during sleep are usual features of the syndrome affecting as much as 3.5% of the male obese population over 40 years of age and as much as 25% over 65 years).

When opioids are given prophylactically without controlling the actual pain state, the incidence of respiratory depression might increase (Gowan et al. 1988).

b) Situations with increased intraspinal pressure and circulation resulting in fluctuations in the CSF pressure or a concomitant increase in systemic drug uptake:

- Increased intrathoracic or intra-abdominal pressure
  . obstruction of the vena cava
  . aorta clamping
  . coughing, vomiting
  . grunting
  . brisk movements
  . mechanical ventilation (e.g.)

c) Drugs:

- hydrophilic opioids
- large opioid doses and volumes

- repeated spinal injections at a short interval
- use of other central depressants by systemic route before, together with or after the spinal opioids
- concomitant use of local anaesthetics (Jensen NH et al. 1985)
- concomitant use of benzodiazepines (Shulman et al. 1984 b) (e.g.)

d) Technique:

- catheter migration
- inadvertent dura puncture, dura leak
- high thoracic or cervical injection
- Trendelenburg position after injection
- intrathecal administration

e) Indications

- low pain level
- wrong indications for spinal opioids, e.g. sympathetic pain

Most of these situations can be avoided by proper treatment (Zenz 1984 d) (Tab. 28).

Table 28. Delayed respiratory depression after spinal opioids, prophylaxis.

USE   • Lipophilic opioids • Small doses or continuous infusion
AVOID   • Intrathecal route • Concomitant use of parenteral opioids • Drug associations • Adrenaline • High thoracic injection • High volume
• Hyperbaricity, upright position ?
• Survey over 12 - 24 hours is recommended

Reduced risk factors

a) Patients:

- opioid tolerant patients.

b) Drugs:

- lipophilic opioids
- reduced injection volume and doses (Nordberg et al. 1986 d)
- avoidance of drug associations.

c) Technique:

- injection at lumbar level
- hyperbaric solutions (only if intrathecal injection)
- continuous infusion (El-Baz et al. 1982)
- sitting position injection (only if intrathecal injection).

6.2.1.4 Dose response curves

The risk of respiratory depression after spinal administration of opioid agonists increases with the dose administered. The respiratory depression can be demonstrated in most cases by the expiratory PCO_2 elevation and a shift to the right of the CO_2 ventilatory response curves (Piepenbrock et al.1981 a; Piepenbrock 1981 b). This depression generally remains within clinically acceptable limits. Using agonist-antagonists by the epidural route, even, if progressively higher doses of these substances are administered, the severity of the depression is not linearly increased because of a rapidly appearing ceiling effect. However, after dose increase, the duration of the depression becomes always more prolonged (Rein et al. 1985).

6.2.1.5 Prophylaxis

All factors predisposing to the side effects enumerated above can be avoided. For maximal safety the following rules have to be adopted:

- use lipophilic opioid with high molecular weight
- reduce dose by carefully and individually titrating

- use small volumes
- prefer lumbar injection
- avoid association with CNS depressors
- use short acting opioid in infusion
- reduce dose in elderly patients
- administer the drug strictly by epidural route
- provide long lasting supervision (> 12 hours if the patient is not accustomed to opioids)
- place the patient in upright or sitting position (of minor importance).

Preference must be given to the use of *lipophilic opioids* and to substances with a *high molecular weight*. When using such products, it is practically always possible to avoid delayed respiratory depression.

This is the case for buprenorphine (De Castro and Hörig 1981 a) as well as for fentanyl (Lam et al. 1983).

Negre et al. (1985), when using epidural fentanyl in a 1 µg/kg bolus postoperatively after orthopedic surgery, noted only a mild respiratory depression which lasted from 30 min to 120 min immediately after the administration period.

Twenty-one patients were studied during the postoperative period for evaluating of the respiratory effects of epidural fentanyl administered in repeated doses or in continuous infusion 1 µg/kg/h starting 60 min after a bolus injection of 0.5 µg/kg. Following single epidural doses respiratory rate decreased significantly, but end-tidal CO_2 showed an insignificant increase. These changes occurred only within minutes of injection and not thereafter. Low doses of continuous epidural fentanyl infusion had no effect on end-tidal CO_2 concentration or respiratory rate for up to 18 hours (Ahuja and Strunin 1985 b).

A satisfactory technique is provided by the postoperative epidural use of fentanyl given in a bolus 1 µg/kg followed by a continuous infusion of 1 µg/kg/h over a 20 hour period.

This technique produces :

- adequate pain relief
- a mild respiratory depression of rapid onset suggesting a systemic action rather than a spinal rostral spread of fentanyl
- no delayed respiratory depression
- acceptable plasma level of the opioid and of the blood gases (Renaud et al. 1985 a, b).

High doses and high volumes of opiods must be avoided (Nordberg et al. 1986 d). This is especially true with old and high-risk patients.

The influence of position of the patient with respect to the rapid or delayed respiratory depression after 4 mg of epidural morphine was investigated by Molke-Jensen et al. (1984). This study concluded that the adoption of a proclive position of 45 degrees after the epidural injection of morphine did not prevent respiratory depression.

Prophylactic use of opioid antidotes (Tab. 29)

Prophylactic use of opioid antidotes for prevention of respiratory depression induced by spinal opioids is still a controversial problem. Rawal (1985 a; 1986 a) in a double-blind placebo controlled study in 45 postoperative patients demonstrated that naloxone given in a low dose continuous intravenous infusion of 5 µg/kg/h prevents respiratory depression without affecting analgesia depth. However the duration of analgesia was reduced by about 25%.

This result is in contradiction with the results of more recent investigations (Gowan et al. 1987a, b; 1988).

High infusion doses of naloxone (10 µg/kg) reversed analgesia and respiratory depression. Low infusion doses of naloxone (5µg/kg) also reversed analgesia (however, less than do high infusion doses) but was inadequate to reverse the respiratory depression (Guéneron et al. 1988).

Oral naltrexone, 6-12 mg, reduced the side effects of ED morphine (Cullen et al. 1988; Mok et al. 1986) but also reduced analgesia (Norris et al. 1989).

6.2.1.6 Treatment

a) Naloxone

The right treatment for early or delayed respiratory depression consists of the administration of naloxone in repeated intravenous doses of 0.1 mg or of a continuous infusion at a dose rate of 0.4-0.8 mg/h.

The effects of naloxone are rapid, effective and in some cases without important loss of analgesia. In most cases however the effect is shorter than the duration of the respiratory depression (Baskoff et al. 1980; Christensen 1980; Glynn et al. 1979; Jones et al. 1984; Scott and McClure 1979), (Tab. 29, 30).

If necessary, respiratory assistance or mechanical ventilation is instituted.

Table 29. Drugs administered for correction or prevention of side effects produced by epidural or intrathecal opioid analgesia.

INN	RN	Medium dose I.V. mg/70 kg	Authors
NALBUPHINE	Nubain®	20	Baxter et al. 1989 Hammond 1984 Henderson and Cohen 1986 Mok et al. 1985 Penning et al. 1986 Wakefield and Mesaros 1985 Wang JJ et al. 1986
NALMEFENE	–	0.5	Dixon et al. 1984 Gal and DiFazio 1986 Konieczko et al. 1988
NALOXONE	Narcan®	bolus 0.4 inf. 0.35-0.7/h	Brookshire et al. 1983 Gilly et al. 1985 Gowan et al. 1988 Guéneron et al. 1986 Knape 1986 Korbon et al. 1983 Perrot et al. 1983 Petry et al. 1985 Ramanathan et al. 1986 Rawal et al. 1983 a, 1985 b, e, 1986 a Thind et al. 1986
PHYSOSTIGMINE	Antilirium® Anticholium®	1-2	Shulman et al. 1984 a
NALTREXONE	–	oral dose mg/70 kg 6-12	Leighton et al. 1988 Mok et al. 1986 Norris et al. 1989

The pharmacokinetics of naloxone are well known. The effects appear 30-60 seconds after the intravenous and 2-3 min after the intramuscular injection. The antagonistic effects may persist over 45 minutes following intravenous and over 2-3 hours following intramuscular injection, but they can also be shorter living. A continuous naloxone infusion ensures a stable minimal plasma concentration necessary to avoid a return of respiratory depression in some cases without complete reversal of analgesia (Petry et al. 1985) (Tab. 30). In most cases it is difficult to reverse the respiratory depression selectively without also decreasing the analgesic effect (Guéneron et al. 1988).

Anyhow, the long duration of the respiratory depression and the short action of naloxone makes repeated injections or continuous infusion of the antagonist and a surveillance of at least 12 hours necessary.

b) Aspiration of CSF

A recent report presents an interesting solution to the problem of respiratory

Table 30. Treatment of side effects resulting from epidural and intrathecal opioid analgesia.

Side effects	Treatment	Dosage/ 70 kg
• RESPIRATORY DEPRESSION	naloxone IV repeated or infusion	0.1 - 0.4
• URINARY RETENTION	urinary catheter naloxone IV	 0.1 - 0.4
• PRURITUS	antihistaminic drug (not very effective) naloxone IV	 0.1 - 0.4
• NAUSEA AND VOMITING	domperidone PO metoclopramide IV or IM naloxone IV droperidol IV haloperidol PO or IV	10 10 0.1 - 0.4 2.5 - 5 2 - 5
• CONSTIPATION	laxatives	

depression by excessive overdose. The CSF was aspirated and normal saline injected. By this procedure, respiratory and CNS depression was quickly reversed. The authors conclude that the mechanism involved is direct removal of morphine from the spinal CSF, dilution, and displacement of the drug from its receptors by an increase of CSF sodium concentration (Kaiser and Bainton 1987).

c) Opioid agonist-antagonists

In order to avoid the principal drawbacks of naloxone (e.g. short antidote action) and side effects, the use of nalbuphine or butorphanol in place of naloxone has been studied.

Butorphanol

With the association of epidural fentanyl and epidural butorphanol, also significantly higher analgesia with a longer duration was observed (Naulty et al. 1987).

Nalbuphine

Nalbuphine hydrochloride is effective in reversing or preventing respiratory depression associated with epidural morphine without significantly affecting analgesia (Penning et al.1986).

Doran et al. (1987) confirmed the preventive properties of a nalbuphine bolus of 0.2 mg/kg + nalbuphine infusion 0.05 mg/kg/h against respiratory depression produced by 10 mg epidural morphine. The results suggested augmentation of analgesia rather than reversal.

The combination of a μ-opioid agonist (e.g. morphine or fentanyl) and a μ-antagonist/kappa-agonist (e.g. nalbuphine or butorphanol) seems to be capable in producing analgesia with decreasing incidence of μ-mediated side effects via stimulation of both spinal cord receptor types (Naulty et al. 1987). However, the results are not sufficiently controlled to offer a recommendable procedure. A recent report by Baxter et al. (1989) demonstrated the effectiveness of nal-buphine in decreasing the amount of CO_2 retention but could not demonstrate the complete prevention of respiratory depression. Two of 15 patients developed a significant increase in $PaCo_2$ >50 mmHg under continuous nalbuphine infusion.

6.2.2 PRURITUS

Pruritus is the least dangerous but perhaps the most troublesome side effect of spinal opioids.

Aetiology

The explanation of the phenomenon is not very clear, but one is forced to conclude that pruritus is caused by an alteration in the modulations of the sensory system corresponding to a rostral diffusion of the opioids. Histamine release (triggered or not by preservatives in the injectate) in the pathogenesis of pruritus is doubtful for some authors (Berg-Seiter et al. 1985) and evident for others (McLeilland 1986).

Frequency

Frequency, intensity and duration of this phenomenon are influenced by several factors:

- overall frequency: 10 to 50%
- more common in females than in males
- most prevalent in parturient women, 30-90%,
  (Glynn et al. 1987 b)
- more frequent if patient is questioned about it
- increased by the use of adrenaline
  (Douglas et al. 1986 b)
- unrelated to preservatives
  (Cousins and Bridenbaugh 1987)
- less frequent with pure and fresh opioid solutions.

Appearance

It appears 2-3 hours after the injection of the opioid. Duration is variable but always shorter than that of analgesia. It frequently occurs in the beginning of a treatment and may completely disappear after repeated injections (adaptation phenomenon).

Relationship with administration mode of the opioid

Pruritus occurs following the use of opioids whatever the mode of administration. However, its frequency is greater and it is more severe with epidural application than after parenteral use and this is even more the case after intrathecal application (Fischer and Scott 1982).

Dose relationship

Its frequency is directly related to the injected doses: after 10 mg of epidural morphine 28 % of the patients presented a pruritus, opposed to only 1% after a dose of 2 to 5 mg (Lanz et al. 1985). However, in other studies, relationship between dose and frequency of pruritus has not been noted (Martin R et al. 1982).

Product relationship

Pruritus has been observed with all opioids, a possible exception being beta-endorphin (Oyama 1980 c). Authentic comparative studies have not been carried out between the different opioids, but there is a clear agreement that pruritus is most frequent after the use of morphine. Scott and Fischer (1982) recommend to avoid morphine and prefer a combination of bupivacaine with an opioid. Questioning of patients who have been given epidural injections of morphine reveals that 70% to 100% present some form of itching. However this is only the case in 23% of patients after fentanyl and 6% after pethidine (Camporesi and Redick 1983 b).

Not only the frequency but also the severity of pruritus increases to a greater extent after morphine than after other products such as hydromorphone, methadone or pethidine. After morphine the severity of the pruritus can be so great that sleep becomes impossible.

Treatment

In 1% of the cases pruritus is so severe that treatment is mandatory. Antihistaminics or cimetidine are of questionable efficacy. Diphenhydramine (Benadryl ®) tends to sedate patients without really alleviating the symptoms of pruritus. These results indicate also that pruritus is mostly histamine independent.

In some cases naloxone (0.2mg IV) seems to be an effective treatment (Scott PV and Fischer 1982). On the other hand several investigators have obtained poor results in treatment of pruritus by naloxone (McLelland 1986; Samii 1986; Ramanathan et al. 1986) so that successful treatment of this side effect can not be guaranteed in all cases. In a preliminary study the opioid agonist-antagonist nalbuphine was effective for reversal of pruritus secondary to epidural morphine (Wakefield and Mesaros 1985).

Droperidol (12 mg) is also in some cases effective.

6.2.3 NAUSEA AND VOMITING

Aetiology

High concentrations of strong opioids have an inhibiting effect on the vomiting centre and the chemoreceptor trigger zone surrounding the fourth ventricle whereas relative low doses provide stimulating effects.

The chemoreceptor trigger zone is sensitive to dopamine agonists, and other chemical stimuli, and mainly controls the activity of the vomiting centre. Partial occupation of the opioid receptors may facilitate dopamine release. In addition the vomiting center has a neuronal input from other sites in CNS (e.g. cortex, vestibular and cerebellar nuclei). Vestibular stimulation enhanced the emetic effects. Thus nausea and vomiting are relatively common when opioids are given to ambulant patients and are much less frequent in recumbent subjects (Calvey 1987).

Nausea and vomiting occur about 4 hours after the epidural injection of the opioid and last about 3 hours. The time of appearance of these side effects corresponds to the rostral diffusion of small amounts of the opioids to the fourth ventricle.

According to most authors, this side effect has a frequency ranging from 17 % to 24 % (Bromage et al. 1982 a; Camporesi and Redick 1983 b; Lanz et al. 1982; Reiz and Westberg 1980).

Following intrathecal injection of morphine, nausea and vomiting are more frequent than after epidural injections, 75% and 30 to 51%, respectively. In the case of epidural fentanyl, this side effect is observed in only 5 to 10% of the patients. In parturient women nausea and vomiting are quite rare (Perriss and Malins 1981), but more frequent when the intrathecal route is used (Baraka et al. 1981; Scott et al. 1980).

The incidence of nausea and vomiting seems to be much less with repeated epidural dosing and is very low in cancer patients (Coombs et al. 1982 a; Glynn et al. 1981; Howard et al. 1981; Zenz 1981 c). It generally disappears after 2 to 3 weeks of treatment (Zenz et al. 1982 a). The brain becomes tolerant to those side effects as it does to respiratory depression (Cousins and Bridenbaugh 1986).

Treatment (Tab. 30)

Naloxone, 0.4 mg followed by intravenous infusion at a rate of 0.01 mg/kg/h allows a partial reduction of the nausea without a reversal of analgesia (Rawal et al. 1985 a). But this technique is only suitable for bedridden patients. For ambulatory patients, an oral medication must be chosen. In those cases antimuscarinic drugs or dopamine antagonists, e.g. phenothiazines, butyrophenones, metoclopramide or domperidone (3 × 10 mg/d), can be effective.

6.2.4 Urinary retention

Aetiology

Bladder dysfunction is widely observed after the use of spinal opioids. By means of cystometric studies the following observations were made:

- The micturation reflex is inhibited for a long period.
- Urinary retention and micturation difficulties are a source of severe and often prolonged discomfort warranting repeated bladder catheterization.
- Detrusor hypotonicity with continuous filling of the bladder and with bladder overdistension sometimes produce impairment of urethro-vesical function.

- Intraurethral pressure remains unchanged.
- Urine production is not impaired.
- The systemic effects of opioids as the cause of urinary retention can be ruled out (Husted et al. 1985; Rawal et al. 1982; Yaksh et al. 1988 b).

Frequency

The urodynamic effects last 14-16 hours on average after 4 mg epidural morphine (Rawal 1986 b). This action can be reversed by naloxone. It is not evident that a relationship exists for this side effect between dose and degree of urinary retention. Indeed it occurs with the same frequency after epidural morphine doses of 0.5, 1.0, 2.0, 4.0 or 8.0 mg (Martin R et al. 1982; Rawal et al. 1981 b, 1983 a, 1985 a, b, e; Rawal 1986 b). The incidence has been reported to be the same as after intramuscular opioid injection (Petersen et al. 1982). Neither sex nor age of the patient seems to have any influence on the severity of urinary retention.

Urinary retention is very common in male volunteers, less common in postoperative pain therapy, affecting between 22 % and 40 % of patients (Rawal et al. 1981 b) and even up to 80 % (Villalonga-Morales et al. 1984).

After 2-10 mg epidural morphine the incidence of urinary retention observed was 99-100% (Bromage et al. 1982 a; Rawal et al. 1984 a).

It is seldom observed during the treatment of cancer patients accustomed to opioids (Camporesi and Redick 1983 b). In many patients the phenomenon disappears after repeated injections. The incidence of urinary retention decreases during long-term epidural opioid treatment (Glynn et al. 1981). Urinary retention is non-existent after intracerebroventricular opioid analgesia.

Treatment

a) Opioid antagonists
Naloxone restores normal bladder function but also produces a loss of the desired analgesia.

The prophylactic use of a continuous infusion of naloxone in the postoperative period has been recommended (Lanz et al. 1982).

According to Rawal et al. (1981 b, 1986 a) intravenous naloxone 0.4-0.8 mg is the best treatment for urinary retention.

In contrast, intravenous naloxone and neostigmine injections after 4 mg of epidural morphine was only effective in 34.9 % of the cases (Villalonga-Morales et al. 1984).

b) Other substances
Phenoxibenzamine has been proposed by Evron et al. (1984). Following epidural anaesthesia with bupivacaine, at the end of surgery epidural morphine was administered for postoperative pain relief. Oral phenoxybenzamine, 10 mg was applied for prevention of urinary retention, 24 hours and 2 hours before surgery, 8 hours and 16 hours after surgery. Hypotension or any untoward effect was not observed, and the overall rate of urinary retention diminished from 46 % in the control group to 10% in the phenoxybenzamine group. Need for bladder catheterization decreased from 53.3 % to 10 %. Urinary tract infection occurred in 3 patients of the control group and in none of the patients of the treated group. These results indicate that alpha-adrenergic block is useful in alleviating voiding problems after combined epidural local anaesthetic + opioid analgesia (Murray 1984).

Recent investigations of Yaksh et al. (1988 b) have provided further light in this direction. In rats with bladder dysfunction produced by spinal opioids the following statements are made:
- Cholinergic agonists and α-adrenergic agonists stimulate directly the detrusor smooth muscle, and produce an increase in overflow pressure with no bladder emptying and thus may be harmful (e.g. carbachol).
- α-adrenergic antagonists reduce the muscle tone in the spincter, decrease overflow pressure but no bladder emptying and thus may be useful (e.g. phentolamine, metoxamine).
- Dopaminergic agonists produce bladder emptying. Thus they are the drug of choice (e.g. apomorphine).

However, apomorphine has serious drawbacks in the clinic (e.g. emetic and stimulant properties) and cannot be used in this situation. Bromocriptine, another dopamine agonist, is perhaps worth investigating.

c) Use of more selective opioids:
Urinary retention seems more severe after morphine (Camporesi and Redick 1983 b) and the use of lipid soluble opioids seems to produce fewer problems (Brownridge et al. 1983 a).

Inhibition of the micturation reflex is produced only be μ- and δ- but not by κ-ligands. Opioids with relatively more κ-receptor properties would likely cause a less frequent or less severe urinary retention (e.g. pentazocine) (Dray et al. 1988). Epidural methadone is distinguished by its low rate of urinary retention because, unlike morphine or fentanyl, it does not cause bladder relaxation. On the contrary, it increases the detrusor tone (Drenger et al. 1986). Buprenorphine as well has no effect on the bladder (Drenger et al. 1987 a).

Notwithstanding prophylaxis and treatment of this side effect, in some cases it is necessary to catheterize the patient in order to avoid the persistence of a vesical ball. The urinary retention seen after epidural morphine is a serious handicap for the use of such a technique in patients, for whom urinary catheterization must be avoided at all costs.

6.2.5 CONSTIPATION

Aetiology

Opioids increase the resting tone of the small intestine, but propulsive contractions are markedly decreased. In the large intestine peristaltism is diminished or abolished after opioids (Goodman and Gilman's 1985). Constipation is a common side effect of opioid therapy. It occurs during chronic parenteral, as well as during chronic spinal opioid treatment. Even a 100 % incidence of constipation may occur (Krames et al. 1985). Other studies report a lesser incidence, but in those cases a therapy with laxatives was performed (Zenz et al. 1985 a).

Treatment

In any case, when chronic opioid treatment is performed, the frequency of faeces has to be monitored very carefully. A therapy with laxatives is necessary in nearly all patients. No other measures or special antidotes are indicated.

6.2.6 DROWSINESS

Drowsiness may frequently occur after epidural administration of opioids. However, this side effect is seldom bothersome. It is even less severe after epidural administration of opioids than after parenteral injections, where the used doses are generally much higher.

6.2.7 OTHER RARER SIDE EFFECTS

Dysphoria is seldom observed (Bromage et al. 1982 a).

A case of *catatonia* after high doses of epidural morphine was reported by Engquist et al. (1981 a).

Following high doses of epidural pethidine *motor and sympathetic block* can be seen, perhaps due to an injury of the dura mater. All the enumerated side effects are, up to here, reversible by naloxone (Bromage et al. 1982 a).

Crone et al. (1988) pointed out after a retrospective and a prospective study that epidural morphine seems to be a triggering agent associated with reactivation of the herpes simplex virus labialis in obstetric patients.

Some other effects appearing after epidural morphine are mentioned in the medical literature. However, their direct relationship with the opioid administration is not clearly evident.

McDonough and Crannay (1984) observed the delayed occurrence of an epidural abscess 8 days after an injection of morphine.

Wenningsted-Torgard et al. (1982) observed a spondylitis following epidural morphine.

Transient neurologic changes after epidural morphine and also the appearance of a transient bundle branch block and somnolence after a massive overdose were observed (Masoud et al. 1981; Masoud and Green 1982).

Andersen and Eriksen (1984) noted the appearance of an alopecia areata 8 days after epidural morphine.

Robinson et al. (1984) mentioned an accidental epidural morphine overdose (2 x 50 mg) followed by a long lasting depression. After accidental intrathecal puncture, an overdose has produced convulsions in one patient.

In conscious animals it was shown that intra-cerebroventricular injection of short acting opioid neuropeptides (leu- and metenkephalin), results in hypertension and tachycardia. Opiate antagonists abolished this hypertensive response (Schaz et al. 1980). Robinson and Metcalf (1985) observed in a critically ill and old patient a severe hypertensive response to the epidural administration of pethidine 50 mg.

It is really important to realize that for a complete prophylaxis or a complete treatment of all the side effects of epidural opioids it would be necessary to use very high doses of intravenous naloxone.

A Meniere-like syndrome has been reported by Linder et al. (1989). A woman after abdominal hysterectomy was given 2 mg of epidural morphine together with 50 μg of epidural fentanyl. Six hours later the patient complained of Meniere-like syndromes, which reappeared once more after a second dose on the next morning. The symptoms disappeared after naloxone administration.

6.2.8 OVERDOSE, ADDICTION, DEPENDENCE, TOLERANCE AND WITHDRAWAL SYNDROME

Overdose

Overdose after epidural administration of opioids, not only produces all the above-mentioned side effects of opioids but in addition convulsions, spasticity, sympathetic hyperactivity, orthostatic hypotension, transpiration and/or agitation may occur.

In the presence of renal and hepatic insufficiency, a substantial increase in the duration of the opioid action may become evident.

Inadvertent dural puncture, subdural or intrathecal catheter migration may be responsible for overdose symptoms.

Addiction

Addiction is a behavioural pattern of drug use, characterized by overwhelming compulsion to take the drug, securing its supply, and a high tendency to relapse after withdrawal (Jaffe and Martin WR 1985).

Dependence

Dependence is an altered physiological and/or psychological state produced by repeated administration of a drug, which necessitates continued administration of the drug to prevent the appearance of a withdrawal syndrome (Jaffe and Martin WR 1985).

Tolerance

Tolerance is reflected by a shortening of the duration of the drug effect and a need for increasing doses of a drug to produce the same effect.

Addiction is not seen in association with the use of opioids in cancer patients. In many patients receiving regular opioids, however, some degree of physical dependence and tolerance will be seen. Tolerance may be seen as an increase in dose requirements during the first weeks of treatment. However, as treatment proceeds and pain control is achieved, a slower rate of rise in dose, with long periods of dose stability is seen, with even, in some cases, dose reduction (Hoskin and Hanks 1987).

Withdrawal syndrome

It appears in physically dependent subjects when an opioid drug is cancelled abruptly. If during a chronic opioid treatment, oral or systemic opioids are abruptly terminated and replaced by an epidural or intrathecal opioid administration, acute withdrawal symptoms may appear. They respond very well to the conventional treatment with systemic morphine (Messahel and Tomlin 1981;

Tung et al. 1980 b).

A withdrawal syndrome may also become manifest if, in order to replace the pure morphine agonist given by classical routes, an agonist-antagonist is administered by the epidural route (Christensen et al. 1982 b; Weintraub and Naulty 1985).

An exhaustive medical history of the patient is essential to avoid administration of antagonistic opioids to patients addicted to opioids.

6.3 Side effects of intrathecal opioids

Side effects after intrathecal administration of opioids are similar to those following epidural administration, but overdose is more frequent (Tabl. 25, 26, 27). Thus, the incidence and severity of side effects is extremely higher in intrathecal opioid analgesia than in epidural opioid analgesia. The differences are less important in chronic treatment. Spinal headache is a possible side effect particularly seen after intrathecal injections.

6.3.1 RESPIRATORY DEPRESSION

Just as for epidural opioid analgesia the late respiratory depression is the most important danger of this method of analgesia. However, the frequency of this side effect is four times higher after the intrathecal route than after the epidural route. 2.2% (Kossmann et al. 1984 b) and even 3% (Starkman et al. 1984) is still a very high incidence of such a life-threatening side effect.

Respiratory depression seems directly proportional to the dose used, and this depression reaches its maximal depth between 7 hours and 11 hours after the intrathecal opioid administration (Clergue et al. 1984). A dose of 20 mg of intrathecal morphine induced respiratory depression over a period of 20 hours, although a total dose of 30 mg of naloxone was given (Paulus et al. 1981).

Also the use of a hyperbaric solution and the upright position of the patient does not prevent late respiratory depression (Glynn et al. 1979; Liolios and Andersen 1979). Also, reducing the dosage to 0.5 mg of intrathecal morphine is not a completely safe measure (Glass 1984).

Predisposing factors responsible for late respiratory depression

The putative risk of respiratory depression observed after lumbar IT administration of opioids appears to be mainly related to the absorption of the opioid into the systemic circulation and to redistribution back into the CSF (Maurette et al. 1989). Practically the same elements enumerated for epidural opioid analgesia play a role here. The safe dose of morphine is better correlated to age than to body weight (Barrow 1981).

It is evident that acute opioid treatments provide a much higher risk for late respiratory depression than treatment in cancer patients accustomed to opioids. Nevertheless Krantz and Christensen (1987) reported on patients receiving long-term epidural opioid therapy and who had shown tolerance to their effects and who were not protected against respiratory depression after inadvertant intrathecal morphine injection.

After the intrathecal administration of an opioid the problem of crossing the dura mater into the CSF does not exist. But the problem of diffusion and return to the systemic circulation remains for the opioid fraction that is not fixed at the specific receptors. Thus, the choice of the opioid product for intrathecal administration is as important as for the epidural route. With highly lipophilic products, the risk of respiratory depression is significantly reduced. Low lipid solubility of morphine results in a sustained CSF concentration that declines only slowly from an initial high level.

Using the intrathecal route, the hypobaric or hyperbaric density of the injected solution and the choice of the position of the patient after the injection is of much more importance than when using the epidural route (Simionescu 1982). Nevertheless, with intrathecal morphine, the use of a hyperbaric solution and the maintenance of the patient in a half sitting position, even over 24 hours, offer only a relative and temporary protection against delayed respiratory depression.

The risk of delayed respiratory depression is seriously enhanced in cases of repeated intrathecal administration of morphine. King and Tsai (1985) reported this side effect in a 64 year old patient who received only 2 separate doses of 0.4 mg of morphine. Repeated doses facilitate accumulation in the 4th ventricle and subsequently respiratory failure.

If a radiopaque substance is injected intrathecally following previous intrathecal opioid administration the possibility exists that, because of the high hyperbaricity of the radiopaque fluid, the cephalidad flow of the remaining CSF is increased and a delayed respiratory depression may appear.

6.3.2 OTHER SIDE EFFECTS

Pruritus, urinary retention and nausea

These side effects may appear, even after the intrathecal administration of a relatively small dose of 1 mg of morphine.

Convulsions

In animals at very high doses, it is possible for spinally administered opioids to cause either convulsions of a generalized nature or rather localized muscle contractions (Yaksh et al. 1985 b).

In the clinic an overdose may produce convulsions. Such an accident may occur by inadvertence, in the case of the migration of the catheter, in which a primary epidural injection is transformed into an intrathecal administration. Landon (1985) noted such a complication after the administration of 15 mg of morphine epidurally.

Withdrawal syndrome

After the switch over from intravenous to intrathecal morphine a withdrawal syndrome has been observed by Messahel and Tomlin (1981).

Hyperalgic response

In animals at very high doses a bizarre syndrome of *hyperalgesia* (allodynia) has been observed (Yaksh et al. 1986 b). The same phenomenon, an hyperalgesic response in a patient receiving high doses of intrathecal morphine has been reported by Ali (1986) and Stillman et al. (1987).

Tolerance

Yaksh et al. (1986 b, c) speculated that high concentrations of spinal opioids as may be necessary in tolerant terminal cancer patients, could exert an action that physiologically antagonizes the analgesic effects otherwise mediated by the action of morphine on the spinal opioid receptors.

Comparative continuous infusion studies with equianalgesic doses of morphine and sufentanil in rats, indicated that tolerance develops significantly slower from chronic exposure to a high potent opioid (sufentanil) than to an opioid with lower potency (morphine) (Sosnowski and Yaksh 1989).

6.3.3 PREVENTION OF SIDE EFFECTS AFTER INTRATHECAL ADMINISTRATION

The measures to reduce the severity and the frequency of side effects, are similar to those discussed for epidural administration.

Special measures for the intrathecal route are as follows:

- use of an hyperbaric solution
- upright position of the patient after injection
- doses of morphine must be limited to the least effective amounts (0.3-0.4 mg).

For the intrathecal administration all the points to reduce side effects have an even higher importance than for the epidural route.

Thus, dose, product, injection level, volume, density and position are all potential elements reducing or increasing the risk for late respiratory depression. However, just like for epidural opioids in intrathecal administration the risk depends on the presence or absence of previous opioid consumption of the patient. That is the reason why the intrathecal route is frequently used only in cancer pain treatment, and more and more abandoned for acute pain therapy. For the latter the epidural route seems to offer a safer solution.

Brookshire et al. (1983) recommended the intravenous bolus administration of naloxone 0.4 mg followed by a continuous infusion of 0.6 mg/h running during 24 hours. This measure provides a reduction of the side effects from 50 to 15 %.

In our opinion, a dose reduction of the opioid is perhaps a more reasonable decision.

6.4 Tolerance, tachyphylaxis

6.4.1 DEFINITION AND CHARACTERISTICS

Tolerance is defined as the reduction in the magnitude of effect produced by repeated doses of a drug. It requires increasing the dose to achieve a certain magnitude of effect. Tachyphylaxis, desensitization, habituation are synonyms of tolerance.

The time of receptor occupation is very important for the tolerance development. Different hypotheses have been proposed:

- down regulation of receptors (e.g. decrease in number)
- uncoupling of receptor and effector activity
- change in pharmacokinetics.

Tolerance may be assessed by different tests:

- behavioural methods: analgesimetry
- physiological methods: neuronal inhibition
- biochemical methods
- histochemical methods.

Some degree of tolerance can be observed during chronic treatment with all opioids and with all routes of administration.

It is recognized by:

- reduction in duration of action
- reduction in magnitude of drug effect.

Tolerance is partly dependent on the degree of receptor activation. If the dose of the opioid is in excess of that required for adequate analgesia, it is reasonable to assume that such peak levels would contribute to the rapid loss of effectiveness of the administered agent (Onofrio et al. 1981).

Slow tolerance development is one of the most important characteristics in the decision making regarding the most appropriate drug choice for long-term use of spinal opioids. It may be expected that under repeated or continuous spinal administration of spinal opioids, sufentanil, with an high analgesic potency, high lipid solubility, rapid onset of action, high receptor binding affinity, short receptor dissociation time and hence low cumulation tendency, requires low concentration levels at the receptor for efficient analgesia, resulting in slow tolerance development.

Preliminary comparative data obtained in the rat with implanted micropumps and chronic infusion of sufentanil, morphine and other fentanyl analogues provided support for such a hypothesis (Sosnowski and Yaksh 1990).

6.4.2 RAPIDITY OF APPEARANCE

In some cases the appearance of tolerance development may be very rapid. In fact it may already become evident after 10 days of opioid treatment (Milne and Williams 1981).

True tolerance and pseudotolerance

A false diagnosis of tolerance, *pseudotolerance*, is frequent in chronic treatment. Causes can be multiple:

- inappropriate patient selection
- changes in physiologic or psychological status of the patient
- delivery system failure
- development of reflex sympathetic dystrophy
- progression of the disease is the most frequent factor for the need of increased doses (further tumor growth e.g.)
- dura thickening and fibrotic reactions or cocoon formation in the epidural space occur after prolonged use of an epidural catheter and can affect transdural kinetics (Coombs et al. 1985 a), reduced penetration faculty e.g. (Feldstein et al. 1987). Most investigators agree with the statement that development of tolerance appears more slowly after chronic intrathecal opioid treatment than after the use of the epidural route (Coombs et al. 1984 a; Greenberg et al. 1982; Madrid et al. 1987; Ventafridda et al. 1987).

Pseudotolerance caused by dura thickening can be improved by injection of a steroid solution (methylprednisolone e.g.) and lidocaine into the epidural space (Feldstein et al. 1987).

In clinical practice the rapidity of true tolerance development is:
inversely proportional to:
- the duration of the analgesia obtained with a fixed dose of a product
- the time the ligand has been exposed to the receptors
directly proportional to:
- peak effects of repeated high doses.

It was also reported that rapid development of tolerance occurred when the opioid was given in excess of the required dose (Erickson et al. 1984).

Slower development of tolerance may perhaps be obtained by continuous infusion of low opioid doses rather than by intermittent action of repetitive doses.

If tachyphylaxis occurs an increase in doses becomes necessary, finally producing an exhaustion of the effects.

Tolerance development may differ for separate effects of opioids. It appears in greater frequency and rapidity for the side effects of the drug on the CNS (such as sedation, sleep, respiratory depression, emesis) than for the analgesic effect. Tolerance is minimal for miosis and constipation.

In chronic pain conditions, the development of tolerance is extremely slower than in normal pain-free situations (Colpaert 1979). Also, it is to underline that an increase of painful input is more likely to be responsible for any dose increase in cancer patients than will be the development of a strictly pharmacological tolerance (Arnér et al. 1988).

6.4.3 REVERSIBILITY OF TOLERANCE

Tolerance development will also be slow if for a chronic pain treatment program, from the beginning on a ladder of progression in treatment, intensity is followed only step by step. Strong opioids are to be administered only after exhaustion of the minor analgesics. Once the decision to use opioids has been made, careful adjustment of the dose to the individual patient's needs and regularity in drug administration will slacken the tolerance.

Even an initial period of increase in dose requirements may frequently be followed by a long lasting period of dose stability.

Tolerance is a reversible process. Following prolonged application, removal of the drug from the receptor results in the initiation of restarting sensitivity to opioids. So it can be seen that the tolerance phenomenon becomes reversible after the treatment has been stopped for one or two weeks.

6.4.4 CROSS TOLERANCE

Cross tolerance may develop between different kinds of pain treatment (agonists, stimulation, etc.).

The tolerance in the opioid system is a cross tolerance for most of the opioid agonists. It is a cross tolerance between members of a particular drug family, acting upon the same receptor (morphine, fentanyl, sufentanil act on the same μ-receptor). No cross tolerance exists between different classes of agonists (e.g. between μ- and δ-receptor agonists like morphine and DADL). Animals rendered tolerant to morphine show no loss of sensitivity to DADL (Yaksh and Harty 1982 b).

The activation of δ-receptors produces analgesia without inference with pre-existing tolerance of the μ-receptors. This fact indicates that the different spinal opioid receptors react in a different way. Thus, the alternative use of opioids with different receptor affinities may offer a solution to the problem of tolerance.

A recent clinical report indicates that the same can be demonstrated in man (Krames et al. 1986). A patient tolerant to increasing doses of morphine obtained effective analgesia by substituting the μ-agonist morphine by the δ-agonist DADL. The daily dose of DADL was 230 mg.

If real tolerance against spinal opioids has been developed, cancer pain can become unbearable. One approach to overcoming tolerance is to deactivate the μ-opioid receptors while activating alternate non-opioid receptor systems known to mediate anti-nociception. Indeed spinal analgesia may also be produced by non-opioid substances. There are at least eight different neurotransmitter systems involved in nociceptive modulation: enkephalins, epinephrine, serotonin,

GABA, adenosine, etc. Cross tolerance does not develop between the various spinal antinociceptive systems (Tung and Yaksh 1982 b).

Consequently, the following solutions can be considered to overcome tolerance:
1. Enkephalin peptidase inhibitors may influence analgesia prolonging the active life of enkephalins (de la Baume et al. 1983).
2. The use of a drug with similar structure activity which may produce or imitate similar analgesic responses (baclofen or ketamine).
3. Activation of the postsynaptic adrenergic receptors at the spinal level, with either the lipophilic α-agonist clonidine or its analogue ST-91 (Yaksh and Reddy 1981).
4. Co-administration of drugs acting on different systems, such as an opioid associated with clonidine seems to slow the development of tolerance (Yaksh and Reddy 1981; Yaksh and Harty 1982 b).

In spite of the many suggestions, it is practically impossible to completely prevent the development of tolerance during a prolonged treatment.

6.4.5 METHODS OF DELAYING TOLERANCE DEVELOPMENT

If there is a requirement for chronic treatment, the preferential use of one of the following methods is recommended, in order to postpone or reduce the tolerance (Tab. 31):

1. The choice of the opioid is important with reference to the avoidance or delay of a tolerance phenomenon. It is thus accepted that tolerance appears more slowly if agonist-antagonists like buprenorphine or nalbuphine are used (Crawford et al. 1983; Zenz et al. 1982 b).
2. If the epidural or intrathecal opioid administration is carried out in the form of a continuous infusion with low doses instead of bolus injections, the appearance of tolerance might be delayed (Cousins and Mather 1984 b; Glynn and Mather 1982; Müller et al. 1984; Woods and Cohen 1982).
3. The association of an opioid with a local anaesthetic in order to reduce the required opioid doses anticipated may delay tolerance (Chayen et al. 1980; McCoy and Miller 1982). However, the technique is not always successful (Coombs et al. 1982 a; Coombs 1983 b) and carries the risk of hypotension.
4. The stop of the conventional opioid (acting on the μ-receptors) and its temporary replacement by an opioid acting only on the δ-receptors such as DADL (Atchison et al. 1984; Moulin et al. 1985; Onofrio and Yaksh 1983).
5. Injection of methylprednisolone and lidocaine into the epidural space via an

Table 31. Methods for delaying tolerance.

Start spinal opioids only if analgesia obtained by other drugs or routes becomes insufficient
Change the administration route of the opioids: - epidural to intrathecal   - intrathecal to intracerebroventricular $\}$ and reduce the dose

Stop the use of:	Replace by:
- μ - receptor agonists	- δ - receptor agonists (DADL intrathecal) - non-opioid analgesics

Use: - agonist-antagonist opioid (buprenorphine, e.g.)   - continuous infusion   Avoid: - high bolus doses
Associate to the opioid: - a local anaesthetic (bupivacaine) or   - droperidol or   - midazolam or   - baclofen
Replace the opioid by: - local anaesthetics (bupivacaine) or   - AINSA lysine acetylsalicylate infusion: < 7 g/70 kg/d intrathecally) or   - α-adrenergic amine (clonidine 0.3 mg/70 kg/d intrathecally) or   - non-opioid neuropeptides (somatostatin ? calcitonin ?)   - enkephalinase inhibitors (bestatin + thiorphan intrathecally)

epidural opioid delivery system may delay opioid tolerance development as reported by Feldstein et al. (1987). Beneficial effects of steroid treatment in such situations may be explained by reduction of dural thickening processes encountered currently after chronic spinal injection.

6. Co-administration of clonidine by means of a bolus injection of 0.3 mg/d produces an activation of the postsynaptic adrenergic system and allows a rest period for the μ-receptor system (Coombs et al. 1985 a, c).

7. Use of a non-opioid neuropeptide: somatostatin or calcitonin, or an enkeph-

alinase inhibitor: bestatin + thiorphan or kelatorphan.

8. Another method which is still in the experimental stage could be the association of droperidol and morphine intrathecally. This combination slows the appearance of tolerance, at least in the rat (Kim and Stoelting 1980; Bach et al. 1985).

6.5 Side effects due to the technique used

6.5.1 FIBROTIC REACTIONS

During chronic epidural opioid treatment large interindividual variations in opioid concentrations in the CSF were found. Progressively reduced CSF opioid concentrations in spite of the given increased doses have been observed. It is suggested that the variations are due to substantial differences in dura thickening and in transdural opioid diffusion between individuals (Samuelsson et al. 1987).

Epidural catheters remaining for long periods in the epidural space produce non-specific foreign body reactions such as an increase in giant cells and single connective tissue adhesions (Ehring and Boekstegers 1986). These histological changes may reduce or impede the efficiency of the opioid injections.

A case of a fibrous reaction that developed around the silastic catheter tip progressing into a mass was reported (Rodan et al. 1985). This caused a significant displacement of the spinal cord with the development of long tract symptoms. Identification of this abnormality was possible by myelography and computed tomography. Surgical decompression was necessary to improve the patient's condition.

6.5.2 NEURONAL DEGENERATION

Preservative-free morphine or morphine metabolites are not considered to cause neurotoxicity.

However, the post mortem examination of patients treated with chronic spinal opioid infusion for intractable cancer pain revealed posterior column degeneration in some cases (30% of the autopsies performed) (Coombs et al. 1985 e).

On the other hand, it is known that selective demyelinization of the posterior column can occur in cancer patients, even those with minimal neurological findings (Norris 1975). Possible causes of degenerative changes include vitamin deficiency, invasion by tumor, changes caused by radiation or chemotherapy, trauma, etc., so that it can be admitted that neuropathy associated with malignant disease is more likely to be the cause of the observed degeneration (Meier et al. 1982 a).

Dural thickening or fibrotic cocoon formation around implanted epidural catheters is observed. It can effect transdural diffusion kinetics and may lead in time to reduced analgesia but has nothing to do with toxicity.

6.5.3 INFECTION

Infection problems need all our attention. However infection is generally a minor problem in chronic spinal opioid treatment (Meier et al. 1982 b). Signs of contamination are rarely found during bacteriological culture of residual volumes taken from patients treated with drug delivery systems or during incubation of collected samples of the used materials (Müller et al. 1984).

Zenz (1988) noted two cases of reversible spinal infection in a large series of 163 cancer patients on long-term treatment with intermittent administration of epidural opioids in a total treatment period of 11.736 days.

Crawford et al. (1983) reported one catheter tip culture of Staphylococcus aureus among 94 cancer patients with concomitant septicaemia but without symptoms of infection around the spinal cord.

Van Diejen et al. (1987) described during chronic epidural opioid treatment an infection with spinal cord compression. Sensory loss and motor weakness in the legs disappeared after catheter removal and antibiotic treatment.

6.5.4 VIRUS REACTIVATION

Reactivation of the herpes simplex virus labialis by spinal opioids has been reported. Several reports suggest that in obstetric and pediatric patients, an association between a recurrence of oral herpes simplex lesions and the use of epidural or intrathecal morphine exists (Acalovschi et al. 1986 a; Cardan 1984; Douglas et al. 1986 b; Gieraerts et al. 1987; Crone et al. 1988).

Conclusions

It is evident that the spinal administration of opioids is seldom completely free of side effects. It must be underlined that for the more serious of these, such as respiratory depression, nausea, vomiting, urinary retention, pruritus and somnolence, the risk of an overdose (as result of rostral diffusion of the products) is always present. However, the following efficient means of treatment are at our disposal to diminish or prevent the above described adverses reactions:

- the choice of lipophilic opioid

- reduced doses and volumes
- the administration of continuous infusion
- naloxone.

Effective treatment of side effects with naloxone is most easy for the respiratory depression. However, it is difficult to do this without concomitant decrease in quality of analgesia. On the other hand prophylaxis of the side effects other than respiratory depression are not always successful (Gowan et al. 1988; Ramanathan et al. 1986; Samii 1986; Thind et al. 1986).

Following spinal opioid analgesia for acute pain treatment, patients should remain under close supervision in a recovery room, intensive care unit or some appropriate open ward situation and in clear view of the nursing staff.

During chronic treatment, need for increasing opioid doses due to progress and extension of the underlying disease is to be differentiated from real tolerance.

Tolerance may become a serious problem, however in many cases, avoidance or slowing down of the phenomenon is possible if spinal opioids are only used in the right indications (particularly if the benefits of oral and parenteral treatment are exhausted) and if the opioid treatment is scheduled using regular administration in well adjusted doses (see Chapters 14 and 15).

7. Drugs

The choice of an opioid for spinal administration is based not only on pharma-cokinetics but also on some criteria of unequal importance:

- safety index
- speed and duration of action
- immediate and delayed side effects, toxicity
- potency
- existence or absence of an accumulation phenomenon
- response to antidotes
- absence of histamine liberation.

In experimentation the *safety index* is the relationship between lethal and thera-peutic dose. It is the dose producing death in 50 % of the animals divided by the dose producing effective analgesia in 50 % of the animals. In the clinical practice the safety index is evaluated by the ratio between effective doses and the doses producing unacceptable side effects (Tab. 32).

If during anaesthesia the intravenous route is used in ventilated and relaxed patients there exists a direct relationship between analgesic potency and the safety index of the opioids (De Castro et al. 1979 a). The higher the potency the higher is the safety. Under anaesthesiological conditions very high doses of pure potent opioids may be administered without any acute danger, e.g. 100 times the normal dose of fentanyl or sufentanil.

However, the safety found in spontaneous breathing rats and dogs and the relationship between drug safety and drug potency can in man only be applied on intubated and ventilated patients (De Castro 1972). If the same opioids are used for spinal analgesia the clinical situation is not the same. The patient is not under mechanical ventilation and full muscle relaxation. High epidural or intrathecal doses even of the most potent opioid may produce motor block, convulsions or collapse. The clinical safety index of spinal opioids is not higher than twice a full effective dose. For spinal application of opioids a safety increase related to higher potency has not been demonstrated neither in animals nor in man. This particular difference in safety of spinal opioids compared to intrave-nous opioids given during anaesthesia is illustrated by several clinical reports:

Table 32. Comparative physicochemical factors affecting the safety and the efficacy of opioid analgesics.

Drug	Safety index LD$_{50}$/ED$_{50}$ rat, IV	MED IV clinic (mg/70 kg)	MED ED clinic (mg/70 kg)	Analgesic potency ratio IV clinic M = 1	Analgesia ratio MED IV/ MED ED
MORPHINE	70	10	2	1	5
METHADONE	12	10	5	1	2
PETHIDINE	5	100	25 - 50	0.1	2
ALFENTANIL	1080	0.5	0.5	30	1
FENTANYL	277	0.1	0.1	100	1
SUFENTANIL	26716	0.02	0.02	500	1
LOFENTANIL	112	0.005	0.005	2000	1
BUPRENORPHINE	3166	0.3	0.3	35	1

- LD 50 : lethal dose in 50% of animals.
- ED 50 : effective dose in 50% of animals.
- MED IV: medium effective dose (IV route).
- MED ED: medium effective dose (ED route).
- Analgesic potency ratio IV clinic: relative potency by IV route, compared to morphine = 1.
- Activity ratio MED IV/MED ED: relationship of IV to ED doses in order to obtain equianalgesia.
- Safety index: LD 50/ ED 50 rat.
(Adapted from Janssen 1984).

- The 10-fold normal epidural dose of sufentanil produced cardiac arrest in a patient during the postoperative period (Donadoni and Capiau 1987 d), whereas it is generally admitted that the same dose increase of sufentanil given intravenously under anaesthesiological conditions (mechanical ventilation, muscle relaxation) has no effect on the cardiovascular system.

- High doses of intrathecal pethidine (2 mg/kg) may produce cardiovascular collapse (Famewo and Naguib 1985 a, b).

Frequency and intensity of the *side effects* are, evidently, also for spinal treatments, the most essential elements determining the choice of an opioid. The risk of diffusion to the brain and therefore again the lipid solubility and the amount of the un-ionized fraction of a substance, are in this regard of the greatest interest. The *speed of onset of action* has a great importance for acute pain treatment and has no importance in chronic pain treatment.

The *duration of action* of an opioid substance is less important than has been estimated at the beginning of our experience with spinal opioids. At the beginning, a long duration of action was the most interesting property of morphine, but with growing experience it has been shown that morphine also exposes the patients more frequently to delayed respiratory depression than any other opioid. That is the reason why in recent investigations more and more preference is given to other opioids. Today, the interest of many authors is for acute treatment more often concentrated on fentanyl, sufentanil or buprenorphine, products which have shown high efficacy associated with a rarer occurrence of serious complications (Cousins and Mather 1984 b).

Toxicology

It is clear that adequate animal studies must be carried out to determine the acute spinal tissue toxicity of drugs proposed for spinal administration.

Concern about the deleterious effect of chronic spinal opioid administration is also necessary. Although studies in animals and humans after chronic administration of *morphine* have failed to show evidence of demyelinization, necrosis, vascular changes or fibrosis within spinal cord and brain (Abouleish et al. 1981; Meier et al. 1982 a).

Toxicological studies done after chronic spinal use of other opioid compounds than morphine are rather scarce. The *4-anilinopiperidines* administered in repeated daily intrathecal injections in rats and cats were without observable irreversible effects on either behaviour or spinal histology (Yaksh et al. 1985).

For the *non-opioid substances* proposed for spinal use in several pain situations, it has become increasingly apparent that in animals the spinal administration of even apparently benign or physiologic agents (e.g. adenosine, calcitonine, ketamine, lysine acetylsalicylate, somatostatine) have shown significant unexpected anatomopathological nerve degeneration or other spinal tissue pathology, e.g. paralysis and spinal nucleolysis in rats, mice and cats (Ahuya 1983; Amiot et al. 1986; Gaumann and Yaksh 1988; Mollenholt et al. 1987).

7.1 Pure opioid agonists

7.1.1 MORPHINE

Morphine, a μ-agonist, has been the mother-drug of opioids since its introduction into the clinic more than 180 years ago (Fig. 31).

Morphine for spinal use exists on the market under the following registered names:
- Amphiolen Morphinum hydrochloricum ®: morphine HCl; 10 or 20 mg/ml, ampoules 1ml

Morphine

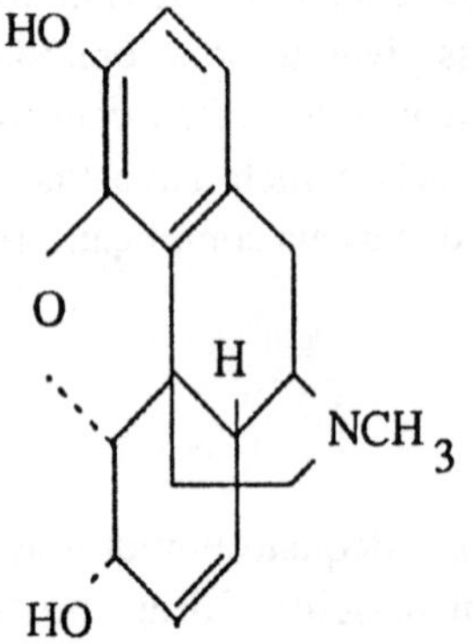

Molecular weight (dalton) 285

Lip. solub. (log P)   0.78

pKa   8.15 - 9.55

	intravenous	epidural	intrathecal
Plasma t $1/2\beta$ (min)	100 - 240	173	70 - 170
Dose (mg)	11 - 20	2 - 5	0.1 - 0.5
Onset (min)	10 - 20	20 - 35	10 - 20
Peak effect (min)	30	30 - 60	20 - 40
Duration (h)	4	8 - 22	8 - 24

Fig. 31. Data on morphine.

- Astramorph ® (Astra): morphine sulfate injection; 0.5 mg/ml and 1 mg/ml; 10 ml ampoules and 10 ml single dose vials.
- Duramorph ® (PF Robins or Elkins-Sinn Inc): microcrystalline aquous suspension of morphine sulphate; 0.5 mg or 1 mg morphine sulfate/ml, ampoules 10 ml.
- Morphine sulfate epidural injection ®:morphine base; 0.2 mg/ml, ampoules 10 ml. (All four forms of morphine are preservative free.)
- Morphine sulfate with preservatives: Eli Lilly, Schein, Wyeth, Astra, Winthrop, Elkins-Sinn, JMS.

Some preparations (Eli Lilly, Wyeth) contain chlorbutanol 0.5%, a preservative that has not been shown to have neurotoxic properties.

Certain morphine products contain toxic preservatives (e.g. phenol or formaldehyde). They should be avoided (Du Pen et al. 1987b).

a) Epidural

The most used effective doses of epidural morphine range from 2.5 mg to 5 mg. The analgesia is selective and produces neither a sympathetic nor a motor block. So, actually the effect of epidural morphine is more an hypalgesia than a complete analgesia.

The onset of action of morphine is the same when it is given epidurally or intramuscularly. Morphine given via the epidural route has a higher vascular absorption rate than morphine given via the intrathecal route (Chauvin et al. 1981 a,b).

The peak effect of analgesia is obtained after 30 to 60 min. The central effects of morphine are less pronounced than those obtained after a parenteral injection. The duration of hypalgesia is in most cases longer than 6 hours and in some cases the patients are pain free over 24 hours.

After the first observation by Bahar et al. (1979), it was largely confirmed that epidural injection of morphine produced analgesia of good quality, notwith-standing the fact that the blood plasma concentrations of the opioid remain far below those necessary for analgesia by the parenteral route.

Epidural morphine produces delayed peak concentrations in the CSF. This is in agreement with the slow onset of action in epidural morphine analgesia (Tamsen et al. 1983). Gustafsson et al. (1982 a) showed that extremely high opioid concentrations are achieved in the CSF during the first five hours following 3.5 mg of epidural morphine (peak concentration: 13.890 nmol/l).

Since the t 1/2 β of morphine in the CSF is similar to that reported in plasma (100-240 min), the long lasting effect following epidural morphine compared to parenteral administration should be related to the high initial morphine concentrations in the CSF. Nordberg et al. (1983) obtained t 1/2 β values of 173,200 and 213 min, respectively, after 2, 4 and 6 mg of epidural morphine. Even after 16 hours, some patients may still have high CSF morphine concentrations and the interindividual differences are very large (Gustafsson et al. 1984). Several factors seem to contribute to the large interindividual differences: supine position, age, decreased elimination through the intravertebral foramen etc.

Comparing plasma and CSF morphine concentrations after epidural and intramuscular application, Bellanca et al. (1985) and Drost et al. (1986) found that the morphine passage into plasma is similar for both routes. The highest values of epidural morphine are attained in the CSF at the end of 90 min and are followed by a slow downsloping; the lowest values are observed 4 hours after drug administration. Given epidurally, morphine is significantly lower in CSF than in plasma 30 min after administration. However, after 60 minutes plasma and CSF concentrations are similar. But in some cases the CSF concentrations are 4 to 8 times higher than those obtained after an intramuscular administration. Such high levels persist for a long time.

Epidural morphine 3.5 mg was more than four times longer lasting than intravenous morphine notwithstanding similar pharmacokinetics (Kossmann et al. 1983). This suggests that the small amounts of morphine diffusing across the dura to the spinal cord remains a long time at the opiate receptors.

The drawbacks of morphine for epidural administration are well established:

- Slow clearance from the CSF: the drug remains available for rostral distribution with potential risk of delayed respiratory depression. Other adverse effects are frequent: pruritus, nausea, sedation, urinary retention. Their severity and the frequency of their occurrence are the reason why many authors, nowadays, prefer other opioids for spinal application.

Morphine was the first opioid in use for intrathecal and epidural administration. It no longer seems the ideal drug for this route. The pharmacokinetic data indicate the ever existent danger of late respiratory depression. Also, the clinical practise confirms those theoretical considerations. Today, the use of epidural morphine can only be recommended for acute pain treatment if sufficient close and long lasting supervision can be provided or, for chronic treatment, in cases of cancer pain.

b) Intrathecal

Wang (1977) was the first to use the intrathecal route for injections of morphine in man. The discovery of this method preceded the epidural administration of opioids.

The doses used intrathecally may be much lower (up to 10 times lower) than the epidural doses. If opioids are administered intrathecally, the fraction of the product that is absorbed into the systemic circulation is clearly lower than by the epidural route.

The studies by Nordberg et al. (1984 a), Nordberg (1984 b) indicate that the most significant pharmacokinetic parameter related to the long duration of analgesia is the high CSF concentration. He found that 0.25 to 0.5 mg of morphine results in dose-dependent CSF concentrations, which are higher than concentrations achieved after epidural administration of 6 mg of morphine. In contrast, plasma concentrations remain very low.

Kinon et al. (1989) demonstrated that 0.1 mg of morphine intrathecally is effective in reducing postoperative pain and is not associated with side effects. Combined with local anaesthetics the minimal effective dose of intrathecal morphine has been found at 0.04 mg (Yamaguchi et al. 1989).

Intrathecal morphine is eliminated from the CSF with a t1/2 β, which is similar to that in plasma after various forms of parenteral administration.

Intrathecal morphine gives sustained pain relief, but there is a considerable time lack before analgesia appears. This is consistent with a rapid transport across the dura, a slow rostral diffusion as well as a slow penetration of the hydrophilic morphine into the spinal cord.

Morphine given intrathecally and intramuscularly has a similar rate of vascular absorption and the pharmacokinetics are the same (Chauvin et al. 1982 a). Such similarity contrasts with the more prolonged analgesia after intrathecal morphine. But the slow resorption of morphine from the CSF, because of its low lipid solubility, may explain the differences.

A plasma morphine level greater than 50 ng/ml is required to produce moderate analgesia (Berkowitz et al. 1975). After 0.2 mg intrathecal morphine plasma concentrations of 42 ng/ml are reached within 60 min. This concentration may contribute to analgesia, but only direct spinal action explains the long duration of analgesia.

One mg of intrathecal morphine produced peak values in the CSF of 4,000-8,000 ng/ml during the first 6 hours (Jørgensen et al. 1981). This suggests that the intrathecal dose of morphine, compared to the parenteral dose should be reduced considerably.

Injected intravenously in a normal adult 100 mg of morphine produces a respiratory arrest in all non-addicted patients (Stanley and Lathrop 1977; Stanley 1980). It can be accepted that out of these 100 mg of morphine only 0.1 % (= 0.1 mg) will appear in the entire brain (Mule 1971). One mg of morphine injected intrathecally is 10 × the amount in the entire brain and probably at least 100 × that found in the region of the medullary respiratory centres following a 100 mg intravenous dose of the drug. Considering the potency of morphine and the free communication in the CSF between the brain and the spinal cord it is surprising that the initially used intrathecal doses of 20 mg of morphine (Samii et al. 1979) did not cause respiratory depression and/or arrest more often (Stanley 1980).

Because morphine is a weak lipophilic product the spinal cord is reached with difficulty. The fraction of the injected drug that is not directly bound at the specific opioid receptors in the spinal cord will linger in the CSF and have the tendency for diffusion from the CSF to the rostral centres for a long period of time. This occurs even if certain precautions (hyperbaric solution, upright position of the patient) are taken.

At present, for intrathecal just as for epidural opioid administration, there is a clear tendency to reduce the opioid doses compared to the early doses of Wang and Samii.

Glass (1984) proposed an intrathecally dose of 0.1 to 0.5 mg of morphine. Nordberg (1984 b) used 0.25 mg of morphine intrathecally, and even these doses correspond to 25-50 mg of morphine administered by the intravenous route (Stanley 1980).

Inherent to intrathecal morphine are CSF concentrations corresponding to a multiple-fold of those obtained by other routes. Consequently, analgesia is highly efficient. But as well, the dangers are extraordinarily high. The place of intrathecal morphine in acute pain treatment is more than questionable. The postoperative course of our patients has indeed been more comfortable with this method. But there is a crucial lack of clinical data indicating a real advantage over conventional analgesia justifying the potential danger of the intrathecal method. Only for cancer pain treatment does the long duration of action and the apparently low danger of respiratory depression in this indication seem to justify the use of morphine.

7.1.2 DIAMORPHINE (HEROIN)

Diamorphine (heroin) or diacetylmorphine (Fig. 32) is rapidly and progressively deacetylated in tissues and blood to mono-acetylmorphine and morphine. It has the same potency as morphine. The oil/water partition coefficients for morphine and diamorphine are 1.5 and 1.7, respectively. Therefore diamorphine acts as a

Diamorphine
(heroin)

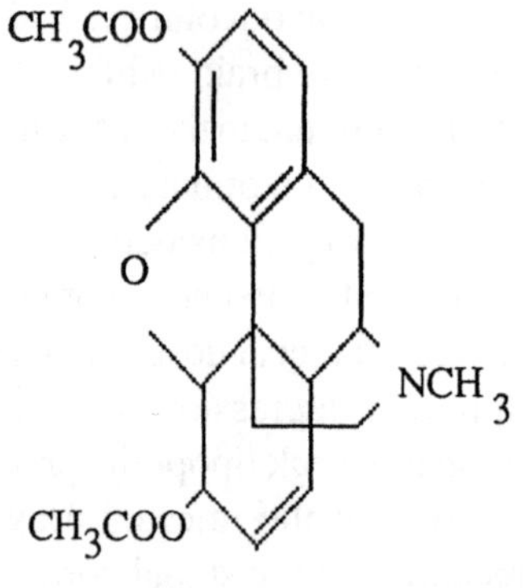

Mol. weight (dalton) 369

Lip. solub. (log P)   0.66

	intravenous	epidural	intrathecal
Plasma t 1/2 β (min)			40 - 50
Dose (mg)	5 - 10	5 - 10	1
Onset (min)	5 - 10	5 - 10	5
Peak effect (min)	30 - 60	30 - 60	10
Duration (h)	4 - 9	6 - 12	12 - 24

Fig. 32. Data on diamorphine.

lipophilic prodrug of morphine (Cowen et al. 1982). Diamorphine, when given by the parenteral route, has the same potency and produces the same duration of action as morphine.

a) Epidural

Comparing diamorphine to morphine, opioid plasma concentrations occur significantly earlier and the peak concentrations are significantly higher.

So, it is estimated that after epidural administration of diamorphine, only 55% crosses the dura (Watson et al. 1984). Notwithstanding the slightly higher lipid solubility epidural diamorphine produces analgesic effects (duration and depth) very similar to those seen after epidural morphine. The side effects after epidural diamorphine are also comparable to those seen after morphine.

In contrast to morphine, with diamorphine, respiratory depression is seen earlier, and delayed respiratory depression has not been noted until now (Phillips et al. 1984; Teddy et al. 1981; Watson et al. 1984).

"Extradural diamorphine appears to be an exotic method of administering a systemic opioid" (Jacobson et al. 1983).

b) Intrathecal

Comparing intrathecal diamorphine (1 mg) to morphine (1 mg) the peak plasma concentrations are significantly shorter (Alexander and Black 1984; Child and Kaufman 1985; Cooper et al. 1982; Cowen et al. 1982; Houlton and Reynolds 1981; Jacobson et al. 1983, 1987; Kaufman 1981; Kotob et al. 1986; Macrae et al. 1987; Malins et al. 1984; Normandale et al. 1985; Paterson et al. 1984).

Barron and O'Toole (1986) compared in 90 postoperative patients 0.15 mg/kg intramuscular morphine to 0.5-1 mg intrathecal diamorphine and 0.5-1 mg intrathecal methadone. With diamorphine significantly better results were obtained than with morphine or than with methadone in terms of duration of analgesia, pain scores, modification of the stress response and in total analgesic requirements.

7.1.3 PETHIDINE (MEPERIDINE)

a) Epidural

The lipid solubility of the μ-agonist pethidine (Fig. 33), is higher than that of morphine. This allows faster penetration into nervous tissues. Consequently, epidural pethidine has a shorter latency of onset of analgesia than morphine (Tamsen et al. 1983). Pethidine has also a shorter duration of action. Epidural pethidine due to the higher lipid solubility compared to morphine seems less likely to induce late side effects.

Pethidine was used epidurally in doses of 20 to 100 mg. With these doses analgesia is generally satisfactory (Bapat et al. 1980 a; Cousins et al. 1979 a; Glynn et al. 1981; Glynn and Mather 1982; Gustafsson et al. 1982 c; Latarjet et al. 1985; Meunier 1984; Perriss 1980a; Perriss and Malins 1981; Raj et al. 1985; Robinson et al. 1986; Rutter et al. 1981; Scott and McClure1979; Skjöldebrand et al. 1982 a; Stoyanov et al. 1981 b; Torda and Pybus 1982).

Albright (1983) observed one respiratory depression among six patients who had received 75 mg of epidural pethidine. Such a depression was not seen after the epidural use of 20 to 25 mg doses.

In obstetrics pethidine produced an analgesia of minor quality than that observed with bupivacaine (Hammonds et al. 1982). The duration of the analgesic action was clearly inferior to that of epidural morphine or buprenorphine. However, the analgesia lasted longer than it did with fentanyl.

b) Intrathecal: spinal anaesthesia with high doses of pethidine

Pethidine given intrathecally at the relative high dose of 100 mg as the sole agent acts not only as an analgesic but also as a local anaesthetic. It produces a spinal anaesthesia adequate for perineal surgery lasting 40-120 min with a transient motor block (2-3 hours) and a sensory block of the lower limbs and lower abdomen. In some cases also a transient sympathetic block has been noted. The surgical analgesia is followed by a prolonged postoperative analgesia (Mircea 1981; Mircea et al. 1982). The observations of Mircea have been confirmed by many investigators (Andrivet et al. 1987; Cozian et al. 1986; Famewo and Naguib et al. 1985 a, b; Fontanals et al. 1986; Janvier et al. 1985; Naguib et al. 1986 b; Ragot et al. 1984 a, b; Saissy 1984 b; Sandu et al. 1981; Tauzin-Fin et al. 1984). Lower doses of 35 mg pethidine have been used by Acalovschi et al. (1986 a, b) for saddle block anaesthesia.

These phenomena are due to the potent local anaesthetic activity of pethidine, which is unique for opioids (Way 1946).

Ragot et al. (1984 a, b) and Janvier et al. (1985) have applied the technique in a total number of 150 patients. They confirmed the possibility of achieving a real surgical anaesthesia with the exclusive use of high doses of pethidine. Advantages of the method compared to a spinal anaesthesia were stable haemodynamic parameters (in normovolemic patients), long lasting postoperative analgesia, possibility to antagonize side effects by naloxone. However, the potential risk of

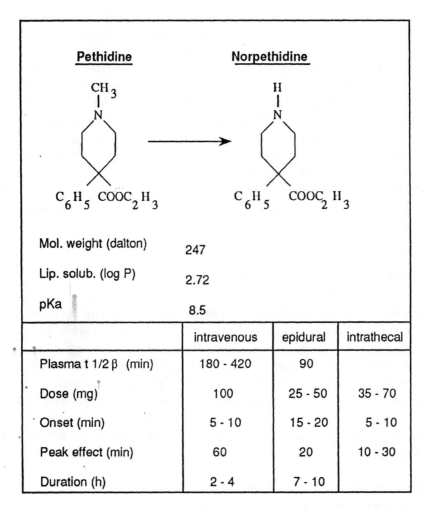

Fig. 33. Data on pethidine.

delayed respiratory depression necessitated a close and long lasting postoperative supervision.

Side effects

The following side effects were noted in the series of Famewo and Naguib (1985 a, b) or Tauzin-Fin et al. (1984):

- bradycardia 20%, vagal collapse 10%, drowsiness 63%, headache 3%, miosis 12%, nausea 30%, pruritus 25%, sphincter relaxation 6%, urinary retention 10%;
- no early or delayed respiratory depression, except one case of severe immediate respiratory depression with cardiovascular collapse and bradycardia. It was produced by an overdose of pethidine (2 mg/kg intrathecally), and necessitated repeated injections of naloxone. Nevertheless, 20% of all severe respiratory depressions were observed in a small series of patients (Andrivet et al. 1987).

After a pethidine saddle block with 0.5 mg/kg pethidine side effects were significantly lower than with the 1 mg dose:
- respiratory depression 0 %
- headache, leg weakness, rigidity 2.7 %, pruritus 6.3 %, nausea and vomiting 4.5 %, urinary retention 1.8 %.

Action-mechanisms of high doses of intrathecal pethidine

Pethidine is a lipophilic opioid, which, after intrathecal injection, penetrates rapidly to the spinal cord receptors and non-specific binding sites producing a high local drug level in the spinal cord. Different explanations have been proposed for the surgical anaesthesia after high doses of intrathecal pethidine (a phenomenon that is not observed after high doses of epidural pethidine):

Rapid passage across the arachnoid granulations and rapid absorption by the arachnoid villi located in the spinal root sleeves, provide anaesthetic blockade and also important systemic uptake (Acalovschi et al. 1986 a; Mather and Phillips 1986).

- The motor block can be explained by:
  . direct action of pethidine on spinal grey matter
  . diffusion into motor fibres
  . local anaesthetic action on axonal membranes in the anterior spinal nerve roots (Cozian et al. 1986).
- The partial sympathetic block and bradycardia may be explained by vascular absorption and ascent of the drug in the CSF and direct action on opioid receptors in the medulla oblongata and the vagal system (Cozian et al. 1986).
- The long duration of postoperative analgesia, long time after the reversal of the motor and sensory blockade, suggests that the intrathecal pethidine also has an effect upon nociceptive synaptic functions in the dorsal horn of the spinal cord (Acalovschi et al. 1986 a). Perhaps due to the synonymous isonipecaine it has not been realized that the local anaesthetic properties of pethidine have been well established since 1946. Way (1946) has demonstrated that pethidine

produces pronounced corneal analgesia, sciatic nerve block and intradermal wheal anaesthesia. The effectiveness was found to be 7/10 of that of cocaine.

For intrathecal pethidine it is essential to note that the substance at 37 °C has a density of 0.998 and is therefore slightly hypobaric (Brownridge et al. 1983 b). An hyperbaric solution is obtained by the addition of 0.3 ml glucose 33 % (Acalovschi et al. 1986 b).

Potential advantages and drawbacks

A high dose of intrathecal pethidine may be effective as the sole agent for anaesthesia and may produce prolonged postoperative analgesia. It may offer an advantage for painful operations, where a prolonged postoperative analgesic effect is desirable. It could also serve as an alternative agent for spinal anaesthesia when a local anaesthetic is contraindicated. However, this technique implicated the necessity of postoperative monitoring during 24 hours after the administration (Tauzin-Fin et al.1987 a, b).

The advantages of high dose intrathecal pethidine seem attractive. However, the method has to be applied with great caution (see toxicology of pethidine). Theoretically, the danger of side effects may increase when the operative pain and stress wear off. On the other hand, the method provides postoperative analgesia only for a limited period of time. Perhaps, an epidural opioid for the postoperative period provides a better alternative. So, the indication for intrathecal high-dose pethidine seems to be quite limited.

Toxicology of pethidine

Nevertheless all these more or less enthusiastic reports about the clinical use of intrathecal pethidine are to be seriously tempered by toxicological considerations about this compound.

Some years ago, in dogs as well as in the clinic, we showed the relatively low safety index of pethidine compared to the more potent opioids (De Castro et al. 1979 a).

More recently, new sensitive analytical methods for measuring opioid metabolites have identified a toxic metabolite of pethidine. Indeed, the major metabolite of pethidine is norpethidine (Fig. 33). It has about half the analgesic potency of pethidine in experimental animals, but it causes toxic convulsions in monkeys and mice (Umans and Inturrisi 1982). Norpethidine is eliminated more slowly than pethidine with a t 1/2 β of 14-21 hours versus 3 hours (Holmberg et al. 1982). The plasma concentration ratio of norpethidine to pethidine is usually less than one.

But, if in man this ratio increases to more than one, the pethidine use is associated with neurological sequelae ranging from shaky feelings to grand mal seizures (Inturrisi and Umans 1986).

In clinical practice the plasma norpethidine/pethidine ratio is often greater than one (liver and kidney disorders, elderly, neonates, etc.). The risk of an accumulation of the toxic norpethidine metabolite makes pethidine a poor choice clinically (Moore et al. 1987).

Thus we can conclude that for toxicological reasons the high doses of pethidine are difficult to justify for spinal analgesia.

7.1.4 METHADONE

D/L Methadone (racemix mixture of (+) and (-) isomers), a μ-agonist widely used in oral cancer pain treatment (Fig. 34), is also used for spinal administration. The analgesic activity is the property of (-) methadone which is some 8-50 times more potent than the (+) isomer. The analgesic potency is equal to that of morphine. But the lipid solubility is much higher. This advantage is counteracted by the unpredictable half-life time of methadone, which can exceed two days. After a single intravenous dose, mean values of multiple dosing are about 18 hours (although with large interindividual variations) and 36 hours in patients with moderate to severe liver disease (Novick et al. 1981).

Epidural methadone offers the advantages of relatively short latency, moderately long duration of analgesia and low incidence of side effects (Barron and O'Toole 1986; Beeby et al. 1984; Bromage et al. 1980 c; Eimerl et al. 1986 a, b; Evron et al. 1985; Magora et al. 1986 b, 1987 c; Max et al. 1982; Torda and Pybus 1982; Welch and Hrynaszkiewcz 1981 b). It is distinguished by its low rate of urinary disturbances because, unlike morphine, it causes no bladder relaxation (Drenger et al. 1987 a).

Eimerl et al. (1986 a, b); Magora (1987 b) proposed a continuous plus on-demand epidural infusion of methadone for postoperative pain relief: loading bolus of 2 mg of methadone, continuous infusion of 0.4 mg/h, and an additional bolus of 0.2 mg by self-administration. Effective analgesia needed 9 to 21 mg methadone epidurally for the first-operative day and 4 to 10 mg during the second and third days. Serious side effects have not been observed in a limited number of treated patients.

Experiences with intrathecal methadone are limited and demonstrate no advantages for this drug (Barron and O'Toole 1986).

The major clinical difficulty with methadone lies in the unpredictable duration of action of a spinal injection which is in some patients not really longer than that seen after intramuscular injections.

Methadone			
Mol. weight (dalton)	309		
Lip. solub. (log P)	2.06		
pKa	8.3		

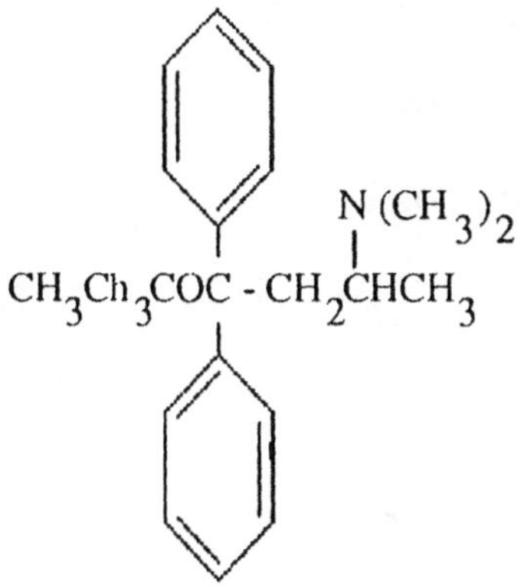

$$N(CH_3)_2$$
$$CH_3Ch_3COC - CH_2CHCH_3$$

	intravenous	epidural	intrathecal
Plasma t 1/2 β (min)	500 - 5220		
Dose (mg)	10	5	
Onset (min)	10 - 20	10 - 15	
Peak effect (min)	30	20 - 30	
Duration (h)	4 - 6	7 - 9	

Fig. 34. Data on methadone.

7.1.5 HYDROMORPHONE

Hydromorphone, μ-agonist (Dilaudid), is available as a preservative free preparation (Fig. 35). Because of its long duration of analgesia clinically it appears to be, a useful epidural opiate for postoperative analgesia, even when used in a single dose technique.

In a recent study, 1 mg of preservative free epidural hydromorphone resulted in a pain free period of 19 hours until the first supplemental analgesic was required, whereas 2 mg of intramuscular hydromorphone lasted only 5 hours (Henderson et al. 1987).

Other investigators reported a shorter duration of action with epidural hydromorphone (Albright 1983; Bromage et al. 1980 c; Chestnut et al. 1985, 1986). But pruritus is reported to have a high incidence (Chestnut et al. 1986; Coombs

Hydromorphone

Mol. weight (dalton) 286

Lip. solub. (log P)

pKa   8.05

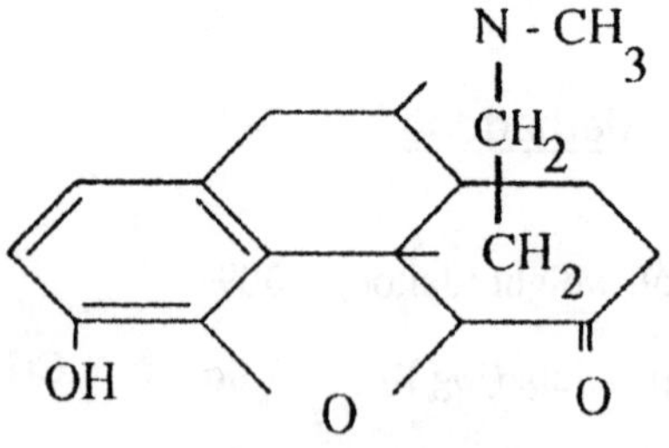

	intravenous	epidural	intrathecal
Plasma t $1/2\beta$ (min)			
Dose (mg)	1 - 2	1	
Onset (min)	15	10 - 20	
Peak effect (min)	60	20 - 30	
Duration (h)	4 - 6	6 - 19	

Fig. 35. Data on hydromorphone.

et al. 1986 b; Henderson et al. 1987; Horan et al. 1985; Matthew et al. 1987; Moon and Clements 1985; Parker et al. 1985; Wakerlin et al. 1986).

Respiratory depression was observed (12% of the cases) if doses up to 2 mg were used (Shulman et al. 1984 b). Delayed respiratory depression was noted by Wust and Bromage (1987) in a patient receiving, after an adrenalectomy, hydromorphone through a thoracic epidural catheter.

7.1.6 NICOMORPHINE

Nicomorphine, a µ-agonist is a lipopilic opioid; the dinicotinoyl ester of morphine probably acting as a prodrug to morphine. It is reported to be equipotent to morphine (Fig. 36).

(Nicomorphine, t $1/2\beta$ 3 min, 6-mononicotinoylmorphine t $1/2\beta$ 15 min, morphine t $1/2\beta$ 180 min)

Nicomorphine was used in epidural doses of 5-10 mg (Dirksen and Nijhuis 1980 a). The duration of analgesia is relatively long (6-18 hours). Higher doses produce a high incidence of side effects.

Hasenbos et al. (1985 a, b, 1987) used in 163 patients 4-6 mg epidural nicomorphine at thoracic level (T3-T4) after thoracic surgery. Analgesia was rapid and effective. Severe respiratory depression was not seen, but nausea and vomiting occurred in 20 and 11%, respectively, pruritus in 7% and urinary retention in 71%. In a recent study, the effects on ventilatory and airway occlusion pressure responses to CO_2 were minimal, indicating no significant respiratory depression (Hasenbos et al. 1986). Postoperative epidural nicomorphine allowed better ventilation and diminished the number of postoperative pulmonary complications (Hasenbos et al. 1987).

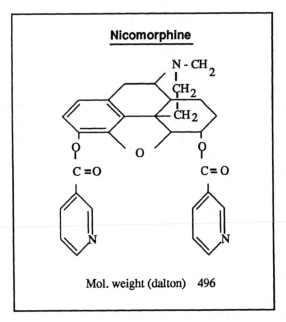

Fig. 36. Chemical structure of nicomorphine.

7.1.7 FENTANYL

Ampoule-packed fentanyl is a preservative free solution. In contrast, the vials contain preservatives so that the vial preparation should not be used for spinal administration (Fig. 37, 38, Tab. 33, 34).

After an epidural injection of fentanyl (a μ-agonist) there remains only a small amount of the highly ionized liposoluble drug in the CSF. The substance will penetrate rapidly to the spinal cord receptors and non-specific binding sites . But fentanyl is also characterized by a rapid regression, unless the drug has a particular affinity for lipid tissues and a high receptor binding.

Shipton et al. (1984 b) investigated the plasma pharmacokinetic profile of 0.1 mg epidural fentanyl in comparison with the data obtained after 0.1 mg intravenous fentanyl. By the epidural route the same amount of fentanyl did not lead to plasma levels, which could be dangerous in respect of respiratory depression.

The use of epidural fentanyl in place of morphine becomes more and more current practice for acute pain treatment (Arcario et al. 1987; Bormann et al. 1983 b; Chrubasik et al. 1987 b, 1988 b; Dietzel et al. 1982; Estok et al. 1987; Fierro et al. 1982; Frings et al. 1982 a, b; Garcia Guasch et al. 1982; Gessler et al. 1983; Herrera Hoys 1983; Houlton and Reynolds 1981; Lomessy et al. 1982, 1984, McQuay et al. 1980; Negre et al. 1985; Pandit et al. 1987; Parker et al. 1985; Pierrot et al. 1982; Piva et al. 1982; Rutter et al. 1981; Severgnini et al. 1982; Shipton 1984 a, c; Shipton et al. 1984 b, 1986; Stoyanov et al. 1981 a, b).

A recent survey performed by Mott and Eisele (1986) in 104 American anaesthesia departments revealed that for postoperative and posttraumatic pain treatment 32 anaesthesia departments currently used fentanyl against 57 departments currently using morphine.

Most authors agree with the observation that the analgesic effect of fentanyl has only a latency of 4-6 min after the epidural injection. The maximal effect is reached after 10 to 20 min (Fig. 37). Effective analgesia is provided for 2 to 3 hours. The duration of action of this opioid is clearly shorter than that observed with several other opioids. The significance of this disadvantage, however, is only relative. It is outweighed by the reduced number of side effects and the possibility of administration in continuous infusion.

If the doses administered are not greater than 50 µg/h and if the association with other central nervous system depressors or opioids is avoided, severe delayed respiratory depression has not yet been reported after the epidural use of fentanyl (Bowen-Wright and Goroszeniuk 1980; Ahuja and Strunin 1985 a, b). Nevertheless, a mild early respiratory depression (1-2 hours after the injection) with bradycardia and a slight transient rise in PCO_2 was observed (Samii 1986). Only with doses as high as 5 µg/kg was respiratory depression demonstrated (Pierrot et al. 1982).

The quality of the postoperative analgesia after one administration of 50 µg fentanyl is satisfactory for 2 to 3 hours. After the administration of fentanyl in epidural doses of 100-200 µg it has been noted that also the pain produced by coughing disappears.

This postoperative treatment produced a significant increase in vital capacity, allowing an earlier institution of more intensive physiotherapy than after conventional analgesic treatment (Lomessy et al. 1984).

Nausea and pruritus were side effects observed after the epidural injection of fentanyl. Nausea and vomiting were more frequent if a continuous infusion of

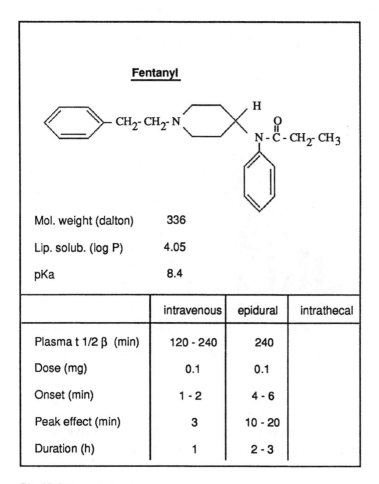

Fentanyl

Mol. weight (dalton)	336
Lip. solub. (log P)	4.05
pKa	8.4

	intravenous	epidural	intrathecal
Plasma t 1/2 β (min)	120 - 240	240	
Dose (mg)	0.1	0.1	
Onset (min)	1 - 2	4 - 6	
Peak effect (min)	3	10 - 20	
Duration (h)	1	2 - 3	

Fig. 37. Data on fentanyl.

epidural fentanyl in a dose 50 to 60 µg/h was given. But these effects generally disappear if the doses were reduced to 25 µg/h.

Many authors recommend the use of epidural fentanyl in a bolus of 0.001 mg/kg, followed by a continuous infusion of 0.001 mg/h for postoperative analgesia (Ahuja and Strunin 1985 a, b; Bailey and Smith 1980; Bowen Wright and Goroszeniuk 1980; Chrubasik et al. 1987 b; Guéneron et al. 1986; Renaud et al. 1985 a, b; Skerman et al. 1985 a, b; Steppe et al. 1983; Welchew and Thornton 1982 a; Welchew 1983 e.g.). This technique provides an effective analgesia without clinically significant respiratory depression. Plasma fentanyl levels reach a plateau below 2 ng/ml.

For postoperative treatment the best results can be obtained if fentanyl is given in continuous plus on-demand infusion (Bell et al. 1987).

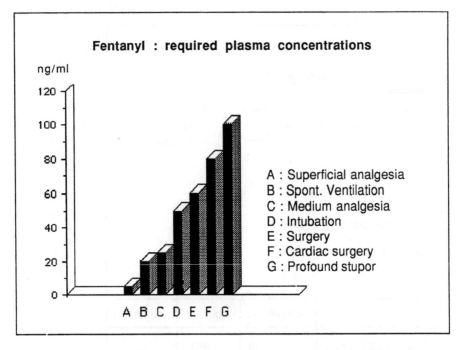

Fig. 38. Required plasma concentrations of i.v. fentanyl for various anaesthesiological events. (Adapted from Hug and Chaffman 1984 a)

The advantages of this technique are summarized as follows:
- continuous infusion of fentanyl avoids the drawback of short activity
- considerable reduction in total fentanyl doses (0.025 mg/h) is achieved
- high efficacy
- patient alertness, mobility, ability to cough
- absence of hypotension or fecal incontinence
- slow tolerance development (Bowen-Wright and Goroszeniuk 1980; Mc Quay et al. 1980). The method is reserved for inpatients only.

The most effective fentanyl doses are:
- loading dose of 0.5 µg/kg
- maintenance dose with 1 µg/kg/min in a solution of 10 µg/ml
- on-demand bolus injections of 0.1-0.2 µg/kg, when necessary.

After abdominal or thoracic surgery this method provides effective and continuous analgesia without significant respiratory depression. Urinary retention is seldom seen and pruritus is noted in only 15 % of the cases.

The association of bupivacaine (0.5%) with fentanyl 50-100 µg provided excellent surgical analgesia (Bromage et al. 1987; Camara et al. 1984; Garcia

Table 33. Comparative properties of four pure opioids for spinal opioid analgesia.

Properties	Fentanyl	Alfentanil	Sufentanil	Lofentanil
- Molecular weight (dalton)	336	416	387	409
- Stable in saline and glucose solution	+	+	+	+
- Preservative free preparation	+	+	+	+
- Can be mixed with a local anaesth.	+	+	+	+
- Highly lipophilic properties (n-heptane/H_2 O log Pi-Pu)	2.98	2.11	3.24	3.16
- Dose bolus (mg/70 kg bw) continuous inf. (mg/h) on - demand bolus (mg)	0.050 - 0.1 0.250 - 0.075 0.001 - 0.002	0.15 - 0-03	0.050 0.005 0.005	0.05 - 0-01
- Analgesia onset (min) peak effect (min) duration (h)	5 - 10 20 - 30 2	10 15 1 - 1.5	7 - 10 15 6	20 - 30 50 6 - 10
- Antagonism by naloxone	+	+	+	–
- Tolerance development	+	+	+	+
- Drowsiness	–	–	–	–
- Low risk of delayed resp. depression	+	+	+	+
- Common properties	- analgesia | onset more rapid | longer lasting - remain more segmental - rostral spread less likely			

+ = yes, - = no

Guasch et al. 1982; Lecron et al. 1979; Maione et al. 1983; Milon et al. 1983; Poupard et al. 1984; Rucci et al. 1985; Salvetti et al. 1983; Servergnini et al. 1982; Solanki 1987). Such a technique is currently used in obstetrics where the association of a local anaesthetic and an opioid realizes maximal analgesia with a minimum of drug amount (Bagley et al. 1987; Bohannou and Estes 1987; Chestnut et al. 1987; Cohen at al. 1986; Grice et al. 1987; Preston et al. 1987). The technique will be explained in detail later.

Respiratory function following simple bolus doses as well as continuous in-

Table 34. Comparative properties of fentanyl, alfentanil and sufentanil.

Alfentanil (AF) or sufentanil (SF) compared to fentanyl (F)		
	AF versus F	SF versus F
Hepatic extraction	↑	↓
First pass effect	↑	↓
Peripheral sequestration	↓	↓

(Adapted from Bovill et al. 1984; Hug 1984 b)

fusions of epidural fentanyl were studied in 21 patients by Ahuja and Strunin (1985b). End tidal CO_2 showed an insignificant increase following single doses of 0.0015 mg/kg. These changes occurred within minutes of injection but could not be attributed only to rapid systemic absorption of fentanyl from the epidural space. Continuous epidural infusion (0.0005 mg/kg/h) starting 60 minutes after the bolus dose had no effect on end tidal CO_2 concentration for up to 18 hours, although the respiratory rate became slower. Infusions were continued for up to 9 days during which there was no clinically significant respiratory depression.

Nevertheless, if fentanyl (100 µg) associated with bupivacaine and adrenaline is followed by intravenous midazolam (2.5 mg), nalbuphine (2.5 mg) and droperidol (1 mg) it is not surprising that in such a case profound nervous system depression may occur as exemplified by the recent report of Wells and Davies (1987 b).

Also the intrathecal route has been studied with fentanyl doses of 0.05 mg (Cabo Franch and Marti 1981; Guerin et al. 1983; Otteni et al. 1982).

The results of more than 60 clinical studies (> 5000 patients) demonstrate clearly that the risk of delayed respiratory depression following epidural or intrathecal fentanyl is minimal. Notwithstanding these results, close monitoring of ventilation is always necessary (Samii 1986).

A relatively safe drug like fentanyl given in the wrong dose and in a wrong indication can even lead to death. From Germany a case has been reported where epidural fentanyl was given after a vaginal hysterectomy for postoperative pain control. Close supervision was omitted and the patient died after severe respiratory depression (Zenz 1988, personal communication).

Fentanyl has no active or toxic metabolites and is not associated with clinical problems when administered to patients with renal or hepatic dysfunction (Glynn et al.1987 b).

The compound undoubtedly deserves a substantial place in spinal opioid therapy.

7.1.8 ALFENTANIL

Alfentanil, a μ-agonist, has a weaker potency and shorter duration than fentanyl (Fig. 39 to 45, Tab. 33, 34).

Chauvin et al. (1983), Cookson et al. (1983), Levron et al. (1983) investigated the plasma pharmacokinetic profile of alfentanil after 0.015 and 0.03 mg/kg epidurally or 0.015 mg/kg intramuscularly. The results indicated that the half-life and clearance parameters of alfentanil were similar to those reported in other studies, in which the intravenous administration was used (Bower and Hull 1982).

Alfentanil administered epidurally easily crosses the haematomingeal barrier and rediffuses rapidly into the systemic circulation. It produces an analgesia of rapid onset and short duration (Levron et al. 1983).

Chauvin et al. (1985 a) treated 18 patients for postoperative pain with

Alfentanil

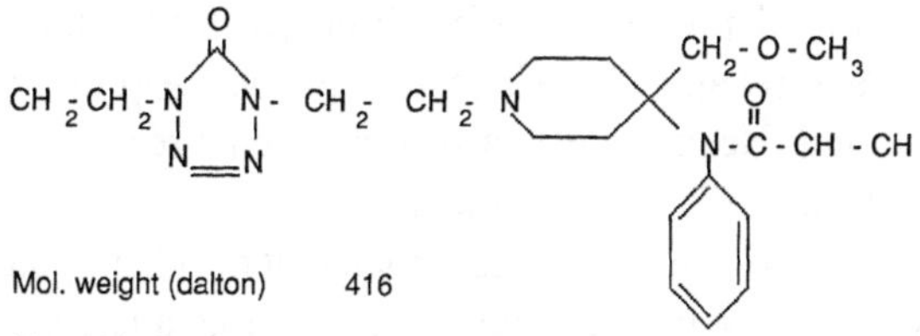

Mol. weight (dalton)	416
Lip. solub. (log P)	2.16
pKa	6.25

	intravenous	epidural	intrathecal
Plasma t 1/2 β (min)	70 - 110	89.4	
Dose (mg)	0.5 - 1	0.5 - 1	
Onset (min)	0.5 - 1	5	
Peak effect (min)	3	15	
Duration (h)	0.5	1.5	

Fig. 39. Data on alfentanil.

154

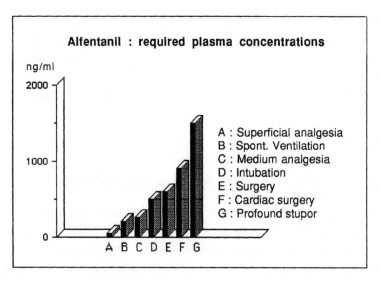

Fig. 40. Required concentrations of i.v. alfentanil for various anaesthesiological events. (Adapted from Ausems et al. 1986; Bovill et al. 1984; Sebel et al. 1985; Stanksi 1982)

injections of alfentanil in epidural doses of 15 to 30 µg/kg. Alfentanil rapidly produced effective analgesia but analgesia of relatively short duration (90 to 100 minutes). The side effects were acceptable; they were slightly more severe and frequent for the 30 µg/kg dose. The dose of 15 µg/kg therefore seems to be the most appropriate dose for epidural alfentanil.

A slight respiratory depression may be observed 45-90 minutes after epidural administration (Penon et al. 1988). Up to now delayed respiratory depression has never been observed. Nevertheless, also for patients receiving epidural alfentanil, close monitoring remains necessary.

The greater clearance rate of alfentanil than that of other opiates suggests that it may be a safe drug to be used for the epidural opioid analgesia (Matsumoto et al. 1983; Penon et al. 1986).

Nevertheless, the pharmacotherapeutic parameters of alfentanil may present abnormal values for t 1/2 β, VDss, clearance (Fig.42,43,44,45), so that in several patients, the duration of action of this opioid may be longer than normal. Age and extracorporeal circulation are typical situations presenting after alfentanil a longer lasting analgesia.

The short duration of action and the pharmacokinetic data favour alfentanil for the treatment of acute pain. However, facing the short duration of action, which corresponds to conventional systemic analgesia, it seems that there is no place for spinal bolus administration of this compound. The theoretical security index of alfentanil favours this drug for a continuous epidural infusion.

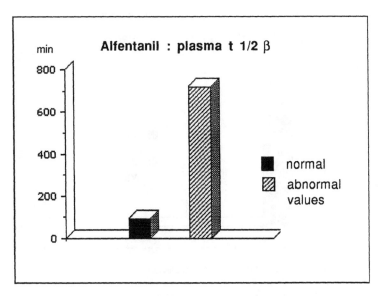

Fig. 41. Comparison of plasma half-life time β of alfentanil in normal pathological patients.
(Adapted from Ferrier et al. 1985; McDonnel et al. 1982)

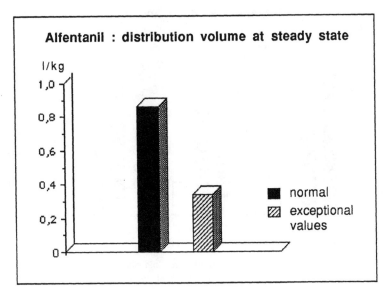

Fig. 42. Comparison of distribution volume of alfentanil in normal and pathological patients.
(Adapted from Ferrier et al. 1985; McDonnel et al. 1982; O'Connor et al. 1983)

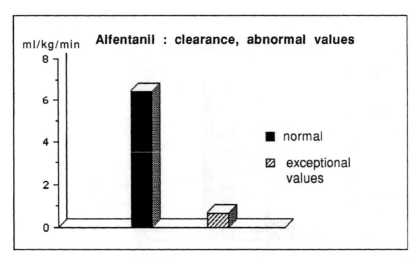

Fig. 43. Comparison between normal and abnormal clearance values for alfentanil in normal and pathological patients.
(Adapted from Ferrier et al. 1985; Shafer et al. 1985; Yate et al. 1986)

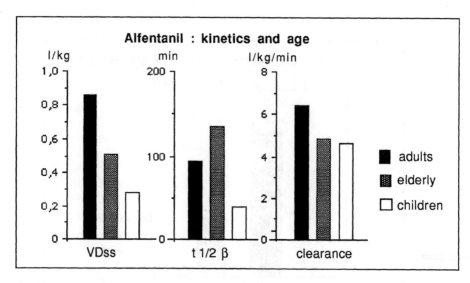

Fig. 44. Age-dependent variations of alfentanil kinetics and clearance.
(Adapted from Helmers et al. 1983, 1984 ; Levron et al. 1983; Hug and Chaffman 1984 a)

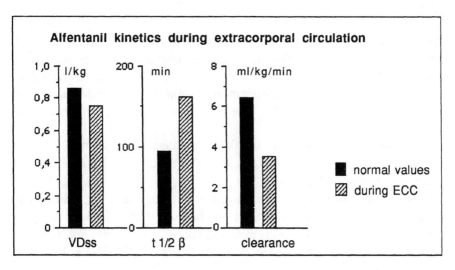

Fig. 45. Variations of alfentanil kinetics and clearance in normal patients and patients during ECC. (Adapted from De Lange and De Bruijn 1983)

7.1.9 SUFENTANIL

Sufentanil® ampoules and Sufentanil forte® ampoules are preservative free preparations (Fig. 46-49, Tab. 33, 34).

Animal studies

Sufentanil is a highly selective μ-ligand in vivo with a receptor affinity 10 times higher than that of fentanyl (Leysen and Gommeren 1983).

Sufentanil has, in animals, an extremely high safety index, nearly 100 times that of fentanyl. Administered epidurally in rats analgesic doses showed extensive μ-receptor binding in the lumbar cord. Apparent binding in the cervical or thoracic spinal cord or in the brain was only seen after high doses. (Colpaert et al. 1986).

Sufentanil has a lipid solubility quotient double of fentanyl and 1000-fold higher than morphine. This results in a less drug depot remaining in the CSF, thus reducing the potential hazard for respiratory depression.

Colpaert et al. (1986) studied in rats the comparative safety index for thoracic rigidity appearing after intravenous or epidural administration of sufentanil. The epidural route allowed 3 times higher doses before side effects appear.

158

Clinical studies

The clinical pharmacokinetics of epidural sufentanil were studied by Camu et al. (1985). In a dose of 50 µg sufentanil analgesia had a rapid onset (latency 7 min), a peak effect after 10 min and a duration of action of 330 min. Discrete respiratory depression was observed between 5 min and 30 min after the injection, and slight sedation was observed during 2 hours. Delayed respiratory depression was absent.

The association of adrenaline 1/200.000 to sufentanil 50 µg resulted in an intensification of segmental analgesia with longer duration (5 hours) and less side effects (Klepper et al. 1987).

Epidural sufentanil is particularly suited in obstetrics for labour, delivery and postpartum pain relief (Fanard 1988; Leicht et al. 1986 b; Little et al. 1987; Madej and Strunin 1987 b; Naulty et al. 1986 d; Noueihed et al. 1984; Tan et al. 1986 a, b; Van Steenberge 1986; Van Steenberge et al. 1987 a, b) and in

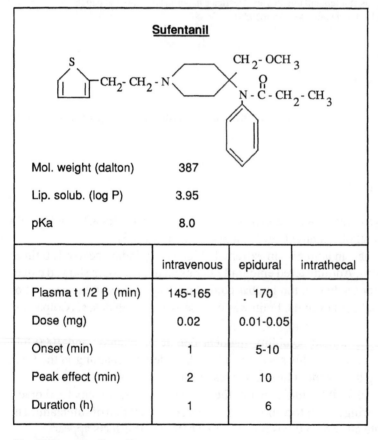

Sufentanil

Mol. weight (dalton)	387
Lip. solub. (log P)	3.95
pKa	8.0

	intravenous	epidural	intrathecal
Plasma t 1/2 β (min)	145-165	170	
Dose (mg)	0.02	0.01-0.05	
Onset (min)	1	5-10	
Peak effect (min)	2	10	
Duration (h)	1	6	

Fig. 46. Data on sufentanil.

postoperative pain treatment (Camu et al. 1985; Diesbecq 1986; Donadoni et al. 1985, 1987 c; Donadoni and Rolly 1987 b; Donadoni and Capiau 1987 d; Duckett et al. 1986; Noueihed et al. 1984; Parker et al.1985; Philips 1987 a, b, c, 1988; Rosseel et al. 1987 a, b; Stanton Hicks et al.1987; Strutigi et al. 1987; Van den Hooger 1987 a, b, c; Van Droogenbroeck et al.1985; Van der Auwera et al. 1986, 1987; Verborgh et al. 1986; Vercauteren and Hanegreefs 1986, 1987; Whiting et al. 1986). The optimum epidural dose is 50 µg diluted in 10 ml saline. In obstetrics, if the substance is associated with bupivacaine 0.25% and epinephrine, the dose may be reduced to 15 µg. Even a dose of 5 µg sufentanil + 10 ml bupivacaine 0.25 % in labour reduced the onset time of analgesia and improved the quality of the epidural block for 30-60 minutes without an increase of side effects (Little et al. 1987). For the postoperative period higher doses of sufentanil or an association with bupivacaine or epinephrine may be beneficial.

However, if the epidural dose of sufentanil is high (75 µg) and repeated too rapidly (2-3 hours interval), severe respiratory depression has been observed (Whiting et al. 1986; Sanford 1988). Blackburn (1987) reported two patients who suffered respiratory arrests following 4 to 7 doses of ED sufentanil 50 µg over 20-22 hours. Dose of 75 µ-injected at Th5-Th6 level produced 4-5 hours after injection a reduced respiratory rate (Verborgh et al. 1988). Doses of 50 µg

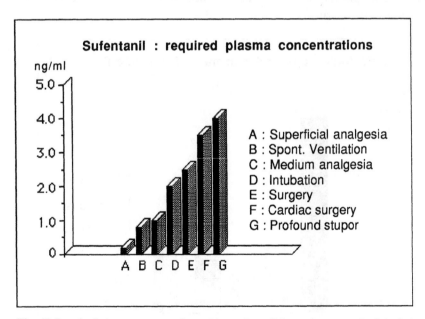

Fig. 47. Required plasma concentrations of i.v. sufentanil for various anaesthesiological events.
(Adapted from Hug and Chaffman 1984 a)

produced an acceptable degree of respiratory changes occurring during 10 to 40 min after the sufentanil injection. If after 4-6 hours patients complain of pain an additional bolus injection of 50 μg may be given (Duckett et al. 1986; Van Droogenbroeck et al. 1985). Delayed respiratory depression was not noted. However, in animals the degree of naloxone reversal seems less with sufentanil than with fentanyl (Aoki et al. 1986).

The pharmacokinetic parameters of sufentanil are nearly identical in renal transplant patients as in healthy surgical patients. Renal function plays little if any role in the elimination of sufentanil during the first hours after administration; this suggests that liver function, the primary determinant of sufentanil clearance, is well maintained during surgery (Fyman et al. 1987).

Sufentanil is most useful when given in intermittent or continuous epidural infusion (Cheng et al. 1987; Duckett et al. 1987; Madej et al. 1987 a, b, c).

Also in children, epidural sufentanil has been used successfully. Doses of 0.75 μg/kg have been used for pain relief after urologic surgery (Benlabed et al. 1987).

High lipid solubility and high receptor affinity of sufentanil provide the explanation for rapid analgesic effect and limited CSF sequestration, limited rostral spread and slight transient vascular uptake, resulting in minimal risk of delayed respiratory depression.

The duration of action of sufentanil is significantly modified by the age of the patient, e.g. the plasma t $1/2$ β is increased in neonates and the clearance is highest in children (Fig. 48, 49).

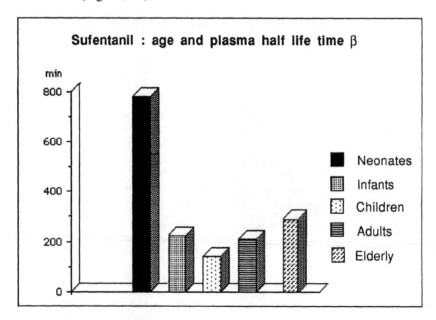

Fig. 48. Age-dependent variations in sufentanil plasma half life time β.
(Adapted from Greeley 1986; Hug 1984 b)

The important *advantages* for epidural sufentanil can be summarized as follows:

- strong segmental hypalgesia
- duration is volume related (optimum = 10 ml)
- low accumulation tendency during continuous infusion
- side effects for the 50 μg dose are relatively low and mild compared to morphine.

Advantages of sufentanil versus fentanyl:

- lipid solubility: higher
- un-ionized plasma fraction: higher
- receptor affinity: higher
- risk of delayed respiratory depression: the same or lower for the 50 μg dose
- onset of analgesia: more rapid
- duration of analgesia: longer
- side effects: the same or lower.

Considering physiochemical, pharmacodynamic and pharmacokinetic parameters sufentanil is theoretically the opioid with the most appropriate properties for intraspinal administration (Aoki et al. 1985; Kitahata and Collins 1984 a; Leysen and Gommeren 1983; Meert and Noorduin 1988; Noueihed et al. 1984).

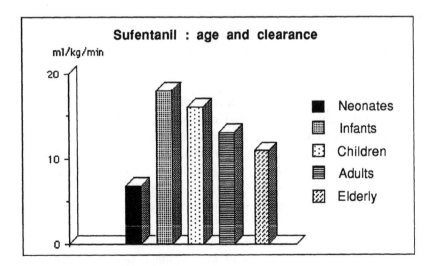

Fig. 49. Age-dependent variations in sufentanil plasma clearance.
(Adapted from Greeley et al. 1986; Hug 1984 b)

However, epidural doses higher than 50 µg of sufentanil are not completely free from danger. A cardiac arrest has been reported after an erroneous spinal administration of 100 µg epidural sufentanil + bupivacaine instead of 10 µg sufentanil (Donadoni and Capiau 1987 d). The error was due to a mistake with the two commercial solutions of sufentanil, which contain 5 µg/ml and 50 µg/ml, respectively. Here again it is shown that the clinical safety margin of spinal opioids is probably not higher than two times the correct dose.

Also intrathecal sufentanil in a dose of 7.5 µg + 1.5 ml lignocaine 5%, has been studied but no beneficial effect of this route has been noted (Donadoni et al. 1987 c).

Taking into account the good pharmacokinetic properties and excellent clinical results obtained with optimal dosages, it might be that sufentanil becomes one of the future drugs for epidural analgesia.

Sufentanil is not available in all countries (e.g. Germany). Epidural sufentanil was also used in continuous infusion for relief of cancer pain on an out-patient basis. Thirty-five patients were studied during a period of two years. Mean sufentanil doses necessary for good pain relief during 24 hours were 350 µg (200-640), no serious side effects were observed (Boersma et al. 1988).

7.1.10 LOFENTANIL

Lofentanil is a pure µ-agonist derived from fentanyl. It is the most potent opioid to be administered to humans, about 500-1000 times more potent than morphine (Fig. 50).

The un-ionized fraction of the molecule at pH 7.4 is greater than that of fentanyl (27% versus 9%). The deposit of the drug in the lipophilic sites of the epidural space is substantial. Lofentanil provides a higher affinity quotient with longer dissociation times for the µ-receptors than fentanyl, 80 and 280 as against 7.5 and 1.2, respectively (Mather 1983 b).

Lofentanil produces, after epidural administration, an analgesia of longer duration than that obtained with epidural fentanyl: 5-10 hours compared to 2-3 hours. In comparison to buprenorphine there was a stronger pain suppression and longer duration of activity with epidural lofentanil (Bilsback et al. 1982, 1985; De Castro et al. 1980 a; Lecron et al. 1980 b; Rolly et al. 1984; Van Steenberge 1983 c; Waldvogel and Fasano 1983). However, the duration of analgesia obtained with this drug after spinal injections is not necessarily longer than that after parenteral use.

Notwithstanding potential qualities, the practical use of spinal lofentanil is limited. During acute treatment, fear of long lasting respiratory depression, impossible to antagonize with naloxone, is always present. For chronic treatment unpredictability and inconsistency in the results are current observations.

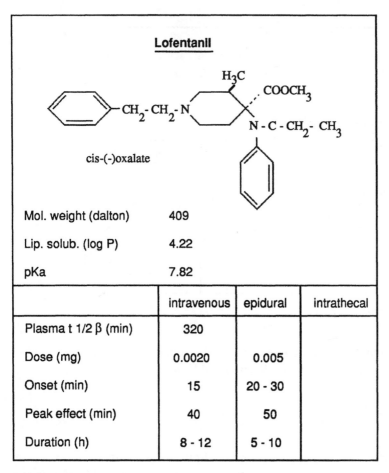

Lofentanil

cis-(-)oxalate

	intravenous	epidural	intrathecal
Mol. weight (dalton)	409		
Lip. solub. (log P)	4.22		
pKa	7.82		
Plasma t 1/2 β (min)	320		
Dose (mg)	0.0020	0.005	
Onset (min)	15	20 - 30	
Peak effect (min)	40	50	
Duration (h)	8 - 12	5 - 10	

Fig. 50. Data on lofentanil.

7.1.11 DADL

D-ala-D-leu-enkephalin (DADL) is a synthetic opioid peptide with dominant δ-receptor affinity producing profound analgesia after intrathecal administration (Fig. 51). DADL has a higher molecular weight than morphine. The lipid solubility of the compound is unknown, but it is suggested that DADL and morphine are comparable in this respect (Moulin et al. 1986 b; Krames et al. 1986). DADL has respiratory depressant effects similar to morphine.

All side effects are naloxone-reversible (Atchison et al. 1984; Onofrio and Yaksh 1983 a).

There is a lack of cross tolerance to δ-agonists in animals already tolerant to the μ-agonist (e.g. to morphine), (Yaksh et al. 1986 a).

Preliminary findings suggest that intrathecal use of DADL in doses of 0.5-1 mg restore analgesia in patients tolerant to morphine. Chronic alternating

DADL			
D-Ala-D-Leu-Phe-Gly-Gly-Tyr			
Mol. weight (dalton)　　569			
	intravenous	epidural	intrathecal
Plasma t 1/2 β (min)	115		115
Dose (mg)			0.25 - 1
Onset (min)			17
Peak effect (min)			35
Duration (h)			5 - 11

Fig. 51. Data on DADL.

infusion of DADL and morphine appears to prevent tolerance to either drugs but additional studies are essential (Krames and Wilkie 1987).

7.1.12 METENKEPHALIN

Metenkephalin with dominant δ-receptor affinity is a naturally occurring opiate peptide (Fig. 52). It is subject to rapid metabolic breakdown. FK 33-824 is a synthetic analogue of metenkephalin, which is less susceptible to enzymatic breakdown.

Andersen et al. (1982 a) administered metenkephalin (FK 33-824) in epidural doses of 0.02-0.5 mg for postoperative pain treatment. Results have shown that the analgesic effects provided by this substance are poor, unpredictable and short acting.

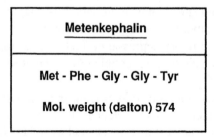

Metenkephalin
Met - Phe - Gly - Gly - Tyr
Mol. weight (dalton) 574

Fig. 52. Chemical structure of metenkephalin.

7.1.13 BETA-ENDORPHIN

This neuropeptide of 31 amino-acids (molecular weight 3300 daltons) with μ/δ-receptor affinity isolated from the pituitary gland is the most potent endogenous opiate. It provides prolonged pain relief after a single intrathecal administration (Fukushi 1981; Havliecek et al. 1980; Max et al. 1982; Oyama et al. 1980 a, b; Oyama 1980 c; Oyama et al. 1982; Van de Woerd et al. 1985).

Doses: Synthetic β-endorphin is used in a dilution of 1 mg/ml saline, in doses of 1 to 1.5 mg/day, administered by infusion.

Side effects: Transient mental disturbances. They decrease by a reduction in the delivery rate (Oyama et al. 1985).

Potential advantages and drawbacks of intrathecal β-endorphin used in doses of 1-2 mg/day:

- it produces longer lasting analgesia than morphine
- it produces all the side effects of morphine: e.g. respiratory depression and tolerance
- once the administration of the β-endorphin treatment is stopped, oral opioids can be given and they produce more profound and longer lasting effects (Van de Woerd et al. 1985).
- it is a very expensive drug.

These results need further confirmation.

7.1.14 SPIRADOLINE 5 U-62,0066E

Spiradoline mersylate is a potent selective κ-agonist producing, in animals, in epidural doses of 45 to 120 μg/kg good analgesia and sedation during 2 to 4 hours without evidence of respiratory depression (Lander et al. 1987 a). Further studies are continuing.

7.2 Mixed opioid agonist-antagonists and partial agonist-antagonists

7.2.1 BUPRENORPHINE

Buprenorphine is a partial agonist-antagonist at the μ-receptor (Fig.53, Tab.35). It has a very high receptor binding affinity. The pharmacokinetic data of buprenorphine indicate that diffusion into nervous tissue is comparable to morphine. But, in contrast to morphine, the danger of rostral diffusion is less due to its higher lipid solubility. Although buprenorphine is highly liposoluble, it is relatively slow to reach the peak analgesic effect after injection. After a slow onset the duration of analgesia is long lasting. This discrepancy of pharmacokinetics and dynamics is due to slow dissociation from the μ-receptor (Boas and Villiger 1985).

Calculations indicate that only 0.2 % of an epidural dose of buprenorphine (due to the high molecular weight) would cross the dura, compared with 20 % for epidural morphine (McQuay et al. 1986; Moore et al. 1982). Nevertheless, this lipid soluble drug is well reabsorbed into the spinal cord by villi and nerve roots, so that good analgesia can be obtained by parenteral as well as by spinal routes.

Epidural buprenorphine has been used in various situations:

- in postoperative pain (Alexander and Black 1984; Andersen et al. 1981; Andersen 1983; Bilsback and Rolly 1983; Bilsback et al. 1985; Cahill et al. 1983; De Castro 1979 b; Gerig and Kern 1983; Gundersen et al. 1986; Hartung et al. 1986; Kierkegaard et al. 1981; Lanz et al. 1984 b; Louis et al. 1982; Müller et al. 1983 b; Petit et al. 1986; Rolly et al. 1984; Raudamanska et al. 1980; Ruppert et al. 1982; Zenz et al. 1981 d, 1983 a, 1984 f; Zinck and Fritz 1982 a; Zinck et al. 1982 b; Zinck 1983 e.g.)
- in cancer pain (Crawford et al. 1983; Crawford and Ravio 1986; Nicosia et al. 1984; Zenz et al. 1985 a, e.g.)
- in obstetrics (Srivastava 1982).

The analgesia is generally satisfactory. The onset of action is observed after 5 to 10 min, with a duration of action lasting from 4 to 10 hours. In most cases a very comfortable painfree period is induced, lasting 6 hours. Some authors, comparing buprenorphine either in saline solution or in 5% glucose solution, have pointed out that the results with saline are better. This view is corroborated by the experimental work of Snyder (1977), indicating that the receptor binding of antagonists is increased if the receptor is in a sodium state.

However, on the contrary to most other opioids, the duration of analgesia produced by epidural or intrathecal buprenorphine is not significantly longer than that obtained by intramuscular or intravenous administration of the compound (Tab. 21). This is not necessarily evidence that buprenorphine does not have a significant spinal effect as was recently proposed by Glynn et al. (1987 b). It rather indicates that with buprenorphine the duration of analgesia is predominantly determined by a long lasting receptor-binding activity (independent of the administration route) and only for a smaller part determined by the absorption, distribution and elimination parameters. Such a situation is an exception compared to most other opioids which show important differences according to their use by parenteral or spinal routes.

The side effects are acceptable: delayed respiratory depression has not, up to now, been observed. However, urinary retention, pruritus, nausea and drowsiness are noted.

These side effects occur in the same frequency as those seen after the parenteral use of buprenorphine but less than those seen with epidural morphine (Piepenbrock et al. 1981 c; Zenz et al. 1981 d; Zenz and Piepenbrock 1982 c). Buprenorphine produces drowsiness more frequently. The duration of analgesia is shorter and more inconstant than that observed after morphine.

A drawback of buprenorphine is the difficulty in antagonizing this substance by naloxone. So, if respiratory depression should occur, extremely high doses of naloxone are necessary to correct this effect.

Finally, buprenorphine like all other partial agonists shows ceiling effects at doses not far in excess of the effective doses. So, repeated injections with a short interval or high doses of buprenorphine sometimes may not produce a further

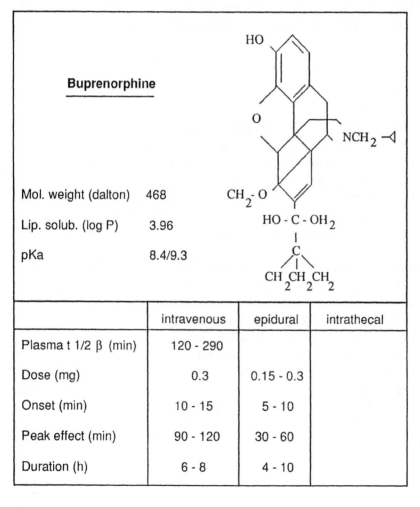

Buprenorphine

Mol. weight (dalton)	468		
Lip. solub. (log P)	3.96		
pKa	8.4/9.3		

	intravenous	epidural	intrathecal
Plasma t 1/2 β (min)	120 - 290		
Dose (mg)	0.3	0.15 - 0.3	
Onset (min)	10 - 15	5 - 10	
Peak effect (min)	90 - 120	30 - 60	
Duration (h)	6 - 8	4 - 10	

Fig. 53. Data on buprenorphine.

increase in analgesia.

But even minimal doses of epidural buprenorphine (0.06 mg), repeated when necessary, are effective in postoperative pain treatment (Murphy DF et al. 1985).

A recent study, comparing 3 mg epidural morphine with 0.3 mg epidural buprenorphine demonstrated significant alterations in a number of respiratory function indices in the buprenorphine group in the immediate period until 90 minutes after injection (Pasqualucci et al. 1987). But contrary to morphine, there was no respiratory depressant effect after 6 and 18 hours. The authors conclude that the early effects are due to a systemic uptake of the lipophilic substance, and that there is no danger of late respiratory depression with epidural buprenorphine (Pasqualucci et al. 1987).

Although it is shown that epidural buprenorphine has fewer side effects than morphine, it seems, for several investigators, illogical to give a drug epidurally when a similar result can be achieved intramuscularly (Shah et al. 1986; Glynn et al. 1987 b).

7.2.2 NALBUPHINE

Chemically, nalbuphine, a partial agonist, is related to oxymorphone and to the pure antagonist naloxone (Fig. 54, Tab. 35). Nalbuphine is reported to be highly specific for κ-opioid receptors in the spinal cord, where it acts agonistically. At the μ-receptor nalbuphine acts as an antagonist.

Nalbuphine has been administered epidurally and intrathecally for the treatment of postoperative pain. The doses were 5 to 10 mg and 0.4 mg, respectively (Blaise et al. 1986; Mok and Tsai 1984 a; Mok et al. 1985; Wang et al. 1984, 1986).

Analgesia occurred after 15 min and reached its maximum effect at the end of 10 to 18 minutes. The duration of analgesia was 9 hours (4-20). Side effects were minimal, respiratory depression, nausea or pruritus have not been seen up to now. Nalbuphine can be antagonized by naloxone.

A low incidence of side effects and long duration of action seem to be typical properties of epidural nalbuphine. Therefore, the substance deserves further studies (Henderson and Cohen 1986).

The antagonist activity of intravenous nalbuphine given after a spinal administration of a pure opioid is effective and of longer duration than that of naloxone. Nalbuphine (10-20 mg intravenously) was studied by Doran et al. (1987), Hammond (1984) and Penning et al. (1986), who reported that intravenous nalbuphine prevents epidural morphine induced respiratory depression. Nalbuphine (10 mg s.c.) has been demonstrated to effectively prevent or reverse *pruritus* induced by epidural fentanyl (Davies and From 1988).

The sedative effect of morphine and nalbuphine were additive, analgesia was not reversed but longer lasting.

Table 35. Comparative properties of two agonist-antagonists opioids used for epidural opioid analgesia.

Properties	Buprenorphine	Nalbuphine
- Molecular weight (dalton)	468	393
- Stable in saline and glucose solution	+	+
- Preservative free preparation	+	+
- Can be mixed with a local anaesth.	+	+
- Lipid solubility	+	+

- Dose
    bolus (mg/70 kg bw)
    continuous inf. (mg/h)
  - on-demand bolus (mg)
	0.15 - 0.3
	0.02
	0.05
		5 - 10

- Dose range	narrow (ceiling effect)	narrow (ceiling effect)

- Analgesia
    onset (min)
    peak effect (min)
    duration (h)
	10 - 20
	40 - 50
	4 - 10
		15 - 20
		30 - 60
		6 - 12

- Antagonism by naloxone	–	+
- Tolerance development *	+	+
- Drowsiness	+	+
- Low risk of delayed resp. depression	+	+

+ = yes, - = no, * slower than pure opioids.

	Nalbuphine		
Mol.weight (dalton)	393		
Lip.solub. (log P)	2.52		
pKa	8.7 / 9.96		

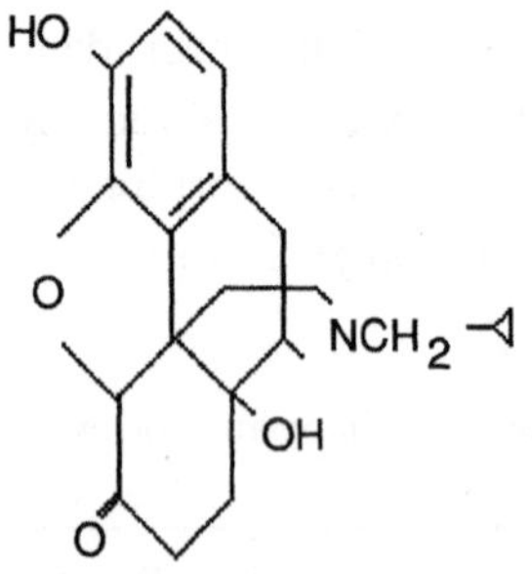

	intravenous	epidural	intrathecal
Plasma t 1/2 β (min)	180 - 306		
Dose (mg)	5 - 15	4 - 6	2
Onset (min)	5 - 15	5 - 15	
Peak effect (min)	30	20	
Duration (h)	3	6 - 18	>24

Fig. 54. Data on nalbuphine.

7.2.3 BUTORPHANOL

Butorphanol is a μ-agonist-antagonist and κ-agonist opioid (Fig. 55).

Epidural butorphanol for delivery pain at doses ranging from 3 to 6 mg, gives effective analgesia of long duration (± 18 hours) (Naulty et al. 1984, 1987). Nausea, pruritus and severe respiratory depression did not occur, but drowsiness sometimes lasted longer than 6 hours.

The respiratory depressant activity of epidural butorphanol is demonstrated by elevation in resting PCO_2 from 3/4 to 2 hours, after 2 mg and from 3/4 to 4 hours, after 4 mg (Rein et al. 1985).

Abboud et al. (1986, 1987) as well as Kartha et al. (1987), Mok et al. (1986) and Tan et al. (1987) concluded that the epidural administration of butorphanol (4 mg) appears to be a safe and reliable method for postoperative pain relief after caesarean section. Epidural doses of 2-4 mg were used by Roman de Jesus et al. (1988) for postoperative pain relief.

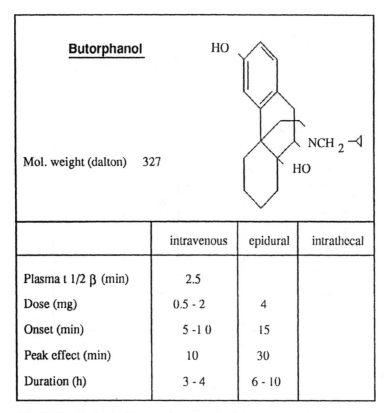

Butorphanol

Mol. weight (dalton)   327

	intravenous	epidural	intrathecal
Plasma t 1/2 β (min)	2.5		
Dose (mg)	0.5 - 2	4	
Onset (min)	5 -1 0	15	
Peak effect (min)	10	30	
Duration (h)	3 - 4	6 - 10	

Fig. 55. Data on butorphanol.

7.2.4 PENTAZOCINE

Pentazocine acts as an antagonist at the μ-receptor and an agonist at the κ- and σ-receptor (Fig. 56). Given systemically it has a high incidence of psycho-mimetic side effects due to its action at the σ-receptor. Pentazocine is a highly liposoluble opioid inducing higher brain/plasma ratios than morphine.

Epidural doses of 20 mg were given for postoperative pain relief. Onset of analgesia was rapid (2.5 min) and maximal analgesic effects were reached at the end of 15 to 25 min. The duration of analgesia was 4 to 24 hours with a mean duration of 10 hours. Good analgesia was obtained in 80% of the cases.

Side effects were minimal: drowsiness 50 %, immediate or delayed respiratory depression or urinary retention have not been observed (Kalia et al. 1983). However, the number of observations is small. Due to the σ-agonistic effect it is hard to recommend pentazocine for spinal analgesia.

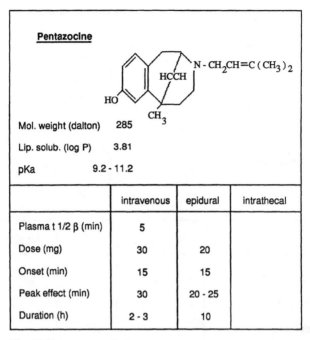

Pentazocine

Mol. weight (dalton)	285
Lip. solub. (log P)	3.81
pKa	9.2 - 11.2

	intravenous	epidural	intrathecal
Plasma t 1/2 β (min)	5		
Dose (mg)	30	20	
Onset (min)	15	15	
Peak effect (min)	30	20 - 25	
Duration (h)	2 - 3	10	

Fig. 56. Data on pentazocine.

7.2.5 MEPTAZINOL

Meptazinol a synthetic hexa-hydroazepine, is a relatively lipophilic agonist-antagonist. So, theoretically it should be less prone to rostral spread. Given intravenously, meptazinol is concluded to have central adrenergic stimulating effects which may account, at least in part, for its analgesic effects (Bold et al. 1987), (Fig. 57).

After 30 or 60 mg epidural meptazinol the postoperative analgesia was rapid in onset (15 min) and had a median duration of 124 and 122 min, respectively (range 70 to 212). The pain relief was satisfying in 95% of the cases, and no drug related adverse effects were observed during the study (Rao et al. 1985). A longer duration of epidural meptazinol is reported by Budd et al. (1983) in 23 patients suffering from spinal lesions and back pain. After several doses the duration of analgesia reached a plateau between 11 and 12 hours. Nausea and vomiting as well as dizziness had an incidence of 25 % with the high dose of 90 mg. Birks and Marsh (1986), Verborgh et al. (1987 b) used epidural meptazinol 90 mg and observed good analgesia within 5 min, lasting 5 hours with minimal sedative effects.

In pain after caesarean section no advantages of meptazinol could be demonstrated. Analgesia was not adequate and side effects were far too high (Francis and Lockhart 1986). In a recent letter Rao et al. (1987) confirmed the short duration of action but did not agree with the high incidence of side effects reported by Francis and Lockhart (1986).

Meptazinol

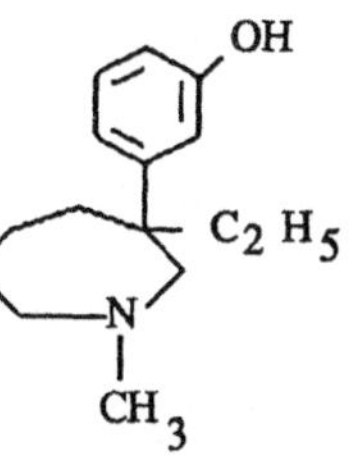

Mol. weight (dalton)	233
Lip. solub. (log P)	2.89

	intravenous	epidural
Plasma t 1/2 β (min)	90	
Dose (mg)	50 - 75	30 - 90
Onset (min)	3 - 5	15
Peak effect (min)	20	30 - 60
Duration (h)	2 - 3	2 - 5

Fig. 57. Data on meptazinol.

7.2.6 Tramadol

The use of epidural tramadol, an agonist-antagonist is only reported once in the literature about spinal opioid analgesia (Chrubasik et al. 1987 c, 1988 a).

Total doses of 330 ± 29 mg tramadol were necessary for adequate analgesia. Serious side effects were not observed, but duration of pain relief was short and analgesic potency of the substance is 30 times less than that of epidural morphine. So, there does not seem to be any advantage for this opioid in spinal analgesia.

Conclusions

- The place of opioid agonist-antagonists in spinal opioid analgesia is limited. All the compounds studied up to now have several common properties:
- Addictive properties are low. However, this consideration should not be a clinical consideration in the management of pain in patients selected for spinal opioid treatment.
- Risk of respiratory depression is reduced. However, other side effects are in the same order of frequency as those seen with pure opioids.

174

- Agonist-antagonists are capable of antagonizing the effects of opioid agonists. This antagonism by itself though is not free of side effects.
- Analgesic effects are relatively inconstant.

7.3 Pure opioid antagonists

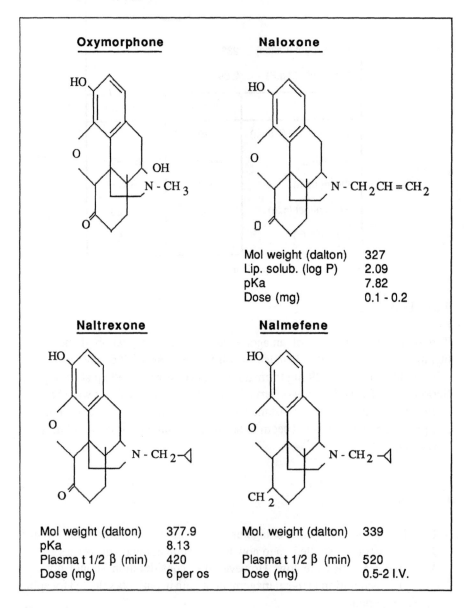

Fig. 58. Chemical structure of oxymorphone, naloxone, naltrexone and nalmefene. (Adapted from Budd 1987)

7.3.1 NALOXONE

Naloxone is a pure antagonist at the μ-, κ-, δ- and σ-receptors (Fig. 58-60). The chemical structure of naloxone is similar to oxymorphone.

Given after an agonist opioid, naloxone reverses the agonistic effects. In this way, analgesia, sedation, nausea, respiratory depression is antagonized. The antagonistic effect of naloxone is dose-dependent, and the effect depends on the receptor affinity of the agonistic drug, e.g. buprenorphine has such a high receptor affinity that even high doses of naloxone can hardly antagonize the effects (Orwin 1977).

However, the pure antagonistic effects of naloxone are not clear cut. Long lasting pain relief was observed when patients complained of pain after buprenorphine and naloxone was given (Schmidt et al. 1985 b). Experimental data and theoretical considerations led to the conclusion that there might exist a peripheral hyperalgesic opioid receptor, which by selective antagonism could induce analgesia (Gillman and Lichtigfeld 1986 a).

Naloxone (0.1-0.2 mg intravenously) is in some cases able to reverse all the side effects of the epidural or intrathecal opioids. The resulting effect is rapid but transient (<1 hour), (Fig. 59-60). In many cases, it is necessary to repeat the injections or to administer naloxone by continuous infusion. Some reports indicate that naloxone infusions are effective in the reduction or prevention of side effects associated with epidural morphine or fentanyl without concurrent loss of analgesia (Brookshire et al. 1983; Pigot et al. 1987; Rawal et al. 1986 a; Thind

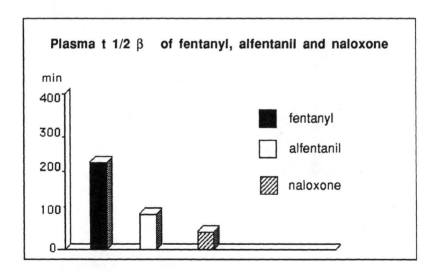

Fig. 59. Comparison between a pharmacokinetic parameter of fentanyl, alfentanyl and naloxone. Naloxone has a much shorter plasma t 1/2 β.
(Adapted from Schuttler et al. 1983)

et al. 1986). However, such results have not been observed by all investigators. Gowan et al. (1987 a, 1988) found in a double-blind study that analgesia was detrimentally affected by prophylactic naloxone infusion and that the side effects of epidural morphine were not always decreased. Even with continuous naloxone infusion 3 cases of respiratory depression occurred in a group of 16 patients (Gowan et al. 1988). The same was demonstrated by Guénéron et al. (1988). Ramanathan (1986) considered that naloxone infusion was ineffective in preventing the side effects of epidural morphine.

In cases of massive overdoses of epidural morphine, continuous naloxone infusion of 2 μg/kg/h may be necessary during 20 hours (Masoud and Green 1982). Nevertheless, it must be stated that naloxone, due to its strongly positive inotropic effects, is to be administered with caution in patients with cardiovascular diseases.

Attempts to synthetize naloxone analogues, pure opioid antagonists with longer duration of action, have resulted in compounds such as naltrexone (Jaffe and Martin WR 1985) and nalmefene (Dixon et al. 1984).

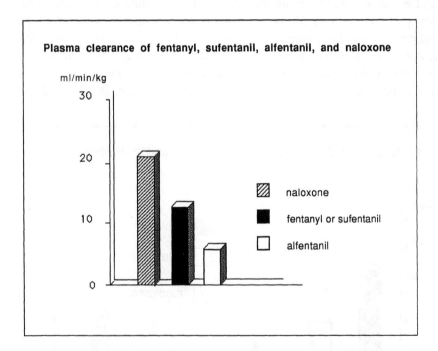

Fig. 60. Comparison of a pharmacokinetic parameter of naloxone and other opioids. Naloxone has a much higher plasma clearance rate than the other opioids so that the duration of the antidote effects of naloxone are short lasting.

The danger of remorphinization can only be avoided by repeated naloxone administration. (Adapted from Bovill et al. 1982; Mather 1987; Stanski 1987)

7.3.2 NALMEFENE

Nalmefene is a pure opioid antagonist (Fig. 58), 0.5 mg has a duration of action of 2-3 hours (3-4 times longer than naloxone). Contrary to naloxone this sustained reversal effect is clearly dose related. In a first clinical study, this new substance has been successfully used after intravenous fentanyl in doses of 0.5-2 mg (Gal and DiFazio 1986). At this moment clinical studies of reversal effect of nalmefene after spinal opioids have not been performed.

7.3.3 NALTREXONE

Naltrexone is a pure opioid antagonist (Fig. 58), which is two-fold more potent than naloxone. The duration of action is much longer. Naltrexone is best acting after oral administration. Six mg pulverized naltrexone in 30 ml water orally together with epidural morphine 5 mg provided a useful means to reduce the undesirable side effects of epidural morphine without significantly diminishing its analgesic activity (Mok et al. 1986).

7.4 Non-opioid drugs

The endogenous opioid system is the main modulator of pain perception. The opioid receptors in the dorsal horn of the spinal cord are the basis for epidural or intrathecal administration of opioids in the treatment of pain. However, opioid administration can be associated with side effects, can provide insufficient pain relief, or good results can become exhausted. Thus, alternative methods perhaps producing adequate analgesia or additive relieving effects with a lower incidence of unwanted complications are worth investigating. Among the most interesting non-opioid drugs, acting on the dorsal horn the following substances are to be mentioned (Fig. 15):

- Substances acting on the serotoninergic system
  . calcitonin
  . droperidol
- Antagonists of acetylcholine, of substance P, of glutamates
  . baclofen
- GABA agonists
  . baclofen
  . midazolam
- Adrenoceptor agonists
  . ketamine

. clonidine
. adenosine analogues
- Prostaglandin inhibitors
. lysine acetylsalicylate
- Neuropeptides
. calcitonin
. somatostatin
- Enkephalinase and aminopeptidase inhibitors
. bestatin
. thiorphan
- Cholecystokinin inhibitors
. proglumide
. xylamide

When patients chronically treated by spinal opioids are not completely pain free, or if tolerance has developed, a trial can be given to use non-opiod drugs parenterally or spinally to rest the opioid receptor and to occupy other pain pathways. Some of them like calcitonin and somatostatin are neuropeptides. The transport of neuropeptides through the dura mater into the CSF is known to be limited (Meisenberg and Simons 1983). Clinical results obtained with several neuropeptides administered epidurally prove, however, that there must be a pathway to reach the intrathecal space (Chrubasik et al.1985 l). The subarachnoid protrusions, described by Welch and Salder (1966), could probably allow for this passage, so that the epidural administration of some neuropeptides appears to be justified.

Nevertheless, the use of new agents in man has to be performed with great care. A clear distinction is to be made between the use of the pure peptides and the commercially available forms due to the presence of additives or preservatives in the latter that may not be compatible with spinal routes of administration. Toxicological investigations have to precede their administration in humans to exclude local nerve damage (Candeletti and Ferri 1989; Gaumann et al. 1989). In some cases this has not been done.

7.4.1 CALCITONIN

The hypocalcemic hormone is a polypeptide isolated from human "C" cells, present in the thyroid, parathyroid and thymus and it can be also totally synthetized (Fig. 61). This regulator of blood calcium is a neuropeptide widely distributed in the spinal cord (Gibson et al. 1984). The substance is involved in the mediation of analgesia via a non-opiate mechanism (Yamamoto et al. 1982). As observed by various authors the systemic injection of calcitonin is followed

Calcitonin			
Mol. weight (dalton)	3432		

	intramuscular	epidural	intrathecal
Plasma t 1/2 β (min)			
Dose (IU)	80 - 160	15	6 - 100
Onset (min)		10 - 30	
Peak effect (min)			
Duration (h)		7 - 8	> 48

Fig. 61. Data on calcitonin.

by analgesic effects in man. However, injections of calcitonin resulted in reduction of pain only, when pain was secondary to bone pathology (Maggi 1978). The mechanism by which calcitonin produces analgesia is much discussed. The substance inhibits cyclooxygenase, thus reducing the production of prostaglandins and thromboxane-A2 (Ceserani et al. 1979). A rise in the plasma endorphin levels follows the administration of calcitonin (Gennari et al. 1981). Also the serotoninergic system may be involved in calcitonin induced analgesia (Miralles et al. 1987).

Fraioli et al. (1982) and Fiore et al. (1983) were the first to observe the analgesic effectiveness of calcitonin in man after epidural and intrathecal administration. The dose of salmon calcitonin (Calcitonin, Sandoz ®) in patients suffering from oncological pain were 15 IU in 6 ml epidurally and 6 IU in 6 ml intrathecally (Fiore et al. 1983). The doses used were markedly lower than those used by Fraioli et al. (1982) and Blanchard et al. (1988) who gave respectively 300 IU and 100 IU salmon calcitonin intrathecally. Analgesia started 10-30 min after injection and was effective over 7-8 hours (Navarro et al. 1986). With 100 IU salmon calcitonin intrathecally a complete pain relief for more than 48 hours was obtained in 60 patients after lower extremity or lower abdominal operations (Miralles et al. 1986).

Side effects were short lasting, vomiting up to 78% in the series of Blanchard et al. (1988) and increased diuresis.

In treatment of chronic cancer pain, calcitonin is only really effective, if used in association with opioids. It allows a dose reduction of morphine so that the frequency and severity of side effects are decreased (Meynadier 1986b; Mitterschiffthaler et al. 1987). However, other clinical investigations with salmon calcitonin in the treatment of acute pain have been rather disappointing (Falke et al. 1986).

Intrathecal salmon calcitonin (100 IU) given in association with spinal anaesthesia (lignocaine 1 mg/kg+adrenaline 0.1 mg) provided effective postoperative analgesia in 30 patients (Miralles et al. 1987). However, in studies using drug associations, it is difficult to evaluate the individual part to be implicated for calcitonin.

In a recent letter Eisenach stressed that animal studies should be performed before any further clinical trial of calcitonin (Eisenach 1988 c). Also Wiesenfeld-Hallin argued against the intrathecal use of calcitonin (Wiesenfeld-Hallin 1988). This argument against calcitonin was given in view of other studies demonstrating a lack of analgesia after subarachnoid calcitonin in rats (Wiesenfeld-Hallin and Person 1984).

Calcitonin gene-related peptide (CGRP)

Recently, a calcitonin-like peptide has been discovered in the dorsal horn of the spinal cord. The novel peptide termed calcitonin gene-related peptide (CGRP) is involved in processing painful stimuli (Rosenfeld et al. 1983). After central administration in relatively high doses in mice, it produced transient antinociception (Bates et al. 1983). It is encoded by the calcitonin gene via tissue specific RNA processing (Rosenfeld et al. 1983). The distribution of CGRP-producing cells and pathways in the brain suggest functions for the peptide in nociception. Clinical investigations with CGRP are now being undertaken (Meynadier 1986 b).

7.4.2 DROPERIDOL

Droperidol is a neuroleptic mainly known from the anaesthesia technique, named neuroleptanalgesia (Fig. 62) (De Castro 1985). Droperidol in ampoules is preservative-free. In contrast, vials with the same drug contain neurotoxic preservatives and should not be used for spinal administration.The neuroleptic agents may increase the analgesic effects of opioids by impairing the dopaminergic impulses at a segmental level of the spinal cord.

In animal experiments the simultaneous intrathecal administration of morphine and droperidol produces a potentiation and a prolongation of the analgesia, as well as a delay of tolerance development (Kim and Stoelting 1980).

Droperidol

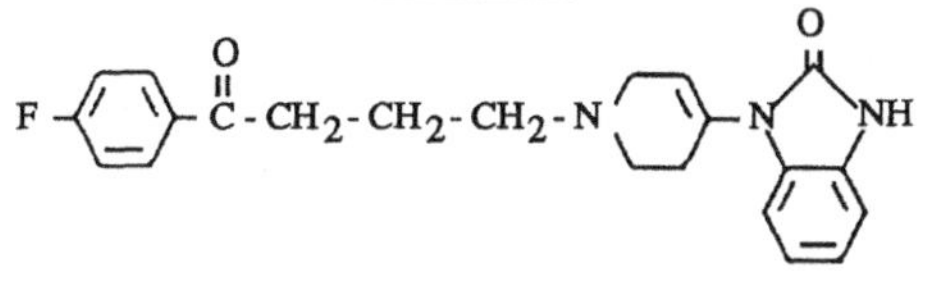

Mol. weight (dalton)	379
pKa	7.68
Plasma t 1/2 β (min)	140
Epidural dose (mg)	2.5

Fig. 62. Data on droperidol.

The addition of 2.5 mg droperidol intrathecally to morphine provided potentiation and prolongation of analgesia and also slowed the development of opioid tolerance (Bach et al. 1985; Kim and Stoelting 1980; Ochi et al. 1985; Tulunay et al. 1976). The combination of 2.5 mg droperidol and 3 mg morphine epidurally prevents postoperative nausea and vomiting. This combination also reinforces and prolongs the analgesic and sedative effects of morphine (Ochi et al. 1985; Bach et al. 1985).

The association of a CNS depressant drug (parenterally or epidurally) with an epidural opioid invariably increases the risk of respiratory depression. The administration of the two drugs in a short interval may produce severe respiratory depression (Cohen et al. 1983 b).

7.4.3 Baclofen

Baclofen, an analogue of aminobutyric acid, is considered to be the prototypic GABA-agonist (Fig. 63). It antagonizes excitatory transmitters, e.g. acetylcholine, substance P, glutamate at the dorsal horn level. It reduces polysynaptic and monosynaptic reflexes leading to muscular hypotonia. It has been used by oral application for the treatment of muscle spasms and rigidity. The systemic application of baclofen results in side effects like drowsiness, sedation and confusion. Given intrathecally the potency of baclofen is increased 600 times.

The regional effect of baclofen has been demonstrated in animals (Wilson and Yaksh 1978; Yaksh and Reddy 1981). Penn and Kroin (1984) were the first to demonstrate the same effects in man. A dose of 5-50 μg given into the lumbar intrathecal space reduced muscle tone and frequency of spasms for about 4-8 hours (Penn and Kroin 1984). Given continuously via a drug pump the daily dose of baclofen ranges from 10 μg/day to 500 μg/day for the treatment of

182

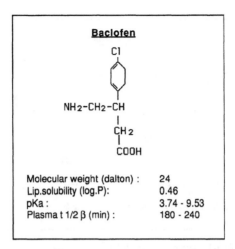

Baclofen

Cl

NH₂-CH₂-CH

CH₂

COOH

Molecular weight (dalton) :	24
Lip.solubility (log.P):	0.46
pKa :	3.74 - 9.53
Plasma t 1/2 β (min) :	180 - 240

Fig. 63. Data on baclofen.

spinal spasticity (Penn and Kroin 1985a). For the treatment of tetanus, doses may be higher (up to 2 mg/day) (Dralle et al. 1985; Müller et al. 1987; Müller-Schwefe and Milewski 1985 a; Penn and Kroin 1985 a). Baclofen is the drug of choice for the treatment of severe spasticity.

7.4.4. MIDAZOLAM

Midazolam is the only water soluble benzodiazepine appropriate for spinal administration (Fig. 64).

Intrathecal midazolam has been shown to interrupt sympathetic reflexes evoked by stimulation of A-delta and C afferents in anaesthetized dogs (Whitwam et al.1982). Midazolam interferes with transmission of nociceptive formation in the dorsal horn (Rigoli 1983 a, b). Goodchild and Serrao (1987) reported that intrathecal midazolam causes spinally mediated analgesia by binding to benzodiazepine receptors in the spinal cord of rats and that this response was blocked by flumazenil (Anexate ®) an antagonist of benzodiazepines (Serrao and Goodchild 1987).

Intrathecal midazolam causes spinally mediated analgesia by binding to benzodiazepine receptors in the spinal cord of the rats (Goodchild and Serrao 1987).

Intrathecal midazolam 1 mg provided deep analgesia for 60 minutes in dogs (Carrasco et al.1985).

In patients undergoing surgery intrathecal midazolam affords analgesia equivalent to diamorphine 2 mg (Cripps and Goodchild 1986). The association of midazolam intrathecal 5 mg with the opiate induces a potentialization of the analgesia as well.

Epidurally, the drug has been used for relief of spinal spasticity (Müller et al.

Midazolam

Mol. weight (dalton)	326
Lip. solub. (log P)	3.94
pKa	6.15
Plasma t 1/2 β (min)	90 - 150

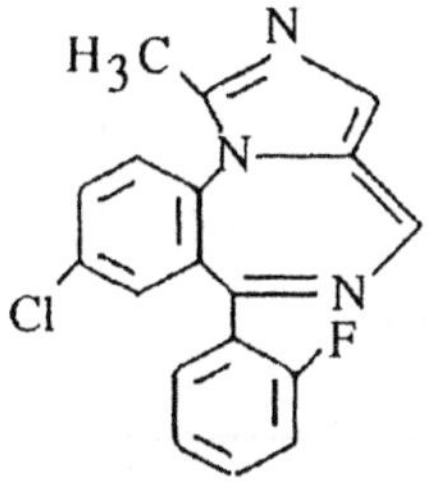

Fig. 64. Data on midazolam.

1985 c). Other investigators have used epidural midazolam as a potentiator of opioid analgesia for the relief of cancer pain (Carrasco et al. 1985).

7.4.5 KETAMINE

Ketamine is a dissociative anaesthetic (Fig. 65). Given intravenously, it leads to sedation, amnesia, analgesia and catalepsia. The mechanism of action is unknown. Ketamine may act as an agonist at the spinal opioid receptors. But it is not fixed at the opiate receptor (Fratta et al. 1980). Action on adrenaline and serotonine systems was also reported by Martin et al. (1982); Lundy and Jones (1983). Other investigators, using decerebrated cats, found that ketamine has a lack of direct supression of pain transmission at the spinal cord dorsal horn. It had only an indirect action exerted through the action on the spinal pain inhibiting system (Mori et al 1981; Mori and Shingu 1988). Nevertheless, analgesia due to ketamine is antagonized by naloxone, a pure opioid antagonist (Ahuja 1983). It has a high lipid solubility and a low protein binding. 4 to 8 mg ketamine epidurally are not adequate for postoperative pain relief (Kawana et al. 1987; Ravat et al. 1987 a, b). The results with 10 to 30 mg epidural ketamine for postoperative pain treatment were satisfying. All patients were pain free within 10 minutes, analgesia lasted about 4 hours. No side effects were recorded (Islas et al. 1985; Mankowitz et al. 1982; Mok et al. 1987; Rubin et al. 1983; Saissy et al. 1984 a; Samaryutel 1986).

Recently, Naguib et al. (1986 a) studied 34 patients for postoperative pain relief. They administered 30 mg of epidural ketamine, a much higher dose than that used by Saissy et al. (1984 a), Islas et al. (1985) or Mankowitz et al.(1982). Forty-five per cent of patients did not require further analgesia after the single ketamine injection. Four patients who received epidural ketamine with benzethonium chloride as the preservative complained of transient burning pain in

Ketamine			
Mol. weight (dalton)	238		
Lip. solub. (log P)	2.18		
pKa	7.5		

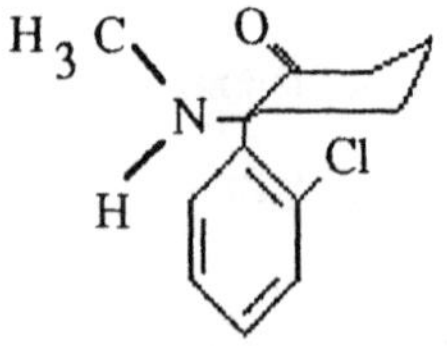

	intravenous	epidural	intrathecal
Plasma t 1/2 β (min)	120		
Dose (mg)	100	10 - 30	
Onset (min)			
Peak effect (min)			
Duration (h)			

Fig. 65. Data on ketamine.

the back during injection. No other side effect, e.g. neurological deficit or psychic disturbance, respiratory depression or cardiovascular hyperactivity, was seen. The authors concluded that 30 mg epidural ketamine used in a single injection was in 54% of the patients an effective method for postoperative pain relief for 24 hours (Naguib 1988).

But an incidence of 10 % of psychotomimetic effects were reported in a series of 40 patients treated with 15 mg epidural ketamine (Mok et al. 1987).

The only advantage of ketamine over opioids seems the lack of respiratory depression.

However, a limiting factor is the observation of nerve degeneration in rats and small monkeys after intrathecal ketamine (Ahuja 1983; Amiot et al. 1986; Brock-Utne et al. 1982, 1985). Until the possible toxicity of ketamine has been investigated more completely, the clinical studies with spinal ketamine should be postponed (Migaly 1986).

7.4.6 CLONIDINE

Clonidine is an α_2-*adrenoceptor* agonist (Fig. 66). It has a direct antinociceptive effect at the spinal cord. It can be administered epidurally or intrathecally.

The preparation is highly liposoluble, preservative free and isotonic with a pH of 4.0-4.5 (Coventry and Gordon 1989). It has no neurotoxicity (Coombs et al. 1984; Tamsen and Gorth 1984).

Yaksh and Reddy (1981) demonstrated both adrenergic and serotoninergic descending inhibitory systems in the dorsal horn of the spinal cord. Activation of the postsynaptic adrenergic receptors with either the lipophilic α_2 -adrenergic agonist clonidine or its more polar analogue ST91 produced analgesia in various laboratory models even in the presence of opioid tolerance.

Clonidine given epidurally or intrathecally in animals and in humans produced analgesic effects occurring predominantly at the spinal level (Calvillo and Ghigone 1986; Coombs et al. 1986 b; Drasner and Fields 1988 b; Ghigone et al. 1987; Gordh et al.1986 a, b, 1988; Hare and Franz 1987; Nalda and Gonzalez 1986 a, b; Strube et al. 1984 b; Tamsen and Gordh 1984). This effect is mediated in the dorsal horn at the postsynaptic terminals of descending inhibitory systems, when activated inhibits the release of substance P and does not produce muscle weakness or tolerance to opioid receptors (Coombs 1989).

In awake sheep, epidural clonidine (25 mg/kg) does not produce dangerous cardiovascular depression or global spinal cord ischaemia (Eisenach and Grice 1988 a).

Epidural clonidine reduces both intraoperative anaesthetic and analgesic requirements (Flacke et al. 1987; Engelman et al. 1989) and potentiates lidocaine block (Veillette et al. 1989).

The antinociceptive effects are reversed by α-receptor blocking agents but not by naloxone.

Glynn et al. (1986) suggested that the spinal noradrenergic system may be as important as the opioid system in pain transmission in patients with spinal cord injury. Epidural clonidine 150 µg in 5 ml of saline had an analgesic effect in 7 patients not responding to epidural morphine (Glynn et al. 1986). The haemodynamic changes were minimal.

In continuous infusion the intrathecal association of clonidine 0.3 mg + morphine allowed a substantial reduction of the opioid dose needed (Coombs et al. 1985 c). The concomitant use of epidural clonidine and morphine prolongs analgesia to more than 15 hours, indicating a synergistic interaction of clonidine with the opioid.

In postoperative pain 75 µg of epidural clonidine had an onset time of 15 minutes and a duration of analgesia of 5 1/2 hours (Nalda and Gonzalez 1986 a). The results support the existence of a significant deposit of the drug in the fat tissue and a high protein binding. In a single-blind study 75 µg epidural clonidine had the same effect as 25 µg epidural pethidine. The duration of analgesia lasted 265 minutes (pethidine 278 minutes), but the time to onset has been slightly longer with clonidine, 44 versus 34 minutes (Tamsen and Gordh 1984).

186

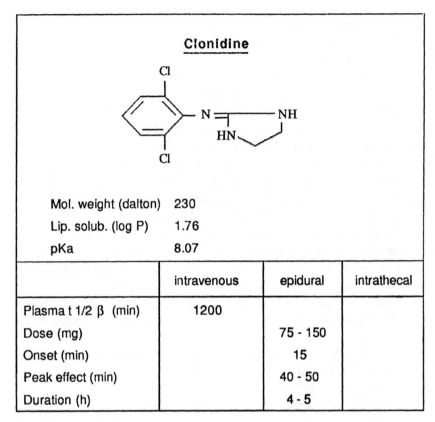

Fig. 66. Data on clonidine.

Epidural clonidine HCI, in total doses was injected using a repeated bolus of 4 µg/kg produced good analgesia, in various severe pain situations, lasting from 4 to 72 hours (mean 6-8 hours).

Side effects:

After epidural clonidine hypotension (without hypertensive rebound), bradycardia, dry mouth, sedation, urinary retention, vomiting, headache may be observed.

Spinal clonidine does not only potentiate the analgesia of opioids, it also enhances markedly the opioid respiratory depression (Penon et al. 1989; Petit et al. 1989). In cancer patients this property is not a practical clinical problem (Coombs 1985; Tamsen 1984) but it may present a danger if clonidine is used in anaesthesia with or after administration of opioids.

Disadvantages

- Chronically hypertensive or atherosclerotic patients are not indicated for epidural clonidine treatment.
- Clonidine hypotension requires close monitoring.
- If used for postoperative pain:
  - . clonidine alone produces only minor analgesia
  - . clonidine + opioid may produce severe respiratory depression
  - . early mobilization is limited by the nature of hypotensive side effects encountered.

Advantages:

- Action mechanism is different from that of opioids, so clonidine can be used in opioid tolerant patients to allow their receptors to rest (Germain et al. 1988).
- In cancer pain, intrathecal clonidine alone or in combination with morphine or hydromorphone may produce successful and long lasting pain relief even in patients with opioid tolerance (Coombs et al. 1985 d; Coombs 1986 c, 1989).
- Doses of 75-800 µg of epidural clonidine every 3 days have been effective in reducing tolerance produced by morphine treatment in cancer patients (Rossignoli et al. 1985; Ranck et al. 1989).
- The results of Coombs et al. (1985 c, d) indicate that in cancer patients intrathecal clonidine might be useful when the opioid action alone is not strong enough.

Glynn et al. (1987 b) reported their conclusions after an epidural clonidine treatment of 52 patients with intractable cancer pain. Hypotension requiring therapy occurred in one patient. Fifteen patients did not obtain analgesia with clonidine. In all other patients analgesia from clonidine was similar to that from morphine. It provided longterm (weeks to months) pain relief in 20 patients. However, side effects were significantly lower.

Epidural clonidine does not always produce good results. In some cases intrathecal clonidine plus morphine resulted in a rebound pain phenomenon limiting the potential utility of such association (Coombs et al. 1987 b). The authors speculate that bulbospinal adrenergic inhibitory pathways may be blocked by clonidine, thus inhibiting morphine analgesia mediated at a higher level. It was suspected that in some cases the molecule may not reach the CSF in sufficient concentration (Strube et al. 1984 b). Personal experiences, however, have shown that the clonidine effects are often limited to 2 to 3 weeks and then cease.

Epidural clonidine may be an acceptable alternative in several painful situations. The procedure could replace or complement the antinociceptive effect of epidural opioids.

Other α₂-receptor agonists

Plus points and weak points of clonidine have been the starting point for the synthesis of new more specific α_2-receptor agonists with potent analgesic and opioid potentiating properties:

- Tizanidine (Lubinov et al. 1989) and
- Dexmedetomidine (D-med, Pharmos) are now under clinical investigation (Flacke at al. 1989).

Adenosine analogues

Intrathecal administration of cyclohexyladenosine, N6-2-phenylisopropylad-enosine (two α_1-agents) or 5′N-ethylcarboxamide-adenosine (an α_2-agent) in doses of 0.3 nmol showed in rats typical antinociceptive effects. Intrathecal doses of 1.0 nmol of these substances produced transient motor impairment (flaccidity) and changes in behavioural characteristics but were without significant changes in heart rate or blood pressure. Effects on nociceptive and motor endpoints were at least partially antagonized by pretreatment with intrathecal caffeine (Sosnowski et al. 1989; Sosnowski and Yaksh 1989).

7.4.7 LYSINE-ACETYLSALICYLATE

Lysine-acetylsalicylate is the injection form of a standard antipyretic ASA (Fig. 67).
  Inhibitors of the prostaglandin synthesis have not only a peripheral analgesic

Lysine-Acetylsalicylate	
Mol. weight (dalton)	326
pKa	5.5 - 5.9
Plasma t 1/2 β (min)	140 - 150

Fig. 67. Data on lysine-acetylsalicylate.

effect, their central action on the nociceptive transmission has been demonstrated (Ferreira 1979). Devoghel (1983 a, b) recommended the intrathecal use of 180 mg lysine-acetylsalicylate (3 ml) for the treatment of severe cancer pain. The analgesic effect was rapid (15 min) and long lasting (1-22 days). This result was obtained without any sign of sensory, motor or sympathetic block.

With 120-750 mg of an intrathecal hyperbaric solution of lysine-acetylsalicylate for the treatment of cancer pain, good results were obtained in 65% of the cases (Pellerin et al. 1986). However, it has been shown in rats that intrathecal lysine-acetylsalicylate may produce radicular demyelinization and other toxic effects (Amiot et al. 1986).

7.4.8 SOMATOSTATIN

Somatostatin is a tetra-deca-peptide (molecular weight 1638 daltons), (Fig. 68). It is a hydrophilic substance that can be found in the central and peripheral

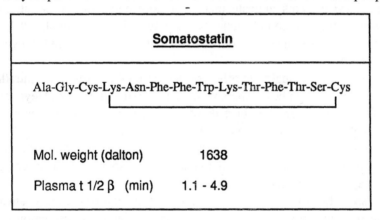

Fig. 68. Data on somatostatin.

nervous system, in the endocrine cells of the pancreas and in some cells of the intestinal tract. In the brain, somatostatin is found in the cortex, in the basal ganglia, the hypothalamus and the brain stem. The highest concentration is found in the hypothalamus. It plays a physiological role in the inhibition of multiple endocrine metabolic and neurotransmitter systems. For potential clinical applications somatostatin has been explored for prevention of ketoacidosis in juvenile types of diabetes, in patients with pancreatic tumors (Goodman and Gilman's 1985).

Intrathecal application causes characteristic changes in the motor system and behavioural aberrations.

Animal toxicity

In animals (rats and rabbits), toxic effects produced by somatostatin at relative low intrathecal doses are severe and frequent. Inflammatory reactions and nucleolysis of the dorsal horn, rigidity, catatonia, paralysis, convulsions, apnea, stupor were noted. Lethality was observed in 4 of 6 animals after 80 μg intrathecal somatostatin. The LD 50/ED 50 ratio of somatostatin was only two (Ackerman et al. 1985; Cohn and Cohn 1975; Jaffe et al. 1978; Kalia et al. 1984; Mollenholt et al. 1987, 1988). In rats, no margin of safety existed between anti-nociception and motor dysfunction (Gaumann and Yaksh 1988; Gaumann et al. 1989). Intracisternal injection of somatostatin produced apnea (Harfstrand et al. 1984).

IT somatostatin produced in cats and in mice focal demyelinization in the posterior column of the spinal cord and reversible flacid leg paralysis (Gaumann et al. 1989).

In dogs, toxicity of spinal somatostatin seems to be more reduced (Chrubasik et al. 1986 a).

Animal experiments indicate that respiratory depression after intrathecal injections of this compound cannot be excluded (Harfstrand et al. 1984). The development of tolerance after somatostatin is also to be considered (Meynadier et al. 1985 b).

In man, the acute analgesic effect of one dose of 250 μg/70 kg intrathecal somatostatin seems to be comparable to that of 10 mg morphine (Meynadier et al. 1986 c). However, the short duration of action necessitates continuous infusion of somatostatin, if prolonged analgesia is required.

Epidural somatostatin does not readily cross the dura mater. Nevertheless, the product is well reabsorbed by villi and nerve roots so that, by this route, good analgesia can be obtained as well.

The association of epidural somatostatin with small doses of diazepam and a muscle relaxant provided surgical anaesthesia. Significant reduction of the anaesthetic doses necessary for surgery and a long lasting postoperative analgesia were noted (Chrubasik 1985 a).

In some cases, tachychardia and hyperglycaemia were observed during anaesthesia. The tachycardia was seen during periods of insufficient surgical analgesia, and the hyperglycaemia is probably due to the stronger inhibition of insulin rather than to glucagon secretion. When somatostatin was used alone, the product elicited neither respiratory depression nor urinary retention, nor euphoria, drowsiness, and nausea. Motor, sensory, sympathetic block or cardiovascular side effects were not registered.

Chrubasik has evaluated that somatostatin has about 1.6 times the analgesic potency of morphine but the plasma half-life time of the product is in the order of minutes (Redding and Coy 1974), so that the use of a continuous infusion is necessary.

Somatostatin was administered by Chrubasik (1985 c, d) via the epidural route by continuous plus on-demand infusion for the treatment of postoperative pain. With the aid of an externally portable infusion device a bolus injection of 0.25 mg of somatostatin was followed by an initial infusion rate of 0.8 mg/h. Supplementary infusion of 0.1 mg and/or supplementary on demand bolus of 0.25 mg were occasionally administered if needed. For constant analgesia the patients required a total dose of 5.7 mg of somatostatin. A comparable series of patients, treated in analogous circumstances with morphine required 11.9 mg of morphine.

Carli et al. (1986) report on the epidural use of somatostatin alone for postoperative pain treatment in 25 patients. They used a loading dose of 250 µg followed by an infusion of 120 µg/h.

The results were as follows:

- onset of analgesia:15 min
- short duration; 1 hour
- segmental analgesia
- no cardiovascular or respiratory side effects
- unchanged respiratory parameters (PET CO_2, $\dot{V}E$, slope $\dot{V}E$/PET CO_2).

In chronic cancer pain Meynadier et al. (1985 c) showed that intrathecal somatostatin was as effective as intrathecal morphine in producing analgesia in patients with intractable cancer pain. Even during intrathecal somatostatin therapy maintained for several weeks side effects are not observed. Whether during long term treatment the increase in somatostatin demand should be attributed to actual tachyphylaxis or to deterioration of the patient's condition, remains to be established.

The mechanism of action of spinal somatostatin is different from that of intrathecal morphine, since the analgesia induced by somatostatin cannot be reversed by naloxone (Chrubasik et al. 1985 j). Acting on different receptor sites, the typical morphine side effects such as respiratory depression, euphoria, dysphoria, sedation, pruritus, urinary retention, and drug addiction, have not been, up to now, observed after somatostatin treatment.

Epidural or intrathecal somatostatin has been proposed as an alternative for pain treatment in morphine tolerant or morphine resistant patients (Chrubasik et al. 1985 a; Dalmas 1986; Meynadier 1986 b), for peroperative analgesia (Chrubasik et al. 1985 a), for treatment of acromegalia (Plewe et al. 1986; Schmidt et al. 1986) and for cluster headache (Sicuteri et al. 1984).

However, on the one hand the serious toxicity of the substance observed in several animal species and on the other hand reports that the commercial solutions are not always free of local toxicity are to be considered. Some

192

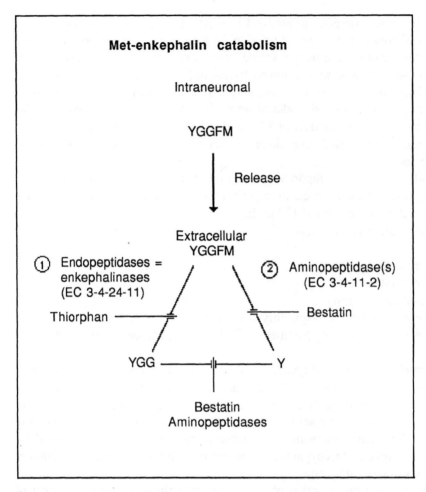

Fig. 69. Pathways of endogenous enkephalin synthesis and degradation with involved neuropeptidases.

Enkephalinase and neuropeptidase inhibition protects metenkephalin from degradation and induces antinociceptive effects in animals.

- YGG = Tyr - Gly - Gly, an extraneuronal metabolite of an opioid peptide derived from proenkephalin A formed in the brain by the action of enkephalinase.
- YGGFM = Tyr - Gly - Gly - Phe - Met, an endogenous enkephalin.

(Schwartz et al. 1986; Meynadier et al. 1987 a)

somatostatin preparations contain disulphide, others contain acetate and mannitol.

SMS 201995 is a long acting preparation of somatostatin. It has been used epidurally for postoperative pain relief in doses of 15 µg/70 kg (Vandalouca et al. 1988).

Extended toxicological investigations should prove that the drug is inert for spinal administration. Further investigations are also necessary to assess the results of very long term treatment with this substance and the price of somatostatin has to be reduced. In the meantime, serious warnings about the clinical use of somatostatin and somatostatin derivates are to be expressed.

7.4.9 ENKEPHALINASE AND AMINOPEPTIDASE INHIBITORS

The endogenous enkephalins are, after their release, inactivated by the peptidase enzymes: enkephalinase and aminopeptidase (Fig. 69), (de la Baume et al. 1983). The use of inhibitors of these enzymes, causing enkephalin accumulation, increases the natural enkephalin activity and inhibits pain stimuli. In this respect, bestatin, captopril, D-phenylalamine and thiorphan have been used for pain treatment in cancer patients.

Bestatin is a specific inhibitor of aminopeptidase B and leucine aminopeptidase.

Thiorphan produces an hydrolysis of enkephalinase.

In animals the administration of both products produces an additive inhibiting effect and this inhibition can be counteracted by naloxone (de la Baume et al. 1983).

Thiorphan or bestatin given alone, intrathecally, in patients suffering from cancer pain produce significant analgesia. Meynadier et al. (1985 c, 1987 a) assessed the intrathecal activity of the associated enkephalinase inhibitors thiorphan 0.0125 mg and bestatin 1.55 mg in 5 patients with terminal cancer pain. A pain relief of 90% occurred and was long lasting (18 hours). The effect was more significant than with each product used alone. It can be speculated that peptidase inhibitors may constitute another new therapeutic approach to pain control in terminal cancer patients.

Kelatorphan is a novel mixed peptidase inhibitor. In rats the compound almost completely prevented the enzymatic degradation of metenkephalin. Compared to thiorphan and bestatin the enzyme inhibiting potency of kelatorphan is much more potent (Bourgois et al. 1986). The intrathecal use of the product in the treatment of cancer pain is now under clinical investigation (Meynadier, pers. communication).

Captopril, the angiotensine converting enzyme, although it is a distinct species, has some similar characteristics with the brain enkephalin degrading enzyme (Swerts et al. 1979). One can assume that the inhibition of the angiotensine converting enzyme by captopril can cause an accumulation of enkephalins in the brain, so that some opiate like effects may occur.

Greenberg et al. (1979) and Ercan et al. (1980) have shown that captopril potentiates the analgesic effects of morphine .

194

Proglumide is a gastrin receptor antagonist known for its inhibitory effect on gastric secretion and used in the treatment of gastritis in daily intravenous doses of 0.5-1.2 mg (Fig. 70). It has been investigated in animals by the intrathecal and the intracerebroventricular route as an inhibitor of cholecystokinin, a physiological opiate antagonist (Watkins et al. 1985 a, b). The animal experiments showed that proglumide markedly potentiates analgesia induced by endogenous opiates. The substance, administered intravenously in doses of 50-100 μg is of clinical value in the treatment of pain and appears to reverse tolerance to opioid analgesics (Price et al. 1985).

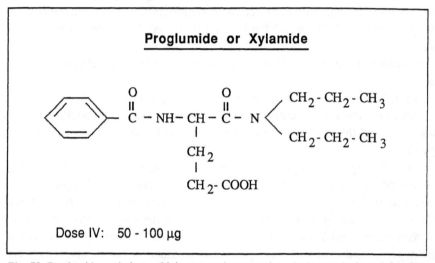

Proglumide or Xylamide

Dose IV: 50 - 100 μg

Fig. 70. Proglumide, a cholecystokinin antagonist, potentiates both magnitude and duration of analgesia produced by morphine and endogenous opiates and appears to reverse tolerance to opioid analgesia.

7.5 Adrenaline (Epinephrine)

In regional anaesthesia, there is general agreement that vasoconstrictors reduce vascular absorption and increase the efficacy of epidural blocks. However, this increase is much less pronounced with the long acting local anaesthetics.

Adrenaline is used as well in combination with spinal opioids (Perriss and Malins 1981; Nordberg et al. 1986 b). The overall effects are not comparable to the use of vasoconstrictors in regional anaesthesia. The effects of the addition of adrenaline to epidural morphine can be summarized as follows:

- depth of analgesia: increased
- blood resorption: reduced
- onset of action: faster
- duration of action: no difference
- level of analgesia: more extended
- supraspinal diffusion: greater
- overall analgesic effect: not significantly improved
- danger of respiratory depression: greater
- side effects: more severe and of longer duration.

The use of adrenaline for epidural opioid analgesia is to be applied with caution. In many cases the disadvantages are in excess of the advantages. However, the addition of adrenaline 1/200,000 (5 µg/ml) to epidural morphine reduces the systemic absorption of the opioid (the plasmatic concentration is three times lower) and increases the rapidity of onset of analgesia and intensity of the effect. However, most of the side effects such as pruritus, urinary retention and respiratory depression are increased as well (Bromage et al. 1982 a, 1983 a; Collier 1984; Fasano and Waldvogel 1982; Martin R et al. 1985; Robertson et al. 1985; Douglas et al. 1986 b). Thus adrenaline increases both the bad and the good effects of spinal opioids (Bromage 1984 a).

However, there seems to exist differences between the different opioids in combination with adrenaline. Whereas the effects in combination with morphine seem disappointing, there are relatively good results in combination with fentanyl or sufentanil. Here, clearly duration and depth of analgesia was improved, while the side effects were decreased by the addition of adrenaline. The risk-benefit ratio the authors concluded to be improved (Klepper et al. 1987). The negative effects of adrenaline seem to be less severe if this product is used in association with lipophilic opioids, e.g. pethidine (Collier 1984), or if the opioid is used in a low dose and in association with a local anaesthetic in order to obtain a better spinal analgesia or an actual surgical analgesia (Bromage et al. 1987).

Adrenaline test-dose
Just like for local anaesthetics, adrenaline in a dose of 3 ml 1/200,000 can be used as a test-dose for exclusion of intravasal position of the catheter.

7.6 Drug-related problems

7.6.1 PHYSICAL PROPERTIES

7.6.1.1 Solutions

The required properties of the opioid solutions for spinal use are as follows:

- aqueous solution
- preservative free
- pH near 7.4
- no opalescence if mixed with CSF.

7.6.1.2 Stereospecificity

Stereospecificity is important since the receptor site must be recognized by the drug. The behaviour of opioids administered by the spinal route is at this point not different from that seen after their use by other routes. Example: the dextrorotatory isomer of morphine is totally inactive. The active morphine is the natural levorotatory molecule.

7.6.1.3 pH

It is essential for receptor binding that the pH of the opioid solution (Fig. 71) is near its pKa values to guarantee a great amount of un-ionized substances.

Although the tissue has an enormous buffer capacity, opioids with a very low

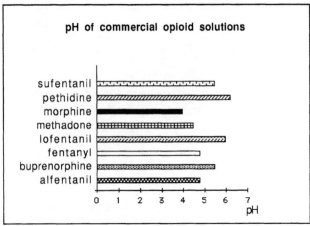

Fig. 71. Comparative values of the pH of commercial opioid solutions.

Table 36. Physicochemical compatibility of opioids and some local anaesthetics with the CSF (in vitro).

	Concentration mg / 10 ml NaCl	pH *	Concentration mg / 10 ml CSF	Decrease in pH of CSF	
Opioids					
- Alfentanil	1.00	5.56	1.00	- 0.15	
- Burprenorphine	0.15	5.93	0.15	- 0.14	
- Fentanyl	0.25	5.73	0.25	- 0.12	
- Lofentanil	0.005	6.39	0.005	- 0.14	
- Meperidine	50.00	6.22	50.00	- 0.12	
- Methadone	2.50	4.52	2.50	- 0.02	
- Morphine	5.00	4.78	5.00	- 0.22	
- Opium (Pantopon)	10.00	3.38	10.00	- 0.08	opalescence
- Piritramide	11.00	3.96	11.00	- 1.52 !	opalescence
Local anaesthetics					
- Bupivacaine 0.25 %		5.87		- 0.02	
- Bupivacaine 0.50 %		5.90			
- Etidocaine 0.50 %		4.75		- 0.82 !	crystalization
- Lidocaine 1 %		6.85		- 0.25	
- Mepivacaine 2 %		6.55		- 0.30	
- Prilocaine 2 %		6.66		- 0.32	

Etidocaine, pantopon and piritramide are potentially incompatible with CSF.
*: pH of the commercially available preparation/10 ml saline.
(Adapted from Börner et al. 1980)

pH (e.g. piritramide) have been demonstrated to induce opalescence in the CSF (Börner et al. 1980) (Tab. 36).

7.6.2 Preservative-free products

For all opioids it seems to be necessary to select a pure preservative-free, pyrogen-free preparation, e.g. for morphine Amphiolen morphinum hydrochloricum ®, Astramorph ® or Duramorph PH ®. Some commercial solutions are unacceptable as they contain additives such as antiseptics and antioxydizing agents (chlorocresol, formol, methylhydroxybenzoate, methyl or propyl parasept, etc.) which are toxic products for nervous tissues (Du Pen 1987 b). Multidose vials of opioids always contain preservative substances. Therefore, their use for spinal analgesia has to be avoided.

The effects of storage of preservative-free morphine have been investigated (Orr et al. 1982). It was demonstrated that the drug could be stored in glass for up to 9 months and autoclaved. However, after the storage of the solution in a plastic syringe for only 20 minutes, a degradation product (possibly apomorphine) was identified. Therefore it was suggested that preservative-free morphine should only be drawn up immediately before use. However, these findings were recently doubted (Bray et al. 1986). In contrary to the previous investiga-

Table 37. Presentation of opioids used for regional opioid analgesia.

Products	Concentration		Volume	Dose (mg/70 kg)		Registered name
	mg	ml	ml/amp.	ED	IT	
Alfentanil HCl	0.5	1	2 10	0.50 - 1	0.1	Rapifen
Buprenorphine HCl	0.3 0.6	1	1 2	0.15 - 0.3	0.1	Temgesic Buprenex
Butorphanol tartrate	2 4	1	1 2	2 - 4		Stadol
Diamorphine	10	10	10	5	1	Heroin
Fentanyl citrate	0.05	1	2 10	0.100	0.05	Fentanyl, Leptanal
Lofentanil	0.005	1	10	0.005		R-34995
Pethidine HCl * low dose high dose	50 100	1	1 2	25 50	35 70	Pethidine Roche Dolosal, Dolantine
Methadone HCl	10	1	1	5		Physeptone
Morphine sulfate	0.5 1	1 1	10 10			Duramorph
	2	10	10	2 - 4	0.2 0.5	MS epidural inj.
	10 20	1 1	1 1			Amphiolen
Nalbuphine HCl	20	2	2	5 - 10	0.4	Nubain
Naloxone HCl	0.4	1	1	0.4	0.2	Narcan
Phenoperidine HCl	1	1	2	1 - 2	0.5	Phenoperidine, Lealgine, Operidine
Pentazocine lactate	30 60	1	1 2	20		Fortal, Fortral, Sosegon, Talwin
Sufentanil citrate	0.05 0.005	1 1	5 10 2	0.01 to 0.05		Sufenta forte, Sufenta

* high dose: local anaesthetic effects.

tions (Orr et al. 1982) quantitative measurements were performed showing no loss of morphine concentration over a period of 36 hours. As most epidural morphine injections clinically show no loss of efficacy, and as apomorphine, if present, must induce a significant degree of vomiting, the conclusion of Orr seems questionable.

7.6.3 DOSES

What is the correct spinal opioid dose ? According to various authors the useful morphine doses range from 2 mg to 20 mg/70 kg bw for administration by the epidural route and from 0.1 mg to 5 mg/70 kg bw, for the intrathecal route (Tab. 37,38). For safety reasons there is a clear cut tendency nowadays in favour of the

Table 38. Opioid and non-opioid drugs used alone or in association for spinal opioid analgesia.

Drugs	Dose (mg / 70 kg)		Registered	Manufacturer
INN	ED	IT	names	
- Endorphins				
β - endorphin		0.15 -3		
DADL		0.5 - 1		
dynorphin				
metenkephalin	0.02 - 0.5			
- Pure opioids				
alfentanil	0.5 - 1	0.1	Rapifen	Janssen
dextromoramide	20		Palfium	Janssen
diamorphine	5	1	Heroine	
fentanyl	0.1 - 0.2	0.05	Fentanyl	Janssen
hydromorphone	0.5 - 1		Dilaudid } Hydromorphan	Knoll
lofentanil	0.0025 - 0.005		Lofentanil	Janssen
methadone	5		Polamidon } Physeptone	Hoechst / Wellcome
meperidine } pethidine	25 - 75	35 - 70	Dolantine } Dolosal	Bayer / Specia
morphine	2 - 4	0.05 - 0.5	Duramorph	Robins
nicomorphine	5		Vilan	Nourypharma
phenoperidine	1	0.5	Phenoperidine	Janssen
sufentanil	0.05		Sufenta	Janssen
- Agonist-antagonists				
buprenorphine	0.1 - 0.3	0.1	Temgesic Buprenex	Reckitt & Colman
butorphanol	4 - 6		Stadol	Bristol
meptazinol	30		-	Wyeth
nalbuphine	4 - 6	0.4	Nubain	Dupont de Nemours
pentazocine	20		Fortral	Winthrop
tramadol	200		Tramal	Grünenthal
- Pure opioid antagonists				
naloxone	0.4	0.2	Narcan	Dupont de Nemours
- Neuropeptides and non-opioid drugs				
ACTH				
clonidine	0.3		Catapressan	Boehringer (Ingelheim)
droperidol	5		Inapsine	Janssen
ketamine	4		Ketalar	Parke Davis
L-baclofen		0.05	Lioresal	Ciba
midazolam	10		Dormicum	Roche
somatostatin	0.25		Somatostatin Modustatin	Curamed Serono Sanofi - Labaz
- local anaesthetics *				
bupivacaine 0.125-0.25 %			Marcaine	Astra
etidocaine 0.5-1 %			Duranest	Astra
lignocaine 1-2 %			Xylocaine	Astra

* with or without epinephrin 1/200 000

reduction of the doses, even if this means a greater frequency of injections. That means for morphine the right dose is 3 to 5 mg/70 kg bw by the epidural route and possibly less than 0.1 to 0.5 mg/70 kg bw for the intrathecal route.

However, in special cases with long term treatment, doses may increase extremely due to whatever reason. One case is reported with an epidural dose of 540 mg morphine in a patient with terminal cancer (Samuelsson et al. 1987).

The spinal doses used for hydrophilic opioids have to be much lower than the parenteral doses proposed for the same product. For lipophylic opioids the spinal doses are close to those used by parenteral routes.

7.6.4 DRUG INTERACTIONS

All drugs with a depressant activity on the CNS given concomitantly to spinal opioids, intensify and prolong mutually the depressant effects (Tab. 39). Several cases of delayed respiratory depression can be explained by such interactions. It is a current but dangerous practice, in cases where the administration of a spinal opioid has not produced the desired effect, to complete the analgesia by a complementary intravenous analgesic injection. When this is done, patients must be closely supervised for many hours.

Compatibility of opioids and local anaesthetics with CSF
Spinal opioids or local anaesthetics have to pass neuronal membranes and CSF before reaching their specific action sites. So, compatibility is an essential point as long or short-time neurotoxicity must be excluded. All opioids and local anaesthetics are acidotic in relation to the pH of the CSF. Piritramide, opium and etidocaine (high concentration) have the lowest pH values, and just those three substances are incompatible with CSF. After piritramide, a deproteinization of the CSF is observed, whereas opium leads to opacity. Etidocaine reacts with CSF by a crystallization of the substance. Consequently, piritramide or opium should not be used for spinal administration (Börner et al. 1980). The reason for the quoted reaction is not discussed in the report. It seems most likely that in fact the low acidotic pH might be the reason for the incompatibility. Over a certain time the CSF certainly will buffer the reaction. But it is unknown whether the sudden crystallization or deproteinization might lead to local reactions at the nervous tissues. Pain by injection may be an indicator for such a reaction.

7.6.5 DRUG ASSOCIATIONS

Aquous solutions may be associated with opioids for epidural or intrathecal administration if absence of incompatibility and neurotoxicity is guaranteed, e.g.:
- low acidity
- pH near pKa values (great amount of un-ionized molecules)
- absence of crystallization or turbidity
- absence of nerve irritation
- absence of pain during injection.

Substances used until now in this field are listed in Tab. 37, 38.

To those, if necessary, can be added:

- antibiotics (ampicillin, cephaloridin, cephalothin etc.)
- antifungals (miconazol)
- antineoplastics (cytosine arabinoside, methotrexate, vincristine etc.)
- radiopaque substances (metrizamide= Amipaque ®)
- steroids (methylprednisolone, dexamethasone)

A more extended list of substances that can be used by the intrathecal route is presented by Allinson and Stach (1978).

7.6.5.1 Local anaesthetics

In some situations spinal opioids alone may provide slow, insufficient, or too short lasting analgesia (Tab. 40). In some situations also local anaesthetics if used alone may provide slow, uncomfortable or too short lasting analgesia. Association of a spinal opioid and a spinal local anaesthetic producing mutual additive or potentiating effects will develop more rapid, more adequate and longer lasting analgesia. Quality of analgesia will be improved by the association. Side effects, however, will also change.

Related to the selected doses of the two substances, side effects will be less frequent or less severe, but they can also become increased, changed or more delayed. In any case close survey of the patient cannot be avoided.

The following combinations are to be considered:

- *Low concentrations* of a local anaesthetic added to low opioid doses in the same syringe increase the analgesic effect, the rapidity of analgesic onset and the duration of analgesia. Several reports have produced evidence that in many situations these advantages may be obtained without increasing the side effects (Abouleish et al. 1987; Bagley et al. 1987; Bromage et al. 1987; Chestnut et al. 1987; Drenger et al. 1987 b; Grice et al. 1987; Hjortsø et al. 1986 b; Little et al. 1987; Naulty 1986 a; Naulty et al.1987; Pandit et al. 1987; Preston et al. 1987).
- *Medium concentrations* of the local anaesthetic added to the opioid result in an even more pronounced analgesia but with the risk (or the advantage) of a more intense sensory, motor and sympathetic block. It has to be kept in mind that giving spinal opioids on top of local anaesthetics might increase the risk of respiratory depression (Hanks et al. 1981).
- *High concentrations* of local anaesthetics with an opioid will give rise to a longer and better surgical analgesia but also with an increased risk of remnant effects on the sensory, motor and/or sympathetic system.

Table 39. Factors changing the analgesic potency of opioids.

Increase in effects	Decrease in effects
- Rapid bolus injection - Alkalosis - Urine alkalisation - Anuria, renal insufficiency - Biliary obstruction - Hepatic insufficiency - Decrease in body O_2 demand - Hypothermia - Low plasma catecholamines - High plasma Mg level - Hypoproteinaemia - Muscle atrophy - Hypothyroidism - Hypoventilation	- Slow, diluted injection - Acidosis - Urine acidification - Forced diuresis - Drug addiction - Enzyme induction - Increase in total body O_2 demand - Hyperthermia - High plasma cathecholamines - Low plasma Mg level - Hyperproteinaemia - Muscle hypertrophy - Hyperthyroidism - Hyperventilation
Synergism or potentiation by means of drug interaction	
- CNS depressants	- Benzodiocepines, tranquillizers - Neuroleptics - Hypnotics, barbiturates - Tricyclic antidepressants - Antiepileptics - Antiparkinson drugs - Antihypertensive drugs
- Drugs acting on the autonomous nervous system	- Parasympathomimetics - Sympatholytics - Ganglionic blocking agents - α_2-receptor agonists
- Neurotransmitter substances	- Serotonin antagonists - Dopamine antagonists - Antihistaminics - ACTH agonists - GABA agonists
- Various compounds	- Aprotinine - Cystostatics - Ecothiopaque - Ketamine - Lithium salts - Magnesium sulfate

The net risk/benefit ratio of the association has to be put in balance for each clinical situation.

The general use of a spinal opioid-local anaesthetic association cannot be recommended, but this association may be justified in certain cases where the isolated use of one of the two products is expected to be inadequate.

7.6.5.2 Other drug associations

The simultaneous association or the successive use of *different opioid agonists* must be avoided because the final results are difficult to foresee.

The epidural association of μ-agonists (e.g. morphine or fentanyl) used together with an intravenous μ-antagonist / κ-agonist (e.g. nalbuphine or butorphanol) can produce an increase in analgesia with longer duration and fewer side effects (Naulty et al. 1987; Doran et al. 1987). However, such an association cannot be recommended for routine use because final results are variable and not easy to predict.

Several investigators have associated epidural fentanyl with *droperidol* or with *ketanserine* (an antiserotonine substance) or with *midazolam*.

Other combinations include the association of an opioid with calcitonin, clonidine, ketamine or somatostatin. All these associations may significantly increase the depth and the duration of the epidural analgesia (see Part II: Clinical Practice).

Table 40. Physicochemical properties of local anaesthestics currently used in association with opioids.

	Bupivacaine	Etidocaine	Lignocaine	Mepivacaine	Prilocaine
Molecular weight (base)	288	276	234	246	220
pKa (25 ° C)	8.1	7.7	7.7	7.6	7.7
Partition coefficient	27.5	141	2.9	0.8	0.9
Usual concentration (%)	0.25 - 0.75	1 - 1.5	1 - 2	1 - 2	1 - 2
Usual onset (min)	10 - 20	5 - 15	5 - 15	5 - 15	5 - 15
Usual duration of surg. anaesth. (min)	120 - 140	120 - 140	60 - 120	60 - 150	60 - 150

(Adapted from Covino and Scott 1985)

The drowsiness observed after epidural morphine can be treated by the intravenous administration of physostigmine without reduction in the analgesic effect (Shulman et al. 1984 a). However, the central stimulating effects of physostigmine are not without any danger.

Finally, some investigators have proposed an intravenous injection of *naloxone* before the epidural administration of the opioid in order to prevent the systemic effects of the morphinomimetic (Rawal et al. 1986 a); but this procedure results mostly in other side effects (e.g. cardiovascular stimulation) and reduced analgesia (De Castro and Andrieu 1980 c).

7.6.6 DRUG ADMINISTRATION MODALITIES (TAB. 41)

7.6.6.1 Patient's position

The position of the patient is only important after an intrathecal injection of the opioid. The use of an hyperbaric solution in a sitting position slows the diffusion of the product to the higher centres. However, the use of such a technique does not offer a complete guarantee that respiratory depression will be avoided.

7.6.6.2 Injection volumes

Volumes of 2 ml to 10 ml of the opioid solutions are used for the epidural route. Without any doubt, the least volume is the best one in respect of possible side effects (Nordberg et al.1986 d; Chrubasik et al. 1985 m). In the postoperative period a volume of 5 ml is efficient in many cases and can be recommended (Lanz et al. 1986 a). Mok et al. (1984 b) demonstrated that a volume of 4 ml is sufficient for an epidural injection in postoperative pain treatment.

On the other hand, it is evident that the volume must be sufficient to allow a diffusion across biological membranes. But if the volume is too great, the risk of respiratory depression by rostral diffusion of the opioid is increased especially in small, slight or older patients with a reduced size of the epidural space.

The effect of volume of an epidurally administered opioid on rapidity of onset and duration of analgesia seems to be different for hydrosoluble and liposoluble substances.

1. Morphine
Chrubasik et al. (1985 m) reported that in dogs an epidural injection of a bolus of 2 mg of morphine diluted in 10 ml of saline produced concentrations at the level of the cisterna magna, which accumulated more rapidly and were higher than those measured after bolus injection of 2 mg of morphine only diluted in

Table 41. Technical specifications relevant to the evaluation of spinal opioid analgesia.

A - Injection technique	Depth	Intrathecal or Epidural
	Height	Segmental level of the injection
	Patient position	Upright position (only important for IT) or Horizontal
	Solution	Diluent: dextrose or saline Iso- or hyperbaric (only important for IT) Quantity pH
	Dose	Repeated bolus doses or Continuous infusion alone or Continuous infusion + on demand bolus
	Catheter	Yes or no
B - Drug association	Drugs added to the opioid	Local anaesthetic Epinephrine 1/200 000 Clonidine etc.
	CNS depressant used by other route	Before Together After
C - Physio-pathology	Age Venous congestion Sclerosis of ligaments Intraspinal pressure Previous opioid treatment	
D - Investi-gation	Double-blind or no	

1 ml. He advises the epidural use of morphine in the following way: bolus of 2 mg diluted in 2 ml followed by a continuous infusion of 0.16 mg in a solution providing 0.06 ml/h via a pump device. However, other clinicians stated that the epidural opioids administered in such a low volume are not efficient in any case.

Nordberg et al. (1986 d) presented a clinical comparison of epidural morphine 2 mg given either in 2 or in 10 ml either at the L3-4 level or at the T7-8 level. The spread in the epidural space and the CSF was significantly delimited by the use of smaller volumes. He suggested that major side effects could be avoided by the use of small volumes.

These findings are also consistant with the data provided by El Baz et al. (1984).

However, there are no significant differences in the plasma concentrations, whether epidural morphine is given in a volume of 3 or 30 ml (Scheinin et al. 1986). Nevertheless, postoperative analgesia was slightly better with the 30 ml volume. The volume of 5 or 10 ml had no influence on the duration of analgesia (Phan et al. 1987).

Lanz et al. (1986 a) performed a randomized double-blind study in 161 postoperative patients with 3 mg morphine in 2.5, 10 or 15 ml saline. The results showed that the dose of 3 mg morphine given in a volume of 5-10 ml is the best compromise providing adequate analgesia with the lowest frequency and intensity of side effects.

Completely different conditions may exist in the treatment of cancer pain. In most of our patients (author M.Z.) a low volume regimen was insufficient to control pain. Those patients with up to 240 mg morphine epidurally per day needed high volumes of 10-15 ml per injection to obtain sufficient analgesia. So, in cancer pain treatment the volume is dictated by the severity of pain and not by theoretical considerations (it will be discussed later that a lot of the "low volume"-patients possibly could be treated by simple oral opioids instead of by pumps, ports and spinal opioids).

2. Lipid soluble drugs
Increasing the volume of normal saline for epidural fentanyl or sufentanil injections produced significantly faster onset and longer duration of analgesia than that obtained with low volume injections (Arcario et al. 1987; Donadoni 1987 a).

7.6.6.3 Level of administration

Opioids may be administered at different levels of the spine: caudal, lumbal, thoracic, cervical, intracisternal or intracerebroventricular.

The most frequently used level is located between L2-L5. It seems logical that the level of administration should be chosen as a function of the localization of the pain. However, the matter has not yet been completely resolved. For some authors, the thoracic epidural injection is the method of choice to obtain good results for thoracic or upper abdominal pain treatment. However, it is also accepted that opioids administered at a thoracic level lead more frequently to delayed respiratory depression (Gustafsson et al. 1981, 1982 d).

In contrast to regional anaesthesia with local anaesthetics spinal opioids diffuse in any case in rostral direction (Bromage et al. 1982 b). So, it is a function of time until the opiate receptors above the injection level are reached. It has been demonstrated that no difference in analgesic outcome is obtained whether the epidural catheter is placed at the thoracic, lumbar or even caudal level (Brodsky et al. 1988; Højkjaer-Larsen et al. 1985; Nordberg 1984 b).

In respect of security, we would advocate to start with a lumbar injection or catheter position for all pain locations below the cervical dermatoma. In most cases the lumbar level will be the safest and also the easiest route and the relief of pain (even thoracic pain) will be in most cases effective enough.

In children (2-12 years old) caudal morphine 1 mg provided good thoracic pain relief after cardiac surgery (Rosen et al. 1987). Jensen (1981) and Krane et al. (1987) reported also that caudal opioid injection (e.g. morphine 0.5 mg/ml, 0.1 mg/kg) was a simple technique to perform in children. It provided good postoperative pain relief with rapid onset and longer lasting duration (8-24 hours) than that obtained with caudal bupivacaine. However, urinary retention, pruritus, and nausea appeared with slightly greater frequency. Delayed respiratory depression may occur (Krane 1988; Krane et al. 1988).

Also in patients with cervical or facial pain the rostral migration of the opioid from the lumbar epidural space provided sufficient pain relief (Gourlay et al. 1985; Sullivan and Cherry 1987). Only in the case of insufficient analgesia in the thoracic region a thoracic placement of the catheter was indicated (Zenz et al. 1982a ; Zenz and Piepenbrock 1983 b; Zenz 1983 c).

However, in some patients with cervical cancer the pain is not sufficiently relieved by lumbar or thoracic administration of spinal opioids. Apparently, the opioid concentration in the affected area is not high enough. In those cases, cervical administration of epidural opioids may be necessary and safe for effective pain control.

Recently, the cervical administration of epidural opioids using portable or implanted delivery systems has been proposed (Waldman et al. 1987 b). With such a device 1-2 mg epidural morphine provided excellent and safe analgesia in the management of upper body pain.

7.6.6.4 Injection routes

a) Epidural versus intrathecal administration

The intrathecal route seems to be the more logical one. Opioids are placed near to their receptor sites, less dosage is needed, and as a result, systemic side effects should be fewer (Tab. 42). Epidural opioids results not only in less "selective spinal analgesia" but give rise to a higher systemic uptake of the drug. A higher dosage and a higher volume are needed. On the other hand, the fact that the dura mater is not punctured with the consecutive possibility of postspinal headache is in favour of the epidural route.

208

Table 42. Potential advantages and drawbacks of spinal opioid analgesia.

	E D O A	I T O A
- Technical difficulties	possible	fewer
- Dosage	low	very low
- Analgesia		more rapid more effective more reliable duration longer

- Side effects (global)
  • Severity
  • Frequency
	less severe
	less frequent
		more severe
		more frequent

- Respiratory depression
  • Early (1 - 2 h)
    (systemic route)
  • Delayed (6 - 24 h)
    (migration in CSF)
	+
	
	+
		+ +
		
		+ +

- Headache - CSF hygroma	rare non existent	possible possible
- Sedation - Nausea, vomiting - Urinary retention - Pruritus - Miosis - Withdrawal syndrome	± + + + ± possible	+ + + + + + + + possible
- Infection risk	low	meningitis possible
- Tolerance: frequency rapidity of onset	+ +	+ + + +

± = very rare, + = frequent, ++ = very frequent.

However, all these arguments are very theoretical ones. Clinically, the side effects and the technical difficulties are clearly higher in the intrathecal route. But the most important point: the right dosage for the intrathecal route seems not yet to have been found.

Even 0.1 mg morphine given by the intrathecal way can result in severe side effects. Perhaps the right intrathecal dose is extremely low. Only when the right dose is found, should the theoretical considerations favour the intrathecal over the epidural route. Until that time we would recommend for routine use the epidural administration of opioids.

b) Intracisternal versus intracerebroventricular injection

In patients with severe cervical or facial pain an opioid injection into the lateral ventricle can be performed (Leavens et al. 1982). More recently for the same indications morphine injections into the cisterna magna have been applied with excellent results, see Section 14.8 (Schoeffler et al. 1987 a, b).

Conclusions

Up to now, clear cut pharmacokinetic or pharmacodynamic arguments are lacking to justify the choice of a well specified opioid compound as the best product for spinal analgesia. All authors share the opinion that morphine, although it is the most used substance, is not the opioid of choice for spinal use. Notwithstanding its low cost and long duration of pain relief, it has undoubtedly the highest incidence of serious side effects and it must be replaced in so far as this is possible by an opioid with high lipid solubility.

Intrathecal *pethidine* has found a particular application in saddle block analgesia and in intrathecal anaesthesia techniques for low abdominal surgery. However, the safety of high doses of intrathecal pethidine is not supported by toxicological studies performed in animals.

More extended experience with epidural *methadone* has to be performed in order to provide further evidence of the particular properties of this opioid.

Among the fentanyl family, the results obtained with *fentanyl* itself and *sufentanil* are promising and it is to be noted that the place of these substances in spinal opioid treatment is expanding.

The *neuropeptides* used up to now have found little practical application.

The place of the opioids agonist-antagonists in this field is presently not well defined. Among them, *nalbuphine* and *butorphanol* (with a relative rapid and long acting analgesia, minimal respiratory depression and reduced activity on the urinary system) justify further clinical trials.

The non-opioid drugs are up to now only to be considered as complementary drugs in spinal opioid treatments. Among them *clonidine* and *midazolam* are perhaps the most promising substances.

8. Equipment and drug delivery systems

The technical data and illustrations of special regional opioid analgesia equipment mentioned in this chapter, as well as the Tab. 79 to 89 and Fig. 89 to 122 are arranged in groups in Chapter 20. In Chapter 8 are only reported the clinical problems and results due to the equipment and drug delivery systems.

8.1 Equipment

Spinal opioids have to be administered into the neighbourhood of the spinal cord via a single shot technique or via a catheter for long-term application. For the single shot technique the equipment is nearly the same as for the standard intrathecal or epidural blocks. But for the long-term administration the evaluation of equipment, delivery systems and techniques play a major role, because the spinal opioid analgesia may necessitate extremely long treatment periods. So, since the introduction of spinal opioids a number of new techniques and equipment have been developed, and other techniques have been modified and adapted for the special needs of spinal opioid therapy. Spinal infections, catheter problems (kinking, clotting), and/or pump problems have been observed and gave rise to these modifications.

The development of various opioid delivery systems has facilitated the expanded role of perineural opioids for pain treatment. However, it will be seen that the "right" technique is still to be found. The different technical possibilities have to be adapted for different indications. The main point seems to be the right evaluation of the equipment for a given situation and a given patient.

8.1.1 EPIDURAL, INTRATHECAL NEEDLES

Different needles for epidural and intrathecal injection or catheter placement are available.

All needles used for spinal blocks should have a close fitting removable stylet. This prevents coring of the skin (Fig. 89, 90, 91).

a) Epidural

For the single epidural shot many needles have been introduced, but only the *Crawford needle* is widely distributed and used. It is a short-bevelled needle (40°) with smooth edges to prevent dura puncture. The needle is available in 14, 16, 18, 19 gauge. The minor sizes of 18 or 19 gauge are preferred, because the tissue trauma is minor and the possible hole by accidental dura puncture is minor. Disposable needles with centimeter calibrations have our preference (Fig. 90).

For catheter introduction the *Tuohy needle* is used. This is a needle with a Huber point. It is available in 16, 17, and 18 gauge. Again, we prefer a disposable needle with centimeter markings. To prevent the catheter from kinking when introducing into the needle, Scott has made a modification (Fig. 91). The same is achieved by the disposable introduction aid fitting closely between needle and catheter (Fig. 93).

b) Intrathecal

For subarachnoid techniques different needles with different "philosophies" exist.

The standard spinal needle is the *Quincke-Babcock* spinal needle. It has a sharp point with a medium length cutting level. The *Pitkin needle* has a sharp point but is short-bevelled with cutting edges and a rounded heel. The *Greene* spinal needle has a rounded non-cutting bevel and a rounded point. The *Whitacre spinal needle* has a completely different design. It has a solid tip which is rounded with a non-cutting bevel. The side hole is 2 mm proximal to the tip (Fig. 89).

The size of the needle has a direct relationship to postspinal headache (Renkl and Dittmann 1984; Kortum et al. 1982; Eckstein et al. 1982; Barron and Strong 1984 b). The size should be as small as possible. Needles from 20 to 29 gauge are produced. However the handling of the small 29 gauge needles is very difficult, even for the well-trained. The ideal size seems to us the 25 or 26 gauge needles. They have to be used with an introducer. The 22 gauge needle can be used without an introducer, but the incidence of postspinal headache is significantly higher with this size.

8.1.2 CATHETERS

To obviate repeated access of the epidural or intrathecal space a catheter can be inserted via a Tuohy needle.

Different catheters and catheter materials have been developed (Fig. 92, 93, 94, 95).

The following properties for the ideal spinal catheter are postulated (Bromage 1978; Coombs 1985 f):

- biochemically stable
- non-irritant
- low friction, relatively soft
- good tensile strength
- resistant to kinking and traction
- radiopaque with markings.

8.1.2.1 Materials and models

PCV (Polyvinylchloride) is composed of 45% di-2-ethylhexyl-phthalate (DEHP), a substance necessary for softening of the material. DEHP due to its high lipid solubility diffuses easily in the blood and hydrolyzes in mono-2-ethylhexyl-phthalate (MEHP). This substance is toxic.

When the PVC catheter is in sîtu for a certain time it loses the flexibility and is going to be stiff. Due to the toxic reaction and to the possible stiffness PVC catheters should no longer be used (PVC is the typical material for grounds).

A *Teflon®* catheter provides mechanical dangers: its high rigidity increases the risk of perforation of the dura mater or the vessels and may also be responsible for neural lesions. The plasticity of a Teflon catheter may be deformed by changes in body T° (Riegler et al. 1984).

Polyurethane and even better polyether-urethane, has been substituted for polyesther-urethane, because of its higher stability against hydrolysis. Polyurethane catheters due to their high biocompatibility have real advantages for chronic use (Gebert 1983). However the high flexibility of polyurethane is responsible for problems of migration and notching.

Polyethylene and polyurethane catheters have a smoother surface than PVC, silicone-rubber or Teflon catheters. Polyethylene becomes harder with age due to the loss of the softener. This is a serious drawback of this material.

Polyamide and *nylon* are soft materials by themselves with a low content of softener. The material is well tolerated over long periods without losing its flexibility. We use exclusively polyamide catheters for long-term treatment.

Silicone is a material with a great biocompatibility. The material is extremely soft so that a silicone catheter has to be introduced with an inner guide wire. Possibly, this is a drawback, because the guide wire can perforate the catheter at the tip when used without caution. The other drawback of a silicone catheter is the ease of kinking and obstructing.

Spetzler catheters are special catheters made also in silicone rubber. They are radiopaque, non-collapsible, have a multi-hole tip and remain supple even after many months of use.

Hickman or Broviac catheters can be used to reduce the risk of infection. These catheters are provided with two Dacron felt cuffs on the portion designed for tunnellization. Once the catheter is in place, the cuffs are colonized with subcutaneous tissue cells, ensuring firm fixation of the catheter and serving as a barrier infection, at least theoretically (Douard et al. 1985).

Double lumen catheter: Amaki et al. (1982) developed a double lumen epidural catheter in Teflon. The internal lumen opens at the distal end. The external lumen opens at the proximal port 5 cm from the distal port. Each lumen can be injected separately. The objectives of this special catheter are: to provide a greater analgesic flexibility in particular situations such as during labour and to provide a deeper analgesia with a smaller injection volume. However, the catheter is expensive, and the cost/benefit ratio for acute pain treatment seems more than questionable.

Theracath (Racz ®) is a spring wire reinforced epidural Teflon catheter with non-kinking characteristics, and with a spring-like tip to help prevent inadvertent dural puncture. This catheter has been specially designed to be used without a removable guide and to be left in the epidural space for extended periods of time. The catheter wall is similar in construction to an armoured endotracheal tube (Racz et al. 1982, 1986). However, this catheter seems to present serious drawbacks, e.g. leakage, difficulties in removal and high price (Coombs 1985 b; Coombs et al. 1985 e; Ellis and Ramamurthy 1986; Frankhouser 1986; Lingenfelter 1983; Riegler et al. 1984). Coombs (1985 b) reported a case of catheter disruption 8 cm from the tip. As well, he described from his clinic four other events with Racz's catheter, e.g. cracked catheter and catheter with leakage.

The Du Pen catheter is a new exteriorized epidural catheter prepared from radiopaque silicone rubber. The device consists of three pieces:

1. an epidural segment that is placed through a needle into the epidural space
2. an exteriorized line equipped with an external Luer connector and a subcutaneous Dacron cuff
3. a small spliced segment to join the two other segments (Du Pen et al. 1987 c).

A *radiopaque* catheter has the disadvantage of the admixture of, e.g., wolfram to the relatively inert catheter material. In this way it is not as inert as the catheter itself. On the other hand, the injection of radiopaque fluid enables sufficiently the identification of the catheter position. Radiographic control of the catheter position is always recommended, especially if the injections are to be repeated during several days.

The *tip* of most catheters exists in two different designs. The catheters have either an open end or a rounded tip with side holes. The closed end catheter is less traumatic when advancing in the epidural space. But it has the disadvantage of possibly being introduced in different spaces with the different holes (Beck et al. 1986). In this way, a catheter with side holes can have access to the subarachnoid space with one hole and to the epidural space with the other one, or simultaneously to a vessel and to the epidural space. This is not possible with a catheter with a single open tip. We recommend catheters with an open tip.

8.1.2.2 Catheter problems

Complications may be due to mechanical, pathological or rejection phenomena (Tab. 43):

- *Displaced catheters (migration)* can have access to bloodvessels or to the area of nerve roots. This may lead to bleeding or to impaired analgesic effect. To avoid migration it is recommended that the catheter must never be pushed forward for more than 3 cm.
- *Clogged kinked catheters* suppress drug delivery with a resulting loss of pharmacological action.
- *Dural or neuronal penetration* produces increased pharmacological action.
- A *leak* may induce a hygroma (in intrathecal techniques).
- *Acute tissue reactions*, for example an arachnoid reaction, induces localized swelling, heat and pain.
- *Haematoma formation* may impede diffusion.
- *Difficulties during removal:* this problem is usually resolved by flexing the patient's back and applying steady traction to the catheter. Knotting rarely occurs, it may be related to the insertion of too much catheter into the epidural space. Removal may exceptionally necessitate a laminectomy (Blass et al.1981, Riegler and Pernetzki 1983).
- Danger of *infection* after a simple epidural injection is <1/30,000 (Bromage 1978). However repeated epidural opioid administration and long lasting catheterization increases infection risk and the quality of the nursing becomes most important (Iversen 1985; Koch and Nielsen 1986; Zenz et al.1981 g).
- *Abcess and fistula formation* following an epidural catheter has surprisingly been observed in one case by Wanscher el al. (1985). In this case the catheter was in place only for 2 days. Clinical signs of such a complication elicit further examinations: skin culture, blood culture, cerebrospinal fluid examination, radiography of the spine and myelography. According to the actual experience, in such a situation, laminectomy should be performed without delay.

Use of disposable equipment, adherence to aseptic techniques and single use preparations of preservative-free injectable drugs have reduced the risk of an epidural abcess as a result of epidural catheterization to an extremely rare condition (Fine et al. 1988).

Table 43. Potential catheter complications

Mechanical catheter complications	Pathological catheter complications
- Clot formation	
- Leakage	- Fistula formation
- Curling up, knot formation	- Infection
- Displaced (slip out)	• heat, pain
- Haematoma formation	• localized swelling
- Kinking	- Reinjection pain
- Migration of catheter	- Tissue reactions
- Misplaced	
- Plugged catheter	
- Removal difficulties	

(Bromage 1978; Brown and Rein 1985; Brownridge 1984; Carl et al. 1984; Duffy 1981 b-c; Ellis and Ramamurthy 1986; Frankhouser 1986; Hartrick et al. 1985; Lingenfelter 1983; Macintosh 1985; Nielsen et al. 1985; Ravidran et al. 1979; Wanscher et al. 1985).

- *Accidental drug injection* of toxic substances through the epidural catheter or infusion errors into the epidural space have been reported (e.g. Lin et al. 1986: injection of potassium chloride after disconnection of the infusion set and erroneous connection with the other infusion bag). The possibility of such complication is certainly underestimated and requires all our preventive attention. To avoid such accident with regional opioid analgesia treatment:

- use for epidural injection only special microbore tubing sets
- use a Luer lock connection between infusion set and catheter
- tape securely all the connections
- identify the epidural tubing with a particular color code.

8.1.2.3. Externalized or tunnelled catheter

The simplest system to use is a catheter brought out from the spinal space onto the skin.

a) A spinal catheter may be externalized through the midline posteriorly and *taped percutaneously* in position. The catheter should be connected to a bacterial filter. This is the current situation for postoperative and obstetric patients receiving spinal drugs.

For chronic treatment an externalized percutaneous catheter can also be taped over the skin (Zenz 1985 c), (Fig. 72 a, b; 74).

b) A catheter can also be *tunnelled subcutaneously* away from the insertion site to a more comfortable position for the patient laterally to the region of the antero-lateral chest wall where the catheter exits from the skin.

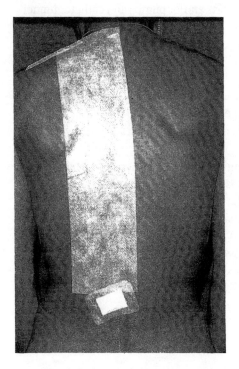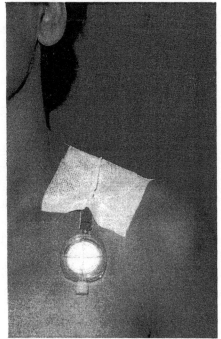

Fig. 72 a, b. Epidural opioid analgesia with a percutaneous catheter.

a) The catheter is fixed on its entry with a dressing.
b) The free part of the catheter is conducted externally to the intraclavicular region and fixed with a stretch dressing.
(Zenz et al. 1985 c)

The last solution is more comfortable for the patient and a reduction in the risk of spinal sepsis may be expected. Both systems are relatively inexpensive and simple to implement. Topping up of the catheter is straightforward. The patient or their relatives can readily be educated in the principles relating to aseptic technique, decreasing for long term use the requirement for medical and nursing supervision. Two bacterial filters in series are recommended with regular renewal of the distal filter and less frequent changing of the proximal filter. In one series of 150 patients treated with such externalized systems, there were no cases of spinal infection (Cherry 1987 d).

8.1.2.4 Open or closed systems

Repeated administration of intraspinal opioids are necessary for chronic pain treatment. The use of open or closed administration systems are to be considered. *Open systems* use external syringes, reservoirs or pumps charged with the opioid solution. *Closed systems* use implanted ports and/or pumps and catheter tunnelling.

The following important parts emerge in two recent surveys presented by Benedetti (1987) and Ventafridda (1987 a):

- As well with epidural as with intrathecal administration, the closed systems showed that they can be used for longer periods of time.
- With both systems, the advantages of continuous infusion rates allowed better and more uniform pain control.
- Apparently with closed systems, an higher rate of tolerance development may appear. This however, is debatable: it is not the use of a continuous and closed system that induced tolerance but the longer duration of treatment (closed systems are more frequently used in patients with higher life expectancy).
- Patient acceptance is greatly increased if the entire administration system can be housed subcutaneously (Cherry 1987 d).
- Side effects and complications are expected to be higher in open systems compared to closed systems both with epidural and with intrathecal delivery (Cherry et al.1987 c). However, this is not always reality.

8.1.3 MICROPORE FILTERS

The use of micropore filters to prevent spinal infection is controversial (Fig. 96). Most infections in the extradural space result from haematogenous spread. However to exclude the injection of particulate matter from ampoules, filter use can be recommended (Stanton-Hicks 1985).

The disc-type filter is not ideal for fixation on the skin and can cause the catheter to kink if not properly splinted. The flat filter lies flat against the patient's skin, ensuring both comfort and full flow through the catheter. Intrathecal catheters are recommended always to be connected to a micropore filter.

8.2 Drug delivery systems (Tab. 44)

8.2.1 PORTS

If chronic treatment frequently requires reinjections into the catheter the subcutaneous implantation of an injection port will facilitate nursing and possibly decrease the risk of infection (Fig. 97- 103, Tab. 81). The goal of these "access sites" is:

- to transform a spinal or intracerebroventricular puncture into a simple transcutaneous injection for repeated use
- to provide an easy to reach internal reservoir for connection and continuous perfusion via an external pump.

Cherry (1987 b) has summarized the required properties of an injection port for repeated opioid administration:

- high biocompatible material, corrosion and polymerization-free, inert, easy to mould in complex shapes (e.g., titanium, stainless steel, polysulfoneresin, Teflon, or medical grade silicone elastomer);
- easily sterilized;
- simple to implant and to anchor under local anaesthesia;
- relatively inexpensive;
- simple to use by non-medically trained personnel;
- simple to connect with the standard spinal catheter;
- readily palpable percutaneously;
- easy to inject into (with definite end point to injection);
- leak proof after >1000 punctures (resealable membrane);
- able to cope with high pressure associated with injection through a narrow bore catheter;
- not become occluded by foreign material;
- not to be subject to inadvertent disconnection from the catheter.

Different ports from various manufacturers are available.

Apart from size and design, ports are always composed of a plastic or a metal chamber and a membrane. Both metal and plastic chambers have advantages and

Table 44. Delivery systems for epidural or intrathecal opioid administration.

1 - Externalized catheter

2 - Externalized catheter
  + subcutaneous catheter tunnelling

3 - Subcutaneous catheter tunnelling
  + implanted reservoir bag or port
  + external manual infusion pump

4 - Subcutaneous catheter tunnelling
  + implanted reservoir bag or port
  + stationary or portable pump

5 - Subcutaneous catheter tunnelling
  + implanted pump

6 - Subcutaneous catheter tunnelling
  + implanted pump
  + external programmer

(Adapted from Waldman and Coombs 1989)

disadvantages. In particular the metal base of the port affords reassurance to the inexperienced injector that the needle is correctly sited. To avoid microemboli being injected into the catheter some ports have a filter incorporated at the exit. The quality and thickness of the membrane must allow that a needle remains implanted in the port over a period of at least 2 weeks.

Ports are punctured with special *Huber point needles* to prevent coring membrane material (Fig. 97 in Chapter 20). Those needles also exist in a special design for continuous infusion. They are 90°-angled with an adhesive area to be taped on the skin over the port.

The port situated on the anterior chest wall is in a position which can be easily reached and is in a direct line of vision. Top up injections are initially made by the hospital nurses. After an initial period the patients and their close family are instructed in self-administration of the top ups. Details of necessary sterile precautions are given.

Advantages and drawbacks of implanted ports

The implanted injection ports have advantages, they provide injection facilities and can also be used in connection with continuous external pump-infusion.

- If there are no external ports or no catheter exit site, theoretically the infection risks are reduced.
- Nursing during long-term medication is easier.
- A more normal quality of life can be maintained (e.g. bath facilities).
- Injection ports are relatively simple, effective, and economical devices compared to implanted pumps.
- They provide an efficacious progress for cancer pain relief.

The combined use of an external portable pump infusor and an implanted port allows for transfixing the port membrane only once every second week. Leaks are easier to avoid by the epidural route than by the intrathecal injection. Abou-Hatem et al. (1985) reported on more than 1000 injections administered in a port system during 410 days without infection or skin damage.

However ports also have some *disadvantages:*

- if it is required to carry out multiple punctures there is a higher infection risk than with a fully implanted pump device
- injections at frequent intervals necessitate nursing constraints, and interfere with the mobility and independence of the patient
- the device is, in some cases, less effective than continuous infusion (Muller 1985 a)
- several mechanical complications are possible
- rejection phenomenon
- the port can be difficult to palpate (Coombs 1985 f)
- port infection
- disconnection port-catheter

Reports on different models

- *AHS Spinalgic* ®: Dumas et al. 1985; Findler et al. 1982; Laugner et al. 1985 a, 1986; Leavens et al. 1982; Malone et al. 1985; Meynadier et al. 1986 a, 1987 c; Muller et al. 1982; Muller 1985 a; Muller and Laugner 1986; Schoeffler et al. 1986 e.g.;
- *Cordis Secor* ®: Husebo 1986; Lazorthes et al. 1980, 1985 a; Gestin 1987; Motsch et al. 1987 d, e.g.
- *Unidose* ®: Gonzalez et al.1985; Meglio et al.1985; Saunders and Coombs

1983; Wang 1985; e.g.

- *Pharmacia, Port-A-Cath* ®: Abou-Hatem et al.1985; Cherry et al.1987 a, b, d; Descorp Declere and Begon 1986 a; Descorp Declere et al.1987; Madrid et al.1986; Motsch et al. 1987 d; Nicaise et al.1983, e.g.;

8.2.2 SPECIAL DRUG DELIVERY SYSTEMS

8.2.2.1 Roquefeuil's self-administration system

The system consists of a plastic bag (200 ml container, Terumo blood bag) with an uni-directional Hakim-type valve, an A.H.S. Spinalgesic-type injection port and a tunnelled catheter (Tab. 45). The bag is filled with the opioid solution. It is worn externally in the subaxillary region and provides up to two months' opioid supply for the intrathecal route. With each squeeze of the bag the valve allows the injection of 0.1 ml drug. Between the injections the catheter is clamped near the bag avoiding unwanted injections as a result of accidental pressure on the bag (Roquefeuil et al. 1982).

With this system the patient has at his disposal a substantial quantity of an opioid, so that the risk of drug abuse must be taken into consideration (Batier et al. 1983).

Due to the low volume of 0.1 ml per squeeze the unit is only useful for intrathecal administration. The relationship between the single deliveries of 0.1 ml and the total volume of the bag of 200 ml (=2000 shots) is not realistic but economic.

This system is not distributed.

8.2.2.2 Muller and Laugner's self-administration device

A device of an intermediate type was proposed by Muller and Laugner (1986), (Fig. 73).

The fully implantable device consists of:

- a large implantable silicone reservoir (50 ml), A.H.S.
- a separate filling and an emptying port
- a metered dose valve (MDV)
- a tunnelled catheter.

The MDV valve is operated through the skin by finger pressure.
Each bolus delivers a volume of 0.2 ml. The activation of this one way valve, is indicated by a tactile sensation.

Table 45. Comparison between 3 devices developed for self-administration of opioids during regional opioid analgesia.

	System of Roquefeuil *	System of Muller *	Secor system
- Administration route	ED or IT	IT	IT
- Tunnelled catheter	yes	yes	yes
- Injection port	external	implanted	implanted
- Uni-directional valves	1	1 MD 4	3
- Port capacity (ml)	1.2	25 50	12
- Dimensions of implanted material (mm)			65 x 15
- Bolus volume delivered at each finger press (ml)	0.1	0.2	0.1
- Separate filling port emptying port	no no	yes yes	yes no
- Implanted material	A.H.S. port	reservoir + 2 ports A.S.H.	reservoir filling and dosing system
- External material • external bag capacity (ml) • external Hakim valve • clamp	200 yes yes	no no no	

* These prototypes are not on the market.

During self-injection through compression of the MDV the opioid travels through the catheter into the intrathecal space (Muller and Laugner 1986).

The device has the drawback of being not fully controllable by the doctor, whereas the patient can administer as often as he wants to.

This system is not distributed.

8.2.2.3 Self-administration device Secor

Secor (Cordis) ® (Fig.103, Tab. 45, 46) is an implantable multidose reservoir for manually operated administration of opioids. The device is specially designed for the intrathecal administration of a morphine solution.

224

The system consists of a manually operated implantable dosage device with reservoir.

The dosage device itself consists of three functional entities:
- a filling system
- a reservoir
- a dosage system.

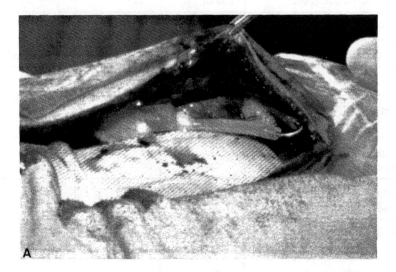

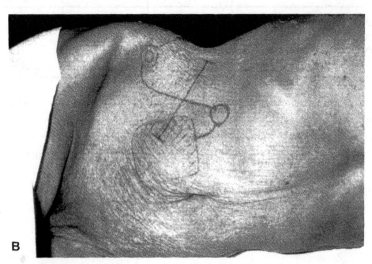

Fig. 73. Subcutaneous implantation of MAD-MDA injection port and reservoir (A.H.S.)
a) implantation
b) abdominal position

Table 46. Secor Cordis ® infusor system used for repeated bolus administration of Sufentanil forte ® (SFf).

- Basic solution: Amp. SFf = 50 µg/ml   5 ml = 250 µg SF - Cordis reservoir = 12 ml Reservoir is filled with 12 ml SFf = 600 µg SF. Each push on the button delivers 0.1 ml = 5 µg SF
Settings for the Secor cordis device **(3 steps regimen for ED infusion)**
- Loading dose   = 10 x push button = 50 µg SF - Maintenance dose = 1 push button/h   = 5 µg SF - Supplemental dose = 1 push button   = 5 µg SF

The filling system consists of a self-sealing silastic dome over a needlestop disc. To prevent reflux from the reservoir, a valve is positioned between the entrance site and the reservoir. The reservoir is filled by introducing a 25 gauge needle into the dome pushing the needlestop disc downward and thus opening the valve underneath. The reservoir consists of a dome-shaped polyester reinforced silicone rubber membrane held in position by a polysulfon ring, thereby keeping the system watertight. The reservoir capacity is 12 ml, dimensions: 6.5×1.5 cm.

The dosage system: by manually pressing two buttons in a certain sequence, a fixed quantity (bolus) of drug is transferred from the reservoir to the catheter. Any incorrect handling such as inverse sequence, pressing one of the buttons several times, pressing two buttons at the same time or pressure on the device itself, does not result in liquid release. The bolus quantity is 0.1 ml.

However, the system has some drawbacks:

- The push-buttons must be sequentially pressed in the correct order. But once the device is implanted the buttons are not always easy to locate.
- Precise patient dosage records are mandatory in order to know exactly the date of refill. A follow-up report in the form of a pain diary, written by the patient, is the best way to maintain satisfactory results.
- The implantation requires a relative large wound incision, so that pressing the buttons can be painful for the patient during the first post-implantation period.

226

Table 47. Choice between external worn pump and implanted pump devices.

	Externally worn pumps + implanted port	Implanted disposable pumps
- Investment	relatively low	very high
- Reusable	multiple use	only one patient
- Treatment • Adaptation possibilities • Infusion rate • Bolus • Refill volume • Drug association	higher variable PCA by patient 100 ml possible	reduced constant by MD bolus septum relatively small possible
- Dimensions	miniaturization becomes possible	small, heavy
- Infection risk	higher	lower

Table 48. Potency / Volume ratio of opioids for intravenous and epidural administration.

Drugs	Potency Acute equipotent doses µg/70 kg		Volume Volume of commercial solutions necessary to obtain one dose ml/70 kg	
	IV	ED	IV	ED
- Pethidine HCl - Morphine sulfate **	100 000 10 000	50 000 2 000	2 0.5 1 2	1 0.125 0.25 0.4
- Phenoperidine HCl - Alfentanil HCl - Buprenorphine HCl - Fentanyl citrate - Sufentanil citrate - Sufentanil citrate forte	1 000 500 300 100 10 10	500 100 - 500 * 300 100 25 - 50 * 25 - 50 *	2 1 * 1 2 2 0.2	1 0.2 - 1 * 1 2 5 - 10 * 0.5 - 1 *

* Author dose differences
**According to commercial solution
The table shows that the selection of a strong opioid available in low volume may be easier adapted to epidural needs.

These problems are partly solved in the new model: the MPAP Cordis (Multi-purpose access port), standard (44 mm) or miniport (31 mm) model. This is a simplified self-administration device of reduced volume, providing a bolus administration of 0.5 or 0.09 ml. However the volume capacity of the device is so low that only the use of the intrathecal or intracerebroventricular route can be considered.

8.2.3 PUMPS

Many different models of pumps can be used for pulsatile or continuous opioid infusion.

On the basis of the different modalities of their use, the pump devices may be divided into:

- external or implantable
- programmable or operating on a fixed rate
- continuous or pulsatile
- stationary or portable
- peristaltic or mechanically driven
- manual, self-powered or battery operated
- equipped for the use of a syringe or a reservoir
(Tab. 85 - 89 in Chapter 20).

The greatest difference between internal and external pumps is the price. The decision depends on the prognosis of the patient, the general conditions, mobilization possibilities, the life expectancy of the patient and the price (Tab. 47).

The opioid volume that is to be infused is another important parameter for the choice of the required pump device. It is determined by the selected drug and its concentration, by the infusion mode and by the indication (Tab. 47, 48, 49, 50).

8.2.3.1 Pros and cons of pump devices

Constant infusion offers the advantage that there should not be the peaks and troughs of pain relief associated with bolus injections.

Table 49. Opioids used for infusion analgesia

a) PRESENTATION			
	µg / ml	ml	Pack
- Alfentanil	500	10	5 amp.
- Fentanyl	50	10	5 amp.
- Sufentanil	5	2 - 10	5 amp.
- Sufentanil forte	50	5	5 amp.
b) DOSES AND VOLUMES						
	Sufentanil forte		Fentanyl		Alfentanil	
Dose, volume	µg / 70 kg bw	ml	µg / 70 kg bw	ml	µg / 70 kg bw	ml
Loading dose	50	1	250	5	750	1.5
Maintenance dose / h dose / 24 h	5 120	0.1 2.4	25 600	0.5 12	250 6 000	0.5 12.0
Supplemental dose 4 supp. doses	5 20	0.1 0.4	25 100	0.5 2	250 1 000	0.5 2.0
Total volume / 24 h		4		20		16.0

The table shows that small insuline pumps which can accept only syringes of 1 to 3 ml cannot contain an opioid dose sufficient for 24 hours even if the strong sufentanil solution is selected.

Table 50. Infusion settings for the use of sufentanil (SF) with the Travenol infusor.

- Basic solution:	Amp. SF 10 ml 5 µg/ml = 50 µg SF
- Infusor solution:	3 amp. SF 10 ml = 150 µg SF/30 ml 3 amp. 10 ml NaCL 0.9% = 30 ml $\}$ SF 2.5 µg/ml
- Infusor delivers:	2 ml/h or 5 µg/h SF
- Syringe solution:	2 amp. 10 ml SF = 100 µg/20 ml or 5 µg/ml
Settings for the Travenol infusor device (3 steps regimen for epidural infusion)	
- Loading dose with syringe → 10 ml = 50 µg SF	
- Maintenance dose with infusor → 2 ml/h = 5 mg SF	
- Supplemental dose with syringe → 1 ml = 5 µg SF	

A three-way stoprock is mounted between the Travenol Infusor and the syringe.

- Nursing is easier than with repeated injections (Müller et al. 1984). Refill of the pump needs a medical visit only every 2 to 4 weeks.
- The pump devices actually at our disposal become more and more miniaturized, have a high working precision, a high safety degree and are relatively simple to use.
- External or implanted pumps are well adopted by the patient who feels himself less treatment-dependent than the patients requiring 2-3 top ups per day.
- Patients receiving mostly lower total opioid doses are more alert and also show a higher lucidity (Steppe and Camu 1982).
- Most pump devices need high financial investment and there is an urgent need for more simple and more economical systems.

8.2.3.2 External pumps (Tab. 51 and 84-87)

a) Portable mechanical syringe drivers

These pumps are designed to be connected to a percutaneous catheter or to an implanted port via a special needle. They deliver a certain drug amount per hour, which can be adjusted to the patient's need. The more simple models (e.g. *Graseby MS 26* ®, Fig. 107 in Chap. 20) are easy to handle (Chrubasik et al. 1985 k; Eimerl et al. 1986 a, b) but they allow only continuous infusion with a fixed rate. Costs are low when often used for many patients; they also become low when once used for a single patient over a long period.

Other pumps have more complicated programmes, e.g. *Acta-A-pump* ® (Chrubasik 1984 e; Chrubasik et al. 1985 h-j; Meynadier et al. 1985 c; Motsch et al. 1987 b; Müller et al. 1985 d,f, 1988; Reig et al. 1986); *Graseby MS 2000*®; *PCAS Graseby*®, *Harvard mini-Infusor (Bard)*®, (Fig. 106 in Chap. 20) but they require a higher investment.

b) Portable volumetric reservoir infusors

These devices are battery-driven peristaltic or roller pumps. The pump delivers the opioid solution at a continuous fixed rate with additionally possible bolus injections. There is a refractory period between each bolus. The pumps are quite easy to handle and they are convenient portable models, e.g. *CADD* ® and *CADD PCA* ® (Computerized Ambulatory Drug Delivery system Patient Controlled Analgesia, Pharmacia, Fig. 110), *Chronomat* ® (Fresenius, Fig. 114).

However, their price is quite high because they are much more sophisticated than the simple syringe drivers (Du Pen 1987 e; Eimerl et al. 1986 a, b).

Table 51. Advantages and disadvantages of external infusion devices.

Advantages or disadvantages	Externally stationary pumps	Externally worn pumps	Implanted pumps
- Investment	+	+ +	+ + +
- Miniaturization	+	+ +	+ + +
- Reservoir volume limitations	+	+ +	+ + +
- Mobility of the patient	–	+	+ +
- Infection risks	+ +	+ +	+
- Refill problems	–	–	+ +
- Catheter connection leakage	+	+	+ +

- = nonexistent
+ = number is proportional to high intensity, importance or frequency.

c) The Baxter Travenol Infusor ® (Fig. 111, 112, Tab. 50)

This plastic and disposable infusion system is simple, compact, lightweight, free of motor driven or external energy sources and relatively cheap. The infusor is designed to provide a continuous flow of medication for over about 24 hours. The total content is 60 ml. The delivery rate is 1.8-2.4 ml/h. The medium delivery volume over a whole day is 2.2 ml/h. So, the volume is sufficient for at least one day (Benahmed et al. 1985; Caballero et al. 1986; Ingemar et al. 1987; Krynicki and Hjelmerus 1985; Mok et al. 1986; Pozzi and Caravatti 1985).

Use of the Travenol Infusor for chronic pain treatment:
The infusor regime is initiated in the hospital. The pump is connected to a tunnelled catheter and a microfilter. A test injection with the opioid solution allows an evaluation of effect and duration of pain relief so that the most convenient opiate concentration to meet the requirements for 24 hours can be selected. The patient and a relative are to be instructed in the use of the infusor. Pump refill can be done by a nurse.

After an observation period of 3-4 days, the infusor can be used for home treatment.

Advantages:

- Fluctuations in the pain relief are minimal, due to the mechanical flow at 2ml/h the daily dose of opioid solution is easy to keep constant. Hazardous excess of the administered volume is impossible.
- Progress of the disease or tolerance may necessitate dose increase. This can be done easily by the use of higher opioid concentrations in the same volume.
- The epidurally administered volume each day is relatively high, implying a relative great extension of the pain relief (Ingemar et al. 1987).
- The device is light, easy to carry and handle, the patient is not limited in performing daily functions.
- The opening of the catheter system via a three way stopcock is reduced to once a day instead of several times as required for intermittent injections.
- The same infusor can be used during several days in order to keep treatment costs to acceptable limits.

d) The Pen Pump Infusor®

It is a wearable, lightweight, compact infusor without battery or electronic device (Fig. 113). The solution is delivered with the precision of a micrometer by a simple manual clicking device at the top of the infusor. Each click delivers 0.025 ml of the solution. The dosage knob turned clockwise through 360° produces four clicks and delivers 0.1 ml. The Pen Pump ® is appropriate for multiple daily auto-injections and was initially designed for subcutaneous injections (Henry et al. 1985) .

Advantages:

- low price
- simple to use
- portable.

Drawbacks:

- not programmable
- no alarm
- no security valve
- volume of the syringe is very small (3 ml).

The device is convenient for intrathecal or epidural use of a potent opioid as Sufentanil forte ® (De Castro 1986).

8.2.3.3 Implantable pumps

For longer periods of treatment completely implantable systems have been developed (Tab. 88, 89, Figs. 115-119). Connected to an epidural or intrathecal catheter they deliver certain drug amounts over periods of 1-3 weeks until the next refill.

Theoretically, the complete implantation should reduce the infection rate. Practically, these systems certainly increase the patient's mobility and make care and daily life easier.

Required properties of implanted pumps:

- high biocompatible material
- corrosion- and polymerization-free
- inert, durable
- resistant to autoclave (121°C)
- resistant to ethylene oxide sterilization
- easy to mould in complex shape
- easy to handle
- antibacterial filter must be included
- its life expectancy must be sufficient
- the working mechanism should avoid all risks of involuntary administration
- the price should be acceptable (Lazorthes and Verdie 1988 a).

Up to now, the cost of these devices, which are not reusable, exceeds 5000 US $.

a) The Infusaid system: full implantable non-programmable pump

The Infusaid® system (Fig. 118, 119), is as yet the only completely self-powered implantable device designed for continuous infusion of opioids.

The system consists of :

- a drug chamber (50 ml)
- a charging fluid chamber.

The two chambers are seperated by a metal bellow. The charging fluid chamber is filled with a two-phase (gas-liquid) fluorocarbon which generates a vapour pressure on the drug chamber. The constant pressure of the charging fluid (freon) exerted on the reservoir expels the drug causing it to flow through the bacterial filter, flow restrictor, and out of the outlet catheter.

The pressure in the fluid chamber varies with the temperature and filling conditions (because of the recoil force of the bellows). A change of 1 C° induces a difference of internal pressure of ±4%. The flow rate is fixed with small variations as a function of the filling level. The flow difference beween a full and an empty drug chamber is ±7% (Franetzki 1984).

It is impossible to change the flow rate after implantation.

The device is refillable by percutaneous puncture through the inlet septum. During each refill procedure the act of forcing a drug into the pump's reservoir simultaneously reenergizes the charging fluid.

Several models of the basic Infusaid pump are available. These models are distinguished by the size of the drug chamber and the optional presence of a side mounted auxiliary drug injection septum. The infused flow rate is 1-6 ml/day corresponding to maximal 20-120 mg morphine per day (Greenberg 1986; Harbaugh et al. 1982; Krames et al. 1985; Lazorthes et al. 1985 c; Lazorthes and Verdié 1988 a; Müller et al. 1985 g; Onofrio 1983 b; Paice 1986; Penn and Paice 1985 c; Shetter et al. 1986; Weigel et al. 1986, e.g.). The flow rate is related to the osmolality and thus to the concentration of morphine. With higher concentrations the flow is decreased (Rippe et al. 1984).

b) Implantable programmable pumps

Three models were experimentally used:

- Promedos ID1 ® (Fig. 115 in Chap. 20): implantable delivery device, DFA-1-S, combined with the external programming and control device PFA-1, manufactured by Siemens (withdrawn from market).
- Synchromed; not yet introduced (Penn et al. 1984; Penn and Kroin 1985 a; Penn 1985 b).
  These two pumps facilitate the telemetric coupling with an external programmer monitor device.
- Pacesetter (only an experimental model is available).

The implantable multi-programmable system
(Synchromed ® or Medtronix's DAD-mod 8600 or 8610) (Fig. 116, 117 in Chap. 20).

The system is composed of two parts.

- An implantable infusion pump (DAD) which consists of:
  - a lithium thionyl chloride battery
  - a radio frequency receiver and antenna
  - a microprocessor

- a reservoir (20 ml) with rubber septum and catheter
- a bacterial retentive filter (0.22 μm)
- a rotary pump (peristaltic)
- a titanium enclosure.
- An external non-invasive programmer for the individual pump prescriptions.

The programmer is the external non-invasive component of the system and controls the administration functions of the DAD by telemetry. Establishing a two-way radio frequency link the programmer transmits interrogation to the DAD and receives status information concerning the pump (battery status, volume, dose). The programmer can also modify the delivery profile.

The implantable programmable infusion pump DAD No. 8610 allows for different programmable parameters:

- measurements in micrograms, milligrams, milliliters
- infusion rates from 0.009 ml/hour to 0.9 ml/hour
- delivery as bolus, multi-step bolus, continuous, continuous-complex, bolus delay.

At the moment the pump device can only be connected to Medtronic Silastic catheters.

Adaptation possibility to individual needs of the patient is the great advantage of this programmable system.

Programmable implantable pump Infusaid ® Model 1000

This programmable implantable pump is powered by positive pressure (freon), while the drug flow rate is governed by battery powered electronics. The pump consists of the same parts as the constant flow pump, and additionally an electronic port connected to a valving system. The vapour pressure of freon forces the drug from the reservoir through a filter to a first valve. When this valve opens, fluid passes into an accumulator in the valving system. According to the programming, a second valve opens, allowing a certain volume of the drug to flow from the accumulator through the catheter.

The valve accumulator electronics are controlled using a hand-held programmer with display. The programmer programs the pump into a constant flow, periodic flow, multiple rates flow or single bolus mode. The flow rate can be adjusted from 0.001 to 0.5 ml/h.

The pump allows for alarm function and self-diagnosis. The programmer has an interface for connection to a computer, plotter or modem.

The implantable pump has a usable volume of 22 ml and a sideport for bolus injections (Fig. 119 b, c). The battery life time extends from 5 to 8 years.

c) Intracerebroventricular injection devices

The use of injection devices for intracerebroventricular administration of opioids have been studied by many authors, e.g. Batier et al. (1985; Batier (1986); Blond et al. (1986); Lazorthes et al. (1985 b); Lefebvre et al. (1985); Lenzi et al. (1985); Lobato et al. (1983, 1985, 1986); Meynadier et al. (1985 a); Nurchi (1984); Obbens et al. (1987); Roquefeuil et al. (1984 a); Roquefeuil (1986 a); San Emetrio and Izquierdo (1985); Serrie et al. (1986); Thiebaut et al. (1985); Weigel et al. (1985 a, b; 1986).

8.2.4 DRESSINGS

For the fixation of the catheter on the skin every dressing can be used, but for the puncture site itself the characteristics of the dressing are essential for long-term use. (Fig. 72, 73)

8.2.4.1 Transparent dressing

Aplicat (Beiersdorf), Bioclusive (Johnson), Ensure (Goedecke), Opsite (Braun) or Tegaderm (3M) dressings.

Advantages:
Transparent dressings have interesting properties (Duffy 1981 c):

- thin, transparent, elastic
- adherent for several days
- low allergic potential
- moisture, vapour and air permeable.

The dressing is placed over a simple loop of the catheter:

- providing a good anchorage
- allowing direct inspection.

Not all those properties have been clinically confirmed.

Drawbacks:

- not completely moisture permeable
- cannot be combined with unguent at the puncture site. After some days, the skin

may be affected, the dressing loosens, so it cannot be tolerated at the same place over a long period
- expensive.

8.2.4.2 Cross elastic wound dressing:

(Hansapor ® steril)

Advantages:

- air and moisture permeable
- allows povidone-iodine-unguent at the puncture site
- is tolerated over many months without skin reactions
- less expensive.

Drawbacks:

- not transparent
- not waterproof.

8.2.4.3 Unguent

The only existing disinfectant unguent is povidone-iodine-unguent. For cover of the puncture site povidone-iodine-unguent (Braunovidon, Betaisodona) is recommended (Zenz et al. 1981 g). Contrary to most others, this unguent is not an antibiotic with limited spectrum and possible resistance development (Fig. 74).

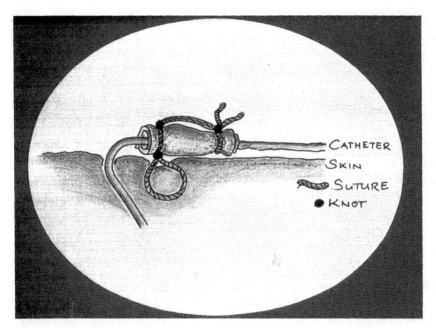

Fig. 74. Catheter fixation with' a non-resorbable subcutaneous suture, sleeve and povidone unguent (Zenz 1981 j).

8.3 Drug administration techniques

Before puncture of the skin a careful disinfection is performed with povidone-iodine solution. The skin over the interspace as well the ligamenta are infiltrated with prilocaine 2% (total amount 2-3 ml).

8.3.1 SINGLE SHOT TECHNIQUE

Spinal opioids due to their long duration of action can be given as a single injection for acute pain treatment. However, indications for such a single shot spinal opioid application seems at least questionable in view of the possible side effects.

8.3.1.1 Epidural

With a 18 gauge *Crawford needle* the epidural space is identified in the usual way by loss of resistance (Covino and Scott 1985; Zenz et al. 1985 c; Macintosh

1985). The level of injection is in the lumbar region. Preferentially, a lipophilic opioid is injected, e.g. 0.3 mg buprenorphine or 50 µg sufentanil in 10 ml saline 0.9 %.

8.3.1.2 Intrathecal

A 25 or 26 gauge *Quincke-Babcock* needle is advanced through an introducer until the subarachnoid space is reached. The stylet remains in place until a feeling of puncturing the dura (a very fine click) is recognized. Diamorphine 0.5 mg or morphine 0.2 mg in 10% glucose solution (hyperbaric) are injected.

8.3.2 Catheter placement

Different indications have been proposed for intrathecal or epidural catheters in acute pain treatment. We cannot fully agree with these differential indications, because in acute pain therapy the rate of side effects is clearly higher in the intrathecal route (Zenz 1982 f). So, for postoperative pain treatment we exclusively use epidural catheters. In contrast, for chronic treatment, e.g. in cancer pain, both the epidural and intrathecal route of administration are justified. These indications are rather based on previous failures or differences in local situations.

Indications for an epidural catheter:

- pain localization below the diaphragm
- patient does require very high doses of opioids by the systemic route for pain control
- side effects of systemic opioids.

Indications for an intrathecal catheter:

- patient has had previous back surgery
- patient has a cancer related spinal block
- patient requires high doses of opioids by the epidural route
- patient's pain is not localized above the diaphragm.

Indications for an intracerebroventricular catheter:

- patient's pain is localized above the diaphragm
- pain not controllable by oral, epidural, or intrathecal opioids.

Method

The method of catheter placement is the same for the epidural and intrathecal space. For both methods a disposable18 gauge Tuohy needle with centimeter markings to identify the depth is introduced. The catheter is introduced through the needle. We use a polyamide catheter with an open tip and centimeter markings. The catheter is advanced 3 cm into the adjacent space, and no further than 3 cm.

Before fixation of the catheter identification of the correct catheter position is performed. For the intrathecal space we use 1.5 ml hyperbaric mepivacaine 4%. For the epidural space we inject first 4 ml mepivacaine 2% with epinephrine 1/200,000 to (relatively) exclude intrathecal or intravasal catheter position. Within five minutes we control heart rate, blood pressure and sensible block. When no signs of spinal anaesthesia or intravasal drug action are seen, the test dose is completed to verify the epidural catheter position using about 5 ml of prilocaine 2%.

After correct catheter placement povidone-iodine-unguent is applied on the puncture site. The catheter is taped with a little sloop around the puncture site, and over the back to the infraclavicular groove. At the catheter end a micropore filter is connected.

8.3.3 PERCUTANEOUS CATHETER FIXATION

For longer periods of treatment we perform a percutaneous catheter fixation (Zenz et al. 1981 j). We make a skin suture about 1 cm distally to the puncture site with 2/0 mersilene and a triangular needle. An air knot is made. A short piece of adhesive tape (Leukoplast) is closely rolled around the catheter directly at the place leaving the skin. Around this tape the suture is fixed. The tape prevents catheter obstruction by the suture or the suture from being loose around the catheter (Fig. 72, 73).

8.3.4 SUBCUTANEOUS TUNNELLING

Subcutaneous tunnelling is an alternative means of catheter fixation for long-term treatment (Carl et al. 1984; Campailla 1985; Cherry 1987 a, d; Meier 1982), (Fig. 75, 76).

Theoretical *advantages* and disadvantages of tunnelling compared to percutaneous introduction (Tschirner and Zeuner 1987):

- infection risk is expected to be lower
- possibility of catheter displacement is lower
- nursing problems are more simple
- patient's comfort is increased especially in personal hygiene
- tunnelling and extunnelling need a surgical intervention.

Implantation methods

The Carl and Crawford method:

- A catheter is inserted to the lumbar region, using a Tuohy needle.
- After removal of the needle, an incision is made in the adjacent skin.
- A local anaesthetic solution (e.g. prilocaine 1%) is injected subcutaneously using a 120 mm needle along the line chosen for the tunnel.
- The tunnel extends from the midline posterior to the left or right iliac region.
- A small incision is made approximately 11 cm lateral to the original midline incision.
- A tunnelling needle is passed posteriorly, so that the catheter tips emerges through the original midline incision.
- The catheter is passed through the tunnelling needle and the needle is removed.
- This procedure is repeated once or twice and the incisions are closed with nylon sutures.
- The catheter is anchored in the iliac region in the following way.

The catheter is passed through a 2 cm length of plastic tubing from a 23 gauge "Butterfly" infusion set and fixed to the skin with a non-absorbable suture. The catheter and the "Butterfly" tubing are then glued together. The suture and catheter are passed through a short piece of tubing (3 mm) and a knot is tied around this. The advantages of the latter method are that catheter-kinking is relatively impossible and the fixation to the skin is very stable.

The part of the catheter protruding through the skin is covered by a colostomy bag for protection. A micropore filter (Sterifix) is attached to the end of the catheter.

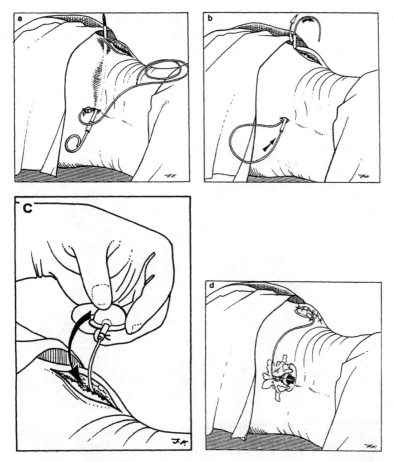

Fig. 75 a, b, c, d. Schematic representation of the implantation technique of a tunnelled catheter and an injection port.

a) The catheter is in IT or ED position, the metallic guide covered by a plastic sheath (A.H.S.) is in subcutaneous position.
b) Withdrawal of the plastic sheath positioned the catheter under the cutis of the anterior chest wall.
c) Introduction of the injection port in the subcutaneous breast pocket and connection with the tunnelled catheter.
d) Port connected with the implanted spinal catheter.
(Adapted from Laugner et al. 1985)

The Campailla method:

- The tunnelling is performed using a 15 cm long 16 G (Longdwell B D) intravenous cannula.
- The cannula (plus needle) is inserted through the skin after a weal is raised 15 cm lateral to the insertion site (incision in the midline should be made before

242

the extradural catheterization); local anaesthesia of the tunnel is performed while the cannula is advanced under the skin, a syringe filled with local anaesthetic being attached to the needle.

- Once the insertion site is reached, the needle is withdrawn and an external catheter is passed through the cannula (which is removed at the end of the procedure). This procedure is repeated until the desired site is reached.

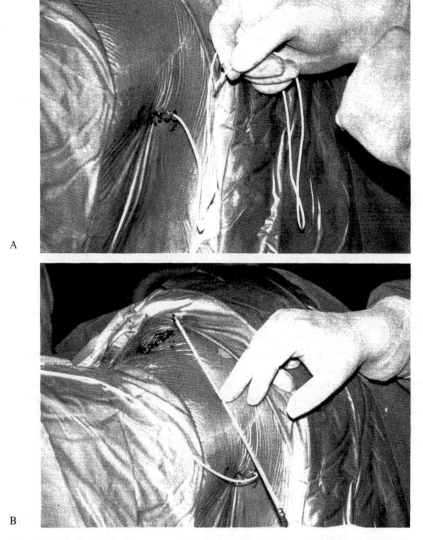

A

B

Fig. 76 a, b, c, d. Surgical sequences of the implantation of a tunnelled intrathecal catheter and an A.H.S. injection port.
(Blond et al. 1985 c)

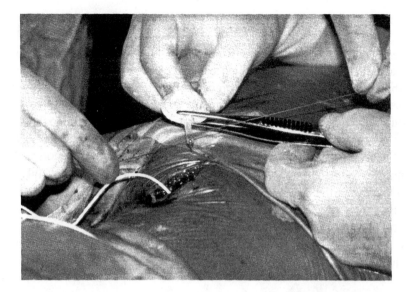

C

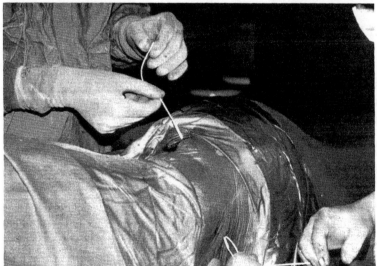

D

Fig. 76 c, d.

- With this modification the length of the tunnel is shorter, the iliac region is reached with a couple of tunnellings (the catheter needle can be bent during the insertion to follow the curves of the patient's skin).

8.3.5 PORT IMPLANTATION

The implantation of the port is performed in the operation room using surgical aseptic conditions under regional anaesthesia. The patient is lying in a lateral decubitus position. A skin pocket is prepared in the anterior chest wall on the 10th rib or on the fascia of the upper abdomen.

Four non-absorbable ligatures are prepared to fix the port close to the ribs in order to avoid migration. In a second step the catheter is tunnelled subcutaneously to reach the pocket. Then the catheter is cut near to the port and the connection is made. The catheter is inserted into a metal screw tube and connected via a thin metal tube and a silicon buffer with the port. After a test injection with saline the portal is finally fixed. The wound is closed and a test injection of opioid can be given (Abou-Hatem et al. 1985).

Fig.75 and 76 give a schematic representation of the implantation technique of a tunnelled spinal catheter and an injection port.

8.3.6 PUMP IMPLANTATION

8.3.6.1 Implantation technique for the Infusaid ® pump

The implantation is performed in the operation room under thoracic epidural anaesthesia (0,5% bupivacaine) or general anaesthesia (Fig.77, 78). The patient is lying in a lateral decubitus position. The implantation procedure is performed in 3 stages:

The first stage: preparation of the pump:

- The pump in the closed container is put on an electric warming pad (30-40°C) for 30 minutes.
- The electric warming pad is covered with a sterile cloth.
- The pump (without container) is placed on the sterile cloth.
- The patency of the pump is tested through the side port.
- Five ml saline are injected into the drug chamber via an extension tube.
- Free reflux of the injected 5 ml is controlled.
- Fifty ml drug containing solution are injected.
- Needle and extensive tube are removed.
- After 15 minutes there must be free flow out of the catheter end.

The second stage: placement of the epidural or intrathecal catheter:

- The skin is incised until the supraspinal ligament.
- The Tuohy needle is advanced through the skin incision into the epidural or intrathecal space.
- The catheter is introduced through the needle and advanced 3 cm into the adjacent space.
- Correct placement of the catheter is confirmed by contrast medium radiography.
- The Tuohy needle is withdrawn.
- The catheter is armed with a 2 cm piece of another, bigger catheter (e.g. jugularis interna catheter).
- The armed piece of the catheter is fixed with a non-absorbable suture to the superficial ligament.
- Free patency through the catheter is documented by a new contrast medium injection.

The third stage: implantation of the pump:

- A transverse incision of the lateral abdominal wall is made under the ribs.
- The pocket must be great enough to accommodate the pump.
- The pocket must go down to the fascia to guarantee good fixation.
- The Infusaid reservoir is implanted into the pocket.
- The catheter from the pump is subcutaneously tunnelled to the back incision, where it is connected to the epidural catheter with a straight metal connector.
- Contrast medium injection through the side port of the pump confirms free patency.
- All incisions are surgically closed without drains.

Following the surgical procedure the patient remains under observation in the hospital for 3-5 days to assess the opioid response. Prior to discharge, patient and family are informed on the implanted system and the possible side effects.

According to the pump profile (ml/day) the next hospital visit is arranged with the patient to perform the next refill.

8.3.6.2 Implantation technique for the Synchromed ® pump

The catheter placement and the product preparation are the same as in the above mentioned case of the Infusaid pump. There are only differences in preparation of the pump.

Under sterile conditions the pump is filled with 20 ml of the opioid solution. The pump is covered by a sterile cloth. The programmer is held over the pump and the pump status is programmed. Then, a delivery rate of 0.9 ml/hour is programmed. It has to be waited until free patency from the catheter end is documented.

The pump is now programmed in the stop position and implanted. After implantation the pump can be programmed for the individual parameters of the patient.

8.3.7 INTRACEREBROVENTRICULAR PORT IMPLANTATION

For the administration of opioids by the intracerebroventricular route Leavens's technique is applied (Leavens et al. 1982). The operation is performed under local anaesthesia. A rectangular Holter catheter is inserted in the lateral ventricle. With the aid of a trepan hole in the skull the cannula normally used for the measurement of intracraneal pressure is inserted. The catheter is connected with an injection port (1.3 ml) and completely implanted under the scalp. The port is refilled transcutaneously with an insulin syringe and a hypodermic needle.

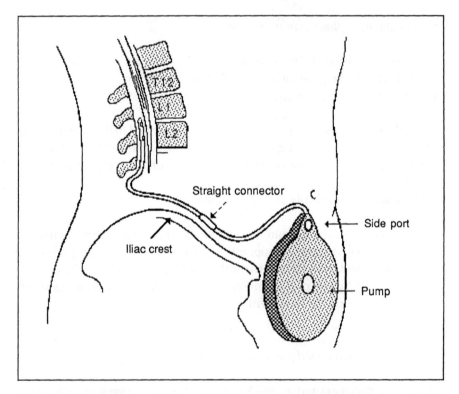

Fig. 77a. Schematic diagram of the Infusaid pump with catheter in the epidural space at L1-L2. The pump is emptied and refilled using a Huber needle. The side port of the pump can be used for bolus injections of the opioid if needed.

(Adapted from Greenberg 1986)

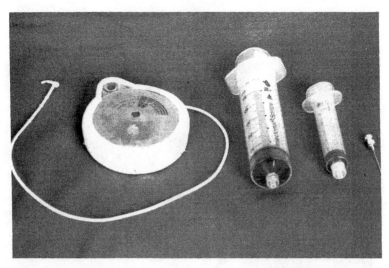

Fig. 77b. Preoperative preparation and control of the Infusaid pump.
Material needed: pump,
50 ml syringe for pump filling,
10 ml syringe for side port injection,
Huber point needle.

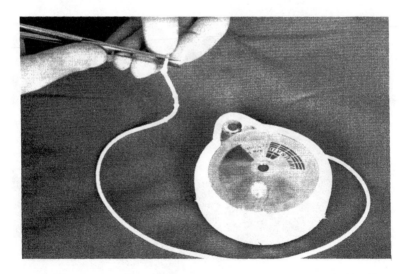

Fig. 77 c. The catheter tip is opened.

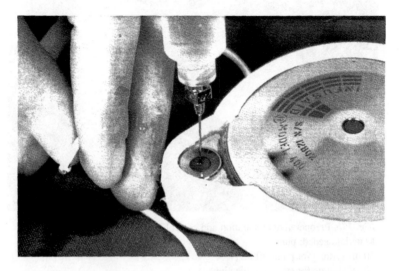

Fig. 77 d. Injection into the side port for control of patency.

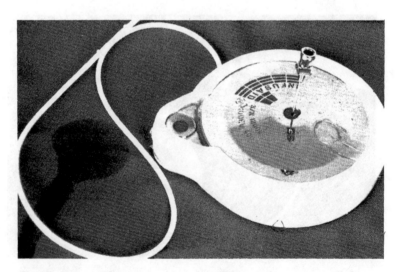

Fig. 77e. Puncture of the pump with an open Huber needle to evacuate all air.

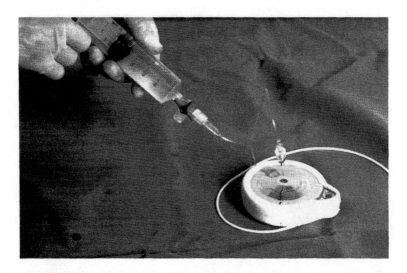

Fig. 77 f. The pump is filled with 50 ml of the opioid solution.

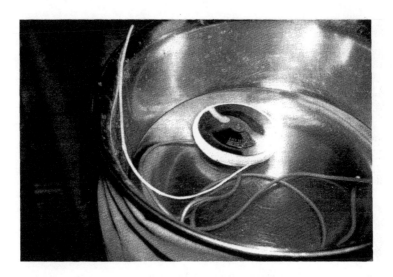

Fig. 77g. Upwarming of the pump in sterile water of 38°C.

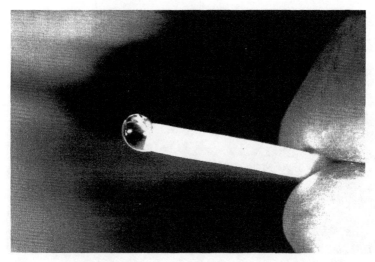

Fig. 77h. As soon as a drop appears at the catheter tip, the pump is ready for implantation.

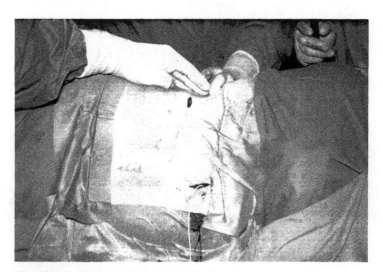

Fig. 78 a. Surgical sequences of pump implantation.
The catheter is injected to the epidural or intrathecal space and visible at the midline incision.

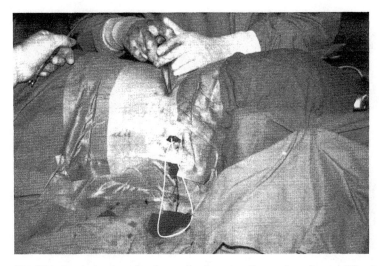

Fig. 78 b. Surgical sequences of pump implantation. Preparation of a tunnel for the catheter.

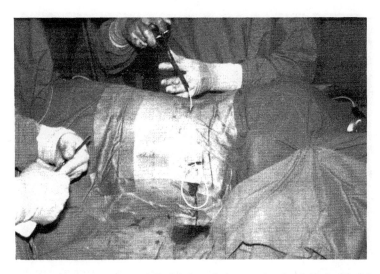

Fig. 78 c. The catheter is carefully led through the tunnel to the abdominal incision.

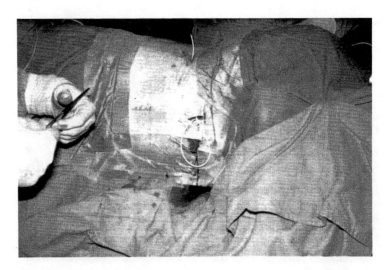

Fig. 78 d. Surgical sequences of pump implantation. The catheter tip has passed the tunnel.

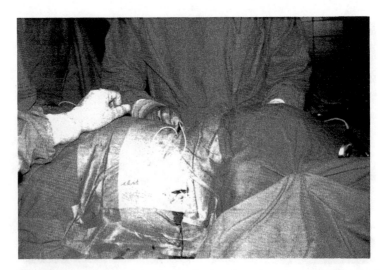

Fig. 78 e. The midline incision is closed, when the catheter is positioned correctly within the tunnel.

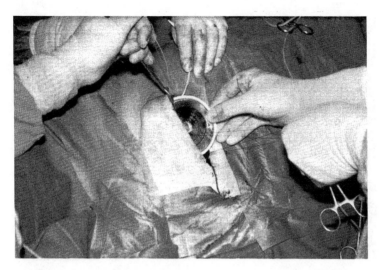

Fig. 78 f. Surgical sequences of pump implantation. A pocket for the pump is prepared.

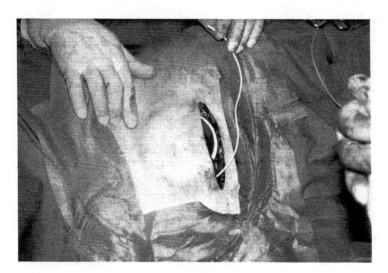

Fig. 78 g. Control of correct pump position.

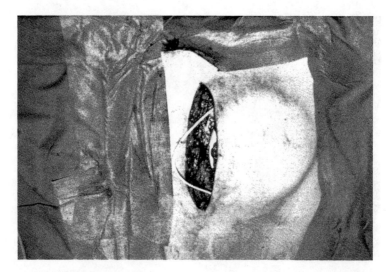

Fig. 78 h. Surgical sequences of pump implantation. After connection of pump and catheter the pump is fixated with 4 sutures to the abdominal fascia.

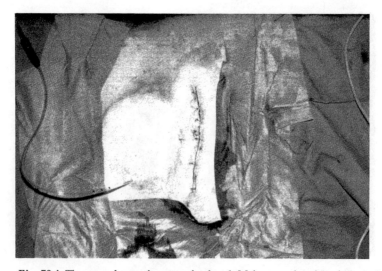

Fig. 78 i. The wound over the pump is closed. Make sure that there is enough distance between incision and pump septum.

8.3.8 Injection into a port, refill of a pump

Injections into ports or pumps always have to be performed under sterile conditions (Fig. 79):
- The port/pump position is palpated.
- The skin over the port/pump is widely and carefully disinfected (povidone-iodine).

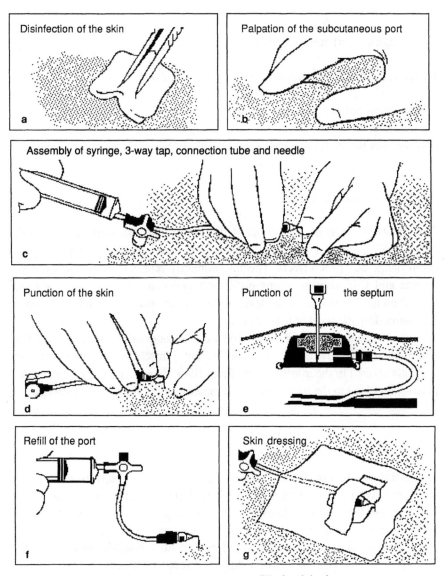

Fig. 79a-g. Nursing sequences for the percutaneous refill of an injection port.

- The centre of the port/pump is injected percutaneously with a Huber point needle.
- The rest volume of the pump can be withdrawn for verification of proper needle position.
  It is very important to be absolutely sure about the right needle position before injecting an opioid.
- The port/pump is filled with the calculated amount of opioid solution.
- After the procedure the skin is carefully washed once more with a disinfectant.

8.3.9 INJECTION-INFUSION TECHNIQUES

Three types of administration of opioids can be chosen:

- intermittent bolus injections
- continuous infusion
- continuous infusion plus on-demand bolus (Fig. 80, 81).

Intermittent bolus injections

They can provide good pain relief if the reinjections are well-adapted to the duration of action of the selected opioid. The doses must be small enough to avoid dangerous peak effects. The intermittently repeated doses must provide plasma and CSF concentrations oscillating between a narrow security band, limited on the lower side by the level of insufficient pain relief and on the upper side limited by the level of toxic effects.

During chronic treatment bolus injections in outpatients are performed by home nurses, family physicians, the patient himself or relatives who are specially trained in the injection technique, filter change and catheter care. All persons involved in the treatment have a schedule over the actual treatment.

Continuous infusion

The technique of continuous infusion provides a very effective analgesia, sometimes with lower doses. It is anticipated that this technique produces less frequent and less severe side effects. It is anticipated as well that continuous infusion induces a lower risk for the development of tolerance (Harmer et al. 1985; Cousins and Mather 1984 b; El Baz et al. 1984; Müller et al. 1988). Nevertheless, continuous infusion during chronic treatment is not always as

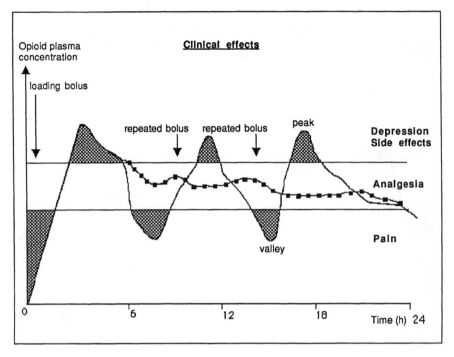

Fig. 80. Analgesia methods: comparison of the opioid effects obtained with a repeated bolus method and with a continuous infusion method.

Continuous infusion: - no peak and valley effects
                         - more comfortable analgesia
                         - with lower doses
                         - with less side effects

Conventional opioid therapy
Continuous infusion

ideal as theoretically anticipated. The suggested higher effectiveness is not always documented by the reality. So, Coombs et al. (1985 a) reported that in some cases even continuous intrathecal morphine plus clonidine was not effective enough and requested additional oral narcotics (Coombs et al. 1985 a).

Continuous infusion is performed with implantable pumps or with external pumps connected to a percutaneous catheter or to a port.

For the postoperative use of continuous epidural infusion with small pumps it is essential to count the minimal effective volume before deciding for one pump model, e.g. the volume of most insulin pumps is too small for this indication.

In Tables 48 and 49 several lipophilic opioids are presented as an example of the volumes needed.

258

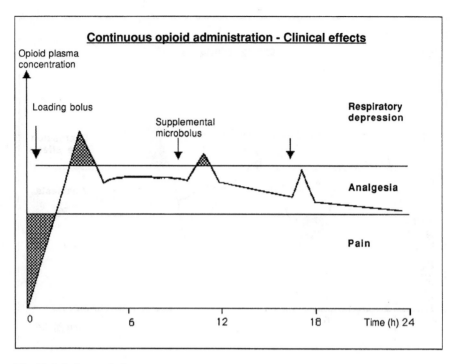

Fig. 81. Infusion methods:

Three-step method for continuous infusion regimen:
a) loading bolus
b) maintenance infusion
c) on-demand supplement microbolus

The graph shows the theoretical relationship between:
- plasma/opioid concentration
- clinical analgesia effects
- dosing interval

Continuous infusion plus on-demand bolus

This administration modality is an attempt to combine the advantages of the continuous infusion with those of the intermittent injections, which are possibly necessary during pain peaks.

The best results are obtained with a *three-step method:*

1. loading dose
2. continuous infusion at a relatively low basal rate in order to avoid any risk of overdose by accumulation
3. intermittent bolus, given on-demand, as soon as pain relief becomes insufficient.

The danger of this method is that the patient has a certain amount of opioid at his/her disposal. To this end, possibly the danger of abuse is increased.

Advantages and drawbacks of the different injection modalities will be discussed in more detail later.

8.3.10 PROS AND CONS OF CONTINUOUS INFUSION

Optimal analgesic results are only achieved by adequate, constant but not excessive CSF levels of the opioid. Such a situation, can best be obtained by a sustained release of the opioid solution near the opioid receptors. To achieve this objective, infusion pumps are used (Tab. 52).

Table 52. Advantages and disadvantages of continuous infusion for epidural or intrathecal opioids.

1 - ADVANTAGES
- Analgesia is more stable, more constant depth and efficacy are increased
- Opioid blood concentration is more stable
- Volume is lower without loss of efficiency
- Total opioid dose is reduced (- 30 %)
- Use of short acting opioids is possible
- Side effects are lower in severity and frequency

respiratory depression
nausea and vomiting
drowsiness
urinary retention
pruritus

- Tolerance develops slower
- Nursing is easier
- Patient is less treatment-dependent

2 - DISADVANTAGES
- Over- and undertreatment may be possible
- Risk of overdose by self-medication exists but is very low
- Cost of pump devices is high
- Refilling problems may occur
- Mechanical failure is always possible
- Spontaneous pain remission may not be noticed

8.3.10.1 Advantages:

- Low-flow continuous opioid infusion produces more stable direct local effects than repeated bolus administration (Chrubasik 1984 a, c; Motsch and Robert 1987 a).

- Pain relief is more complete. Increased depth and efficacy are noted (Sagnard et al. 1987; Blanloeil et al. 1987).

According to Raj et al. (1985), continuous opioid infusion installed over a 3 day period after a major surgical intervention provides 33% more pain relief than that obtained by more conventional methods of pain treatment.

- Pain relief is more constant, without peak CSF levels and peak effects or interruption of the pain control due to delay in administration of analgesics as seen with intermittent dose schedules (Müller et al. 1985 b, d; Nordberg et al. 1983).

- The opioids can be given in a lower volume and the reduction of the injection volume does not result in a loss of analgesic efficacy (Chrubasik et al.1985 f).

- Side effects are lower in severity and frequency. The short, but high, peak concentrations produced by bolus injections are responsible for higher vascular reabsorption and more intensive spread to higher cerebral structures (Müller et al. 1985 f, g). Respiratory depression, sedation, drowsiness, urinary retention, (<20%), pruritus and nausea are rare, infection risk might be lower than with repeated injection (Eimerl et al. 1986 b; Delhaas et al. 1984).

- It has been stated that continuous epidural infusion, compared to intermittent bolus injections, allows a reduction of 30% of the total opioid doses (Coombs et al. 1982 b, d; El Baz et al. 1984). Comparable studies have been done for continuous intravenous infusion of opioids by numerous authors. For continuous epidural administration only El Baz et al. (1984) performed an investigation that allows a comparison between the doses needed for different administration modalities. The results were indeed in favour of continuous infusion.

- Continuous infusion of opioids allows the use of short acting lipophilic substances, e.g. buprenorphine, fentanyl, sufentanil, providing a lower risk of late respiratory depression (Donadoni et al. 1985; Frings et al. 1982 a; Parker et al. 1985).

During chronic pain treatment, also several advantages may be expected:

- Lower incidence of catheter complications can be expected if a closed infusion system is adopted.
- Lower risk of delayed respiratory depression: the long-term infusion of low concentrations of opioids ensures that the absolute level of the analgesic in the spinal space will be low at any given moment, compared with the concentrations

that are achieved in the CSF when a dose sufficient for long-term pain relief is administered in a single shot. It seems reasonable to assume that the CSF concentrations of an opioid infused in low concentrations over a long period of time will be as such that a bolus redistribution rostrally becomes unlikely (Onofrio et al. 1981). However these are theoretical considerations. Clinical data clearly show that a respiratory depression has never been developed in a cancer patient after pure epidural opioid treatment given by the epidural lumbar route, even in high concentration, in high volume and in a single shot.

- Slower development of tolerance? This statement is however not always evidenced by well-controlled investigation. But it can be admitted that the continuous infusion of opioids, in quantities just sufficient to produce a degree of receptor activation associated with adequate analgesia, can minimize the frequency of late respiratory depression and tolerance produced by oversaturation of the receptors.

Tung et al. (1980 a and 1982 a) and Yaksh (1983 a), showed that in animals, intermittent bolus injections provide repeated and short occupancy of the opioid receptors with rebound opiate effects and activation of tolerance development and hyperalgesia. The risk of tolerance development can be reduced by giving the opioid in continuous infusion. Cousins and Mather (1984 b); Delhaas et al. (1984); Glynn and Mather (1982); Müller et al. (1984, 1986 a, 1988); Motsch and Robert (1987 a); Onofrio et al. (1981); Reig et al. (1986) and Weigel et al. (1985 a), reported that the same phenomenon is true in the clinic.

Muller et al. (1982) noted three weeks after bolus opioid administration, a clear cut appearance of a tolerance phenomenon in 15% of 150 patients. He replaced the intermittent bolus injection technique by a continuous infusion with external or implanted pump devices. After such a treatment in 20 patients with a carcinoma he noted the same 15% opioid tolerance but now only after 4 or 6 months. The opioid increase in these patients was of the same importance but the phenomenon was transient and the problem could be solved by a temporary substitution by local anaesthetics.

Unfortunately, the reduction of tolerance by continuous opioid infusion does not occur in every case. Rawal and Tandon (1985 d) e.g. failed to confirm the opinions expressed above. Indeed, their ICU patients receiving epidural opioids notwithstanding continuous spinal infusions already required increasing opioid doses after 2 to 3 days.

A withdrawal syndrome may occur during the initial period of the change from a parental or oral opioid regimen to a regimen of continuous infusion. The diagnosis of such a withdrawal syndrome may be misinterpreted as a tolerance phenomenon against the opioid.

8.3.10.2 Drawbacks

Disadvantages of continuous infusion of opioids are mainly limited to pump investment problems. Technical problems can mostly be resolved.

Nothwithstanding continuous opioid infusion during acute pain treatment closely monitoring of the patient during several hours remains indicated.

Patient controlled analgesia (PCA) treatment added to a low background continuous infusion also provides marked advantages; however, also with potential disadvantages. Limitations and contra-indications of each solution must be taken into account.

8.3.10.3 Drug selection for continuous infusion

Most opioids used for intravenous analgesia can also be administered in continuous spinal infusion, but it is important to avoid drugs with long onset latency (buprenorphine), poorly lipid soluble agents equilibrating slowly (morphine) or high accumulation tendency (methadone).

Preferences are to be given to opioids with some particular properties (rapid and short acting) making adaptation to individual responses easier.

Fentanyl, alfentanil, sufentanil are certainly the three most convenient opioid substances for continuous infusion techniques (Tab. 48, 49, 50).

8.4 Nursing

During the use of implanted catheter, ports or pumps, the following potential complications may occur:

- decubitus over reservoir
- skin infection at reservoir
- infection along subcutaneous catheter
- leakage of CSF
- intraspinal infection
- catheter erosion
- catheter tip displacement
- catheter disconnection
- catheter leakage
- reservoir erosion
- reservoir displacement
- reservoir leakage
- reservoir function failure

- difficulty in refilling the reservoir.

Daily nursing
For the nursing of patients wearing percutaneous epidural or intrathecal catheters the following recommendations of Zenz et al. (1980) should be applied:

- Every two days:
    . povidone-iodine scrub bath
    . povidone-iodine-unguent on the puncture site
    . hansapor steril tape
    . millipore filter.
- Every week check control of:
    . the puncture site
    . the opiate consumption
    . the efficacy.

Opioid injection in a percutaneous or a subcutaneous tunnelled catheter
The opioid injections can be performed by home nurses or family physicians. After special instructions the injections can also be done by the patient's family or by the patient himself. The opioid concentration and the lockout time between injections is determined by the primary physician. The injections are performed under the normal conditions of sterile injections through the bacterial filter.

8.4.1 CATHETER PROBLEMS

The insertion of an epidural or intrathecal catheter is usually simple and safe.
   Properly placed and properly managed, epidural catheters can be left in place for prolonged periods. However, from time to time difficulties arise such as:

Possibility of the catheter entering a vein
The possibility of the catheter entering a vein is well known. Usually this occurs at the initial insertion and blood appears in the syringe during aspiration. However a multiple hole catheter can be positioned in a vein without showing blood by aspiration (Bause 1985).

Possibility of the catheter entering the subdural space
The subdural space is the potential space between the dura and the arachnoid membranes. Opioid solutions entering this space can be expected to spread greatly. Unlike the epidural space, which is obliterated above the foramen magnum by the fusion of the dura with the periosteum of the cranium, no limit

is imposed upon the subdural space (Hartrick et al. 1985). Consequently, opioids injected subdurally can produce a substantial and quick rostral diffusion. This hazard, with the possibility of progressive respiratory depression after opioid injection, must be distinguished from the intrathecal migration of the catheter with the risk of sudden apnea or even convulsions.

The respiratory depression appearing after a subdural opioid injection lasts rather longer than after an intrathecal injection.

If placement of the epidural catheter is uncertain, needle and catheter should be simultaneously withdrawn.

Radiographic checking of the catheter with injection of contrast medium may be necessary to make the right diagnosis (Taveras and Wood 1976).

Possibility of the catheter entering in intrathecal space
Given the physical nature of the plastic catheter and the toughness of the dura, migration would appear most unlikely.

Catheters initially placed within the epidural space have, however, been reported to migrate subsequently to intravascular subarachnoidal or even intrathecal positions (Bromage 1985; Hartrick et al. 1985; Landon 1985; Ravindran et al. 1979; Robson and Brodski 1977).

Many of these cases however, can be explained by the design of the catheter, in particular of those with multiple holes. It is quite possible for the distal hole to be in the subarachnoid space (or a vein) while the proximal holes are into the epidural space. As there is a positive pressure in the intrathecal space it is easier for the injected drugs to escape through the holes in the epidural space, especially if a slow injection is given.

A forceful and rapid bolus will lead to a much greater quantity of the drug leaving the distal hole into the intrathecal space. This is a good reason for using a catheter with a single hole (Covino and Scott 1985).

Kinking and clotting
Occasionally it will be found impossible to inject into a catheter. This is due either to kinking or clot-forming in the catheter. The former will usually respond to the withdrawal of 1 cm of the catheter. If the obstruction is due to a clot, there is no solution except to remove the catheter and insert another (Covino and Scott 1985).

Infection
Superficial infection is evaluated to have a frequency of 6%, meningitis is reported in 1%. The overall catheter failure, with percutaneous catheter technique, inadvertent removal included, is evaluated to reach 20% (Coombs 1986 c).

The catheter must be removed in case of:

- dislodgement
- difficulty in injecting the required volume
- pain caused by fluid injection
- redness, irritation or infection of the skin (Müller et al. 1985 a).

Carl et al. (1984) reported the results of a study performed on 100 patients treated for chronic pain with epidural opioids administered by means of subcutaneously tunnelled catheters. Seventy-three per cent of the patients needed only one catheter and 15% had a catheter in place for more than 100 days, the longest period of time having been 434 days. In only 18 patients, was the catheter displaced accidentally from the extradural space. There were no instances of extradural infections although in three patients the tunnel became infected.

8.4.2 PORT PROBLEMS

Incidents and complications due to the implantation:

- catheter disconnection
  . the diagnosis can be made after observing the subsequent inefficiency of the injections
  . the leak can be visualized through opacification
  . surgical repair will arrange this complication
  . prevention by overlapping the catheter ends and by suturing the metal connector to the fascia
- local infection
- transient meningitis
- haematoma
- skin necrosis.

These potential complications impose *preventive measures:*

- eliminate patients with underlying infection
- ensure a thorough subcutaneous hemostasis
- select an implantation site where cutaneous and subcutaneous layers are adequate
- observe strict aseptic precautions during puncturing, emptying and refilling the reservoir (22 gauges angled needles are to be used) (Lazorthes and Verdie 1988 a).

8.4.3 PUMP PROBLEMS

For epidural or intrathecal administration of opioids the ratio of potency to volume has more importance than for intravenous treatments because of the limited volume of portable or implantable devices.

Tab. 46, 48, 49, 50 indicate that the use of a concentrated morphine solution or sufentanil forte provides the possibility of reaching the necessary analgesic levels with the lowest injection volume.

The syringes or reservoirs that can be used with several pump devices are presented in the Technical Addendum (Chap 20).

Early postoperative problems with implanted pumps:

- device and surgery related problems:
    seromas: blood clots in the pocket
- medication related difficulties:
    mild withdrawal symptoms on removing oral or parenteral opioids can be
    well-controlled using oral clonidine.

Patients can leave the hospital within 3 days of implantation. The sutures at the pocket site have to be removed after 7 days. Depending on the factory preset flow rates and other factors, the refill of a 50 ml reservoir (in case of an Infusaid pump) is carried out in the hospital, every 14-20 days.

Pump refill procedure

In any case, the pump refill has to be performed under absolutely sterile conditions:

- disinfection of the skin
- sterile preparation of the injection solution
- local anaesthesia on the injection septum
- puncture of the septum with a Huber point needle
- connection of the needle on a 3-way stopcock to an empty syringe
- reflow of the residual volume, control of pump function and proper needle
    position
- injection of 50 ml of the opioid solution
- sterile dressing (povidone-iodine-unguent).

Supervision

The patient is instructed to control his/her body temperature carefully, because increase in temperature increases the flow rate of the Infusaid pump.

During visits to the clinic the pocket site of the pump is controlled for potential infections, dislocations, seroma.

Conclusions

Progress in biocompatible materials, in electronics and in miniaturization have allowed the development of a great variety of viable drug delivery devices for spinal opioid therapy. Highly sophisticated and very expensive systems have been proposed but also relatively simple and cheap equipment is at our disposal.

The selection of a complicated system may provide perhaps more comfort for the patient but necessitates a high investment, whereas potential infection and mechanical problems cannot be excluded anyhow.

Thus, the most simple settings applied with rigorous care and devoted supervision will often provide the best solution.

Part II

Clinical practice of spinal opioid

administration

9. Clinical applications, generalities

Since the first reports on the successful administration of spinal opioids for pain treatment, the literature has given access to a wide variance of clinical situations, where the new method has been investigated. One of the great dangers of a fascinating method is the extreme extent to which it possibly may be used. Posttonsillectomy pain, sexual dysfunction, postspinal headache are some of the strange indications seen off and on in the literature. Situations, where spinal opioids may act, other methods act as well and are perhaps less dangerous. We have to realize that spinal opioids are not the treatment of choice for all clinical cases with severe pain.

Indications

The different indications for spinal opioids can be divided into different classes:

Very good indications:

- postoperative pain
- severe acute pain (thoracic trauma, polytrauma)
- prostaglandin abortion
- severe chronic pain (cancer pain); especially if this pain does not respond properly to conventional treatment (if oral opioid treatment is insufficient or results in severe side effects)
- intensive care unit patients under mechanical ventilation

Good indications:

- obstetrical analgesia in association with bupivacaine for the first phase of the delivery
- analgesic potentiation of spinal anaesthesia with local anaesthetics
- extracorporeal shock wave lithotripsy

Questionable indications:

- myocardial infarction
- severe vascular pain
- enuresis
- hyperreflexia of the autonomous nervous system
- intraoperative use as analgesic component of general anaesthesia
- differential diagnosis of a pain syndrom
- causalgia
- neurotic pain
- chronic non-malignant pain.

Contra-indications:

- toxicomania, dependence
- technical difficulties
- spinal injuries
- coagulation disorders
- allergy to opioids
- difficulty in supervision of the patient.

Furthermore, the conventional contra-indications for spinal opioids are the same as those for spinal anaesthesia.

10. Intraoperative use

Spinal opioids (with the exception of high doses of intrathecal pethidine) are not able to provide surgical anaesthesia. Nevertheless, they can be used peroperatively in two situations.

1. To provide the analgesic component of:
   general or intravenous anaesthesia
   neuroleptanalgesia.
2. To potentiate spinal anaesthesia with a local anaesthetic.

Epidural as well as intrathecal techniques have been proposed for this goal. However, these techniques may produce an uncontrollable potentiation of the anaesthetics used concomitantly so that they will induce an increased risk of long-lasting postoperative depression.

10.1 Epidural administration

10.1.1 OPIOIDS IN ASSOCIATION WITH GENERAL ANAESTHESIA

The combination of epidural opioids and general anaesthesia has been proposed by Adu-Gyamfi et al. (1983) and Cousins and Mather (1984 b).

Twenty mg epidural morphine for surgical anaesthesia associated with a thiopentone drip 0.04 to 0.1 mg/kg/min and pancuronium 0.1 mg/kg was studied in 33 patients. All patients had satisfactory anaesthesia intraoperatively and postoperative analgesia was lasting from 13 to 24 hours, but respiratory depression was observed in 3 patients (Adu-Gyamfi et al. 1983).

Epidural administration of 250 µg of fentanyl 20 min prior to surgical incision was compared to a same fentanyl dose provided by IV injection. The ED route allowed a reduction of 30% of the isoflurane requirements during thoracotomy. This reduction lasted at least 2 hours (Grant et al. 1989).

Epidural fentanyl combined with a regular neuroleptanalgesia did not prevent the stress-induced increase of ADH (von Bormann et al. 1982 a).

Interindividual dose response variability of ED opioid administration during anaesthesia is a serious weak point for the technique (Ionescu et al. 1989).

In our opinion, epidural opioids are neither indicated nor well suited for combination with general anaesthesia.

10.1.2 EPIDURAL SOMATOSTATIN

Intravenous opioids were replaced by the epidural administration of the neuropeptide somatostatin in 8 patients during major abdominal surgery (Chrubasik et al. 1985 g). An initial epidural bolus of 250 µg followed by continuous infusion of 1 mg/hour was necessary for stable anaesthesia together with pentobarbital 500 mg (for induction), diazepam 5-35 mg, N_2O 66% and regular pancuronium doses. Side effects of somatostatin were not observed and patients were immediately awake and responsive after extubation. Respiratory difficulties were not registered. Associated with the general inhibiting effects of the somatostatin a state of full surgical anaesthesia was obtained. Notwithstanding the absence of opioids in this anaesthesia protocol, the total amount of the used anaesthetics is not neglegible. As the report was not a controlled study, it is not evident whether the results are more a consequence of the relatively great diazepam dose, the N_2O and the relaxant added or of the supplement of epidural somatostatin. The concluded opioid-sparing effect is in no way to be considered as an advantage, as long as clinical results do not support this statement.

At the moment, the intraoperative use of epidural somatostatin remains an experimental setting. Clinical advantages demonstrating a benefit for the patient are lacking. Further investigations must confirm the usefulness before the epidural somatostatin can be recommended as a short-term analgesic.

A recent paper by Desborough et al. (1989) has clearly demonstrated that epidural somatostatin in a dose of 3 mg failed to provide any postoperative analgesia.

10.1.3 EPIDURAL OPIOIDS IN ASSOCIATION WITH LOCAL ANAESTHETICS

Presently, many investigators are becoming increasingly interested in a combination of spinal opioids and local anaesthetics. There is a dual objective with this trend: faster and better analgesia (this is of particular value in obstetrical analgesia), reinforcement and prolongation of the conventional regional anaesthesia by a small dose of a longer acting opioid. The association technique was first presented in 1979 by Lecron at the Congress of the Association of Latin-American Anesthesiologists in Guatemala City. The opioids proposed by Lecron et al. (1980 b) for the epidural association technique are in the order of preference: sufentanil 0.025 mg, buprenorphine 0.15 to 0.3 mg, fentanyl 0.1 to 0.2 mg, alfentanil 0.5 mg, morphine 1 to 2 mg, lofentanil 0.001 to 0.002 mg. One of these opioids may be associated with one of the following local anaesthetics: bupivacaine 0.25%, 0.50%, etidocaine 1%, lignocaine 1%, mepivacaine 2%.

Examples
- Central sedation and an adequate level of anaesthesia during surgery with high

frequency ventilation (HFV) (100% oxygen) may be obtained with 5 mg epidural morphine, small doses of intravenous morphine infusion (0.1 mg/kg/h) and bupivacaine for sympathetic block (El Baz et al. 1983 b). The mean doses given in 15 cases of major thoracic surgery were:
- morphine epidurally 5.7±2.1 mg
- bupivacaine epidurally 47±1.3 mg
- epidural infusion 7.3±1.9 ml/h
- morphine intravenously 7.9±3.2 mg

All patients required the administration of naloxone (mean dose 0.25± 0.23 mg) for reversal of central depression and to re-establish adequate spontaneous breathing. Additional naloxone (0.1 mg) was necessary in 3 patients during the first 24 hours after operation. The authors stated that this anaesthesia technique successfully eliminated the high incidence of awareness frequently observed during HFV. The method, however, presents a high risk of postoperative respiratory depression, and can therefore only be used for ICU patients.

- An experience with 1000 administrations of epidural fentanyl 2 µg + etidocaine 1% with epinephrine was reported by Barré et al. (1984) for hip surgery. Regulary, this type of anaesthesia produced satisfying results.
- Epidural fentanyl 0.09-0.12 mg + etidocaine 1% or bupivacaine 0.5% was also used by Camara et al. (1984) in hip surgery. The results were generally satisfactory. In respect of side effects, there was little difference in the hemodynamic effects between the two local anaesthetics used in association. Etidocaine caused a greater motor block than bupivacaine.

Potential advantages
The combination technique has several advantages:

- analgesia is more constant and deeper
- drug association allows a significant dose reduction for both substances; the necessary doses are reduced by 30% compared to the necessary mean doses needed if the same drugs are used alone.
- onset of analgesia is faster (15 to 30 min) and longer acting (13 to 24h)
- protection against stress is enhanced
- the association might provide a correction of some weak points of the local anaesthetic
- in the case of bupivacaine its slow onset of action is neutralized
- in the case of etidocaine, the action becomes more constant and the sensory block is reinforced
- mixtures of bupivacaine and fentanyl may improve the quality of analgesia without causing a motor block. This may have a practical interest especially in labour (Justins et al. 1982 b).

Potential disadvantages

An improved quality of analgesia and comfort for the patient by the use of a drug association of an opioid and a local anaesthetic is widely admitted.

However, improved safety of the patient is questionable. Safety can only be guaranteed if lower doses of each compound are used.

- If the opioid dose is not reduced, risk of postoperative respiratory depression is increased.
- If the local anaesthetic dose is not reduced peroperative cardiovascular instability may be higher and a rest of motor and/or sympathetic block may persist during the postoperative period.
- Pruritus, nausea and vomiting, and urinary retention are still potential side effects of the association.
- Controlled studies indicating an improved safety of the peroperative use of an association technique do not exist.

Despite the fact of a better and more comfortable pain relief, a better outcome of the patient has not yet been demonstrated with a combination technique. The need of naloxone in all cases reported in the study group of El Baz et al. (1984) indicates that the possible dangers are in excess of the benefits.

A method necessitating the routine antagonization of the administered drugs seems to be at least very questionable in its logical design. It is to point out that the method of El Baz is the association of an epidural block with a local anaesthetic together with an epidural opioid and an intravenous opioid. Facing the potentially dangerous effects induced by the antagonist naloxone and the lack of clear advantages of the combination method, a well-performed balanced anaesthesia seems preferable.

For all the reported indications exist routine techniques which are not involved with such a high incidence of theoretical and practical dangers.

10.2 Intrathecal administration

Administration of 0.75 mg of morphine intrathecally produced a significant higher reduction in anaesthetic requirements than those produced by the same opioid amount given by intramuscular route. The MAC of halothane after intrathecal opioids was 60% of that determined after intramuscular opioids (Drasner et al. 1988 a). However, the postoperative need for naloxone administration was also increased, so that the real advantages of the technique are not clearly established (Drasner et al. 1988 c).

10.2.1 INTRATHECAL MORPHINE IN ASSOCIATION WITH THIOPENTONE ANAESTHESIA

Open heart surgery
Intrathecal morphine (2 and 4 mg) was used in 60 patients undergoing open heart surgery under general anaesthesia (Aun et al. 1985). Patients were electively ventilated postoperatively, so that respiratory depression was not a problem. Intrathecal morphine has provided useful postoperative analgesia. 4 mg was the most effective dose. Patients with peroperative intrathecal morphine appeared during the postoperative period to be more alert and cooperative when performing pulmonary function tests.

Major abdominal surgery
Intrathecal morphine 1 mg given prior the induction of general anaesthesia, allowed in one series for more rapid extubation of the patients and provided longer postoperative analgesia (Chester et al. 1987).

Scoliosis surgery
Intraoperative intrathecal morphine for postoperative pain control following corrective scoliosis surgery with the Harrington rod instrumentation, was used in children by Broadman et al. (1987). The opioid was injected prior to closing into the intrathecal space under direct vision. Profound postoperatory analgesia lasting 8 to 25 hours was obtained in 90% of the cases. No patients required ventilatory support. Pruritus and nausea were frequent. Monitoring during 18 hours in the ICU was required.

10.2.2 INTRATHECAL PETHIDINE FOR SPINAL ANAESTHESIA IN HIGH DOSES (1 MG/KG)

Intrathecal pethidine occupies, in the practice of some clinicians, a special place for intraoperative use because used in high doses it is able to produce surgical analgesia with sympathetic, sensory and motor block (see Section 7.1.3.).

The use of intrathecal pethidine injections of 1 mg/kg, in a water solution of 50% was first proposed for abdominal surgery by Mircea et al. (1982) and Sandu et al. (1981). With this relatively high opioid dose not only real surgical analgesia was obtained but also a motor block, a sensory block and even a sympathetic block (lasting 92 to 120 min) was produced. Such a high dose produced all side effects of local anaesthetics (e.g. hypotension). These effects appeared 20 to 30 min after the injection of pethidine. Intubation of the patient, respiratory assistance and/or administration of vasopressor drugs was in some cases necessary. However, analgesia by itself was of long duration (14 to 20 hours) and delayed respiratory depression was not observed.

Many other investigators have confirmed the initial observations of Mircea in a large number of patients reported in extended observations.

Examples

- The technique was applied in 150 patients. The possibility of performing by the intrathecal route a real surgical anaesthesia with only the use of high doses of intrathecal pethidine was confirmed (Ragot et al. 1984 a, b, c; Janvier et al. 1985).
- One mg/kg intrathecal pethidine was used in 30 patients for surgical interventions on the lower abdomen, perineum or lower extremities. The anaesthesia obtained was similar to that after local anaesthetics with a sequential appearance of sympathetic, sensory and motor block in a mean time of 7.2 min and with a duration of 100-140 min. Side effects were minimal but hypotension was frequent. The duration of postoperative analgesia was 18 hours, on average (Fontanals et al. 1986).
- For major urological surgery of long duration and in high risk patients 1 mg/kg of intrathecal pethidine in hyperbaric solution associated with a very light general anaesthesia was recommended. After the addition of only very small doses of flunitrazepam and fentanyl intubation and mechanical ventilation was possible (Tauzin-Fin et al. 1984, 1987 a).
- Twenty male patients undergoing surgery of the perineal or inguinal area were treated with intrathecal pethidine, in a dose of 1 mg /kg as the sole anaesthetic agent. There was a sensory and a motor block within ten minutes and surgery was performed under complete analgesia. The duration of surgical analgesia was 40 hours (Tauzin-Fin et al. 1984, 1987 a). Analogue results were reported by Cozian et al. (1986); Naguib et al. (1986 b); Saissy (1984 b).
- The same dose of pethidine was also associated with prilocaine 0.5 mg /kg, for a spinal anaesthesia allowing neurological interventions of 1 hour (Famewo and Naguib 1985 a, b; Tauzin-Fin et al. 1987 b).

Particular application: Saddle Block Technique (Tab. 53)

Hyperbaric pethidine 0.5 mg injected intrathecally at L4-L5 or L5-S1 with the patient in a sitting position produces a saddle block within 5-6 min. Sensory block is achieved in the sacrocoxygeal area of the perineum, buttocks and posterior surface of thigh and is followed 1-2 min later by a motor block. The sensory block lasts 2 1/2 hours and is followed by a postoperative analgesia of 6-7 hours (Acalovschi et al. 1986 a, b).

Table 53. Differences between a saddle block with hyperbaric intrathecal pethidine 0.5 mg/kg and hyperbaric intrathecal lignocaine 4%.

	After pethidine: 0.5 mg/kg
- Time of latency until block develops	Longer
- Extension to sensory and motor block	More limited
- Duration of anaesthetic block	No difference
- Postoperative ambulation	Earlier allowed
- Postoperative analgesia	Longer

Side effects

The following side effects were noted in the series of Famewo and Naguib (1985 a, b) and Tauzin-Fin et al. (1984):

- No early or delayed respiratory depression, except one case of severe immediate respiratory depression with cardio-vascular collapse and bradycardia. It was produced by an overdose of intrathecal pethidine (2 mg/kg) and necessitated repeated injections of naloxone.
- Other side effects were: bradycardia 20%, vagal collapse 10%, drowsiness 63%, headache 3%, miosis 12%, nausea 30%, pruritus 25%, sphincter relaxation 6%, urinary retention 10%.

After an intrathecal pethidine saddle block with 0.5 mg/kg side effects are significantly lower than these noted after the high doses: respiratory depression 0%, headache, leg weakness, rigidity 2.7%, pruritus 6.3%, nausea and vomiting 4.5%, urinary retention 1.8%.

Advantages

Reported advantages of the method compared to the intrathecal use of local anaesthetics are:

- Relative stable haemodynamic parameters (in normovolemic patients).
- Sympathetic block with reduced bleeding.
- The technique provides good surgical conditions to perform major perineal interventions in patients in supine position thanks to the excellent motor and sensory block.
- Prolonged postoperative analgesia is obtained and some patients do not require additional opioid analgesics during the postoperative period.
- Possibility to antagonize most side effects by naloxone.

Disadvantages:

- The low safety index of pethidine does not justify the use of high doses of this compound.
- Potential risk of severe hypotension exist.
- Intubation and mechanical ventilation are necessary.
- Peroperative side effects may be serious.
- Possibility of delayed respiratory depression and hypotension necessitates a close and long-lasting postoperative supervision.

It is concluded that intrathecal pethidine, given in a dose of 1 mg/kg may be effective as the sole agent for intrathecal anaesthesia and produces prolonged postoperative analgesia. It may offer an theoretical advantage for painful operations where a prolonged postoperative analgesic effect is desirable.

Significant advantages of the method compared to spinal lignocaine anaesthesia were not always observed (Sangarlangkarn et al. 1987) and above all, the high toxicity of pethidine (see Chapter 7.1.3.) does not allow recommendation of methods using high doses of this compound.

10.2.3 Intrathecal association of opioids with local anaesthetics

Also, the intrathecal combination of an opioid and a local anaesthetic has been recommended. Most clinicians apply the technique proposed by Lecron et al. (1980 a, b, c). In acute pain a combination of an opioid and a local anaesthetic is able to realize an optimal efficacity/safety ratio for peroperative intrathecal pain treatment, if for both classes of drugs the doses are kept low (Cousins 1987 a). The opioids used in association are the same as those used alone by the epidural route.

Doses are as follows :

- morphine 0.2 to 0.5 mg, or
- fentanyl 0.05 to 0.1 mg, or

- buprenorphine 0.1 to 0.2 mg.

The opioid can be associated with 2 ml of a local anaesthetic :

- bupivacine 0.5%, or
- prilocaine or lignocaine 1%, or
- tetracaine 1% (with or without adrenalin 1/200,000).

In order to obtain a hypertonic solution of 4 ml 10% glucose may be added to the drug association.

Examples with positive results

- The association of morphine 2.5 mg and cinchocaine 7.5 mg intrathecally was used for surgery of the hip. With this association postoperative analgesia lasted for more than 22 hours. If cinchocaine was used alone, the analgesia mostly lasted not longer than 8 hours. Side effects of the association were acceptable. Late respiratory depression has not been reported (Moore et al. 1984 b).

- Surgical anaesthesia and postoperative analgesia was obtained with intrathecal morphine 1 mg and amethocaine 12-14 mg for transurethral resection of the prostate. The addition of the opioid to the local anaesthetic produced excellent surgical conditions and significantly less postoperative pain than in patients receiving amethocaine alone. However, the associated side effects were high, e.g.: respiratory depression, nausea, vomiting and pruritus. In the local anaesthetic group no side effects occurred. In contrast, in the combination group 31 side effects were recorded in 12 patients, 50% of the patients had respiratory depression. The authors conclude that 1 mg intrathecal morphine provides excellent analgesia, but due to the danger of respiratory depression the patients have to be returned to an intensive care unit (Cunningham et al. 1983).

- With an intrathecal isobaric preparation containing fentanyl 1 ml (0.005 mg) and bupivacaine 0.5%, 3 ml and glucose 10%, 1 ml results were successful in 96% of the cases. Respiratory depression was not observed and side effects were minimal (Trinh-Duc and Fontes 1987).

Examples with negative results

For other authors neither the epidural nor the intrathecal association of a local anaesthesia with an opioid have provided significant advantages over the common techniques for intraoperative analgesia.

Spinal amethocaine 14 mg in 10% glucose plus morphine 1 mg was used by

Cunningham et al. (1983) for transurethral resection of the prostate. The association compared to amethocaine alone provided better surgical anaesthesia and longer postoperative analgesia. However subtle respiratory depression, nausea, vomiting and pruritus were more frequent.

Personal opinion (M. Zenz)

The needle in place is absolutely no indication to administer a second drug through the needle, even when each single drug might seem advantageous. "Since these patients were already having a needle inserted into the theca, it was decided to inject the morphine through the same needle" (Gjessing and Tomlin 1981). The result can be seen later in the article. "A number of patients developed respiratory depression and two patients went into carbon dioxide narcosis with associated hypertension, tachycardia, sweating and diminution of consciousness." Regional anaethesia with local anaesthetics has been good enough for decades, the combination of local anaesthetics and opioids for intraoperative analgesia is perhaps not better but more dangerous. When postoperative analgesia should be necessary (and certainly it is necessary in most cases), the analgesic for the postoperative period can be given on-demand postoperatively through a catheter. However, in acute pain like in postoperative pain the prophylactic administration of analgesics may be dangerous.

Conclusion

The patient's comfort during the postoperative period is certainly increased by the use of these associations. But no other profits can be demonstrated. On the contrary, side effects may increase by the combination of two drugs.

Further, it has to be evaluated, whether a combination of a peripheral acting analgesic and a well-titrated systemic opioid does not obtain the same analgesic result without the danger of respiratory depression and the need for intensive care surveillance.

10.2.4 INTRATHECAL ASSOCIATION OF AN OPIOID AND CLONIDINE

In order to reduce the required doses of opioids or local anaesthetics and to enhance depth and duration of analgesia, oral, ED or IT clonidine 300-450 µg have been studied (Boico et al. 1989; Engelman et al. 1989; Penon et al. 1989; Veillette et al. 1989). With such an association analgesia is indeed significantly increased and prolonged. However, marked sedation, hypotension and respiratory depression were inacceptable side effects.

Administering an intrathecal association of 0.1 mg morphine + 0.1 mg clonidine to laminectomy patients, the postoperative morphine requirements were significantly decreased during a first 12 hour period (Coombs et al. 1987 b). However, real arguments for the routine use of this method are lacking.

10.3 PARTICULAR PROBLEM: EXTRACORPOREAL SHOCK WAVE LITHOTRIPSY

Particular peroperative analgesia problems arise with extracorporeal shock wave lithotripsy. This method is an acutely painful procedure, often followed by abdominal discomfort, colics, low back pain, nausea and vomiting. The shock wave by itself, although providing a relatively non-invasive method is not completely harmless: air-containing organs (long-bowel) appear particularly prone to damage. Air injected into the epidural space may predispose this area to injury as well. Additionally the epidural catheter, like air, provide an acoustic transmission interface which may result in energy release to the surrounding tissues. It may be a source of neurologic contusions and radiculopathies (Lander et al. 1987 b).

The procedure requires the immersion of the patient in warm water, in a sitting position . The intervention sometimes needs to be repeated and it is often done during an outpatient program. For all these reasons the required anaesthesia technique must ensure:

- rapid onset of deep analgesia
- haemodynamic stability
- absence of motor weakness
- low rate of urinary disturbances
- rapid recovery
- good postoperative analgesia without risk of delayed respiratory depression.

If regional blocks or general anaesthesia have certain limits for this indication, spinal opioids alone or in association with other substances may be considered.

Examples:

- Relative high doses of epidural fentanyl (200 µg) studied in this indication provided good analgesia but also pronounced respiratory depression.This depression could be prevented or reversed by high doses of intravenous naloxone. However, this was only possible with a concomitant decrease in the quality of analgesia. A low dose infusion of naloxone was inadequate to reverse the respiratory depression after epidural fentanyl (Guéneron et al. 1988).

- Lower epidural fentanyl doses (150 μg) with small doses of intravenous midazolam were initially proposed and strongly recommended by Pandit et al. (1987). They reported excellent or good results in 97% of 105 cases. However, after more extended experience (200 cases) the same authors disclaimed their method, not because of the fentanyl by itself but because of technical failures resulting in inadequate lithotripsy results (Pandit et al. 1988).
  ED fentanyl 100 μg in saline 10 ml were compared with ED lignocaine 1.5% + adrenaline for anaesthesia during extracorporeal shock wave lithotripsy. Both techniques were satisfactory for the majority of patients but the fentanyl group had less cardiovascular changes (Silbert et al. 1989).

- The association of epidural bupivacaine 0.125 or 0.25% (respectively 30 or 45 mg) combined with epidural epinephrine (2.5 μg/ml) and epidural fentanyl (100 μg) together with intravenous diazepam (0.06-0.3 mg/kg) provided successful analgesia and patient's satisfaction (Bromage et al. 1987).

- The association of epidural bupivacaine and methadone was recommended by Drenger et al. (1987 b). Postoperative analgesia was maintained efficiently and safely using a continuous infusion of epidural methadone completed by a patient controlled bolus administration (PCA) of the same opioid.

Repeated extracorporeal shock wave lithotripsy utilizing local anaesthetics alone (e.g. lidocaine 1.5% + adrenaline 1/200.000 is not reliable (Korbon et al. 1987). It produced an incidence of failure in about 50% for fifth and sixth time lithotrypsies (Korbon 1988).

These investigations demonstrate that it is not easy to obtain with epidural opioids alone deep surgical analgesia without respiratory depression. Using opioids associated with other drugs the problem is certainly not easier to solve.

The above proposed solutions are attractive but further investigations and perhaps also more technical refinements are needed before final conclusions about the best anaesthesia technique for this new indication can be made.

Conclusions

Spinal analgesia for surgical interventions or painful diagnostic procedures is not a good indication for opoids. In most situations classical anaesthesia techniques will offer the best choice. In exceptional cases, spinal opioids may have a complimentary role for the patient's comfort. However, the increased comfort must also be accompanied by increased security measures and close surveillance and only then the results may be gratifying.

11. Postoperative pain

11.1 Potential advantages and drawbacks

It is generally accepted that pain following operation is treated inadequately and that most methods of postoperative analgesia are in many cases unsatisfactory (Rawal et al. 1986 a; Scott and Fischer 1982 c).

Unrelieved postoperative pain is associated with abnormal reflex responses conducting to:

- circulatory and metabolic dysfunctions producing an increase of vasoconstriction, cardiac output, blood pressure, O_2 consumption
- nausea, vomiting, abdominal distension and risk of ileus
- pulmonary dysfunction with risk of atelectasis and hypoxemia
- limitation of motion with abnormal muscle metabolism and progressive atrophy
- emotional stress
- increased risk of thrombosis formation (Bonica 1987).

In most patients severe postoperative pain is managed with opioids but unfortunately these are often given in insufficient amounts with vague prescription formulation, wrong informed nurses, etc., so that pain remains locally or altogether unrelieved (Prithvi and Rai 1967).

Indeed, spinal opioids are capable of relieving both visceral pain and also somatic pain so that their application may be considered after:

- thoracic (Chayen et al. 1980, Welch et al. 1981 b)
- cardiovascular (Mathews and Abrams 1980, Bromage et al. 1980 a)
- abdominal (Crawford RD 1981, Magora et al. 1980 a)
- gynaecological (Mc Clure et al. 1980)
- anal and urological (Boskovski et al. 1981)
- orthopedic surgery (Johnston and McCaughey 1980).

Spinal opioids have improved significantly the interest in postoperative analgesia and care. Whether the method also has improved the postoperative analgesia itself is a matter of debate.

The spinal route is inherently more invasive and perhaps needs closer supervision. Nevertheless, it was hoped that by using small analgesic doses near to their site of action, remote from the brain and free of sympathetic or motor effects it would be possible to avoid many of the common side effects associated with the classical administration routes of postoperative opioids.

However, such expectations are unfortunately not completely achieved so that a closer confrontation with the clinical reality and an examination of the pros and cons of the method is to be done.

11.1.1 Better pain relief?

Is there really an intrinsic superiority of spinal opioids in quality, extension or duration of analgesia? Superiority characterized by improved pulmonary function, reduced side effects or at least better outcome over spinal local analgesics or local blocks, over intravenous opioids given by repeated bolus, by patient controlled analgesia (PCA), or by continuous intravenous infusion, or even over intramuscular opioids?

Many authors provided arguments in these directions (Cousins and Bridenbaugh 1986; Cullen et al. 1985; El Baz et al. 1984; Lanz et al. 1982; Rawal et al. 1984 b and 1986 a; Shapiro et al. 1981; Shulman et al. 1984 b; Zenz et al. 1981 b and 1982 a; Zenz 1982 f).

Higher efficacy, more extended and more comfortable pain relief
If used "in the right way, with the right drug and dose, given at the right moment" conventional systemic analgesia provides not only effective analgesia but produces also a very similar and not inferior degree of analgesia. However, compared to spinal opioids the systemic drugs have to be given more often and in higher doses.

The notion that spinal opioids give higher quality analgesia than opioids by conventional routes is very difficult to test. Cullen did it: much smaller epidural doses of morphine (0.4 mg/h) have been shown, in a well-controlled study, to produce safe pain relief superior to that found with conventional opioid use (Cullen et al. 1985).

Several studies documented the high efficacy of epidural opioids (Busch and Stedman 1987; Henderson et al. 1987; Rawal et al. 1981 a; Rawal et al. 1982; Shulman et al. 1984 b).

A controlled study in 100 patients showed that following abdominal surgery, postoperative pain was better controlled by the epidural regimen of bupivacaine 0.5% 5ml/4h for 24 hours plus morphine 4 mg/12h for 72 hours than by systemic morphine. However the achievement of more effective pain relief, postoperative mortality, mobility and convalescence were similar in both groups (Hjortsø NC 1985 a).

Reduced doses

Pain relief from epidural administration of morphine in morbidly obese patients is highly satisfactory and these patients require with this method significantly less opioids than with parenterally methods (Brodsky and Merrell 1984, Rawal et al. 1984 b).

The total epidural dose of morphine to provide a pain-free postoperative period during the first day after current abdominal surgery is only about 4 mg morphine which can be given in repeated bolus doses (Zenz et al. 1981 b; Zenz 1981 h), (Fig. 82, 83, 84).

If lipophilic opioids are used the reduction is as much as a factor of 7 (Chovaz and Sandler 1985).

Longer action

Sixty-six patients were treated with a simple injection of epidural morphine, 4 mg for post-hemorroidectomy analgesia. 83% of the patients needed no other analgesics and 16.6% required only mild analgesics (Kuo 1984).

Following spinal operations the administration of 2.5 mg epidural morphine through a small catheter 4-5 cm above the laminectomy just prior to the wound closure was adopted as a standard protocol to obtain postoperative analgesia. All patients treated in this manner needed no analgesics in the first 16-24 hours after the operation (Grabow et al. 1982 b; Rechtine et al. 1984).

Epidural morphine provided a longer duration of analgesia than that obtained with bupivacaine (Graham et al. 1980; Torda and Pybus 1984; Purves et al. 1987).

Comparing in 41 patients postoperative pain treatment with intramuscular meperidine 50 mg or 100 mg epidurally, similar side effects in both groups were noted. Analgesia was more intense and of a longer duration and the level of consciousness was better with the epidural opioid (Payne 1983 a).

Better appreciated by patients and/or surgeons

The patients' reactions have generally been of high satisfaction with epidural opioids and even more so if the technique is used in continuous infusion (Anderson et al. 1981; Brownridge 1983 a; El-Baz et al. 1982; El-Baz and Goldin 1983 a; El-Baz et al. 1983 b; Harrison et al. 1988; Modig and Paalzow 1981 b).

Also the surgical colleagues strongly supported the epidural opioid analgesia and favoured the method over conventional regimes.

Negative results

Certainly, in most studies the analgesic effect of epidural opioids is better than that of parenteral opioids. However, one study indicates that opinions about the superiority of epidural opioids might be wrong. Rawal and Wattwil (1984 a) have shown that with both epidural and parenteral opioids the same degree of pain relief can be obtained despite the fact of huge differences in the doses needed.

Some authors have not observed any difference in the frequency and the severity of vascular thromboses noted after epidural or intramuscular opioid analgesia (El-Baz et al. 1984; Rawal et al. 1984 b; Shulman et al. 1983).

Other authors stated also that epidural morphine compared to epidural local anaesthetics provided no better pain relief (Scheinin and Rosenberg 1982).

Onset of pain relief is slower; if rapid pain relief is mandatory, intravenous opioids are certainly a better choice than spinal opioids.

11.1.2 Improved pulmonary function?

Comparing epidural morphine with intravenous morphine and epidural local anaesthetics, an advantage of epidural over parenteral opioids could be demonstrated (Rawal et al. 1984 b; Zenz et al. 1982 a; Zenz 1982 f). But no difference between epidural local anaesthetics or opioids was found. The forced expiratory volume in 1 second (FEV_1) improved to 67% by epidural morphine, to 68% by epidural local anaesthetics and only to 45% by intravenous morphine (Bromage et al. 1980 a), (Fig. 82, 83).

In patients following gallbladder surgery, 4 mg epidural morphine produced more favourable changes in blood gases and peak expiratory flow rate than intramuscular ketobemidone 5-7.5 mg, or intercostal block with 0.5% bupivacaine (Shulman et al. 1983).

The pulmonary function of two groups of patients were investigated during the postoperative period. The first group received 5-10 mg of intramuscular morphine; the second group 10 mg epidural morphine. Patients treated by the epidural route distinctly showed fewer signs of pulmonary dysfunction (21%) compared to those treated with IM morphine (67%). However, it should be noted that given the routes of administration, the doses of the opiate were not exactly equipotent. The opioids given in the epidural group having been higher (Rybro et al. 1982).

By contrast, other investigators were unable to demonstrate any improvement in pulmonary function in the postoperative period (Bonnet et al. 1984).

The same conclusion was drawn in another study comparing postoperative pain relief and respiratory performance after thoracotomy using either epidural morphine or subcutaneous nicomorphine. No differences could be demonstrated between the two groups (Højkjaer Larsen et al. 1985).

Indeed, during the postoperative period there exists a dysfunction in the ex- and

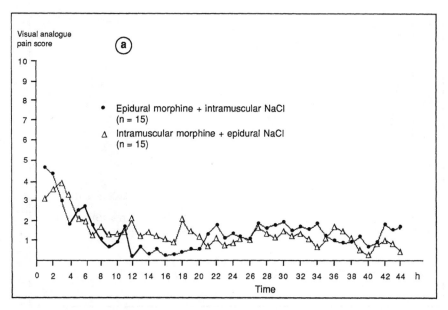

Fig. 82 a, b, c. Comparison of analgesia, necessary morphine doses and respiratory function tests in obese patients.

a) Both analgesia techniques gave effective analgesia.

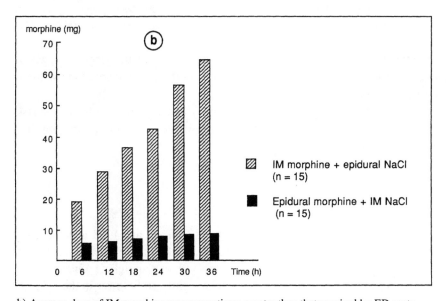

b) Average dose of IM morphine was seven times greater than that required by ED route.

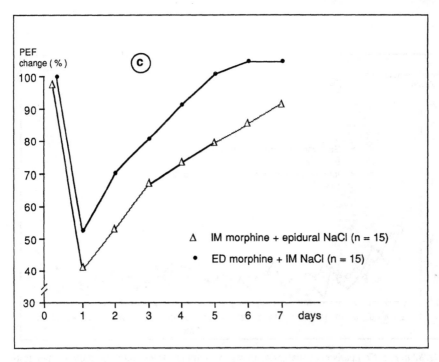

c) Peak expiratory flow values with ED or IM morphine: the results reported by Rawal et al. in a randomized double-blind study of grossly obese patients undergoing gastroplasty for weight reduction and receiving IMOA or EDOA with morphine for postoperative analgesia were clearly in favour of EDOA. A larger number of patients receiving EDOA postoperatively were able to sit, stand or walk unassisted within 6, 12, 24 hours, respectively. Being alert and more mobile, patients in this group benefited more from physiotherapy, which resulted in better pulmonary function, in fewer pulmonary complications and shorter hospitalization time (Rawal et al. 1984 b).

inspiratory muscles which cannot be neutralized even with the deepest analgesia. Nevertheless, deep analgesia allows early physiotherapy and coughing without pain (Simoneau et al. 1984).

It must not be forgotten that the respiratory insufficiency by itself is a risk factor increasing the development of late respiratory depression after administration of opioids.

11.1.3 REDUCED SIDE EFFECTS?

Covering a surgical programme of two years Zenz et al. (1983 a) have compared the overall side effects in 470 patients (221 with epidural opioids, 249 patients with parenteral opioids for postoperative pain relief). Side effects, pneumonia, subileus and mortality have been significantly lower in the epidural group (Fig. 83, 84).

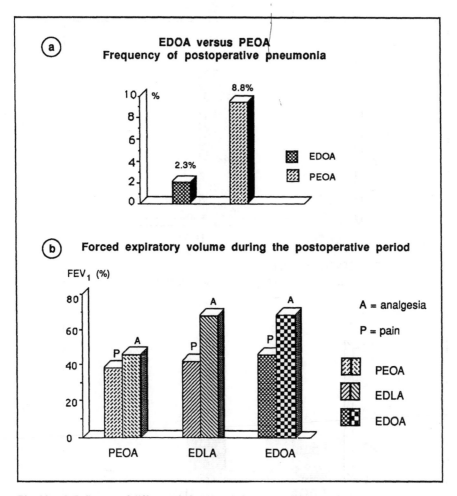

Fig. 83 a, b. Influence of different analgesia techniques on pulmonary function.
(a) - Zenz et al. 1982 a;
(b) - adapted from Bromage 1984 a

Respiratory depression
Risk of immediate respiratory depression is lower after epidural opioids and higher after intrathecal morphinils (Tab. 25, 26, 27, Fig. 84). In contrast, the risk of delayed respiratory depression is higher and more serious. Its frequency after the use of morphine is estimated to be 0.1% after epidural, and 0.4% after intrathecal administration (Rawal et al. 1986 a; Sandler and Chovaz 1986; Stenseth et al. 1985 a).
lipophilic opioids compared to hydrophilic compounds (Cousins and Bridenbaugh 1986).

292

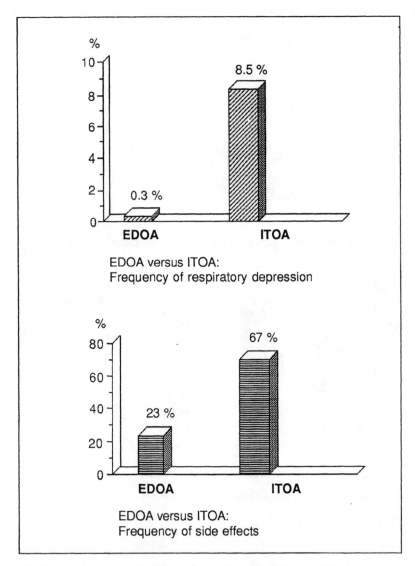

Fig. 84 a, b. Comparative frequency of side effects after EDOA and ITOA.
(Zenz 1982 f) (Bibliography 1979-1981, 68 authors: EDOA: n=2642, ITOA: n=313)

Pulmonary complications

Fewer pulmonary complications have been demonstrated in the epidural morphine group (Rawal and Wattwil 1984 a).

The incidence of pulmonary complications in the postoperative period after
abdominal surgery was significantly reduced by epidural morphine compared
with intramuscular morphine (Rybro et al. 1982). The incidence of pulmonary

infections could be insignificantly reduced by epidural local anaesthetics plus morphine as compared to intramuscular morphine (Hjortsø et al. 1985 a). Comparing the effects of intravenous morphine, epidural lidocaine, and epidural morphine there was a clear advantage of the epidural methods but no difference between the two different epidural methods. So, it is clearly difficult to evidence an advantage of epidural opioids in postoperative pain therapy (Benhamou et al. 1983).

In a double-blind randomized cross-over study epidural morphine 4-8 mg was compared with 4-8 ml bupivacaine 0.5% following abdominal and orthopedic surgery. Peak expiratory flow rate was improved equally and pain relief was similar for the two methods. However, three patients had significant hypotension following epidural bupivacaine (Torda and Pybus 1984).

Pruritus

Pruritus is a side effect that occurs following the use of opioids, whatever the mode of administration. However, pruritus although dose related is more frequent and more severe with the epidural or intrathecal applications than after the parenteral use of opioids (Bromage et al. 1982 a; Douglas et al. 1986 b; Fischer and Scott 1982; Hales 1980; Shipton 1984 c; Nelson et al. 1987). Frequency of pruritus after epidural morphine was 28% in a study of Lanz et al. (1982).

Nausea and vomiting

Frequency and severity of nausea and vomiting after spinal opioids are comparable to those seen after other analgesia methods (Cousins and Bridenbaugh 1986; Lanz et al. 1982).

Drowsiness

Drowsiness is less severe after epidural opioids than after parenteral opioids where the used doses are generally higher (Bromage et al. 1980 c).

Urinary retention

The most common and distressing complication of opioids is perhaps acute urinary retention. After postoperative use of epidural opioids this side effect seems to be more severe than after parenteral application (Camporesi and Redick 1983 b).

Frequency is reported to be largely different according to authors and indications:

- <20% (Chrubasik et al. 1985 f; Sjöström et al. 1985)
- 23% after lower abdominal or leg surgery (Mihic et al. 1982)

- 62% after hip surgery (Barré et al. 1983)
- 80% (Villalonga et al. 1984).

The use of spinal morphine is certainly not the technique of choice in patients for whom urinary catheterization must be avoided.

Constipation
It is also a common side effect of opioid therapy. It occurs during parenteral as well as during spinal opioid treatment. Nevertheless, after spinal opioids passing of flatus and faeces occurred significantly earlier (Rawal and Wattwil 1984 a).

11.1.4 BETTER IN SELECTED GROUPS OF PATIENTS?

It was stated that epidural administration of morphine is a useful adjunct in the postoperative care of morbidly obese surgical patients (Busch and Stedman 1987; Rawal et al. 1984 b). In a recent report comparing intravenous with intrathecal morphine after coronary artery bypass operations 0.5 mg morphine intrathecally provided significantly better analgesia. The intrathecal group needed significantly less sodium nitroprusside in the postoperative period (Vanstrum et al. 1988). However, the authors state as well that heparinisation presents a theoretical risk for lumbar intrathecal blocks.

11.1.5 SUPERIOR TO OTHER ANALGESIA METHODS?

Superior to local anaesthetics?

Examples with positive results:
In a double-blind study, after thoracic and abdominal surgery, the postoperative analgesia induced by the epidural injection of morphine or bupivacaine were compared. Epidural opioid analgesia with morphine produced virtually no change in the physiological parameters. After epidural local anaesthetics with bupivacaine 30% of the cases treated showed hypotension sufficiently severe that medical treatment was required. The quality of analgesia was slightly superior after epidural local anaesthetics than after epidural opioid, but for the epidural opioid analgesia patients the analgesia lasted longer.

The author recommends epidural opioid analgesia for postoperative analgesia, particularly if patients present cardiovascular disorders or if there is a high risk factor with regard to hypovolemia (traumatized patients), (Torda and Pybus 1984).

During the first three postoperative days different types of analgesia treatment using an epidural catheter were compared (Tab. 54).

The patients were treated as follows:

- group a: on-demand bupivacaine
- group b: on-demand bolus injections of epidural morphine
- group c: continuous epidural morphine infusion, completed by an on-demand intravenous bolus of morphine.

In all three groups, all the patients had undergone thoracic surgery. In addition, in all three series the epidural analgesic injection was given at a high spinal level (level T4-T5).

The resultant analgesia and comfort were of virtually the same depth for all the patients in the three groups. Nevertheless, in groups a and b, the duration of effective analgesia was significantly shorter than with the combined infusion technique used in the group c. In the first group, reinjections were more frequently required. The total doses of morphine required in the infusion group (group c), were significantly lower (4.2 mg ± 1.3 mg/24 hours versus 21.7 ± 5.7 mg/24 hours in the bolus group, group b) as well as the plasma concentrations of the opioid. This probably provides an explanation of the fact that the side effects noted in group c were less severe than those observed in groups a and b. The patients in group a in particular presented weakness and numbness of the hands, which was for them a source of anxiety. They also sometimes showed severe arterial hypotension, bradycardia and decrease in cardiac output. Severe side effects were absent in the two other groups. Urinary retention was very frequent in groups a and b and rather rare in group c.

Depressed vigilance and respiration were significantly higher in group b (27%). They were so severe that it was generally necessary to administer repeated doses of naloxone. Such side effects were absent in group a and were without clinical importance in group c.

The conclusions of this comparative study are as follows :

a) The three methods provide comparable analgesia results after thoracic surgery.
b) High dose of epidural bupivacaine (a) or morphine on demand injections (b) produced serious nursing problems and side effects which were unacceptable both in quantity and severity.
c) The best technique, which is both effective against thoracic pain and not too constraining for the nursing staff, producing a minimum of side effects, is the method used in group c in which the continuous epidural opioid infusion was combined with complementary intravenous opioid injections (El-Baz et al. 1984).

Such conclusions are only valid if high levels for the epidural route are used. If the same products and the same doses had been administered in group a and b, but at the lumbar level and for abdominal surgery, markedly fewer problems would have arisen. Nevertheless, it should be pointed out that the number of side effects ran parallel with the size of the doses administered. With the method used in group c, an analgesic base was provided by the epidural route, and according to the patients' requirements, the analgesia was strengthened by the administration of additional intravenous doses. By so doing, it was possible to obtain the same analgesia with a significantly smaller amount of drug and with less frequent side effects. The method used in group c had not shown clinical respiratory depression notwithstanding the combined intravenous and epidural opioid application. Close supervision was always necessary.

- It should be noted that thoracic catheters are mostly unnecessary for opioid application in thoracic pain (Fromme and Gray 1985 a; Fromme et al. 1985 b).
   One of the great advantages of epidural opioid analgesia compared to epidural local analgesia is the possibility to guarantee thoracic analgesia from lumbar puncture site (Höjkjaer-Larsen et al. 1985).

- In 81 patients treated for postoperative pain a double-blind study was performed comparing:

a) epidural opioid analgesia with morphine 0.1 mg/ml infusion
b) epidural with bupivacaine 0.1% infusion
c) epidural analgesia with opioid + local anaesthetic same ratios as above.

The results showed clearly: the group that received the epidural analgesia with a combination of an opioid + a local anaesthetic enjoyed the best pain relief. He was followed closely by the group that received epidural opioid analgesia (Cullen et al. 1985) .
- A comparative study on postoperative nitrogen loss and stress hormones production was performed after:

a) intermittent parenteral morphine for pain treatment
b) prolonged epidural analgesia with local anaesthetics
c) epidural morphine administration.

Urinary nitrogen excretion during the first three postoperative days was significantly less in group b and c than in group a and the lowest in group b. Adrenaline and noradrenaline excretion was almost completely abolished in group b and significantly inhibited in group c but increased during 2 days in group a. These results suggest that the elevated sympathetic activity elicited by painful

Table 54. Postoperative analgesia after thoracic surgery. Comparison of three different analgesia techniques using the ED administration route.

Series	Series A EDLA n = 30	Series B EDOA n = 30	Series C EDOA n = 30
Products used by ED route	bupivacaine on-demand 5 mg/ml	morphine on-demand 1 mg/ml	morphine infusion 0.1 mg/ml/h + morphine IV suppl: 2 mg
Total dose (mg/kg/24h) mean dose during 3 days	-	21.7 ± 5.7	4.2 ± 1.3
Duration of Analgesia (h)	4.9 ± 1.9	5.8 ± 2.3	
Reinjections (24h)	5.1 ± 2.4	4.3 ± 1.4	1 - 2
Analgesia	good	good	good
Muscular weakness (%) (numbness of fingers)	40	0	0
Sympathetic Block (%) (hypotension, bradycardia)	23	0	0
Pruritus (%)	0	40	3
Urinary Retention (%)	100	100	7
Drowsiness (%)	0	27	0
Resp. Depression (%)	0	27	0
Repeated need for Naloxone (%)	0	27	0

(Adapted from El-Baz et al. 1984)

nociceptive and sympathetic nerve afferents, responsible for the postoperative nitrogen loss can be best inhibited by epidural analgesia, but that local anaesthetics are in this field more efficient than opioids (Tsuji et al. 1987).
- Compared to epidural local anaesthetics the duration of spinal analgesia was significantly longer in patients after total hip replacement. Nevertheless the authors reported that one case of respiratory depression occurred after

thoracic epidural morphine in a patient after thoracic surgery (Modig and Paalzow 1981 b).

- In cases where hypotension is to be avoided spinal opioids may offer a better choice than local anaesthetics (Graham et al. 1980).
- On theoretical grounds patients with overt or covert hypertension would be managed more safely with epidural opioids rather than local anaesthetics (Cousins and Bridenbaugh 1986).

Example with negative results:

- For other authors however, epidural morphine compared to epidural local anaesthetics provided no better results in pain relief (Scheinin and Rosenberg 1982).

Superior to local blocks?

The method has been found superior to analgesia produced by intercostal blocks (Rawal et al. 1982).

Superior to intercostal blocks?

Side effects are lower and pain relief is longer lasting.

Superior to intravenous or intramuscular opioid

Examples with positive results:

- Notwithstanding greater invasiveness and currently recognized complications, the method has been found superior to other forms of pain relief such as parenteral opioid administration (Cousins and Mather 1984 b; Harrison et al. 1988; Zenz 1984 a).

- Epidural morphine 3-4 mg versus intramuscular morphine given in the same dose were compared. Results indicated that the epidural route provided an analgesia 4 times more potent and of longer duration than that obtained by the intramuscular route (Torda et al. 1980 b).

- Epidural morphine 3.5 mg were compared to intramuscular morphine 7 mg. Significantly better and longer pain relief was noted after the epidural route than after the intramuscular route. However there was a higher incidence of side effects in the epidural group (Schildt et al. 1982).

- Referring to the pain treatment of 163 thoracotomies performed under balanced intravenous anaesthesia, the results of intramuscular versus epidural nicomorphine given on demand were compared (catheter tip at the T3-T4 level). Postoperatively, analgesia was effective and of rapid onset for both groups. There was no major difference in postoperative pain assessment, neither by the patient nor by the team. However, patients in the epidural group required significantly less nicomorphine for effective pain relief (29 mg over a period of 3 days compared to 52 mg over the same period in the intramuscular group). Significantly fewer pulmonary complications in the epidural group were observed (9 atelectasis in the epidural group, compared to 24 in the intramuscular group). No signs of severe ventilatory depression were evident, but the respiratory function in the epidural group was significantly better than in the intramuscular group (Hasenbos et al. 1985 a, b).

- Four groups of 20 patients were treated for postoperative pain after surgery of the upper abdomen:

a) group a: intramuscular opioid analgesia, with oxycodone, 10-12 mg
b) group b: intercostal block with bupivacaine 0.5%
c) group c: epidural opioid analgesia with morphine 4 mg
d) group d: continuous intravenous infusion of fentanyl 0.54 µg/min + on-demand bolus 7.2 µg, total dose 0.81-2.23 mg during 171 min.

The four groups of patients experienced satisfactory pain relief but the result was slightly better for the fourth group of patients treated with fentanyl and the ODAC (On-Demand Analgesic Computer) intravenous infusion pump (Rosenberg et al. 1984).

- The most important and clear study was presented by Rawal and Wattwil (1984 a). In a double-blind investigation on 30 patients he compared intramuscular and epidural morphine for postoperative analgesia in the grossly obese. This study differs from all others in one main point: the comparison of the two groups is made on the basis of identical pain scores. For this result a seven-fold dose of morphine was necessary in the intramuscular group. Although the same degree of pain relief was obtained with both methods the clinical results were in favour of the epidural opioids. Most importantly, the incidence of pulmonary complications was lower in patients receiving epidural morphine. Passing of flatus and faeces occurred significantly earlier, and the patients of the epidural group could be ambulated earlier. Those positive clinical results stress the importance of the spinal opioids for postoperative pain therapy and clinical outcome after abdominal surgery (Fig.82).

- In an uncontrolled study on 14 patients after laminectomy epidural morphine (3 mg) hastened recovery in comparison to parenteral opioids (Dagi 1984).

- In a double-blind cross-over study 80% of the patients clearly preferred postoperative analgesia with epidural morphine over intramuscular morphine. Pain scoring documented a better analgesia in the epidural morphine group (Anderson et al. 1981).

- Caudal epidural morphine (10 mg) following anal surgery produces better pain relief than intramuscular morphine.

- Significantly better pain relief for 20 hours postoperatively was obtained with epidural morphine compared to intramuscular morphine (Schildt et al. 1982).

- In a carefully performed study of pain relief with epidural or intramuscular morphine in an elderly population undergoing abdominal surgery, Klinck and Lindop (1982) showed that the main difference was less sedation when epidural rather than intramuscular morphine was used. Specifically respiratory mechanics were equally affected in both groups.

- In a comparative study following 45 cases of cardiac surgery, intrathecal morphine (1 or 2 mg) provided better postoperative pain relief and better ventilation than did a conventional intravenous regimen of 30 mg morphine (Fitzpatrick and Moriarty 1988).

- There is only one study, which investigated the effect of different methods under condition of the same degree of pain relief (Fig. 82). With a significantly larger dose of intramuscular morphine the same pain relief could be obtained as with epidural morphine. But importantly, under identical analgesic effects of both methods epidural morphine resulted in fewer pulmonary complications and a significantly shorter hospitalization (Rawal et al. 1984 b). The authors concluded that improved removal of pulmonary secretions in patients receiving epidural morphine appeared to be responsible for a lower incidence of pulmonary complications after abdominal surgery in grossly obese patients.

There seems to be no doubt that regular intravenous or intramuscular injections or continuous infusion or patient controlled infusion of opioids provide effective postoperative analgesia less invasively and perhaps with a lower rate of complications (Cousins and Mather 1984 b). Nevertheless, continuous epidural infusion of a lipophilic opioid as well as of local anaesthetics have been used successfully. We believe that one of the clear benefits of ED opioid administration over conventional IV or IM routes is greater and longer analgesia with less sedation (Bledsoe and Ready 1988). Continuous epidural infusion of lipophilic opioids (e.g. fentanyl or sufentanil) seems to have great appeal (Cousins and Bridenbaugh 1986). However, up to date controlled studies have not been reported and precise definitions of the relative merits of each of these methods awaits further investigation.

11.1.6 BETTER CLINICAL OUTCOME?

Postoperative analgesia may have two aims: to increase the patients' comfort and more importantly to reduce postoperative morbidity, mortality and hospitalization time. The first aim is obtained without any doubt with spinal opioids. The second aim however, is a theoretical possibility that is not obtained by spinal opioids in all cases.

Examples with positive results:

- Well-controlled clinical studies suggested that epidural opioid analgesia reduced morbidity (Shulman et al. 1984 a) and perhaps mortality in high risk surgical patients (Yeager et al. 1987).

- Patients who received epidural morphine were ambulating earlier than patients treated conventionally (Brodsky and Merrell 1984).

- Treated with epidural opioids patients could be mobilized significantly earlier than patients given intramuscular morphine. All these factors, effective analgesia, early ambulation, early normalization of gastrointestinal functions and minimal respiratory complications contributed positively to a shorter hospitalization time. Particularly, improved removal of pulmonary secretions appears to be responsible for a lower incidence of pulmonary complications after abdominal surgery in grossly obese patients. However, the influence of chest physiotherapy, active early ambulation and well-trained nursing should not be underestimated (Rawal et al. 1984 b).

Conclusions

Covering all the available literature there is only limited evidence that the use of spinal opioids increases the clinical benefit, and decreases the postoperative morbidity and mortality. In view of the impressive analgesic effect of spinal opioids this fact seems to be surprising. But it has to be realized that methods using spinal opioids are not more than practical alternative methods providing longer lasting and effective analgesia. It appears that satisfactory postoperative analgesia is dependent on an adequate plasma level of the opioid irrespective of the route of administration (Estok et al. 1987). It certainly has to be realized that most methods in pain control can help for the patients' benefit if the method is applied with care and caution. In this way, very similar results can be obtained if different methods (epidural local anaesthetics, patient controlled analgesia, or epidural opioids) are compared to a standard regimen. For all these methods used in optimal conditions an improvement over the "standard" may be reported. But it is questionable, whether the improvement is due to the method itself or to the greater care, with which the new method is applied. As an example, in our own study possibly the improvement in the epidural group is more a consequence of the greater care, presence of the staff, regular questioning of the patients, and interest in the new method than a result of the method itself. Perhaps the same result can be obtained with the standard intravenous technique, when only more time for care and a greater dose of opioids is given to our patients in the postoperative course (Zenz et al. 1983 a).

So it may be concluded that the use of spinal opioids for postoperative pain relief is today a widely adopted procedure but that real critical evaluations on the superiority of these methods based on very different working conditions and applications remain difficult.

Risk/benefit ratio will further be discussed in their relationship with drugs, doses, routes of application and particular indications.

11.2 Selection of patients

The postoperative use of spinal opioids (epidural or intrathecal) can be particularly recommended after interventions which are generally followed by long-lasting and severe pain e.g.:

- major abdominal and thoracic surgery
- major gynecologic and urologic surgery
- major orthopedic surgery
- intervention requiring early mobilization
- obese patients
- high risk patients
- patients with chronic respiratory insufficiency
- elderly patients.

11.2.1 *Spinal opioids in children* (Tab. 55)

The administration of epidural opioids is a useful analgesic method for treatment of postoperative pain in children and there is no reason that children should not be selected to benefit from it. As a result of the prevention of postoperative pain, physiotherapy is facilitated and the nursing staff will find children easy to manage (Ecoffey 1986; Glenski et al. 1984; Jensen 1981; Parkinson et al. 1989; Shapiro et al. 1984). However, epidural morphine in children provides not only effective analgesia but also prolonged respiratory depression so that close monitoring for at least 24 hours is needed (Attia et al. 1986).

The technique is particularly indicated for children suffering from:

- obesity
- cystic fibrosis
- anticipated respiratory difficulties
- severe emotional reactions.

Table 55. EDOA in children for postoperative pain treatment: results of 5 studies with morphine.

Authors	Jensen et al. 1981	Shapiro et al. 1984	Glenski et al. 1984	Finholt et al. 1985	Ecoffey et al. 1985	Attia et al. 1986
Number	22	5	15	7	16	20
Dose mg/cm body height		–	–	0.024 - 0.031	–	–
or mg/year 3 - 7		1				
8 - 10		1.5	–	–	–	–
11 - 14		2				
or mg/kg bw	0.5	–	0.03	–	0.05	0.05
Position of catheter	–	T4 - 5 T7 - 8		L2 - L3	lumbar thoracic	L2 - L3 / T9 - 10
Onset of analgesia (min)		–		–	˙30 ± 5	30 ± 12
Duration of analgesia (h)	10 - 16	11		16	49 ± 6	20 ± 8
Side effects (%) Pruritus	–	–		–	18	20
Nausea	–	–		–	36	40
Urinary retention	–	–		–	25	70
Respir. depression	0	0		0	0	0

An epidural catheter is easy to insert in children, in view of the increased elasticity of soft tissues, and the enlarged epidural space, especially in the thoracic region.

A 18-19 g Tuohy needle and a loss of resistance technique can be used; level: L3-L4.

One or two ml of 1% lidocaine with epinephrine 1/200,000 is used to test the position of the catheter.

Useful doses of epidural morphine are: 0.03-0.05 mg/kg in a 2 ml solution.

Most side effects are minor and of the same nature as those seen in adults. However, severe respiratory depression has (up to now) not been observed .

The side effects with the exception of drowsiness can be diminished or abolished by means of a titrated intravenous naloxone infusion:10 µg/kg/h. If unwanted side effects of morphine appear 1 µg/kg naloxone in a bolus may be added to a continuous infusion of naloxone (Finholt et al. 1985).

Table 55 summarizes the results of 6 recent clinical studies on epidural opioid analgesia in children.

Caudal administration of opioids was also recommended for postoperative use in children by Jensen (1981); Krane et al. (1987); Rosen et al. (1987) (see paragraph 7.6.6.3).

More recently, excellent results were reported in children with caudal administration of an association of an opioid and a local anaesthetic. Caudal injection of morphine 0.05 mg/kg or fentanyl 1 µg/kg + bupivacaine 0.25% produced adequate analgesia without side effects for more than 24 hours in children undergoing urologic surgery (Wolf et al. 1989; Hoffman et al. 1989; Moine and Ecoffey 1989). The association of an opioid with a local anaesthetic allowed reduction of the opioid dose and provided longer duration of analgesia than with a local anaesthetic alone. Better control of bladder irritability was also observed.

11.3 Selection of drugs and routes of administration

A decision for the selection of the injection route (epidural or intrathecal) is mainly influenced by:

- the catheter already in place
- the possible side effects
- the personal experience of the anaesthetist in spinal injection techniques.

The epidural route has our preference. The thoracic level can be used but in most cases the epidural opioids are injected at the lumbar level. Even for thoracotomy pain the lumbar level ensures satisfying pain relief (Steidl et al. 1984).

Caudal epidural opioids may be considered for postoperative analgesia after abdominal and/or thoracic surgery when the alternative lumbar or thoracic epidural routes cannot be used (Brodsky et al. 1988).

Many opioid substances alone and/or in association with other drugs have been studied for epidural or intrathecal administration (Fig. 31 to 70, chap. 7). The most appropriate opioid for postoperative pain relief is still a debatable matter.

11.3.1 MORPHINE

After spinal opioids a dose relationship with a steep dose-response curve followed by a plateau and a dose related analgesia duration has been observed (Martin R et al. 1982; Nordberg et al. 1983).

Morphine by epidural route

Up to date, the most widely used drug is still morphine: it is characterized by an effective long-lasting analgesia but at the expense of a high incidence of side effects (Hallworth 1984; Rawal et al. 1987; Slattery and Boas 1985). Our files contain more than 500 bibliographic references of use of epidural morphine for postoperative pain treatment.

At present, it can be noted that the high doses of epidural morphine (10 to 20 mg) from earlier publications have become progressively reduced in order to reduce the danger of delayed respiratory depression. Busch and Steidman (1987) used 5 mg doses but the most commonly used doses are now 2 or maximum 4 mg epidural morphine. Nevertheless, also with the reduced doses of 2 mg epidural morphine respiratory depression has been reported (Rawal et al. 1987).

Large interindividual dose response variations make it impossible to recommend a standard dose for ED morphine (Morgan 1989). In view of the known very wide variation in the individual response, it would seem much more rational to titrate the dose until the desired effect is reached (Bromage et al. 1980). Recently, also patient controlled analgesia has been recommended for ED route. Morphine in increments of 1 mg, with a minimal interval of 30 min between doses, produced satisfactory analgesia (Sjöström et al. 1988).

Caudal ED morphine (0.075 µg/kg) was used for control of postoperative pain following open cardiac surgery in children and was found to be safe and effective (Rosen and Rosen 1989).

Morphine by intrathecal route

The intrathecal administration of morphine has also been studied by many authors in the treatment of postoperative or posttraumatic pain (e.g. Andrews et al. 1989; Attig et al. 1985; Aun et al. 1985; Barron and Strong 1981; Barrow 1981; Bengtsson et al. 1983; Blacklock et al. 1986; Chauvin et al. 1981 b, 1982 a, b; Clergue et al. 1984; Dickson and Sutcliffe 1986; Downing et al. 1985; Drasner et al. 1989; Fitzpatrick and Moriaty 1988; Fromme and Gray 1985 a; Fukushima and Nakamura 1989; Gebert and Sarabin 1980 a; Gebert et al. 1980 b; Gjessing and Tomlin 1981; Glass et al. 1985; Glynn 1987; Gray et al. 1986; Harris 1986; Jacobson et al. 1987; Jones et al. 1984; Katz and Nelson 1981; Kennedy 1985; King 1982; King and Tsai 1985; Kirson et al. 1989; Kossmann et al. 1984 b; Lanz et al. 1984 a; Loubser et al. 1986; Mathews and Abrams 1980; Nelson and Katz 1980; Rawal and Tandon 1985 d; Rawal et al. 1987; Rukavina et al. 1986; Samii et al. 1981; Stoelting 1989; Tung et al. 1980 a, b).

Nearly in all the observations postoperative intrathecal morphine produced effective analgesia. However, the doses have ranged from 0.04 mg (Yamaguchi et al. 1989) up to 20 mg (Samii et al. 1979).

Examples
- IT methadone 1 mg versus IT morphine 1 mg was used postoperatively: morphine analgesia was superior to methadone analgesia (Jacobson et al. 1989).
- An age related dose was proposed: 1.5 mg IT for patients of 18 to 55 years and 1 mg up to 75 years and 0.5 mg >75 years (Barrow 1981).
- High doses (1.5-4 mg) were used e.g. after open heart surgery or major abdominal surgery (Chauvin et al. 1981 a, b; Gebert et al. 1980 b; Jones et al. 1984; Mathews and Abrams 1980).
- Low doses (0.1-0.5 mg) were recommended by Glass et al. (1985); Glynn (1987); Kalso (1983); Nordberg (1984 b).

Valid comparisons of the obtained results by different authors and in different situations are difficult to make:

- High intrathecal morphine doses (1-2 mg) provided excellent analgesia but were accompanied by high incidence of respiratory depression. In a series of 56 children treated for postoperative pain after open heart surgery 6 cases of respiratory depression occurred (Jones et al. 1984).
- Low doses intrathecal morphine (0.3-0.5 mg) were associated with inconsistent duration of analgesia and irritating side effects (Drasner et al. 1989).
- The best intrathecal morphine dose probably lies between 0.6-0.7 mg, providing good analgesia, associated nevertheless with irritating adverse effects, e.g. pruritus, nausea, vomiting, urinary retention (Jacobson and Chabal 1988).

Some respiratory depression certainly appears in all the cases, but according to most authors seldom requires treatment. It can appear very late, even after 16 hours (Gray et al. 1986). This does raise an important point: how severe may respiratory depression be before it must be treated? There certainly exists an acceptable degree of postoperative respiratory depression, but the limits of tolerance are so difficult to quantify that it is perhaps wiser to avoid intrathecal morphine for postoperative treatment (Zenz 1982 f) or at least to use this treatment method only for patients where security can be guaranteed by diligent postoperative observation and care (Downing et al. 1985).

11.3.2 EPIDURAL LIPOPHILIC OPIOIDS

At present also another trend can be seen in more and more publications: more and more frequently lipophilic opioids are reported to be used for epidural administration.

Short-acting lipophilic opioids: alfentanil and fentanyl or longer acting lipophilic opioids: buprenorphine, butorphanol, hydromorphone, lofentanil, methadone, nalbuphine, sufentanil are used more and more.

The last opioids are preferred due to their longer duration of action. However, the use of an epidural catheter allows for repeated injections to sustain analgesia. Thus duration of action if no longer the critical factor in the choice of an opioid.

Alfentanil (0.5-1 mg)

The short-acting alfentanil can be best used in continuous infusion: bolus 0.5-1 mg followed by a continuous infusion of 0.25-1 mg/h.

When pain is assessed as zero for at least 2 hours the infusion rate is to be reduced by 50%. If pain exceeds 3 on the VAS a supplementary injection of 0.1 mg of alfentanil may be administered.

The total postoperative opiate consumption during 50 hours after abdominal surgery was for 20 patients 8.8 ± 0.8 mg of alfentanil. Analgesic potency of epidural alfentanil compared to morphine (=1) or fentanyl (=10) used in equivalent pain situations was about 1/10 and 1 respectively (Chrubasik et al. 1988 b).

Lema et al. (1989) studied an ED association of alfentanil 0.5 mg and morphine 4 mg for postoperative analgesia and obtained with the opioid association a seven-fold decrease in onset and a two-fold increase of duration of analgesia when compared with morphine alone. Adding alfentanil to morphine eliminated nausea but produced more pruritus and euphoria.

Buprenorphine (0.15-0.3 mg)

Epidural buprenorphine is a useful opioid for postoperative analgesia (Tab. 56). The results of Lecron et al. (1980 a) were confirmed, e.g. by Carl et al. (1981); De Castro et al. (1982); Gerig and Kern (1983); Gundersen et al. (1986); Petit et al. (1986; Murphy and MacEvily (1984 b); Rondomanska (1980); Zenz et al. (1981 d); Zenz and Piepenbrock (1982 c); Zenz et al. (1982 d); Zenz (1984 d, e); Zenz et al. (1984 f).

ED buprenorphine may produce excitatory effects and hallucinations (MacEvilly and O'Carroll 1989).

The number of reinjections necessary ranges from 1 to 3 daily. Drowsiness frequently occurs as well as transient bradypnea. Delayed transient respiratory depression has never been observed (Tab. 56). However, early respiratory depression has been reported in two cases (Knape 1986). The events coincided with nausea and miosis and occurred 12-17 min after epidural administration of buprenorphine. Both patients did not respond to intravenous naloxone (Knape 1986). The importance of continuous respiratory monitoring also for epidural lipophilic opioids is demonstrated by these two cases. Also, this report highlights one of the few drawbacks of buprenorphine, the limited antagonism by naloxone due to the strong receptor affinity of this partial agonist-antagonist.

Butorphanol (2-4 mg)

There is only a limited experience with epidural butorphanol. Relative low incidence of side effects were reported (Naulty et al. 1987 e.g.). Epidural butorphanol 4 mg provided pain relief with rapid onset (15 min) but relative short duration 5-6 hours (Lipmann and Mok 1988; Mok et al. 1986).

Fentanyl (0.1 mg)

Epidural fentanyl has been successfully used for postoperative analgesia due to high lipid solubility and rapid tissue uptake. However, this opioid has the drawback to provide analgesia of short duration (2-3 hours), (Bormann et al. 1983 b; Dietzel et al. 1982; Melendez et al. 1988; Stoyanov et al. 1981 b). The only improvement for such a situation is the use of continuous infusion techniques (Badner et al. 1989; Bailey and Smith 1980; Bell et al. 1987; Blanloeil et al. 1987; Chrubasik et al. 1987, 1988 b) or patient controlled analgesia (PCA), (Estok et al. 1987).

Table 56. EDOA with buprenorphine (0.3 mg) for postoperative pain treatment: results.

	Number of cases	% N = 72
- Technical failure	1	1.4
- Pain relief: - no	2	2.8
- poor	6	8.3
- excellent	63	87.5
- Pain relief: - duration > 3 h	3	4.1
> 6 h	9	12.5
> 12 h	25	34.7
> 24 h	29	40.2
> 48 h	6	8.3
- Pain relief: - onset (min)	15 (10 - 30)	
- peak effect (min)	30	
- Side effects: - art. hypotension (-25 %)	4	5.5 *
- bradycardia (-25 %)	1	1.3 *
- muscle relaxation	4	5.5 *
- transient bradypnea	31	43.0
- severe respir. depression	0	0
- transient sleepiness	5	7.0
- transient drowsiness	29	40.0
- euphoria	1	1.3
- nausea	3	4.1
- vomiting	3	4.1
- urinary retention	10	14.0
- pruritus	10	14.0
- headache	0	0
- dizziness	0	0
- agitation	0	0
- pupillary modifications	0	0

* 33%, 8% and 33% respectively, of the 12 cases treated with lignocaine before the administration of buprenorphine.
(Rondomanska 1980)

Continuous epidural infusion technique with fentanyl

Bolus of fentanyl 50 µg (to be repeated in 20 min if needed) and followed by a continuous infusion of 80 µg/h. The dose is to be titrated by a correction bolus of 0.1 µg. This allows an optimal pulmonary toilet thanks to a maximal respiratory compliance.

Epidural PCA technique with fentanyl

Bolus fentanyl : 50 µg (to be repeated until effective analgesia is reached), followed by self-administration according to selected settings via a PCA pump. Delivery dose: 20 µg (10 µg/ml) with dose intervals of minimum 6 min. Nevertheless cumulation of the fentanyl doses may be observed so that for long-lasting treatment periods progressive dose reduction is indicated.

Hydromorphone (1.5 mg)

Hydromorphone was first studied by Bromage et al. (1980 c). The drug was compared in a double-blind study with morphine used in equivalent doses. The relatively long duration of analgesia, typical for hydromorphone was nevertheless shorter than that of morphine. Side effects were the same in frequency and severity. Finally, no particular advantage could be attributed to epidural hydromorphone used for postoperative pain treatment (Matthew et al. 1987).

Ketamine (10-30 mg)

Ketamine used at 4-8 mg doses produced inadequate postoperative pain relief (Kawana et al. 1987; Ravat et al. 1987 a, b). Relatively high epidural doses of 30 mg were satisfying and long-acting in 54% of the patients (Naguib et al. 1986).

Lofentanil (0.005 mg)

Analgesia was rapid and relatively long-acting but these effects were too inconsistent to offer practical advantages compared to other opioids (Bilsback et al. 1985).

Methadone (5-10 mg)

- Epidural methadone combined rapid onset, moderately long duration of analgesia and low side effects (Barron and O'Toole 1986; Bromage et al.1980 c; Magora and Shir 1987 c). A continuous infusion plus on-demand analgesia was proposed: a bolus of 2 mg followed by a continuous infusion of 0.4 mg/h and a further bolus of 0.2 mg if needed (Eimerl et al. 1986 a, b).
- Intrathecal methadone 1 mg was compared to IT morphine (Barron and O'Toole 1986; Jacobson et al. 1989). Analgesia provided by methadone was significantly shorter-acting and less consistent in quality.

Nicomorphine (5-10 mg)

- Epidural nicomorphine was estimated to provide a lower risk of delayed respiratory depression compared to morphine (Dirksen and Nijhuis1980 a; Hasenbos et al. 1985 b, 1987).

Nalbuphine (5-10 mg)

- Epidural nalbuphine used after an analgesic anaesthesia provided a relatively long-lasting analgesia with low side effects (Blaise et al. 1986; Mok et al. 1984, 1985; Wang et al. 1986, 1989).

- Epidural nalbuphine 10-20 mg provides good postoperative pain relief (Etches and Sandler 1989).

- The comparative epidural analgesic efficacy of nalbuphine 10 mg, butorphanol 2 mg, pethidine 50 mg and morphine 5 mg was studied in 80 patients after abdominal surgery. With the 3 lipophilic opioids analgesia was of rapid onset and of relative short duration. With morphine analgesia was slow in onset and of long duration. Respiratory depression was not observed in any group, however, incidence of adverse effects was significantly higher after morphine and was most reduced in the nalbuphine group.

- Nevertheless, if ED nalbuphine 10-20 mg was administered at the end of thoracic surgery, the postoperative analgesic efficacy was significantly lower than that provided by ED morphine 5 mg given in analogous situations (Baxter et al. 1989; Etches and Sandler 1989).

Pethidine (10-25 mg)

Pethidine was studied for postoperative pain relief for reasons of faster onset in action and lower risk of delayed respiratory depression if compared to morphine. Most studies with this compound appeared between 1979 and 1982 (Bapat et al. 1980 a; Cousins et al. 1979 a). However, today the interest for this compound for use by epidural route seems to be low.

Sufentanil (0.05 mg)

This opioid has now captured the interest of many investigators.

Examples using epidural sufentanil:

- After abdominal surgery, onset of analgesia occurred at the end of 6 min, total analgesia was reached after 10 min and the peak effect was reached at the end of 12 min. In most cases reinjections were necessary at the end of 6 1/2h. Respiratory depression, quick in onset, was maximal between 5 and 10 min after administration but remained in most cases very discrete. The cardiovascular changes were minimal but sedation lasted sometimes more than 2h (Camu et al. 1985).

- Postoperative sedation was also frequently seen during the first hours. Pruritus was mild and occurred in 15% of the cases (Donadoni et al. 1985).

- After abdominal surgery (19 cases) in a double-blind study the results were compared with epidural sufentanil given either at thoracic level or at lumbar level in volumes of 20 or 10 ml. The patients received excellent analgesia after epidural sufentanil injection, regardless of the site of catheter placement or the volume injected. Duration of analgesia, however, was greater after thoracic versus lumbar epidural injection. However, side effects were surprisingly decreased when the injected volume was 20 ml (Duckett et al. 1986, 1987).

- After abdominal surgery 30 patients received in a double-blind comparative study either epidural morphine 5 mg or epidural sufentanil 50 mg. Sufentanil provided pain relief for a shorter period as compared to morphine. However, pain relief was better with remarkable cardiovascular stability and improved lung function tests allowing adequate pulmonary physiotherapy (Verborgh et al. 1986, 1987 a, b, 1988).

- Whiting et al. (1988) administered 30-50 or 75 µg ED sufentanil after thoracotomy and repeated doses were given as required but at intervals of not less than 30 min. In all groups $PaCO_2$ was significantly elevated at 30 minutes. Severe respiratory depression developed in the group receiving 75 µg sufentanil.

- The addition of epinephrine to lipophilic opioids will reduce the valvular uptake of ED sufentanil, e.g. with as a consequence a reduction of the systemically mediated side effects. In addition a greater mass of drug will be available for its local action on neuroaxial structures. (Bromage 1983; Cousins 1984).

- The duration of postoperative analgesia produced by ED sufentanil infusion is statistically prolonged with the addition of epinephrine (Dickerson et al. 1988; Verborgh et al. 1988).

- Hasenbos et al. (1988) demonstrated that ED sufentanil 50 µg + epinephrine 5 µg/ml in 10 ml saline provide effective analgesia when administered at a high thoracic level. The addition of epinephrine reduces the potential for early respiratory depression and prolongs the duration of analgesia.

- Sufentanil 0.05 mg diluted in 10 ml saline offered excellent quality and relative long duration of pain relief. The association of epinephrine with sufentanil, reduced the frequency of a mostly non-disturbing sedation. An association with bupivacaine was not beneficial in this field (Vercauteren and Hanegreefs 1987).

- During and after thoracic surgery epidural sufentanil provided superior analgesia after lung surgery compared to epidural morphine in terms of potency and onset time. However, the duration of pain relief was intermediary between that reported for morphine and that reported for fentanyl. The administration of sufentanil high in the thoracic epidural space did not produce any clinical respiratory depression. Itching was not observed in the sufentanil group (Rosseel et al. 1987, 1988).

- Vercauteren 1988 reported extreme bradypnea and hypercapnia in two patients after thoracotomy following a first dose of 50 μg ED sufentanil given postoperatively. However, these patients received IV morphine 0.3 mg/kg intraoperatively.

- High thoracic epidural use of sufentanil for post-thoracotomy pain was compared with hydromorphone, fentanyl and nicomorphine. The two last opioids provided adequate analgesia while hydromorphone was associated with late respiratory depression.
Sufentanil provided extremely rapid analgesia of moderate duration. In this series only early and acceptable respiratory depression and slight sedation was noted (Stanton-Hicks et al. 1987).

- A continuous infusion of epidural sufentanil (0.3 μg/kg/h in a volume of 8 ml/h) after a starting bolus of 0.3 μg/kg in 8 ml, provided rapid onset and sustained postoperative analgesia with minimal side effects (Cheng et al. 1987).
In the opinion of several authors sufentanil used at a dosage not higher than 50 μg is the opioid of choice for postoperative epidural opioid analgesia.

Tramadol

Epidural bolus, 20 mg followed by continuous infusion, 8 mg/h was used. If analgesia was sufficient later dose reduction to 4 or 2 mg/h was applied with supplemental on-demand doses of 5 mg. The equivalent epidural analgesia potency of tramadol was only 0.03 compared to morphine = 1. Required doses were enormous, about 350 mg/24 h (Chrubasik et al. 1988 a).

11.3.3 ASSOCIATIONS OF OPIOID AND LOCAL ANAESTHETIC

Epidural route

Presently, injections of an association of an epidural opioid and a local anaesthetic are becoming increasingly popular. There is a dual objective connected
with this trend: the reinforcement of the analgesia (this is of particular value in
obstetrical analgesia) and the reinforcement and prolongation of the conventional regional anaesthesia by a longer acting opioid.

The association technique was first presented in 1979 by Lecron. Today, the
technique is adopted by a great number of clinicians, especially for the analgesia
of parturient women or postoperative pain treatment (Cambell 1989; El-Baz et
al. 1984; Guerel et al. 1986; Hjortsø et al. 1986 a, b; Ionescu et al. 1986; Kehlet
et al. 1987; Kehrberger et al. 1986; Lund et al. 1986; Taverne and Ionescu 1986).

The opioids proposed by Lecron et al. (1980 b) for the epidural association
technique are in order of preference:

- buprenorphine 0.15 to 0.3 mg
- fentanyl 0.1 to 0.2 mg
- alfentanil 0.5 mg
- morphine 1 to 2 mg
- lofentanil 0.001 to 0.002 mg.

One of these opioids may be associated with one of the following local
anaesthetics:

- bupivacaine 0.25%, 0.50%
- etidocaine 1%
- lignocaine 1%
- mepivacaine 2%.

Advantages of the drug association (Tab. 57)

1. This type of association allows a dose reduction for the two products. In some
   cases the reduction is more than 30% compared to the necessary mean doses
   needed if the same products are used alone.
2. The association may also provide a correction of some side effects of the local
   anaesthetic:
a) in the case of bupivacaine the slow onset of action is neutralized.

b) In the case of etidocaine, the action becomes more constant and the sensory block is reinforced. The onset of the analgesia is faster (15 to 30 min), deeper and longer-acting (13 to 24 hours).

3. Mixtures of bupivacaine and fentanyl may improve the quality of analgesia without causing motor block especially in labour (Justins 1982 b).

4. Protection against stress is increased by the use of this association. With epidural opioids used alone, the stress protection is relatively weak. On the contrary, the epidural association of fentanyl (150 μg/kg) and etidocaine at 1%, as used as an anaesthesia technique for orthopedic surgery, produced an effective postoperative inhibition of the endocrine stress responses to surgery (Arroyo et al. 1982, 1983; Ponz et al. 1982 a, b).

5. The combination results in a much improved sensory level of analgesia without tachyphylaxis resulting in consistently low pain scores (Hjortsø et al. 1986 a; Hjortsø et al. 1986 b; Gerber 1988).

Drawbacks of the drug association

Some side effects such as urinary retention may be more frequent than after epidural opioids alone.

Table 57. Advantages and disadvantages of epidural analgesia using an association of an opioid and a local anaesthetic.

- Doses: opioid local anaesthetic	} can be reduced
- Analgesia	- more rapid - increased depth potentiation - more stability - longer duration
- Side effects	- reduced because reduced opioid doses - LA side effects, e.g. hypotension, may persist - risk of delayed respir. depression is not excluded
- Motor block	- minimal
- Tachyphylaxis	- lower
- Surgical anaesthesia	- possible with higher doses
- Catheter placement	- can be avoided in some cases due to the longer duration of analgesia

(Adapted from Kawashima et al. 1980, Lecron et al. 1980 a b, Seebacher et al. 1983)

It is obvious that, depending on the indications and on the used doses of the local anaesthetic, it is possible to realize with these associations very different depths of analgesia, starting from analgesia for the treatment of postoperative pain, to a degree of analgesia appropriate for surgery.

Examples:

- In a controlled study, involving 100 patients following abdominal surgery, the postoperative analgesia with parenteral morphine was compared to that with the same epidural opioid associated with an epidural local anaesthetic: morphine 4 mg + bupivacaine 0.5% 5 ml. Postoperative pain was significantly better controlled by the epidural morphine administration every 4 to 6h. However, in contrast to the improved pain alleviation the epidural regimen had no clinically important influence on the overall postoperative morbidity, and only an insignificant reduction in infectious pulmonary complications was noted (Hjortsø et al. 1985 a, b).

- In a double-blind study in 81 patients after major abdominal operations using epidural analgesia with morphine plus bupivacaine, it was concluded that the drug association did best on all controls. It was safe and easily managed. Pain relief was superior to that provided by other opioid administration techniques (Cullen et al. 1987).

- In a randomized double-blind study in 139 orthopedic patients, the postoperative analgesia obtained during the first 24h, with different bolus doses of morphine (1, 2, 3, 4, 5 mg) with bupivacaine 0.75% was compared. The results indicated that the dose of 3 mg epidural morphine with bupivacaine 0.75% was the best compromise providing reduced pain intensity for the longest time together with an acceptable low frequency and severity of side effects (Lanz et al. 1986 a). It must however be noted that the recommended bupivacaine concentration of 0.75% is high and is not absolutely safe.

- Continuous epidural infusion using diamorphine 0.5 mg/15 ml mixed with bupivacaine 0.125% at a rate of 15 ml/h for postoperative analgesia provided significantly superior analgesia compared with either bupivacaine or diamorphine alone. The technique had a high level of patient acceptability and there were no major side effects (double-blind study in 60 patients, Lee et al. 1988).

- For postoperative analgesia, a bolus dose of epidural pethidine of 35 mg, plus a continuous infusion of 0.125% bupivacaine plus 0.1% pethidine administered at a rate of 6-15 ml/hour was recommended by Raj et al. (1985).

- Epidural buprenorphine 0.2 mg was used for postoperative pain in association with bupivacaine (Louis et al. 1982) (Tab. 58).

- An experience with 1000 epidural opioid administrations using fentanyl 2 µg/kg plus etidocaine 10% plus epinephrine 5 µg/ml, for hip surgery was reported by Barré et al. (1984). This type of anaesthesia produced regularly very satisfying results.

- A low dose of epidural fentanyl 0.09-0.12 mg plus etidocaine 1% or bupivacaine 0.5% was used for epidural opioid analgesia in hip surgery. The results were generally satisfactory in respect of side effects, and there was little difference in the hemodynamic effects between the two local anaesthetics used in association. Etidocaine caused greater motor block than bupivacaine (Camara et al. 1984).

- Fentanyl 0.2 mg, 0.1 mg, or 0.05 mg mixed with bupivacaine 0.5% and epinephrine 1/200,000 was studied for postoperative epidural opioid analgesia in 80 patients who had undergone lower abdominal surgery. The best results were obtained with the higher dose of fentanyl. The patients with this dose also presented a lower incidence of acute hypotension or shivering and postopera-

Table 58. Epidural analgesia using an association of an opioid and a local anaesthetic, advantages and drawbacks.

```
BUPRENORPHINE:   0.2 mg
        +
BUPIVACAINE:     0.25 %
        20 ml
```

ADVANTAGES:

- Analgesia: onset more rapid
                     comfort increased
                     longer duration (< 10 - 15 h)

- Side effects reduced: no late respiratory depression
                        pruritus rate

DISADVANTAGES:

- Risk of immediate respiratory depression is higher

- Urinary retention is more frequent

- Hypotension may occur

(Adapted from Louis et al. 1982)

tive analgesia lasted longer. Postoperative side effects were mild. The technique was well accepted by the patients (Rucci et al. 1984).

- Local anaesthesia alone sometimes does not prevent tourniquet pain. Epidural lidocaine 2% + epinephrine 1/200,000 combined with fentanyl 100 μg provided effective surgical analgesia (Solanki 1987).

Comments by Dr Zenz

Especially in bone surgery, the patients have to be selected very carefully because pain after orthopaedic surgery should actually respond better to local anaesthetics than to opioids. On the other hand, in contrast to abdominal surgery there are no data indicating an improvement in clinical outcome by epidural opioids in orthopaedic surgery. Therefore the only reason left is the patient's comfort. But that reason does not justify an increased danger for the patient. Just like with local anaesthesia hypotension and urinary retention may appear. Possibly, increased dangers of respiratory depression may develop. In a study of Rankin and Comber (1984), 2% of the patients had a mild respiratory depression. Benefits and security may only be expected if the usual doses of the opioid as well as those of the local anaesthetic become significantly more reduced by such drug associations.

Intrathecal route

Just as with the epidural route the association of reduced doses of an opioid with a local anaesthetic may provide good results (Bohannon and Estes 1987).

Technique

Also here most clinicians apply the technique proposed by Lecron et al. (in 1980 a, b, c). The opioids used are the same as those used by the epidural route in the following doses for 70 kg:

- morphine 0.1 to 0.5 mg/1 ml, or
- fentanyl 0.05 to 0.1 mg/1 ml, or
- buprenorphine 0.1 to 0.2 mg/1 ml,
  associated with 2 ml of a local anaesthetic :
- bupivacine 0.5%, or
- lignocaine 1%, or

- tetracaine 1%.
  (with or without adrenaline 1/200,000).

In order to obtain 4 ml of an hypertonic solution 1 ml of 10% glucose may be added to the drug association.

Advantages of the association (Tab. 58):

Just as for epidural opioids the drug combination of an opioid and a local anaesthetic may provide some advantages:

- The analgesia is more rapid and deeper. A surgical depth of analgesia can be reached depending on the total doses used.
- Most authors agree that after the use of a local anaesthetic plus an opioid postoperative analgesia is longer-lasting (Bohannon and Estes 1987).
- The side effects, provided sufficiently low opioid doses are used, may be less severe than those seen after pure intrathecal opioids. However, this is not always the case (Cunningham et al. 1983; Guerin et al. 1983; Lanz et al. 1984 a).
- The method enables a more early postoperative mobilization of the patient.

Drawbacks of the association:

- If the opioid doses are not significantly reduced, then the possibility of long-lasting depression is certainly higher with the association compared to other anaesthetic methods.
- Incidence of itching, urinary retention, nausea and vomiting may be relatively high.

Examples:

- In old patients, 0.2 mg of intrathecal morphine, associated with bupivacaine 0.5% is mostly sufficient and does not produce late respiratory depression. The only side effects frequently mentioned are nausea and urinary retention.

- For treatment of postoperative pain intrathecal morphine 0.5 mg + hyperbaric tetracaine 1% was used (Nelson and Katz 1980).

- A combination of 0.5 mg morphine with hyperbaric tetracaine 1% was investigated in a double-blind study in 42 patients undergoing orthopedic surgery. The postoperative pain relief was more intense and longer-lasting with morphine than without the opioid. However, blood gases were significantly affected and pruritus, nausea, vomiting and micturation disturbances were more frequent in the series receiving the drug association (Lanz et al. 1984 a).

- For surgery of the hip an association of intrathecal morphine 2.5 mg + cinchocaine 7.5 mg was used and a postoperative analgesia for more than 22h was obtained. If cinchocaine was used alone the analgesia mostly lasted no longer than 8h. Side effects of the association were acceptable. Late respiratory depression was not seen (Lanz et al. 1984 a).

- Surgical anaesthesia and postoperative analgesia was provided by intrathecal morphine 1 mg plus amethocaine 12-14 mg for patients undergoing transurethral resection of the prostate. The addition of the opioid to the local anaesthetic produced excellent surgical conditions and significantly less postoperative pain than seen in patients receiving amethocaine alone. However, the associated side effects were high. For example, six of all the patients had respiratory depression. Other side effects were nausea, vomiting and pruritus (Cunningham et al. 1983).

- After orthopedic surgery a satisfying analgesia over 24 hours was obtained with 0.4 mg intrathecal morphine plus isobaric bupivacaine 0.5% (Kalso 1983).

- Using for postoperative pain treatment in 130 patients intrathecal morphine 0.1-0.6 mg, combined with hyperbaric tetracaine 0.5%, the most effective morphine dose was 0.2 mg. Analgesia provided by intrathecal morphine lasted in excess of 20 hours and respiratory depression did not occur if the morphine doses remained below 0.2 mg (Takasaki and Asano 1983).

- The postoperative intrathecal administration of the combination of morphine 0.2 mg with bupivacaine 0.5% provided after orthopedic surgery the longest analgesia with the minimal side effects (Rukavina et al. 1986).
Here again, the trend toward the use of more reduced doses can be seen:

- Gregg et al. (1988) compared analgesia provided by continuous epidural thoracic morphine + bupivacaine versus systemic opioid analgesia in postoperative pain relief. Patients rated their experience with ED morphine significantly better than the control group (50 patients were studied).

- Low doses of IT morphine (0.04 to 0.08 mg) mixed in hyperbaric tetracaine were successful during 34 hours in postoperative pain relief and produced minimal adverse effects (Yamaguchi et al. 1989).

- The combination of low doses of ED fentanyl (50-100 µg) + ED bupivacaine improved postoperative analgesia in surgical patients and required lower total bupivacaine doses (Tewes et al. 1988).

- In 57 urologic patients the intraoperative administration of intrathecal fentanyl 0.05 mg + lignocaine 25 mg produced analgesia but also a sympathetic block, a sensitive block, and a motor block in respectively 17%, 70%, and 6% of the cases (Guerin et al. 1983; Bohannon and Estes 1987).

- Intrathecal buprenorphine plus bupivacaine was used in 50 patients for postoperative pain relief. Synergistic analgesia was noted without appearance of major side or toxic effects (Mattei et al. 1986).

- Analogue results were obtained by Lipp et al. (1987).

11.3.4 NON-OPIOID PRODUCTS

Clonidine and other α$_2$-agonists

Epidural clonidine 15-300 µg administered alone during the postoperative period produced analgesia equivalent to 7 mg morphine (Petit et al. 1989) but with relatively short and variable duration (1h) resembling epidural fentanyl (Boico et al. 1989; Bonnet et al. 1989; Eisenach et al. 1989; Rostaing et al. 1989). Side effects were drowsiness, hypotension, bradycardia. Only for the first 2 hours after injection 150 µg of epidural clonidine was superior to 4 mg of epidural morphine. The authors concluded that clonidine is unsuitable for treatment of postoperative pain in a dose of 150 µg (Lund et al. 1989). Epidural clonidine is not useful in very severe pain (Gordh 1988). Epidural clonidine 150 µg may be associated with low ED opioid doses for increase and prolongation of postoperative analgesia. However, clonidine enhanced also the duration of the respiratory depression induced by the opioid and induced adverse cardiovascular effects (Bonnet et al. 1989; Mok et al. 1989; Penon and Ecoffey 1989; Petit et al. 1989). Further work is needed to determine the most suitable ED opioid and clonidine dose for such combined administration.

Other α$_2$-adrenergic agonists with perhaps more specific and pure potentiating effects on opioids are now under investigation in animals e.g.:
- *Tizanidine* (an analogue of clonidine) has analgesic properties apparently

without the associated hypotensive episodes seen with clonidine (Lubenov et al.1989).

- *Dexmedetomidine* in animals has potent analgesic properties without hypotensive or respiratory depressive effects (Aantaa et al. 1989; Abdul-Rasool et al. 1989; Flacke et al. 1989; Furst et al. 1989; Kendig et al. 1989; Regan et al. 1989; Savola et al. 1989; Vickery et al. 1989; Weinger et al. 1989; Zornow et al. 1989).

Ketamine

Epidural ketamine has been proposed in doses of 30 mg for postoperative pain relief. The substance was effective, but taking into account the neurotoxicological reactions observed with this product after spinal use, ketamine cannot be withheld for spinal analgesia (Amiot et al. 1986; Islas et al. 1985; Mankowitz et al. 1982; Naguib et al. 1986 a; Saissy et al. 1984 a).

Somatostatin

Epidural doses up to 8 mg used by Kawana et al. (1987) were inadequate. Epidural or intrathecal somatostatin has been proposed for postoperative pain relief by Chrubasik (1985 c, d) in continuous infusion. However, the toxicological safety of the compound in man has not been completely cleared and the actual cost of the product makes such a use beyond practical possibilities.

11.4 Selection of injection technique

11.4.1 REPEATED BOLUS INJECTION AND PATIENT CONTROLLED ANALGESIA (PCA)

The most satisfying technique can be applied as follows:

- Preoperative placement of a lumbar epidural catheter.
- The first epidural injection of buprenorphine (0.3 mg) or another lipophilic opioid in 5 ml saline is performed postoperatively in a fully awake patient with moderate pain.
- The injection is to be repeated after 6-8 hours.
- The treatment continues during the first two postoperative days. During this period all sedatives and analgesics are to be avoided. Clinical respiratory depression with this technique was not observed (De Castro and Lecron 1981 b).

Diamorphine, hydromorphone, morphine, pethidine or fentanyl have also been used for epidural postoperative PCA (Bellamy et al. 1989; Walmsley et al. 1989; Wheatley et al. 1989).

Postoperative pain relief was obtained with a programmable PCA pump (Prominject) administering epidural pethidine via an epidural catheter. The pump was programmed to deliver incremental doses of 20 mg of pethidine, 25 mg/ml with a minimum time interval of 30 min between doses. The mean time interval between doses was 84±47 min. Pethidine consumption varied between 5.8 and 35.4 mg/h, mean dose of 18 mg/h. Inter-individual variation in consumption was large but pain relief was very efficient in all patients and no clinical respiratory depression occurred (Sjöström et al. 1988).

11.4.2 CONTINUOUS INFUSION

Epidural opioid analgesia in continuous infusion confers some advantages for postoperative pain treatment.

Recent infusion studies support that the dose response with infused opioids is quite different from that of bolus injection. In a well-controlled study much smaller epidural doses produced safe pain relief superior to conventional opioid use (Cullen et al. 1985; Lee et al. 1988; Mc Quay 1987). Postoperative continuous infusion of epidural morphine plus bupivacaine has synergistic effects (Kehlet et al. 1987). For discussion of pros and cons see Section 11.3.3.

11.4.3 CONTINUOUS, PLUS ON-DEMAND INFUSION

The most convenient method for continuous infusion is the three step infusion technique:

- loading bolus
- maintenance infusion
- on-demand microbolus for correction.

Examples

- A loading dose of epidural morphine, 2 mg/1 ml was followed by a continuous infusion of 0.06 ml/h using a solution of 0.2% morphine. The addition to this basic infusion, of an on-demand microbolus in accordance with the patients requirements, allows individualization of the treatment and provides maximum efficacy notwithstanding the use of low total opioid doses (El-Baz et al. 1984).

- Epidural morphine administered in continuous infusion 0.1 mg/h gave rise to a more effective and constant analgesia than bolus analgesia. A smaller amount of opioids (4.2 mg as against 21.7 mg/24h) was used and fewer side effects (pruritus 3% as against 40%, urinary retention 3% as against 100%) were noted (El-Baz et al. 1984), (Tab. 56).

- A similar technique has been used with continuous buprenorphine infusion. The total postoperative requirements of buprenorphine were not higher than 0.80 mg /d (Chrubasik 1985 a).

- Pain treatment was provided after thoracic and upper abdominal surgery in 43 patients with epidural methadone given in continuous on-demand infusion: loading bolus of 2 mg methadone, connection to an infusion pump set to deliver 0.4 mg/h methadone and a supplementary on-demand bolus as needed. The total amount necessary to produce effective analgesia was 9-21 mg methadone during the first postoperative day and 4-10 mg during the 2nd and 3rd day (Eimerl et al. 1986 a, b).

- Continuous epidural infusion of pethidine 0.25 mg/kg/h was compared with intravenous pethidine bolus 0.8 mg/kg/4h. Continuous pethidine provided post-operative analgesia of better quality with less side effects and significantly lower doses (Sagnard et al. 1987).

- Continuous ED fentanyl provided superior analgesia with minimal side effects either over intermittent ED bolus technique or parenteral morphine (James et al. 1988).

- Continuous ED fentanyl infusion (loading bolus 1 µg/kg, continuous infusion of 1 µg/kg/h) for peripheral orthopedic surgery and postoperative pain relief provided adequate pain relief with moderate ventilatory depression of no demonstrable clinical consequences (Renaud et al. 1988).

- Epidural alfentanil 1 mg, fentanyl ,0.1-0.15 mg or sufentanil 0.05 mg, provided safe and effective pain relief but had a relatively short duration of action: 2-4 h . Administration by continuous infusion of these short-acting opioids is a more appropriate method. For fentanyl the recommended dose is an epidural bolus of 0.1 mg followed by a continuous infusion of 0.02 mg/h and an on-demand supplementary bolus of 0.01 mg. For alfentanil doses of 1 mg, 0.2 mg/h and 0.1 mg respectively may be used. For long-lasting treatment periods a progressive dose reduction is indicated (Chrubasik et al. 1988 b; Parker et al. 1985; Steppe et al. 1983; Wolfe and Davies 1980).

11.5 Selection of equipment: pumps and ports

Portable pumps can be used with excellent results. The technique allows a perfect adaptation to the needs of the patient. Taking into account cost, performance, simplicity and safety we can recommend the following systems:

- the Travenol infusor modified, with a 3-way stopcock syringe
- The Travenol Auto Syringe AS 6H (pulsatile flow)
- the Travenol Auto Syringe AS 2 FH
- the Cadd-PCA, Pharmacia Deltec or the Chronomat infusion Computer
- the Syringe Driver MS 26 Graseby-Fresenius
- the Harvard mini-Infuser mod 950 (only designed for the use of alfentanil).

The pump can be connected directly to an externalized catheter or an implanted port.

11.6 Precautions and surveillance

The use of spinal opioids for treatment of postoperative pain can only be considered in presence of:

- adequate equipment (e.g. pulse oximeter) and drugs
- precise nursing instructions
- detailed written instruction for the recovery room (Tab. 59)
- adequate surveillance for at least 12h after injection.

It is not necessary that these patients should be in an ICU but they do need more nursing care than other postoperative patients, by a nurse who understands the problems and who can apply the adequate treatment associated with these techniques (Ali et al. 1989; Glynn 1987 b).

Table 59. Written nursing orders for patients who are prepared to receive epidural opioids during the postoperative period.

Name of patient [   ]

1 - Initial dose

Drug: [   ]   Dose: [mg] = [ml]   Time: [   ]

2 - For continuing analgesia

Drug: [   ]   Dose: [mg] = [ml]   Interval: [   ]

3 - Maintain IV access for 24 h after the last dose of epidural opioid.

4 - Naloxone 1 amp. = 0.4 mg prepared at bedside (only for emergency use)

5 - Oxygen flow meter and breathing apparatus at bedside

6 - Call anaesthetist for | evidence of airway obstruction,
changes in respiratory pattern,
decreased respiratory effort,
respiratory rate of 10 or below
appearance of unexpected somnolence

7 - Monitoring: respiratory rate and sedation scale / 1 h for first 24 h

/ 4 h after 24 h

Respiratory monitor, pulse oxymeter for first 24 h: yes [   ]

no [   ]

8 - No systemic opioids, sedatives or benzodiazepines are given except

ordered by anaesthesist.

9 - Nausea / vomiting prophylaxis: Metoclopramide 3 x 10 mg / 24 h

Droperidol   2 x 0.25 mg /24 h

10 - Treatment of respiratory depression:

respiratory rate < 10/min = call anaesthetist

< 8/min = naloxone 0.1 mg IV

to repeat after 2 min 3 to 4 times

11 - For inadequate analgesia or other problems related to epidural

catheter call anaesthetist.

Name of the anaesthetist: [   ]

Date of prescription: [   ]

11.7 Side effects

The side effects of spinal opioids have been discussed in Chapter 6 and paragraph 11.1.3. They can be substantially reduced by proper selection of patients, of compound, of administration route, of administration mode, and of doses. Close survey of the patient will allow rapid and effective treatment.

11.8 Indications and contra-indications for postoperative epidural opioid analgesia

Indications:

- severe pain
- epidural catheter in place
- major upper abdominal surgery
- obese patients
- respiratory problems in the postoperative period.

Contra-indications:

- contra-indications to epidural catheter placement
- previous serious adverse reaction (allergy e.g.) to opioids.

11.9 Nursing

Because correct placement of the catheter in the epidural space is essential for postoperative epidural opioid analgesia, neural blockade with a local anaesthetic is to be demonstrated in the operating room.

To minimize the risk of accidental injections of the drugs intended for intravenous administration, a bright coloured injection cap which is distinctly different from intravenous injection ports is placed on the epidural catheter connector and a bright coloured label that reads "epidural catheter" is placed on the catheter near the injection cap (Ready et al. 1988).

The greatest potential hazard in postoperative use of spinal opioids is delayed respiratory depression. Various non-invasive monitors have been suggested, including pulse oximetry, capnometry, impedance plethysmography etc. None of these methods is universally acccepted due likely to their perceived unreliability and their inconvenience, false alarms etc. Thus good nursing care and surveillance following spinal opioids is mandatory during the first 24h.

Conclusions

Postoperative pain must be treated. However, the choice of the method depends on:

- severity and extent of pain

- anaesthesia technique applied
- age and physiopathology of the patient
- nursing, equipment and survey possibilities
- lipophilic drugs, e.g.fentanyl or sufentanil appear to have the best efficacy/ safety ratio and also seem to have a lower incidence of side effects.

For minor interventions minor analgesics may be satisfactory. After more extended surgery intravenous or intramuscular opioids, repeated on-demand or continuous intravenous infusion plus on-demand bolus may offer a good choice. However, spinal opioids applied under optimal care and appropriate monitoring will offer more. This is particularly true in patients with obesity, respiratory insufficiency and hypovolemia.

12. Other applications in acute pain situations

12.1 Post-traumatic pain

In ventilated patients with multiple injuries haemodynamic instability is not unusual and each injection of a sedative analgesic combination may be associated with a fall in blood pressure. This effect can be prevented by the use of intraspinal opioids since this technique has a well-established haemodynamic stability (Rawal 1986). The pain treatment of polytraumatised patients by the epidural administration of opioids has real advantages:

- Compared to the epidural injection of a local anaesthetic, opioids do not produce hypotension with the result that a more objective supervision of the blood pressure values can be made.
- Contrary to epidural anaesthesia with local anaesthetics the epidural opioid analgesia has the advantage that in most cases a lumbar catheter is sufficient even for thoracic pain treatment (Fromme et al. 1985 b; Højkjaer et al. 1985; Shulman et al. 1983).
- Compared to parenteral use of opioids the epidural route does not so much modify the vigilance of the patients. The result is that the clinical changes can be followed more easily.

Morphine

Patients with multiple rib fractures present a good indication for pain treatment with epidural morphine 3-5 mg given at a lumbar level.

The results are uniformly good with an analgesia of 18.8h (5-22) and side effects are greatly reduced (Huesch and Zenz 1981; Kiss and Abel 1982; Petit et al. 1983 b; Reiz 1982).

Fifty cases of chest injury were treated with a regimen of epidural morphine 3 mg plus epidural bupivacaine 0.5% and epinephrine 1/200,000. Forty-three of these patients made satisfactory recoveries without requiring any ventilation support. Six patients were ventilated and among them 3 for respiratory failure. Serious side effects were rare. One patient developed respiratory depression which required withdrawal of morphine and one patient developed an epidural space infection (Rankin and Comber 1984).

For treatment of polytraumatic pain epidural morphine was used in doses of 2 mg. Such a dose produced effective analgesia for at least 6h and the dose could be repeated if necessary (Bahar et al. 1979; Chayen et al. 1980; Johnston and McCaughey 1980; Rawal 1985 c).

Significant differences in patients' outcome could be demonstrated by Ullman et al. (1989). They compared one group of patients with multiple rib fractures treated with systemic opioids with another group treated with thoracic epidural morphine. Patients in the epidural group had less ventilator-dependent time, less time in ICU, and a shorter hostpital stay.

For pain treatment in multiple fractured rib patients good results were reported with intrathecal morphine, 4 mg. Pain relief was complete after 45-60 min and long-lasting. Cough and mobilization were improved (Kennedy 1985).

Dickson and Sutcliffe (1986) did not concur in this opinion. After one year of wide clinical experience with intrathecal opioids they came to the conclusion that the epidural analgesia using bupivacaine still remains the method of choice for chest injuries. However, epidural analgesia with local anaesthetics necessitates for this indication the position of the catheter at a thoracic site.

The advantages of epidural or intrathecal opioids in patients with chest injuries are the possibility of easily inserting a catheter at a lumbar site, the long duration of action, the haemodynamic stability, the stable motor function of the extremities and the consecutive possibility of early mobilization.

Lipophilic opioids

Polytraumatic patients are not accustomed to the use of opioids and frequently they have already received an emergency parenteral injection of an analgesic. Due to these reasons, it is indicated to give preferences to lipophilic opioids such as buprenorphine or fentanyl to avoid delayed respiratory depression.

Buprenorphine

The following technique may be recommended:

- lumbar catheter
- buprenorphine bolus of 0.3 mg in 10 to 15 ml saline; to be repeated each 8 h
- each hour: 15 min CPAP (continuous positive airway pressure) training
- continuation of intermittent buprenorphine bolus and CPAP training according to the clinical needs (Huesch and Zenz 1981).

With this method it was mostly possible to treat patients with multiple rib fractures without continuous mechanical ventilation. However, for maximal security the patient must be transferred into an intensive care unit, so that a continuous, on-demand, epidural opioid infusion can be set up under continuous supervision (McQuay et al. 1980).

Fentanyl

Continuous epidural fentanyl analgesia may be considered as a safe and effective method for routine use in patients with rib fractures or flail chest.

Technique:
- lumbar epidural catheter placement
- fentanyl 100 µg bolus is followed by a continuous infusion in a concentration of 5µg/ml at an initial rate of 50µg/h
- the infusion rate is subsequently titrated based on clinical assessment of the analgesia adequacy.

Results

Mackersie et al. (1987) have applied the method in 40 cases. The use of continuous epidural fentanyl was associated with significant improvement in vital capacity and in maximal inspiratory pressure. Minute ventilatory volumes, end tidal volumes also showed improvement. $PACO_2$ was significantly changed. Full pain relief was obtained in 85% of patients, none of these patients required any other medication. Urine retention 5%, pruritus 15% were the major associated complications. The use of relatively low fentanyl concentration may explain the low incidence of reported side effects.

Lumbar epidural administration provides adequate analgesia even for injuries at the higher thoracic level.

The patients will continue to require vigorous pulmonary care.

12.2 Intensive care unit patients

Analgesia and sedation for patients in intensive care units (ICU) who require mechanical ventilation are most commonly provided by intermittent intravenous injections of opiates and benzodiazepines. However, the technique has a number of disadvantages. In many cases the drugs are inadequate even in large doses. Muscle relaxants may be necessary for patients' respiratory tolerance.

Excellent results with epidural opioids used as an effective method for sedation of ICU patients were confirmed by Rawal and Tandon (1985 d). They studied the analgesic effect of epidural morphine in 24 patients requiring controlled ventilation. In spite of large doses of phenoperidine, diazepam and a number of other analgesics and sedatives all patients were restless, agitated and coordinated poorly with the respirator. Epidural morphine gave potent analgesia and good patient respiratory coordination.

In patients with multiple trauma and in patients where frequent assessment of the level of consciousness are important this technique is superior to parenteral analgesic sedative combinations. The daily analgesic requirement can be reduced about 10 times by the use of epidural morphine.

However, it must be remembered that in ICU patients requiring ventilation assistance the average duration of analgesia after epidural morphine in most cases is not shorter than the duration of analgesia following the same dose for postoperative pain relief (average duration 5h). Rapid development of tolerance seems also to be a particular problem in ICU patients (Rawal and Tandon 1985 d).

The technique of spinal opioids is particularly suited for patients who are to be weaned from mechanical ventilation. The method guarantees pronounced analgesia with a very mild degree of sedation. One danger in this situation has to be considered: the heparinisation which is performed in most ICU patients. Heparinisation may give rise to bleeding within the epidural space. This danger contraindicates an epidural catheter, if other analgesic methods are possible. The same danger is true for patients receiving ASS regularly.

Conclusions

Spinal opioids have gained a definite place in ICU treatments. They are of particular value for weaning a patient from the respirator with a minimum of sedative drugs and to facilitate physiotherapeutical mobilization without pain.

12.3 Myocardial infarction

Epidural morphine (0.5 mg) provided good pain relief in this indication. An initial bolus of 1.2-2.4 mg was given, followed eventually after 30 min by the same dose. Analgesia became mostly effective within 30 min. Total doses needed were 1 to 2 mg morphine, two or three times a day (Skoeld et al. 1985).

However, spinal opioids seem to be a strange method for patients with myocardial infarction. In an acute situation of pain and myocardial dysfunction a catheter has to be inserted and analgesia is not complete before 30 min. Intravenous opioids seem effective and safe enough.

12.4 Visceral pain after arterial embolization

Selective visceral arterial embolization used in cancer treatment provides a severe and long lasting hyperalgesia. Treatment of the pain syndrome by epidural local anaesthetics is not always completely satisfying due to risk of motor block and necessity of frequently repeated injections. Andrieu et al. (1981) treated 11 patients with epidural morphine (7 mg) for this indication. The results were excellent in all cases. A second opioid injection of 6 mg was only necessary (after 18 hours) in one patient. Side effects were not observed, with the exception of urinary retention seen in one case.

Logically the treatment will be started with local anaesthetics. However if motor block problems arise a trial with opioids can be given.

12.5 Acute pancreatitis

Animal studies and clinical experience have demonstrated that block of the afferent and sympathetic supply to the pancreas either by epidural block with local anaesthetics or by epidural opioids not only provide complete pain relief but overcome reflex spasm of the duodenum, the sphincter Oddi and the entire ductal system. So there is a rapid release of extraductal pressure with emptying of the extrabiliary and pancreatic ductal system of toxic fluid. The ileus is decreased and the ventilation increased (Bonica 1987).

Here again the classical therapy of this disease is the sympathetic block by epidural local anaesthetics or by a plexus block. However, opioids may be used if local anaesthetics are contra-indicated or insufficient.

12.6 Headache following dural puncture

Another strange indication for spinal opioids has been proposed: epidural morphine (2-5 mg) for the prevention or alleviation of headache following dural puncture (Boskovski and Lewinski 1982; Thangathurai et al. 1988). The method seems simple but is not safe. To treat an anaesthesia complication with another theoretically dangerous method seems questionable. Imagine a patient with postspinal headache on monday and respiratory depression on tuesday!

Postspinal headache is safely treated with fluids, horizontal position and eventually a dural blood patch.

12.7 Diagnosis of pain aetiology

In order to make a differential diagnosis between somatic and deafferentation pain on the one hand and psychogenic pain on the other hand epidural morphine was given in weak doses. Only when the pain was predominantly of somatic origin (compression neuralgia, spastic paraplegia, traumatisms) the pain relief was rapid and complete (Farcot et al. 1981), (Tab. 60).

In presence of plexus solaris pain the response to epidural morphine was not very good. It took longer for the hypalgesia to become established and duration of relief was relatively short.

In the case of a psychogenic or deafferentation pain (dysesthesia, algohallucinosis, plexic avulsions) there was no pain relief at all. In these cases side effects after spinal opioids were high. This was interpreted as a sign of a wrong indication for epidural opioids.

In the case of neurotic pain, even high doses of the opioid, do not give satisfactory results. These observations provide support for the hypothesis that nociceptive pain and non-nociceptive pain are controlled by different mechanisms (Arner S and Arner B 1985). It is thus apparent that different types of pain will have different responses to epidural opioids (Tasker and Tsuda 1982).

In order to complete the differential diagnosis, anaesthesia with a local anaesthetic given at different levels (e.g. epidural or plexic) may be necessary.

The method of opioid block for the differential diagnosis between pain of a mainly physical and psychogenic origin was refined by Cherry et al. (1985 b). His method was the following: epidural administration of 1 µg/kg fentanyl, followed by intravenous naloxone 0.4 mg and then 15-20 ml of 2% epidural lignocaine. If the visual analogue pain score of the patient decreased following epidural fentanyl and subsequently increased following naloxone, a predominantly physical (organic) base for the pain was likely. In contrast, small changes

Table 60. Criteria for differentiating pain of various origin, on the basis of the response to a test treatment with EDDA.

Type of pain	Pain relief	Dysphoric and other effects
- Somatic pain	+ + +	Ø
- Nerve lesions	+	Ø
- Deafferentation pain	poor	+ +
- Neurotic pain	poor	+

Ø = no + = yes
(Adapted from Cherry et al. 1985 b)

following fentanyl and naloxone suggested a diagnosis of a predominantly emotional basis for the pain. This method may be interesting, however, the intravenous bolus administration of 0.4 mg of naloxone to reverse opioid effects may be dangerous in high risk patients (De Castro and Kubicki 1980 b). On the other hand, it seems likely that in most cases a proper diagnosis can be done by conventional clinical examination.

Conclusions

The use of spinal opioids for treatment of severe subacute pain has found the most valuable applications in Intensive Care Units where close survey of the patients was guaranteed.

13. Obstetrics

13.1 Potential advantages, drawbacks and indications

13.1.1 JUSTIFICATION OF BETTER ANALGESIA

Labour and delivery pain, although it is a result of a physiological process, if unrelieved when it becomes severe may produce deleterious effects on the mother, foetus and newborn:

- severe respiratory acidosis during contractions
- alcalosis-induced hypoventilation between contractions
- maternal and fetal hypoxemia
- marked increase in sympathetic activity
- increase in catecholamine secretion, in metabolism and in O_2 consumption
- increased cardiac output, blood pressure and left ventricle work
- progressive metabolic acidosis
- decreased gastro-intestinal and urinary motility with delayed gastric emptying
- umbilical cord vasoconstriction
- impairment of blood gas exchanges.

All these changes are tolerated by the healthy parturients and the normal foetus who have compensatory mechanisms. However, they may prove deleterious in parturients with heart disease, toxemia, essential hypertension, pulmonary hypertension or severe anaemia. If the foetus is already at risk pain related disturbances in O_2/CO_2 exchange may become a critical factor that increases perinatal morbidity (Bonica 1987). Thus, effective pain control of labour is not only a question of maternal comfort; it may become in many cases of capital importance for maternal and fetal morbidity.

The most simple way for a rapid and well-controlled pain relief is the systemic administration of opioids. However, the potential side effects of parenteral opioids administered to parturients are obvious:

- diminished uterine activity during the first stage of labour

- neonatal respiratory depression
- orthostatic hypotension
- delayed gastric motility and emptying.

In contrast, lumbar spinal analgesia with local anaesthetics may completely block the nociceptive inputs, minimize the reflex responses and thus have beneficial effects on the mother and newborn.

The use of spinal opioids for obstetrics seems particularly attractive because this method offers excellent analgesia without some of the undesirable effects of local anaesthetics e.g. toxic reaction, allergy, non-specific sensory block, motor and sympathetic block.

However, after nearly 10 years experience with the method, it has become evident that spinal opioids are not without problems. So that the role of spinal opioids in obstetrics is today still a subject of controversy. Pros and cons of this topic will be discussed.

13.1.2 Potential advantages

- Spinal opioids compared to local anaesthetics don't produce motor block, sensory or sympathetic block, nor adverse effects on uterine contractility.
- Compared to the parenteral route the deposit of opioids near to the specific receptors in the spinal cord allows the use of smaller doses so that an important reduction in all side effects may be expected.

13.1.3 Potential disadvantages

- Obstetrical patients present an accelerated spread of opioids in the CSF attributable to diminished CSF volume and/or increased CSF circulation so that theoretically the danger of cephalad migration of the opioid might increase (Donnenfeld et al. 1987).
- Special disadvantage: the quality of analgesia is inferior to epidural local anaesthetics and more inconsistent.
- Opioids may cross the placental barrier and produce side effects on the foetus.

13.1.4 Potential indications

Labour and delivery pain
Spinal opioids may be particularly indicated:

- in cases where pregnancy increases the risk of
  . heart failure
  . bacterial endocarditis
  . cerebral thrombosis
- in situations where a decrease in systemic vascular resistance is to be avoided:
  . aortic stenosis
  . tetralogy of Fallot
  . Eisenmenger syndrom
  . coarctation of the aorta
  . toxemia
  . cystic fibrosis
- if regional blocks are ruled out (Hyde and Harrison 1986).

Other obstetrical indications:

- post-caesarean section analgesia
- prostaglandin abortion
- pre-eclampsia
- post-partum episiotomy?

Epidural or intrathecal epinephrine has been reported to improve the intensity and duration of spinal opioid analgesia and to reduce side effects (Malinov et al. 1989). For others, such statements are not evident (Johnson et al. 1989; Moonka et al. 1989; Sharnick et al. 1989).

13.2 Labour and delivery pain

13.2.1 EPIDURAL OPIOIDS

Initially, epidural opioids provided promise as ideal analgesia for labour because of their selective effect on the perception of pain.

13.2.1.1 MORPHINE

In most clinical studies epidural morphine in a dosage of 2 to 10 mg provided relatively poor results.

Examples

- A 2 mg dose of epidural morphine was clearly inadequate (Hughes et al. 1984 b; Martin R et al. 1985; Writer et al. 1981).

- A 4 mg dose of morphine was still inadequate and increased the occurrence of side effects (Husemeyer and Davenport 1980 a; Husemeyer et al. 1980 b; McDonald and Smith 1984; Writer et al. 1981).
- The analgesia obtained with doses of 7.5-10 mg epidural morphine in parturient women was only effective in 64-66% of the cases, only during a medium duration of 6h and only until the end of the first stage of labour (Dick et al. 1983; Hartung et al. 1980 a, b; Knitza et al. 1982; Nybbel-Lindahl et al. 1981).
- In the majority of cases the quality of this analgesia was not as good as that obtained in the first period of the delivery with epidural local anaesthetics (Hughes et al. 1984 b).
- In all patients given epidural morphine, local anaesthesia was needed for the second stage of labour if instrumentation or episiotomy was required (Writer et al. 1981).

When all these observations are taken into consideration it becomes evident that the risk/benefit ratio of epidural morphine in delivery is too high.

The most important disadvantages are :

- variable duration of action
- delayed onset
- pruritus: 80%
- nausea and vomiting
- interference with additional parenteral opioids
- possibility of late respiratory depression
- urinary retention, dysphoria
  (Robertson et al. 1985).

Delayed respiratory depression seems to be a complication which is an unavoidable companion to an opioid with long duration of action and poor lipid solubility. In 1987, Gieraerts et al. reported on increased incidence of oral herpes simplex appearing between days 2-3 postoperatively in patients given ED morphine. Crone et al. (1988, 1989) observed this complication in 14.6% of the parturients. Herpes simplex after delivery is of concern because the virus can spread to the infant and cause herpes encephalitis. The mechanism of reactivation of HSLV is unknown, but may be related to central stimulation of the trigeminal nerve ganglion by ED morphine inducing pruritus (78%) and mobilization of the latent herpes virus (Crone et al. 1989).

Now, most authors have abandoned epidural morphine for delivery (Duffy 1981 a, b).

13.2.1.2 Pethidine

Liposoluble opioids which remain fixed to the spinal cord with little free drug amount available for rostral spread produce a much lower risk of delayed respiratory depression (Bromage 1981 a). They provide a more rapid onset and a better analgesia but are of shorter duration of action (Baraka et al. 1982 a; Hammonds et al. 1982). They are also ineffective in the second stage of labour (Husemeyer et al. 1980 a, 1981, 1982; Malins et al. 1984; Perriss 1979, 1980 a).

Pethidine has been used with little success by most authors. A dose of 25 mg provides an analgesia which is only satisfactory during the first period of delivery and then only in 50% of the cases (Perriss 1980 a).

Baraka et al. (1982 a) obtained a success rate of 84% in primipara using epidural pethidine in the high doses of 100 mg. The addition of adrenaline (1/200,000) sometimes produced an increase in the satisfying results. This point however, is not accepted by all investigators. Skjöldebrand (1982 b), e.g. has not observed any advantage in the use of epinephrine together with pethidine.

After the use of pethidine to the mother during childbirth measurable amounts of the drug are found in the neonate. The neonate will excrete about 0.4% of a maternal dose of pethidine as pethidine or norpethidine in the first 72h of life (Kuhnert et al. 1985). For the toxicity of norpethidine see Section 7.1.3.

13.2.1.3 Fentanyl

Epidural fentanyl was administered at doses of 50 to 100 μg and the results obtained were satisfactory (Carrie 1980; Carrie et al. 1981; Francis et al. 1981; Martin et al. 1983 a, b; Wolfe and Nicholas 1979).

Carrie (1980) and Carrie et al. (1981) found excellent pain relief following epidural fentanyl injections of 0.15-0.2 mg. Although pain scores decreased significantly up to 90 min after the first dose, the second dose caused pain relief only for 60 min, and the third dose was almost ineffective. Thus, both efficacy and duration of action of epidural fentanyl in labour diminished with subsequent doses.

Fentanyl proved more rapid, more effective during early labour than other opiates. Few side effects were reported (Francis et al. 1981; Justins et al. 1982 b). Epidural fentanyl 100 μg produced a significant increase in uterine contractions (Bazin et al. 1989).

Continuous infusion is a possible alternative to bolus application of fentanyl. After the first bolus of 50 μg, continuous epidural infusion of 25 μg/h can be administered. Bailey and Smith (1980); Skerman et al. (1985 a) reported the successful use of this technique.

Conclusions about opioids used alone:

The results in obstetrics with epidural opioids used alone are poor or unreliable (Booker et al. 1980 a, b; Husemeyer et al. 1981). Explanation for the disappointing results of epidural opioids obtained in obstetrics are as follows:

- Increased vascularisation of epidural space:
  . systemic absorption is increased
  . increased abdominal pressure may result in excessive dissemination of the drug.
- Distention of epidural veins:
  . venous re-uptake is increased
  . redistribution is increased
  . hepatic metabolism is increased.
- Endorphins are increased at the end of labour:
  . competition for receptors.
- Uterine contractions are increased by the opioids.

In general, epidural opioids alone have proved to be inferior to even dilute concentrations of local anaesthetics, even when liposoluble drugs have been employed (Skjölderbrand et al. 1982 a, b).

The addition of adrenaline appears to increase the success but not sufficiently to make this a reliable technique. The best results that can be achieved are for the first stage of labour. However, poor analgesia results are frequent for the second and third stage.

13.2.1.4 Morphine + bupivacaine

The association of an epidural opioid with a local anaesthetic was proposed by: Baraka 1982 b; Desprats et al. 1983; Müller et al. 1981; Youngstrom et al. 1984. The analgesia for the first period of delivery was improved and the duration became longer as a result of the association (Niv et al. 1986).

In association with morphine (Hughes et al. 1984 b; Husemeyer et al. 1980 b) the amount of bupivacaine could be slightly reduced. The injection interval was prolonged by about 25%. The patients, however, have shown an increased incidence of nausea and vomiting.

13.2.1.5 Lipophilic opioid + local anaesthetic

Morphine, fentanyl, lofentanil, sufentanil, alfentanil, butorphanol and buprenorphine have been investigated in association with a local anaesthetic.

a) Fentanyl + bupivacaine

Fentanyl 50-100 µg and bupivacaine 0.25%, is the most frequently proposed association for labour (Biehl 1984; Bouvier et al. 1983; Capogna 1987; Celleno and Capogna 1988; Chestnut et al. 1987, 1988,1989; Cohen et al. 1986, 1987; Cousin et al. 1983; Deprats et al. 1983; Celleno and Capogna 1988; Grice et al. 1987; Jorrot et al. 1989; Justins an Reynold 1982 a; Justins et al. 1983; Kavuri et al. 1989; Keruel et al. 1983; Landais et al. 1983; Leveque et al. 1986; Nalda et al. 1982; Seebacher et al. 1983; Skerman et al. 1985 b; Vella et al. 1985 b; Viscomi et al. 1989; Wilhite and Blass 1989; Youngstrom et al. 1984; Younker et al. 1987).

Reported advantages are:

- more rapid onset
- improved analgesia
- improved progress of labour
- significantly shorter first stage of labour
- subanaesthetic doses of both components
- longer-lasting analgesia
- parturients consider motor block with paralysis produced by bupivacaine alone to be unpleasant during labour
- maintenance of full motor function facilitates nursing care (Chestnut et al. 1988).

Examples:

- In a controlled trial, Justins et al. (1982 b) showed that fentanyl 0.08 mg and bupivacaine 0.5% (4 ml) produced an analgesia that was more complete and more rapid in onset than in the control group (saline + bupivacaine 0.5%). The first top-up dose of bupivacaine was needed after 2.36h versus 1.66 h. The epidural fentanyl-bupivacaine association was free from complications, itching being the only clinically significant side effect and even that was mild.

- Van Steenberge (1983 a, b) obtained excellent results with fentanyl (<0.1mg) in association with bupivacaine 0.125%. But, therefore it was necessary that the mother should not receive any parenteral opioid and the concentration of the injected local anaesthetic should be low (Leveque et al. 1986).

- Nevertheless, Deprats (1983 a) observed an elevation of the intra-uterine pressure ensuring fetal bradycardia in 30% of the cases following the administration of fentanyl 0.1 mg plus bupivacaine 15 mg.

- A mixture of low dose bupivacaine and fentanyl slowly titrated can provide excellent analgesia for labour and delivery in parturients with severe pulmonary hypertension and probably in those with other significant cardiac disease, without adverse cardiovascular or respiratory effects (Robinson and Leicht 1988).

- A shorter first stage, better relief of pain and anxiety was reported in women who received a bolus injection of bupivacaine (22.5 mg) and fentanyl (0.05-0.1 mg) compared with women who received either bupivacaine alone (22.5 mg) or bupivacaine (7.5 mg) and fentanyl (0.1 mg) (Cohen et al. 1987).

- The addition of 0.1 mg of fentanyl to epidural bupivacaine did not significantly affect the neurobehavioural scores of newborn infants (Capogna et al. 1987).

- Continuous epidural infusion of 0.0625% bupivacaine with 0.0002% fentanyl produced good analgesia similar to that provided by the infusion of 0.125% bupivacaine alone, but women in the bupivacaine-fentanyl group experienced less intense motor block (Chestnut et al. 1988).

- Parturients who received a continuous epidural infusion of 0.125% bupivacaine plus 0.00025% fentanyl experienced stronger and more profound analgesia than women who received an infusion of 0.125% bupivacaine alone (Skerman et al. 1985 b).

The combination of an epidural opioid with a local anaesthetic administered in continuous infusion can increase the advantages of both drugs. The following method was proposed (Bochenek et al. 1987):

1. First test dose: 3 ml bupivacaine 0.5% + epinephrine 1/200,000.
2. Second test dose: 10 ml bupivacaine 0.125%, in 2 divided doses + fentanyl 50 µg.
3. Continuous infusion: bupivacaine 0.125% + fentanyl 1 µg/ml (1st hour: 10 ml/h, 2nd hour: 8 ml/h, subsequently: 6 ml/h).

This method eliminated the dangerous large boli, allowed the use of lower drug doses due to synergistic analgesic effects and avoided periods of inadequate pain relief for the parturient and detrimental effects for the neonate or on uterine activity (Beneditti 1987; Chestnut et al. 1987; D'Athis et al. 1988).

Epidural fentanyl + bupivacaine infusion compared to epidural morphine + bupivacaine infusion has in the same indication a shorter analgesia but produced clearly less side effects (Fischer et al. 1987). The association of fentanyl and bupivacaine is perhaps today the most widely used analgesic combination in obstetrics. Nevertheless, not all authors reported the same enthousiasm about this association.

Recently a double-blind study was performed with 50-100 µg fentanyl + 3-9 ml of bupivacaine 0.25% in 82 parturients in active labour (Cohen et al. 1987). They did not find any statistically significant difference in analgesia or duration of labour compared to the results with local anaesthetics alone. Hypotension, vomiting, nausea and urinary retention was more frequent with bupivacaine alone but pruritus (30%) and drowsiness was frequent with the association and absent or rare with bupivacaine alone. Neonate condition was similar in all groups. In contrast to previous reports significant potentiation of epidural bupivacaine by fentanyl was not found.

These results do not support the routine addition of fentanyl to bupivacaine. For Cohen et al. (1987), only marginal benefits may result from this technique that justify its use only in certain circumstances, e.g. prolonged labour or pain unrelieved by moderate doses of bupivacaine.

b) Alfentanil + bupivacaine

Alfentanil in continuous infusion of 30 µg/ kg/h + bupivacaine 0.125% was studied by Heytens et al. (1987). The association proved to be unsatisfactory. For others the same association provided excellent results (Ahn et al. 1989; Huckaby et al. 1989; Waldman et al. 1989; Wilhite and Blass 1989).

c) Lofentanil + bupivacaine

The epidural administration of lofentanil 1.25 µg with 0.125% bupivacaine and epinephrine (12.5 µg) was studied by Van Steenberge (1983 a, c). Reinjections, if necessary, were given with the same doses of bupivacaine and epinephrine but only with 0.625 µg lofentanil up to a maximum dose of 2.5 µg lofentanil. An analgesia of inconsistent quality and duration (60 to 120 min) was obtained, nausea and vomiting were frequent.

d) Sufentanil + bupivacaine

As a sole agent, epidural sufentanil is in obstetrics of no value, but when added

346

to bupivacaine and epinephrine the results become satisfying. Compared to bupivacaine alone, the total doses of the local anaesthetic are significantly reduced by the association with sufentanil.

After the use of fentanyl and lofentanil for pain treatment in delivery Van Steenberge has now adopted sufentanil as the opioid of choice. He prepared the following analgesic mixture:

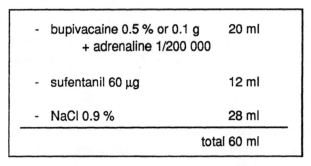

- bupivacaine 0.5 % or 0.1 g + adrenaline 1/200 000	20 ml
- sufentanil 60 μg	12 ml
- NaCl 0.9 %	28 ml
	total 60 ml

According to weight and physical status, the patient received via the epidural catheter, a slow injection of 8 to 10 ml of the solution. Complete pain relief was obtained in 95% of the obstetrical patients. The duration of analgesia after one injection was evaluated between 31/2 hours-41/2 hours.

This drug combination produced only moderate and rare side effects. At total doses of sufentanil lower than or equal to 50 μg, no clinical respiratory depression was noted. Pruritus required no treatment. Dizziness was more bothersome. However it was not long-lasting. Drowsiness was dose-dependent and of variable intensity. It only became really obvious after the delivery, when the stimulus keeping the mother awake has disappeared, and it lasted not longer than 1h. It appeared further that the side effects of sufentanil responded to intravenous injections of naloxone used in doses which did not significantly affect analgesia (Van Steenberge 1983 a, b; Van Steenberge et al. 1987 a, b).

Absence of respiratory depression, acceptable side effects and excellent pain relief with this technique were confirmed by Jorrot et al. (1989); Leicht et al. (1986 b); Little et al. (1987); Mourisse et al. (1985); Naulty et al. (1986 d, 1989); Phillips (1987 a, b, c, 1988 a, b, c); Tan et al. (1986 a, b); Vandermeulen et al. (1989); Vertommen et al. (1989). Sufentanil passed the foeto-placental barrier easily, but penetration into the foetal system was negligible because of its strong plasma-protein binding (92%) and its distribution over the various tissue compartments (Nouheid et al. 1984). The advantages of the epidural association method sufentanil-bupivacaine were recently objectivated by two double-blind studies:

- lower bupivacaine concentrations (0.125-0.25%) were used
- analgesia onset was more rapid
- quality was maintained, residual pain was less frequent

- motor block was less pronouced
- duration of analgesia for one injection was longer (+ 40%)
- fewer analgesic "top-up reinjections" were required (-50%)
- total bupivacaine doses were reduced
- benefits to the mother are not offset by any obvious adverse effect on the foetus
  as evaluated by:
  . neonatal respiratory rate
  . mode of delivery
  . duration of expulsion
  . Apgar scores
  (Phillips 1988 a, b; Van Steenberge et al. 1987 a, b).

The quality of the association (sufentanil and a local anaesthetic) may be improved by continuous epidural infusion. The analgesic solution of Van Steenberge, of 60 ml is then divided as follows:
- loading dose: 10 ml
- continuous infusion: 10 ml/h
- additional bolus if required: 5 ml (Phillips 1988 a, b, c).

e) Butorphanol + bupivacaine

In a double-blind study, epidural butorphanol in doses of 3 mg associated with bupivacaine 0.25% was investigated. Labour and delivery pain was relieved for 6.5h. Somnolence was the only side effect (Abboud et al. 1989; Hunt et al. 1989; Mokriski et al. 1989; Naulty et al. 1986 c; Rodriguez et al. 1989).

13.2.2 INTRATHECAL OPIOIDS

Ideally, analgesia for labour should relieve pain while maintaining maternal expulsive forces of labour and motor tone. Epidural analgesia in some cases fails to meet this criterion because partial motor block at the time of delivery may be present. Intrathecal opioids provide satisfying analgesia in 85% of the parturients (just like do ED opioids) but do not affect motor neurons so that the patient's motor function is unimpaired (Yaksh and Rudy 1977). However, drawbacks of IT opioid analgesia are: lack of perineal analgesia and a higher incidence of side effects compared to ED opioids. In order to prevent the side effects prophylactic administration of opioid antagonists may be considered.

13.2.2.1 Morphine

Several reports indicate that small doses (e.g. 0.5-1 mg) of intrathecal morphine can provide good analgesia for labour (Abboud 1983, 1984 a; Ahmad et al. 1981; Baraka et al. 1981; Bonnardot et al. 1982; Brookshire et al. 1983; Camporesi and Redick 1983 b; Scott et al. 1980; Srivivan 1981).

An intrathecal dose of 1 to 1.75 mg morphine was effective in nearly all the cases and produced very low systemic morphine concentrations in mother and child (Bonnardot et al. 1982).

One mg of intrathecal morphine produced good pain relief after 15-60 min and lasted 12h. This pain relief resulted in a significant decrease in plasma ß-endorphin levels, probably due to alleviation of the stress induced by labour pain (Abboud 1984 a).

Mostly, authors have used doses of 0.5 to 2 mg of intrathecal morphine. This treatment provided in 80-93% of the cases a suppression of visceral pain for several hours.

However, the pain produced by dilatation of the perineum and of the vulva is not blocked. Severe respiratory depression of the mother has been observed. Hyperbaric morphine 1 mg was followed, 7 h after injection, by a respiratory depression requiring the administration of a total dose of 3.6 mg of naloxone (Abouleish 1988).

It is interesting to note that in parturient women, the duration of analgesia with hydrophilic opioids, particularly morphine, is significantly reduced: 5-10h compared to 20h in normal patients (Booker et al. 1980 a).

The following side effects were observed: pruritus 80%, nausea and vomiting 53%, urinary retention 43% (Abboud et al. 1984 a). The use of naloxone became necessary (Brookshire et al. 1983; Dailey et al. 1985).

Intrathecal morphine for labour and delivery has not become popular because of slow onset, side effects, inadequate perineal analgesia or relaxation for delivery and special monitoring requirements for potential delayed respiratory depression (Shnider 1989).

13.2.2.2 Beta-endorphin

Oyama et al. (1980 a) showed that 1 mg of intrathecal β-endorphin relieved first and second stage labour pain in all parturients. Perineal discomfort was absent for 12-32 hours post delivery. However, nausea and vomiting were seen in nearly 30% of the cases. Patients remained alert and there was no respiratory depression. Apgar scores and blood/gas values were normal.

β-endorphin has a high molecular weight, it does not pass the placenta or blood/brain barrier and cannot penetrate the foetal nervous system. This fact makes it necessary to administer the drug by intrathecal route.

The high cost of the product has not allowed its further use.

It has been shown that blood levels of β-endorphin and related neuropeptides rise under stressful conditions such as labour and delivery (Abboud et al. 1984 b).

13.2.2.3 Fentanyl + bupivacaine

After the epidural use of the association of fentanyl and bupivacaine for obstetrical analgesia, the following side effects were noted: hypotension 15%, nausea and vomiting 6%, pruritus 24%, urinary retention 3%. But neither respiratory depression nor headache were observed (Justins et al.1982 b). Johnson et al. (1989) reported that the addition of IT fentanyl to bupivacaine reduced the incidence of spinal headache.

13.2.2.4 Naloxone infusion for reduction of side effects

Naloxone significantly decreased the incidence of pruritus, urinary retention and vomiting. Maternal analgesia was reduced but not completely reversed. Progress of labour and clinical condition of the input at birth or the behavioural status of the baby were not affected.

The efficacy of naloxone in reducing the incidence of side effects after intra-thecal morphine and the effects on the condition of the newborn, were evaluated by Dailey et al. (1985) in 40 patients. Patients in labour were given 1 mg intrathecal morphine and 1h later either a 0.4 mg bolus of naloxone followed by a 0.4-0.6 mg/h intravenous infusion of naloxone, or an intravenous bolus of saline followed by an infusion of saline. Only 50% pain relief was obtained in 78% of the patients given morphine plus naloxone, and good pain relief in 82% of those given morphine alone.

However, the incidence of pruritus during labour and delivery, was signifi-cantly decreased by naloxone without reduction of adversal effects on the maternal or the neonatal status. But there was no significant decrease in the incidence of nausea, vomiting, somnolence, dizziness, or urinary retention in patients given naloxone.

Notwithstanding its partial effectiveness, taking into account the potential danger of naloxone (hypertension, shivering, lung oedema, etc.) the method cannot be recommended.

13.2.2.5 Naltrexone orally for reduction of side effects

Naltrexone, 25 mg, an oral long-acting opioid antagonist attenuates side effects of spinal opioids (Mok et al. 1986; Leighton et al. 1989).

13.2.3 GLOBAL EVALUATION

Considering the risk/benefit ratio of spinal opioids for labour and delivery in all these reports it is no wonder that the opinions in this field remain so controversial. Delivery pain is without any doubt to be treated in most cases. However, several drawbacks of spinal opioids have not been entirely solved.

As well as for the epidural as for the intrathecal use of opioids alone many weak points remain:

- slow onset of pain relief
- inadequate perineal analgesia
- inadequate relaxation for delivery
- pain during the terminal delivery phase
- necessity for special monitoring of the mother for delayed respiratory depression
- frequent side effects e.g. pruritus, nausea, vomiting, urinary retention, drowsiness, dizziness, headache. Respiratory depression (although rare) may occur.

The frequency of side effects are dose related and difficult to avoid if excellent analgesia is required. The respiratory depression of spinal opioids is reversible with a small dose of intravenous naloxone (0.1 mg) without complete reversal of analgesia. Naloxone may help to reduce other side effects and may even prevent deep respiratory depression however, this method provides an awkward solution to the problems.

The routine use of this technique as prophylaxis of side effects cannot be recommended in obstetrics. A method necessitating its own antagonist in conjunction with the agonist is not only theoretically dangerous but also not reliable for current use.

Apart from this, the intrathecal puncture in young patients followed by a high percentage of headache seems at least questionable.

Slow onset of analgesia can be improved by the use of lipophilic opioids and discomfort during the expulsion period can be avoided by complementary local anaesthetic blocks.

The best results seem to be obtained with the association of a very small dose of a lipophilic opioid (e.g. sufentanil) with bupivacaine in a small repeated bolus or administered by continuous infusion. However, this method is best applied in situations where local anaesthetics alone are insufficient or contra-indicated. The association technique may be particularly indicated in treating labour pain in patients with cardiac diseases (Hughes et al. 1984 b).

The use of naloxone for prophylaxis or treatment of side effects is best to be avoided.

13.3 Post-caesarean section

The treatment of postoperative pain after caesarean section with spinal opioids is for many authors currently a standard part of the approach to postoperative pain. However, the necessity of the use of such treatment is to be discussed in each individual situation.

13.3.1 EPIDURAL OPIOIDS

In many clinics conventional epidural anaesthesia with local anaesthetics is used for a caesarean section and the catheter is left in situ for postoperative pain treatment with epidural opioids.

13.3.1.1 Morphine

Many authors (Biehl 1984; Binsted 1983; Brooks et al. 1983; Chambers et al. 1983; Chayen et al. 1980; Cohen and Woods 1983 a; Danielson et al. 1981; Dick et al. 1983; Donchin et al. 1981; Kadieva and Van Hasselt 1982; Parker et al. 1988, Shuider 1989; Zakowski et al. 1989, e.g.) used morphine in epidural doses of 4-5 mg (2 mg were insufficient).

The epidural administration of morphine 5 mg at the end of surgery was associated in 80% of the cases with good to excellent postoperative analgesia lasting 24 to 36 hours (Donchin et al. 1981; Kotelko et al. 1984; Naulty et al. 1985; Phan et al. 1987; Rosen et al. 1983). An analgesia free from sedation and necessity of repeated painful injections enhances early mother-infant contact and maternal mobilisation (Danielson et al. 1981). Side effects however (e.g. pruritus and nausea) occurred frequently, but were usually mild and easily treated.

Leicht et al. (1986 b) reported a prospective study of 1000 patients and found that 85% obtained good to excellent postoperative analgesia lasting 23 hours. The authors noted 4 cases with respiratory rates < 10/min, two of them needed a naloxone injection. In a study of 72 patients Ramanathan et al. (1986) showed that intravenous naloxone infusion given in doses of 0.1 mg/h was effective in prevention of the side effects of epidural morphine in post-caesarean section patients. Cohen et al. (1989) found also a great patient satisfaction (85%) with ED morphine, 4-5 mg, compared to other analgesia techniques.

Nevertheless, in our opinion morphine has a slow analgesia onset and a higher incidence of potentially serious side effects than other opioids. It should be used only if adequate postoperative monitoring is available.

Oxygen saturation in 21 healthy, non-obese post-caesarean patients using epidural morphine 5 mg was studied by Brose et al. (1988). They observed desaturation episodes <85% in 71% of the cases with a minimum SaO_2 mean value of 83% and suggested that all patients receiving epidural morphine should undergo intensive surveillance in the first 24 hours postoperatively.

13.3.1.2 Methadone

Epidural methadone 4 mg was applied routinely, for post-caesarean section, in 178 women (Beeby et al. 1984). The results indicate that methadone is safe and effective for postoperative pain relief (Evron et al. 1985).

13.3.1.3 Hydromorphone

In a double-blind study, the quality of post-caesarean analgesia was reported. Twenty women receiving a single dose of epidural hydromorphone 1 mg were compared with 20 women receiving epidural bupivacaine, 10 ml 0.25%, followed by hydromorphone intramuscular 1-3 mg (Chestnut et al. 1985, 1986) The conclusions of this author were as follows:

- good and long-lasting analgesia
- early return of intestinal transit
- earlier hospital discharge
- but also more side effects (nausea, vomiting, pruritus) than seen after more conventional pain treatment with epidural bupivacaine + intramuscular hydro-morphone.

However, there were no stastistically significant differences between the two groups concerning first ambulation, first void, first passage of flatus, or hospital discharge.

The duration of ED hydromorphone analgesia is significantly prolonged after caesarean delivery with the addition of epinephrine (Dougherty et al. 1989).

- Parker et al. (1989) found after an ED hydromorphone PCA analgesia a higher incidence of side effects than in an IV hydromorphone PCA series of patients.

13.3.1.4 Pethidine

Epidural pethidine 50 mg was effective and had a duration of 4-6 hours (Brownridge 1983 a; Brownridge and Frewin 1985).

13.3.1.5 Fentanyl

Epidural administration of a bolus dose of 100 µg of fentanyl was proposed for routine use after elective caesarean section (Milon et al. 1983; Naulty et al. 1983). The maximum duration of analgesia was 3-7 hours and the side effects were mild: pruritus (41%), nausea (9%), somnolence (9%); respiratory depression was not noted. Because of the short duration of fentanyl analgesia repeated injections through the epidural catheter were to be given. The addition of 25 µg epinephrine to epidural fentanyl 100 µg did not potentiate the speed of onset of analgesia but significantly prolonged its duration of action (from 3 to 4 hours). This result, however, was obtained with an associated increase of pruritus (from 17% to 44%). On the other hand, drowsiness, hypotension, muscular weakness, nausea, vomiting, vertigo, urinary retention and respiratory depression were not observed (Robertson et al. 1985).

The most convenient epidural dose of fentanyl seems to be 50 µg with reinjection in 1 hour intervals (Malinow et al. 1988 b).
- The use of incremental ED fentanyl 50 µg doses titrated by the patient (PCA) is also very satisfying (Yu et al. 1989).
- Another convenient administration technique for fentanyl is the ED continuous infusion: 0.75 µg/kg/h (Ellis et al. 1989).

13.3.1.6 Sufentanil

Sufentanil, due to the high liposolubility is rapidly absorbed after epidural injection. Epidural sufentanil 30-60 µg was compared to epidural morphine 5 mg in 10 ml volume for post-caesarean section analgesia. Sufentanil provided rapid and excellent analgesia for 5 hours with minimal side effects. With morphine, analgesia was slow in onset and long-lasting (26 hours), but side effects (pruritus and nausea) were more frequent (Leicht et al. 1986 b). A minimum dose of 30 µg of sufentanil was found necessary to produce satisfactory analgesia following caesarean section (Rosen et al. 1988).

Increasing the sufentanil dosage to 60-70 μg produced little or no improvement in quality or duration of pain relief.

Increasing the volume of injectate of ED sufentanil without epinephrine had no effect on the duration of analgesia. However, adding 50 μg epinephrine to 20 ml of injectate was associated with a significant prolongation of analgesia (Naulty et al. 1989).

The analgesic effect of sufentanil 30 μg does not appear to be cumulative (Rosen et al. 1988).

The analgesia resulting from 25-50 μg epidural sufentanil appears to be similar to that resulting from 50-100 μg epidural fentanyl. Thus relative analgesic potencies of fentanyl and sufentanil by epidural route seems to be only 1 to 2. It appears to be different from the relative potency when these products are administered by intravenous route (1 to 5 or 10), (Cohen et al. 1988). The use of sufentanil in continuous epidural infusion was suggested as being an improvement against bolus administration (Tan et al. 1986 a, b).

Infusion rates of 10 μg/h ED sufentanil may be required.

13.3.1.7 Butorphanol

Epidural butorphanol 4 mg was administered after caesarean section. It provided effective analgesia within 15 min for a main duration of 51/2 hours and without a significant incidence of side effects (Palacios et al. 1987; Tan et al. 1987).

For the same indication epidural butorphanol 2-6 mg was investigated by Naulty et al. (1984, 1986 b). Butorphanol provided prolonged pain relief, however, somnolence with a mean duration of 6 hours was seen in 92% of the cases.

Abboud et al. (1987) reported on 122 women who underwent caesarean section. They received for the relief of postoperative pain 2-4 mg of butorphanol. Analgesia was effective during 6-8 hours, and produced only minor side effects. Sensitivity to CO_2 was decreased during a period of 1 1/2 hours after the opioid injection.

Good analgesia for 3 hours with minimal side effects was also obtained by Tan et al. (1987).

13.3.1.8 Meptazinol

After meptazinol 30 mg results were poor and side effects far too high so that the study was abandoned (Francis and Lockart 1986).

13.3.1.9 Buprenorphine

Epidural buprenorphine 0.18 mg given after elective caesarean section carried out under epidural bupivacaine provided good pain relief in 80% of the patients. 28% developed urinary retention (Simpson et al. 1988).

13.3.1.10 Opioids associated with local anaesthetics

A local anaesthetic given before or together with the opioid may influence the efficacy of post-caesarean delivery of epidural opioid analgesia.

Bupivacaine has the advantage of long duration of action, high protein binding and hence a low maternal/foetal transfer ratio. However, the drug has also, at high doses or high concentrations, the serious disadvantage of cardiovascular toxicity. Attempts to combine low doses of bupivacaine with low opioid doses seems to be justified. An association with an opioid allows the use of smaller bupivacaine doses and increases the analgesic efficacy as well as the analgesic duration (Van Steenberge 1983 a).

However, also antagonism between two compounds has been reported (change in pH?) with several associations: e.g. lignocaine or chloroprocaine with morphine (Phan et al. 1988 a, b). This seems not true for the association bupivacaine with morphine, fentanyl or sufentanil or with the association lignocaine and fentanyl.

a) Morphine + bupivacaine

Epidural morphine 3 mg + 0.125% bupivacaine used in 100 patients resulted in longer duration of analgesia with lower opioid doses (Douglas and McMorlan 1987 b; Fischer et al. 1987; Hanson et al. 1984).

b) Fentanyl + bupivacaine

The minimum reliable effective dose of epidural fentanyl was 0.05 mg in patients who received 0.75% bupivacaine for caesarean delivery. However, here again it must be noted that bupivacaine 0.75% is a dangerous concentration that should be avoided in obstetrics (Naulty et al. 1983, 1985, 1986 b). Higher doses did not produce longer or more profound analgesia, merely a more rapid onset of the pain relief. The duration of analgesia ranged from 3 to 7 hours. Muscle relaxation at term was always sufficient. Side effects were very mild, of short duration and required no treatment (Bochenek et al. 1987; Fischer et al. 1987; Milon et al. 1985 a, b, 1986; Robertson et al. 1985).

Fentanyl 75 µg + bupivacaine 0.5% decreased significantly the onset of analgesia and improved the overall quality of analgesia (Johnson et al. 1989).

c) Fentanyl + lignocaine

The association of epidural fentanyl 1 µg/kg + lignocaine 2% + epinephrine 1/200,000 provided after caesarean section superior and longer analgesia than epidural lignocaine anaesthesia alone. Adverse neonatal and maternal effects were not observed (Michelangeli et al. 1984; Preston et al. 1987, 1988; Tessler et al. 1988).

d) Fentanyl + chlorprocaine

The addition of fentanyl to ED anaesthesia with chlorprocaine did not facilitate the onset nor improve the quality of analgesia during the immediate period after caesarean section (Phan et al. 1984).

e) Sufentanil + bupivacaine

Epidural sufentanil 25-50 µg associated with bupivacaine and epinephrine was administered for post-caesarean section pain management (Fanard 1988; Naulty et al. 1986).

Advantages of the combination reported by the authors are as follows:

- dose and concentration of bupivacaine can be reduced
- motor block is less pronouced (compared to bupivacaine alone)
- analgesia is more rapid in onset, of better quality and of longer postoperative duration (compared to fentanyl + bupivacaine).

f) Sufentanil + lignocaine

If shivering and hypothermia appeared after ED anaesthesia with lignocaine, the ED administration of 100 µg of sufentanil diluted in 10 ml saline provided cessation of shivering, nausea and hypothermia (case report: Johnson et al. 1989).

13.3.2 INTRATHECAL OPIOIDS

Intrathecal morphine 0.3-0.6 mg provided a similar degree of high quality analgesia as did epidural morphine 3.0-5.0 mg. The duration of analgesia however, was longer with intrathecal administration. (Chadwick and Ready 1988; Zakowski et al. 1989). Stenkamp et al. (1989) noted in a comparative study of 92 patients that the use of IT morphine for pain relief after caesarean section, provided earlier ambulation, reduced morbidity and shorter length of hospital stay than in patients given IV or IM opioids. The lumbar administration of 0.5 mg intrathecal morphine followed by 1.8-2.8 ml hyperbaric 0.5% bupivacaine without epinephrine (the patients being in a supine position) was used by Kadieva and Van Hasselt (1982). The level of anaesthesia reached either the 7th or 8th thoracic dermatome and lasted between 2 1/2-3 hours. All patients were comfortable during surgery and there was no request for additional analgesia throughout the entire postoperative day. Pruritus and nausea were frequent. The intrathecal association of 0.1 mg to 0.2 mg morphine with hyperbaric bupivacaine (0.50%) was a simple, safe and effective method of providing adequate intraoperative and prolonged postoperative analgesia. Neonatal conditions were not adversely affected by this small opioid dose. Nevertheless, close monitoring of the patients during 24 hours was recommended (Abboud et al. 1987, 1988; Abouleish et al. 1987).

IT buprenorphine 0.03-0.04 mg/70kg + bupivacaine was recommended after caesarean section. (Celleno and Capogna 1989).

Real arguments for the intrathecal use of an association of morphine and a local anaesthetic instead of the epidural use are not evident. In most cases the "normal" systemic analgesia is quiet enough to obtain an acceptable pain relief with the minimal risk for mother and child.

13.4 Side effects of spinal opioids in obstetrics

13.4.1 MATERNAL SIDE EFFECTS

Side effects of opioids have been discussed in detail in previous chapters.

Naltrexone 6-12 mg, a long-acting oral opioid antagonist, may slightly decrease the incidence and severity of side effects produced by spinal opioids, however, it also tends to reverse the analgesia (Abboud et al. 1989; Norris et al. 1989).

Total pain relief is seldom a necessity and never free of any risk. The comfort/safety ratio is to be evaluated carefully in each case. If titrated dosage and close survey of the effects of spinal opioids are guaranteed, side effects will be low and the choice of spinal opioids alone or in combination with local analgesics will be justified.

13.4.2 FOETAL SIDE EFFECTS

The magnitude of the foetal effect will be determined by foetal drug exposure and therefore by pharmacokinetic factors governing the disposition of the drug in the mother and foetus (e.g. lipid solubility and protein binding).The placenta, like the blood-brain barrier is a lipid membrane and therefore the opioids that cross the latter rapidly will also cross the former. Hence morphine can be expected to cross the placenta more slowly than the other opioids (Reynolds 1987).

An important determinant of plasma transfer is protein binding, particularly to alpha 1-acid glycoprotein (AAG). Foetal AAG levels are significantly lower than maternal AAG levels. Thus for opioids that are highly bound to AAG such as fentanyl, alfentanil, and sufantanil, the foetal/maternal plasma ratio of drug concentrations will be relatively low (Meuldermans et al. 1986).

A Ratio of around 0.3 has been measured in man following epidural adminis-tration of alfentanil (Gepts et al. 1986). The maternal plasma concentration of fentanyl following epidural administration is low and foetal levels have not been reported (Justins et al. 1983; Vella et al. 1985 b).

13.5 Post-partum episiotomy

With epidural morphine (2 mg) given after post-partum episiotomy the resultant analgesia lasted about 12 hours. If 4 mg of epidural morphine was used the results were not better and side effects were increased (McDonald and Smith 1984).

The use of such method of analgesia seems a questionable indication.

13.6 Prostaglandin abortion

Pain may be very severe and long-lasting in prostaglandin abortion. Also, the difficult psychological conditions of these cases necessitate all our possibilities for pain relief. Epidural opioids by providing long-lasting and strong analgesia seems to be the ideal method of analgesia. However, close supervision in a special ward is a "conditio sine qua non".

A very good indication is the use of epidural morphine 2-3 mg, for prostaglandin abortion during the second trimester of gestation. The dose of morphine is to be repeated according to need. An application of this method over 24 hours was satisfactory in 81.8% of cases. A total dose of 5.25 mg of morphine was required (Magora et al. 1980 a; Tiengo et al. 1984).

13.7 Pre-eclampsia

For a patient with severe hypertension local anaesthetics may present a danger. In such a case, epidural opioids may be indicated.

The epidural opioid reverses the hypertension associated with symptoms of pre-eclampsia and even severe eclampsia (Vincenti et al. 1982 a).

The method is to be considered as supplementary to a classical eclampsia treatment.

13.8 Precautions and surveillance

The use of spinal opioids in obstetrics requires the same precautions as those discussed for their use in surgery. The administration of opioids can only be considered if all the necessary measures are taken for close and prolonged supervision of the patient. The personnel responsible for observing the patients must be aware of the potential complications of the technique and naloxone must be immediately available. Written instructions for surrveillance on the ward are recommended (Tab. 59).

13.9 Survey of the principal clinical reports

Previous data indicate that the efficacy of epidural opioids in obstetrics has been controversial. Results are very different depending on:

- indications
- substances
- doses used.

The authors have surveyed the results obtained by 110 groups of investigators in >4000 parturient women (Tab.61). Among these studies, several are double-blind studies, with respect to both the analgesia technique and the products or the doses used.

Indications for the use of epidural opioids were:

- delivery, first stage: 54 investigations
- post-caesarean operative pain: 54 investigations
- abortion: 2 investigations

Table 61. Multicentre survey of the results in obstetrical pain treatment with EDOA using different opioids alone or in association with a local anaesthetic (N > 4000).

Opioid used	Doses mg / 70 kg bw	Number of studies		Results poor	good	excellent
morphine	2.5 - 5	38				
			43	30	12	1
morphine+ bupivacaine	2	5				
pethidine	25 - 50	6				
			11	4	7	0
pethidine + bupivacaine	25 - 50	5				
fentanyl	0.05 - 01	15				
fentanyl + bupivacaine	0.1	20	37	0	18	19
fentanyl + lignocaine		2				
butorphanol	4	3		0	0	3
diamorphine	5 - 75	2		0	1	1
hydromorphone	1	1	19	0	0	1
lofentanil + bupivacaine	0.00125	1		0	1	0
sufentanil + bupivacaine	0.075 - 0.05	12		0	0	12
total: 110						

The drugs used and doses referred to in this survey are summarized in Tab. 61.

High doses of morphine (7.5 mg) given epidurally for delivery, have provided poor analgesia for 5-6 hours in 66% of the women, and only for the first stage of delivery.

Epidural morphine 2-5 mg was unsatisfactory in more than 50% of patients. In comparison, epidural bupivacaine alone was fully effective in most patients in stages 1 and 2 of delivery. For epidural pethidine 50 mg, associated with epinephrine the results were somewhat better (75% success rate), but still inferior compared with epidural bupivacaine alone (95% success rate).

For pain treatment after caesarean section, 5 mg epidural morphine 0.1 mg fentanyl or 50 mg pethidine, was partially effective, but the reported complications were higher after epidural morphine or pethidine, than those encountered after epidural fentanyl 0.05 mg.

The epidural association of an opioid with a local anaesthetic, permitted better analgesia and significant dose reduction. At present the association of low doses of epidural bupivacaine and sufentanil seems to provide the best and most reliable results.

The overall evaluations of the results have been, for purposes of simplification, classified as poor, good, and excellent. Excellent results are significantly better than those obtained, with non-opioid analgesia techniques.

Although, spinal opioids can provide outstanding analgesia in a wide variety of clinical situations the use of spinal opioids is, at present, also associated with some potentially serious side effects.

The most serious of these delayed respiratory depression (it is also, fortunately, the rarest) leads to a question of safety/analgesia quality ratio, risk versus benefits.

How much risk is the absence of labour or postoperative pain worth? That is the reason why the place of spinal opioids in obstetrics remains limited to particular indications:

- patients with cardiac diseases
- pre-eclampsia or other situations where serious catecholamine or blood pressure increases are to be avoided
- prostaglandin abortion (severe pain and psychological aspects)
- post-caesarean section pain is not a routine indication.

If spinal opioids are to be used:

- the epidural route is the best administration technique
- poor liposoluble opioids are to be avoided

- a lipophilic opioid has our preference.

Until techniques for eliminating serious side effects should be better controlled, adequate nursing surveillance and preparation for reversal of late respiratory depression with intravenous naloxone is mandatory.

Conclusions

Severe delivery pain must be treated. However, neither parenteral nor spinal opioids offer the method of choice.

The local blocks are in a great number of cases superior in this indication. Exceptions are cardiac patients and patients with a specific contra-indication for local anaesthetics.

Lipophilic opioids used in small doses in association with local anaesthetics by epidural or intrathecal route may increase the comfort of mother but such association can only be justified if measures of security and survey are increased at the same time.

14. Cancer pain

Pain is experienced by 60 to 85% of patients with terminal carcinoma and requires effective and consistent therapy (Bonica 1987).

14.1 Analgesic ladder

The first step on the analgesic ladder in cancer patients consists of causal measures in controlling pain e.g. chemotherapy, radiation, surgery (Fig. 85, Tab. 62). Although cancer pain in most patients can be treated by oral medication, the majority of these patients receives analgesics in inadequate amounts or in a wrong way.

The following basic principles (Twycross and Lack 1983; Clarke 1987) are of real value:

- Drugs are given orally wherever possible.
- Drugs are given regularly by the clock .
- No "give-when-required" (p.r.n.) drugs.
- The longest acting drugs are used (the drug of choice is slow release morphine).
- Only one drug in each group is given.
- Only one doctor prescribes.
- Adjuvants are given where required (especially NSAIDS, tricyclics, not phenothiazines or barbiturates, cocaine or amphetamines).
- There is "normal" use of alcoholic beverages.
- Laxatives are taken regularly.
- Antiemetics should be rarely required.

Emergence of side effects after the first few days should initiate search for:

- overuse (rare)
- additional drug use (common where many physicians are involved)
- change in pathology
- affective illness
- new psychosocial stressors.

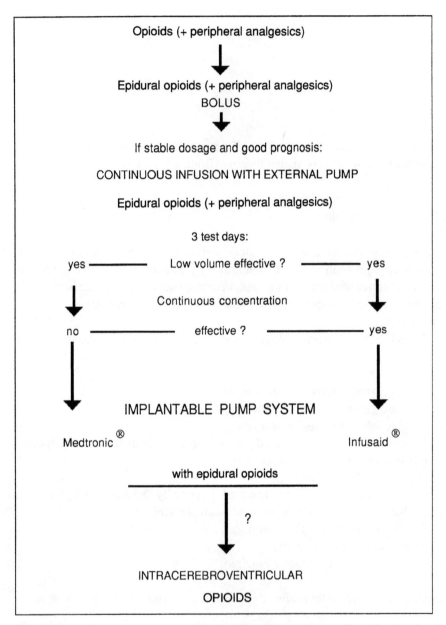

Fig. 85. Schematic representation of technical solutions that may be considered for chronic pain treatment. (Zenz 1988)

Table 62. Sequential analgesic ladder in cancer pain. A suggested 12 step escalation of pharmalogical treatments.

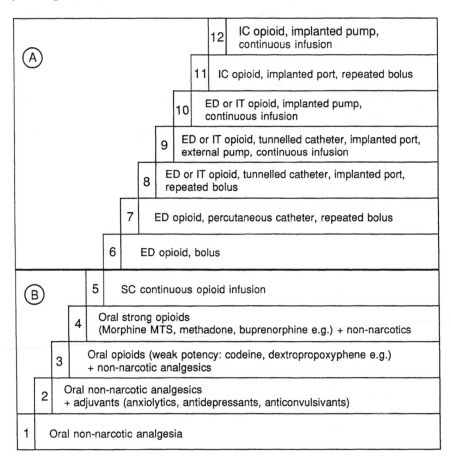

A = RGOA treatments
B = Classical treatments
From step 3: most steps include peripheral analgesic as a basic treatment.
Steps 8, 9, 10: ED or IT is mostly a personal choice of the clinician.

Breakthrough pain should alert to:

- change in pathology
- depressive illness
- new psychological stressors (including pressure from relatives or professional careers)
- inadequate dosage (Clarke 1987).

Treatment starts with peripherally acting analgesics e.g.aspirine 4g/d. As a second step, peripherally acting analgesics are combined with mild centrally acting opioids, e.g. codeine. If this combination also fails, the administration of strong opioids is necessary, e.g. morphine, or buprenorphine. It has been reported that in excess of 85% cancer pain can be effectively managed by use of oral analgesics (Ventafridda et al. 1987 b).

All these analgesics should be given orally whenever possible. The dosage is individually determined. The time course of administration is related to the duration of action. When opioids are given "as required", the incidence of malfunction and side effects will be high and dependence will increase rapidly (Swerdlow 1986; Twycross 1986; Ventafridda et al. 1986; Zenz 1984 a, b), (Fig. 86 a, b).

However, in many patients, conventional opioid therapy does not relieve cancer pain in spite of increasing doses. Other limiting factors may be inacceptable, e.g. sedation, nausea and vomiting.

If cancer pain has become so severe that conventional means of treatment are ineffective and in cases where techniques like chordotomy or neurolysis are not indicated, the administration of opioids by the spinal route is the best suited analgesia technique (Mueller et al. 1983 b; Poletti et al. 1981; Woods and Cohen 1982; Zenz et al. 1982 b).

14.2 Potential advantages

Better analgesia, improved quality of life
Several features of spinal opioids make the treatment attractive in comparison with other modes of pain control, especially when conventional opioid therapy either does not control the pain or is limited by its sedative side effects:

- Opioid doses are reduced.
- Duration of analgesia is increased.
- Side effects (e.g. sedative effects) are reduced.
- Patient sensitivity and mobility are preserved.
- An overdose can be antagonized by naloxone.

In cancer patients, after an initial trial period, post-injection surveillance is not only considered to be unnecessary but many patients can self-administer opioids through an epidural or intrathecal catheter at home.

A treatment with spinal opioids allows a substantial reduction of the daily opioid intake. Patients sedated before this treatment become alert and able to ambulate. Bedridden patients are pain-free, and thus become more manageable from a nursing standpoint. Appetite returns and some patients gain weight and are able to return home, resuming a normal pain-free life style (Malone et al. 1985).

Compared to pain treatment methods using local anaesthetics, the spinal opioid permits the preservation of normal sensitivity and sympathetic function and compared to chordotomy and neurolysis it has the advantage of reversibility (Zenz et al. 1981 a; Zenz 1981 c).

Comparing in cancer pain epidural morphine to peroral morphine, Vainio and Tigerstedt (1988) found as an advantage of epidural morphine: significantly less side effects and slightly better performance and activity level for the patient. However, catheter related technical complications: occlusion, disconnection, local infection, pain on injection are to be taken into account. As well, a certain analgesic ladder has to be followed.

14.3 Selection of patients

Before spinal opioid analgesia is started, the following rules have to be applied for selection of patients:

- intractable pain
- terminal phase
- high opioid consumption by conventional routes
- high degree of side effects with oral or parenteral opiates
- inefficiency of other treatment
- transient treatment, waiting for other solutions
- multiple pain localisation
- chordotomy, neurolysis, peduncular tractotomy, sympathectomy already done, not indicated or impossible.
- opioid sensible pain.

Above all, the indication for spinal opioids in cancer patients is dependent on the response of the actual pain to opioids. Typically nerve compression pain, localized bone pain, ischaemic pain do not respond very well to opioids. In those cases spinal opioids have to be applied very carefully and under close supervision. The danger of respiratory depression is increased in comparison to pain states, where opioids are more effective (Hanks et al. 1981).

For a continuous infusion of opioids for the management of pain related to malignant disease the following recommendation can be given (Tab. 63, 64):

- Prior to the decision to install continuous infusion or implanted devices for spinal opioids, orally administered opioids should be tried in appropriate dosages and schedules.

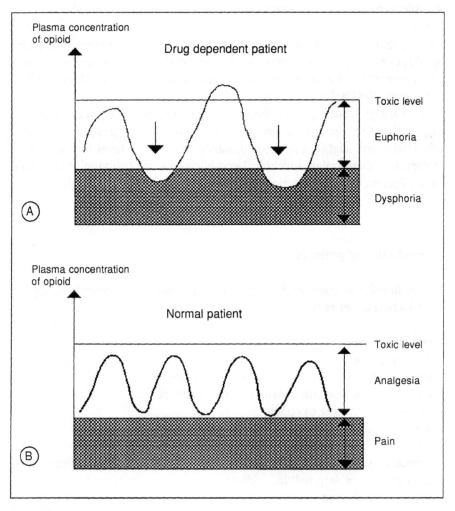

Fig. 86a, b. Schematic representation of the relationship between plasma concentration of an opioid seen after repeated ED bolus administration in patients with chronic pain and "on-demand" ED application.
(Zenz 1984 a)

- Septic patients are to be excluded.
- A pre-pump implantation trial for continuous spinal opioids responsiveness should be done. By doing this test, some patients would be spared the procedure and the expense of pump implantation.
- Myelography and/or computerized axial tomography of the spinal canal to rule out possible tumor encroachment is in certain cases to be performed prior to the implantation decision.

Table 63. Proper patient selection for implantable epidural or intrathecal delivery systems.

```
1 - Oral treatments are no longer efficient or accepted

2 - Indwelling foreign bodies are to be avoided in septic patients

3 - Detailed radiological and tomographic examinations

4 - Necessity of:

            Realistic appraisal of life expectancy
            Evaluation of costs
            Risk-to-benefit consideration

5 - Frank explanation to the patient as well as the family about

    the procedure, the expected goals and the potential side effects is necessary

6 - Repeated pre-implantation trial of spinal opioid is mandatory
```

Table 64. Repeated pre-implantation trial: justifications.

```
1 - Selection of the appropriate opioid

2 - Determination of the appropriate opioid dosage and

    volume of diluent expected to relieve the pain

3 - Selection of route of delivery

4 - Quantification of the results on a flow sheet:

            Duration of pain relief
            Level of activity
            Amount of sleep
            Need for additional analgesics
            Side effects
```

A realistic balance sheet between risk, cost and benefit will provide the right decision in advising implantation devices (Krames et al. 1985; Waldman et al. 1986).

14.4 Selection of drugs

14.4.1 OPIOIDS

For the choice of an opioid for spinal analgesia the duration of action of the substance is a significant factor, in spite of the fact that the use of a continuous infusion pump relegates the duration of action of the selected drug to a lesser importance. The risk of delayed respiratory depression in cancer patients is very low. Therefore, for this indication, the lipophilic or hydrophilic properties of the opioid are not so important as in postoperative treatment. The definite choice of the opioid should only be carried out on the basis of other side effects. With some products urinary retention, nausea and vomiting seem to be less frequent but valuable comparisons are difficult to realize.

Examples:

- One hundred and fifty patients were treated for benign and malign diseases under long-term epidural treatment with morphine and buprenorphine. Satisfactory pain relief was achieved with 45% and 67% of patients respectively treated with morphine and buprenorphine as the sole analgesic. Unwanted side effects with epidural buprenorphine were much less frequent than those seen after morphine. According to the conclusion of Carl buprenorphine was preferable for long-term treatment (Carl et al. 1986).

- During a period of four years, 69 cancer patients were treated with epidural buprenorphine in daily total doses of 1.13 mg (0.6-2.1) given in 2-4 injections over a treatment period of 76 days (3-575). Drug administration was safely managed by general practitioners and district nurses. Satisfactory pain relief was achieved in all patients who managed on buprenorphine as the sole analgesic agent. Infections were not encountered (Boersma et al. 1987).

Fentanyl, sufentanil or buprenorphine enjoy the personal preferences of many authors. Several reports on these opioids used by the epidural route in repeated bolus or continued infusion in cancer patients have been published recently (Boersma et al. 1988; Boersma et al. 1989; Du Pen 1988).

Doses

The necessary dose of the opioid must be adopted to the pain level.

According to a vast experience, mostly doses between 1 and 20 mg of morphine or between 0.15 and 1.8 mg of buprenorphine, per bolus injection, are necessary (Zenz 1984 b). However, the daily necessary dose can vary between 2 and 300 mg morphine or 0.15 and 7 mg buprenorphine, indicating that the high opiate doses that may be necessary in chronic cancer pain treatment are not exceptional.

An extremely high epidural morphine dose is reported by Samuelsson et al. (1987). A patient with cancer of the rectum treated for 366 days received at the end of treatment a daily dose of 540 mg morphine.

14.4.2 Associations of an opioid and a local anaesthetic

If the desired cancer pain control is no longer achieved from epidural opioids alone analgesia may be obtained by the associated continuous infusion of an opioid and a local anaesthetic. Morphine plus lignocaine or bupivacaine was proposed in this context by Du Pen (1987 a, 1988).

The spinal administration of a local anaesthetic (in low doses) with an opioid may provide better pain relief notwithstanding a dose reduction of the opioid. However, blood pressure and motor function have to be controlled more carefully (Vincenti et al. 1982 a).

The combination of an opioid with a local anaesthetic is perhaps on an outpatient basis more dangerous. Nevertheless, Du Pen recommends an opioid-bupivacaine epidural infusion technique for hospitalized and also for home treatment to control resistant terminal cancer pain (Du Pen 1988).

14.4.3 Associations of an opioid and another product

Besides the association of an opioid with a local anaesthetic, many other products have been tried. The goal was either to increase the analgesia of the opioid, or to decrease some of the side effects of opioids or to replace the opioid if its effect has become exhausted.

Clonidine

Epidural clonidine has a pronounced effect on cancer pain in opioid tolerant patients (Lund at al. 1989), while analgesia was dose dependent (ED clonidine 100-800 µg), large doses produced increasing levels of sedation. Continuous infusion of clonidine for prolonged periods eliminated the side effects seen with the bolus dose (sedation, decreased MAP, decreased HR) and maintained adequate analgesia without significant dose escalation. Patients were sent home on continuous ED infusions (basal rate + PCA) of clonidine in conjunction with reduced doses of morphine (Rauck et al. 1989).

Intrathecal clonidine (continuous infusion of 150–800 µg/day) was recommended by Coombs and allowed a stabilization of escalating oral or spinal opioid intake in cancer patients.

Chronic administration of IT clonidine infusion, 400 µg/day, is without evidence of neurotoxicity. It can be given safely using implanted pumps (Coombs et al. 1986; Coombs 1989).

If spasticity aggravates cancer pain intrathecal baclofen may be used to treat severe spasticity.

Calcitonine, droperidol, lysine acetylsalicylate, midazolam and somatostatin have been used alone or in association with opioids in order to improve pain treatment. However, long-term results have been disappointing.

Also inhibitors of physiological opiate antagonists: proglumide and xylamide, and inhibitors of endogenous enkephalinase and aminopeptidase enzymes, all substances susceptible to increase the activity of the natural endorphin system, have been used. Most of these products investigated, in combination with or as an alternative to the opioids, are promising but they are still in an experimental stage.

14.5 Adminstration modalities

14.5.1 INJECTION ROUTE: EPIDURAL OR INTRATHECAL?

Clinical studies with the use of intrathecal morphine for cancer pain have been realized (e.g. by Ali 1986; Benedetti 1987; Blond et al. 1985 c; Cobb et al. 1984; Coombs et al. 1984 a; Coombs et al. 1987 c; Cousins and Bridenbaugh 1987 a; Cunin et al. 1986; Descorp-Declère and Begon 1986; Erickson et al. 1984; Fratkin et al. 1985; Gebert et al.1980 b; Gestin et al. 1985 b; Gestin 1986, 1987; Greenberg HS et al. 1982, 1983, 1986; Hitchon et al. 1987; Jacobson and Chabal 1988; Kiss 1987; Krames et al. 1983; Laugner et al. 1985 a, 1986; Laugner 1985 b; Lazorthes et al. 1980, 1984, 1985 b, c; Leavens et al. 1982; McQuay 1987; Madrid et al. 1986, 1987; Meynadier et al. 1985 b, d, 1986 a, 1987 c; Moulin et al. 1985; Motsch et al. 1987 c, d; Muller and Laugner 1985 b, 1986; Murphy et al. 1987; Nurchi 1984; Onofrio et al. 1981; Onofrio 1983 b; Palme 1981; Penn 1985 b; Penn and Paice 1985 c; Perun 1987; Rawal et al. 1987; Rico et al. 1982; Rodriguez et al. 1986; Shetter et al. 1986; Schoeffler et al. 1987 b; Sjöström et al. 1987 b; Stillman et al. 1987; Ventafridda et al. 1979; Ventafridda 1985; Ventafridda et al. 1986, 1987 a; Wang 1985).

If the intrathecal route is adopted, morphine is the most used opioid.

Opinions about the ideal injection route for treatment of chronic cancer pain are controversial.

Some investigators (e.g. Roquefeuil 1986 a; Zenz 1982 f) are convinced that in this indication the primary intrathecal administration provides higher risks of complications without superior results.

Advantages of the intrathecal compared to epidural route:

- no fibrous tissue reaction in the injection space
- more intense analgesia
- analgesia more constant and more dose dependent
- smaller dosage
- lower volume of the opioid is required (Madrid et al. 1987)
- analgesia is more rapid and longer-lasting
- less systematic uptake
- fewer side effects by systemic uptake (Wells 1987 b)
- direct entry of opioid in the CSF resulting in more direct receptor binding possibilities
- administration is technically easier in most cases e.g. catheter is easier to insert
- known dura puncture: prophylactic therapy of postspinal headache can at once be adopted.

Drawbacks of intrathecal route compared to epidural route are as follows:

- side effects are more severe and more frequent
- postspinal headache is possible (but frequency can be reduced by the use of a small needle and catheter and treated by blood patching (Wells 1987 b)
- the dura seems to act as a barrier to infection (Schoeffler et al. 1986)
- if an intrathecal infection occurs, the consequences are more serious
- effects on nerve tissue is possible.

It can be easily understood that a clear cut superiority of one method on another is rarely present. Real comparative studies have not been done, so that the preferences of most authors are, above all, based on personal experience.

One of the reasons advanced for this dichotomy may be that most clinicians involved in cancer pain treatment are anaesthesists who are more comfortable with epidural catheterterization whereas the majority of papers published on the intrathecal route are written by surgeons (Glynn et al.1987 b).

If for technical reasons or tolerance problems the epidural route becomes ineffective, rather than the intrathecal route, the intracerebroventricular route

is a good alternative (Roquefeuil 1986 b). For many other investigators the intrathecal route is considered the most logical and the best choice currently
employed for relief of cancer pain after all other current therapeutic alternatives
have been exhausted.

From a greater survey, 2 cases were reported where the epidural route failed
to demonstrate sufficient analgesia whereas the change to the intrathecal route
resulted in pronounced analgesia and increase in the corresponding CSF morphine levels. The impairment of a transdural transfer of morphine due to
tumour sheltering or fibrosis accounted for these differences in clinical results
(Arnér et al. 1988).

14.5.2 INTRATHECAL ISOBARIC OR HYPERBARIC SOLUTIONS?

Benefits of intrathecal hyperbaric solutions of morphine (morphine in 7%
dextrose) for cancer pain in the lower half of the body have been reported by
Caute et al. (1988); Lazorthes et al. (1983, 1985); Meynadier et al. (1984);
Onofrio et al. (1983 b).

A hyperbaric morphine solution 2 mg given intrathecally produced the same
degree of analgesia as the isobaric solution (morphine in NaCl 0.9%) but limited
the cephalidad diffusion of morphine, reduced several side effects and reduced
or abolished the central depressant effects of the drug. The duration of analgesia
was significantly longer lasting than after the same morphine dose given in an
isobaric solution (30 hours versus 24 hours), (Caute et al. 1988).

Head up position?
Some authors (Meynadier 1984; Chauvin et al. 1981 a, b) have also reported an
increase in the duration of analgesia in the lower part of the body with hyperbaric
morphine if the patient is maintained in a head up position for several hours.

14.5.3 REPEATED BOLUS OR CONTINUOUS PLUS ON-DEMAND INFUSION?

14.5.3.1 Percutaneous epidural catheter for bolus injection

The percutaneous epidural catheter and intermittent bolus injections are the most
simple procedures in starting spinal opioid analgesia for cancer patients.
The catheter is inserted predominantly at the lumbar level.

Used under severe aseptic nursing conditions, percutaneous epidural
catheterization may be well tolerated for a long time, up to 700 days (Zenz
1988), (Tab. 65).

Table 65. Comparison of complications with different systems of spinal opioids in chronic pain. The incidences are given related to the total amount of treatment days (TD).

Technique	Authors	Treat-ment (days)	Problems expressed in % of treatment days		
			Catheter/ port problems (%)	Local infections (%)	Epidural/ intrathecal space infections (%)
External system					
percutaneous catheter (ED)	Zenz 1988	11 736	0.53	0.18	0.02
Implanted system					
tunnelled catheter (ED)	Du Pen et al. 1988	22 200	0.05	0.01	0.03
	Malone et al. 1985	1 344	0.50		
port (ED)	Andersen et al. 1986 a	303	0	0.33	0
	Vainio and Tigerstedt 1988	970	0.05	0.21	0
port (IT)	Blond et al. 1985 c	4 632	0.09	0.086	0.02
	Schoeffler et al. 1986	37 patients			6 cases
port (IT/ED)	Motsch and Robert 1987 a	1 156	1.04	0	0
pump (IT/ED)	Krames et al. 1984	2 880	0.14	0	0
	Penn et al. 1984	2 152	0.2	0	0
pump/port (IT/ED)	Müller et al. 1988 a	100 patients	16 cases	3 cases	3 cases

From the table it is obvious that the catheter complications are perhaps more frequent with percutaneous systems, but that the rate of meningitis and local infections is not always diminished by the use of an implanted system.

Advantages

- easy to perform
- quickly to perform
- not expensive
- minimal experience is necessary
- in case of infection, the catheter is easy to remove.

Drawbacks

- percutaneous-visible catheter
- increased catheter care
- bathing problems
- frequent injection constraints
- peak and valley concentrations with undulating results in pain control produced by bolus injection.

Du Pen and Ramsey (1988) have preferences for the use of externalized ED catheter for control of terminal cancer pain.

Risk of infection is equal for both internalized and externalized systems. Aggressive antibiotic therapy can be started earlier and catheter replacement is easier.

14.5.3.2 Tunnelled epidural catheter

For protracted treatment (longer than 1-2 months), subcutaneous tunnelling of the epidural catheter from the site of epidural entry to the front of the thorax is indicated (Andersen et al. 1985, 1986 c; Batier 1986; Carl et al. 1986; Cherry 1987 d; Du Pen et al. 1987 c; Malone et al. 1985; Mandaus et al. 1982; Motsch and Robert 1987 a; Muller 1985 a; Muller and Laugner 1985 b; Parker 1989; Roquefeuil 1986 b; Vainio and Tigerstedt 1988; Wyant and Miller 1986).

This is best performed after an initial test period with a percutaneous catheter. During the test period the indication and quality of analgesia can be evaluated.

Advantages:

- care is easier
- bathing problems are solved
- lower infection risk may be expected (but is not proved)

Drawbacks:

- surgical intervention is needed
- catheter is more difficult to change.

Examples of results:

- In 3 of 15 patients the tunnelled catheter had to be changed 7 times (Malone et al. 1985).

- In another series of 100 patients, the tunnelled catheter had to be removed in 44 cases, in 3 cases due to an infected tunnel. In 18 cases the catheter was accidentally removed, which unexpectedly even tunnelling did not prevent (Carl et al. 1984).

- In a case treated with an implantable Holter-Hausner system one pharmacological and two physical complications occurred (Wyant and Miller 1986).

- In 20 patients treated with intrathecal or epidural opioids for chronic cancer pain with tunnelled catheters and ports, 3 systems presented leakage of the port (Motsch and Robert 1987).

- Comparing conventional epidural opioids with tunnelled catheters connected to ports the technical problems were higher in the port group: obstruction, catheter disconnection and infection. Surprisingly, even infection was higher with the tunnelled system (Vainio and Tigerstedt 1988) .

- A severe complication occurred in a cancer patient treated with epidural morphine administered continuously via a subcutaneous access port. Spinal cord compression necessitated a thoracic laminectomy. After the operation the further pain control was instituted by oral indomethacin and nicomorphine (van Diejen et al. 1987).
This case highlights the dangers when not proceeding on an analgesic ladder very carefully. The final treatment with systemic analgesics in this patient with cord compression after spinal opioids should have been performed before the invasive method.

14.5.3.3 Tunnelled intrathecal catheter

For repeated intrathecal injections catheter tunnelling can be recommended. However, this presents, compared to a percutaneous catheter, the same advantages and disadvantages as those enumerated for epidural catheter tunnelling (Benedetti 1987; Blond et al. 1985 c; Cousins and Bridenbaugh 1987 a; Descorp-Declère and Begon 1986; Descorp-Declère et al. 1987; Gestin 1987; Krames et al. 1985; Lazorthes and Verdié 1988 a; Madrid et al. 1987; Motsch and Robert 1987; Muller and Laugner 1986; Ventafridda et al. 1987 a).

14.5.3.4 External unidirectional valves

Twenty-five terminally ill cancer patients were treated with a tunnelled Spetzler catheter with an unidirectional valve (AHS). The catheter was brought out in the epigastric region.
To maintain analgesia the dosage was progressively increased by 100-200%, depending on the duration of treatment. One case of severe respiratory depression occurred in a pneumonectomized patient after the first injection (Gestin

1982). The change of syringes was performed under operating room conditions, but patients lived at home and injections were given by themselves or by their families.

More recently the same author reported successful pain control in 121 cancer patients by bolus administration of intrathecal morphine (0.5 to 1.5 mg x 2/day). He used a lumbo-epigastric silicone catheter placed intrathecally, under mild local anaesthesia. He performed so far 15000 intrathecal morphine injections.

The total follow-up time for all patients treated with this simple and economic equipment was 7869 days, the mean follow-up period was 65 days (3 to 387). All patients experienced a sustained pain relief and could enjoy a good quality of life at home with their family.

A moderate drug tolerance was observed in the majority of the patients. A complete pain relief was achieved in 82% of the patients (Gestin et al. 1985 b).

14.5.3.5 Implanted ports

Leavens et al. (1982), was the first to show that repeated administration of intrathecal morphine, with the aid of a catheter and an injection port can be used effectively for many months without harm.

Excellent results using a Port-A-Cath Orau Ommaya reservoir were reported by Benedetti (1987); Descorp-Declère et al. (1987); Parker et al. 1987; Ventafridda et al. (1987 a, b); Wells et al. (1987 a); Wells and Davies (1987 b). To avoid direct and repetitive lumbar punctures, two solutions for the intrathecal opioid pain treatment in oncologic patients have been proposed:

a) Unidose devices

The most simple method consists in the implantation (after a test treatment) of an intrathecal catheter subcutaneously tunnelled and connected to a subcutaneously implanted port (different models and sizes are available (see Section 20.5). The system needs daily transcutaneous opioid injections. Thus, nursing constraints and/or infection risk may be a problem.

Examples:

- This method was used in 41 patients with intractable cancer pain. The mean amount of morphine needed was 1.48 ± 0.25 mg/day at time of implantation, rising to 6.86 ± 1.47 mg/day after a mean survival time of 65 days. Tolerance became a major problem in 43% of the cases. CSF leakage was another problem in 26% of the cases (Laugner et al. 1985 a, Laugner 1985 b).

- Six patients treated with subcutaneously implanted injection ports were followed up for maximal 150 days. One patient developed infection along the port and the catheter (Andersen et al. 1986 a). So we cannot agree with the authors conclusion that these systems present fewer technical failures and complications.

- Lazorthes (1984) has a preference for intrathecal hyperbaric morphine, using a silicone catheter with or without tunnellisation and an implanted injection port. He treated 49 patients with starting doses of 1 to 3 mg intrathecal morphine. The obtained analgesia had a mean depth evaluated at 90% (60% to 100%), a duration of 24 to 72 hours and a segmental distribution. Transient respiratory depression and urinary retention was seen in respectively 6% and 9% of the cases. Infection was observed in 6% of the patients. Mean duration of treatment was 3.7 months (1 to 14). Morphine was given in repeated bolus, the mean daily doses were 2.3 mg/day (1 to 5).

- The Cordis unidose reservoir (bolus of 2.5, 5, 6, 7.5 or 10 mg) was used according to the individual needs. The bolus was repeated every 2 days in 18 cases, every 3 days in 7 cases, every 5 days in 3 cases or every week (4 cases). Global results were evaluated as poor in 9 cases (27%), good in 19 cases (57%), and excellent in 5 cases (15%). A moderate tolerance appeared in 12% of the cases after more than 4 months of treatment (Lazorthes 1984).

b) Multidose devices

- A more sophisticated method consists in the implantation of the metered dose drug delivery device M 4 D of AHS. A detailed description of the characteristics and the use of this system, developed by Muller and Laugner (1986) is given in Chapter 8.2.2.2.
The treatment can be started with a dose of 1 to 2 ml/day morphine solution (based on the results obtained with a previous intrathecal test treatment). This quantity is further delivered by ± hourly or 2 hourly activation of the valve (each bolus = 0.2 ml).
No tendency for "over auto-administration" was noticed by Muller and Laugner (1986) and Laugner et al. (1986). A progressive tolerance appeared after some days. But with increased doses, satisfactory analgesia could be maintained in all patients (6) until death.
The device is not available on the market.

- Cordis has also developed the multidose reservoir Secor mechanically operated on-demand. The device delivers by transcutaneous action, at each button push a dose of 0.1 ml of the opioid solution. The reservoir of the device contains 10 ml (see Section 8.2.2.3).

This system theoretically avoids the nursing and infection problems inherent to the use of an unidose injection port which allows only a single dose administration and constrains to iterative percutaneous bolus injection. The system has also, compared to implanted pump devices, distinctive properties. It was ensured that the potential quality/safety/cost ratio inclines to the Secor system. However, further clinical investigations are to be done to confirm the preliminary results.

Examples

Thirty cancer patients were treated with self-administration of intrathecal morphine at home using the implanted multidose port Secor Cordis. Boli of 1-4 mg were administered twice a day (daily maximum 12 mg). The results were good to excellent, in 82% of the cases.

The pump was refilled every 30-60 days. The average follow-up was: 2.83 months (ranging 0.1-11 months). Five ports were explanted (17%), due to skin erosion, local allergy, difficulty in push button manipulation, defective pump mechanism. Side effects occurred in 60% of the cases. Tolerance appeared in 50% of the patients (Gestin 1987).

14.5.4 CONTINUOUS PLUS ON-DEMAND INFUSION WITH PUMPS AND PORTS

The efficiency of epidural opioid analgesia can be increased and enhanced by continuous, on demand, infusion, using a portable or an implantable pump system.

The advantages and drawbacks of this technique compared to intermittent bolus epidural opioid analgesia, have been discussed in detail in Sections 8.2.3.1 and 8.3.10):

- avoidance of high peak levels of the opioid in the CSF
- more constant analgesia
- more comfort and independence for the patient are the most outstanding advantages.

These merits are outweighing the drawbacks (Benedetti 1987; Cullen et al. 1985; Magora et al. 1987 a; Oyama et al.1987 b; Payne and Foley 1984; Ventafridda et al. 1987; Wells 1987 a).

After a couple of days of hospitalization for the setting-up and the evaluation of the needs of the patient, the treatment can be followed up by an ambulatory treatment, at home, with the help of a nurse or a general practitioner. Continuous morphine infusion delivers e.g. a 0.25% solution providing 0.06 ml/h (=0.16 mg/h morphine). |

This basic regimen allows an evaluation of the minimal opioid dosage required for a comfortable pain-free condition of the patient so that a stable maintenance regimen for the following days can be established.

Examples:

- Morphine was used by continuous infusion via epidural catheter (tunnelled or not) in oncology patients. Total daily doses were 10-70 mg epidural morphine, the median dose was 20 mg. Treatment ranged from 9-118 days, 75% of the patients had complete relief, while 25% had moderate pain relief. Sixty per cent of the patients became fully ambulatory and 20% resumed work activities (Ausman and Caballero 1985).
- Buprenorphine was used in continuous infusion in 69 cancer patients: mean dosis was 1.13 mg p. 24h (Boersma et al. 1987).
- Sufentanil was administered in continuous infusion via an external portable pump (CADD, Deltec) in 35 terminal cancer patients for a study period of two years: mean dose per 24 hours was 359 µg (200-640). This long-term use of epidural sufentanil provided satisfactory pain relief without serious side effects (Boersma et al. 1988).

14.5.4.1 Portable infusion pump

A portable pump may be connected to an injection port which can be implanted (Welles 1987 a). So infusions, via a tunnelled catheter, may be performed by continuous infusion from an external pump to an implanted port (Abou-Hatem et al. 1985; Beneditti 1987; Cherry et al. 1985 a; Descorp-Declère et al. 1987; Laugner 1985 b; Leavens et al. 1982; Magora et al. 1987 a; Madrid et al. 1987; Malone et al. 1985; Meynadier et al. 1985 b; Müller et al. 1985 e; Muller and Laugner 1985 b; Poletti et al. 1981). For the technique, see Section 8.2.3.2.

Such a solution increases the comfort of patient and nursing but does not necessarily decrease the risk of infection and, exceptionally, the needed doses may increase.

Examples:

- Two of 50 patients had infections at portal site, so that both catheter and port had to be removed (Cherry et al. 1985 a).
- Twenty-four cancer patients were treated with continuous and on-demand intrathecal morphine or fentanyl administered via a portable infusion pump (Act-A-pump 1000 or Deltec CADD) and an implanted port (Port-A-Cath). 18 patients could be treated on an out-patient basis. Duration of treatment ranged from 3 to 77 weeks. The method was very efficient. Good analgesia was achieved until death with initial doses of morphine: 5.3 mg a day, and preterminal doses that reached 22.5 mg (Motsch and Robert 1987 a; Motsch et al. 1987 b).
- To achieve the same degree of pain relief with continuous infusion as with single injections the daily dose had to be increased by at least 50% (Crawford et al. 1983).

14.5.4.2 Implanted infusion pump with epidural catheter

For continuous epidural opioid infusion, implanted pumps (e.g. Infusaid) have been proposed by many authors (see Section 8.2.3.3).

They may be for the patient the most convenient solution with a minimal risk of infection, but the economic investment, required for such an equipment, can be prohibitive.

The side effects and problems observed during the use of an implanted pump are not always minimal. Nevertheless, the most recent reports indicate that increasing experience with the implanted pump goes together with a decrease in the complication rate:

- infection <1%
- pump failure < 0.5%
- no severe respiratory depression (technical error excepted).

Indeed, three non-lethal incidents of respiratory depression are reported after respectively:

- an inadvertent subcutaneous injection of morphine
- an inadvertent catheter flush
- a concomitant agressive use of oral methadone

Even during several months of treatment stable opioid concentrations may be found in CSF (Coombs 1986 c).

Examples:

- During the period 1979-1981, on-demand bolus application of morphine, via external epidural catheter was used for treatment of cancer pain in 150 patients (Müller et al. 1985 b). Since 1982, because of organizational problems, preference of this author goes to epidural infusion systems, with an implanted pump and a tunnelled catheter (n = 18), or external portable pump with implanted port for connection (n = 20). Such a treatment was installed in 5% of the cancer patients and always only after pretreatment with systemic opiates. The daily dose of morphine, initially 12-16 mg, had to be doubled after 3-6 months. In some cases this was due to development of tolerance, but also because of progression of the primary disease and local alterations.
- In some cases the low volume of the pump might be insufficient and volumes between 5 and 10 ml are necessary to control pain sufficiently (Zenz et al. 1985 a). This fact indicates that it is not advisable in the very beginning to start with implanted low volume devices but first to examine the daily needs.

Bacteriological examinations, testing of drug stability, postmortem examinations of the implanted material and histological findings, did not reveal adverse reactions or contra-indications for this method.

14.5.4.3 Implanted infusion pump with intrathecal catheter

If problems arise with cancer patients under epidural opioid analgesia treatment, or if, after a certain time, the results become insufficient, the therapeutic escalation may be pushed further. At this point there is an indication for intrathecal opioid analgesia techniques using a catheter, an injection port and/or a portable or implantable pump device. The use of continuous infusion has advantages and a pump device renders such treatment more practical.

Examples:

- Forty-six patients with intractable pain secondary to cancer of the pelvic organs were treated with intrathecal morphine in initial doses of 0.5-2.0 mg. The patients responding favourably to the test dose were further treated with repeated single injections (14 patients), with an external catheter (28 patients) or implanted pumps (4 patients). No serious respiratory depression was noted (Wang 1985).

- Morphine 0.62 mg/24h provided sufficient analgesia during a period of 10 days. But generally after this point it was necessary to progressively increase doses to obtain an effective intrathecal analgesia. After 3 months of treatment doses were in the order of 1.8 mg morphine/24 h (Onofrio et al. 1981).

- In 26 cancer patients, continuous infusion of intrathecal morphine was applied with a programmable pump. Only 1 case developed significant tolerance (Penn et al. 1984).

- Continuous intrathecal morphine infusion by an implantable system decreased the daily need for opioids and increased pain relief and mobility. However, in this experience, the development of tolerance to intrathecal morphine was at least as rapid as with other techniques (Greenberg 1983).

- A subcutaneous Infusaid pump was implanted in 10 patients with intractable cancer pain. All patients exhibited a good initial response to the intrathecal opioid. All patients with bony metastasis and/or lumbosacral plexopathy developed rapid tolerance. Seventy per cent of the patients could be treated on an outpatient basis after pump implantation. Complications: one pump infection requiring the removal of the implanted system (Dennis and De Witty 1987).

- In 26 cases of chronic intrathecal morphine administration, the use of the Spinalgic subcutaneous injectable reservoir was compared with the use of the Infusaid implanted infusion pump. The two methods gave excellent results with a low complication rate, without clouding of consciousness, no infections and only four catheter blockages (1 by tumor). The implanted pump was considered as a method of choice in patients with a life expectancy in excess of 60 days. Constant morphine levels prevented failure of the method due to intractable nausea and emesis (Brazenor 1987).

If patients have developed a tolerance to intrathecal morphine, it can be attempted to deactivate temporarily the μ-receptor agonists replacing intrathecal morphine by an intrathecal δ-receptor such as DADL 0.5 to 1 mg/d. This delta ligand produced a powerful and long-lasting analgesia in patients showing tachyphylaxis for morphine (Onofrio and Yaksh 1983 a). However, Coombs et al. (1985 a) described cross-tolerance between morphine and DADL after a period of intrathecal morphine.

The morphine and bupivacaine concentrations stored during chronic treatment in pump reservoirs are stable (Müller et al. 1984). Neither examinations of postmortem explanted pumps (inspection for precipitation within the pump and catheters, testing of permeability of filters) nor histological findings of local incompatibility revealed adverse reactions after long-term (>1 year) treatment (Müller et al. 1984).

14.6 Potential drawbacks of spinal opioid drugs

14.6.1 SIDE EFFECTS

The following side effects are observed: constipation, urinary retention, pruritus, nausea and vomiting, dizziness, tachyphylaxis. However, their severity and frequency are greater at the beginning of the treatment. After 2 to 3 weeks of therapy, most side effects wear off, but constipation and urinary retention may persist.

Respiratory depression is very rare in cancer patients. However, the report of Coombs (1986 c) proved that technical faults can always be made, leading to life-threatening danger.

Another case of respiratory depression was due to 5 mg intrathecal morphine 6 hours after the implantation under general anaesthesia (Motsch and Robert 1987). Whenever cancer pain is chronically treated by opioids, it is extremely important to monitor the side effects carefully. This is especially true for constipation as a side effect. The patient has to be instructed to call the doctor as soon there has been no faeces for one day. In many cancer patients there is a high risk of ileus which will additionally be increased by epidural opioid analgesia.

Comparison of side effects observed with spinal opioids used for postoperative pain and for cancer pain (Fig. 86 a, b).
The response on spinal opioids is fundamentally different in acute surgical patients and chronic cancer patients.

In the first group immediate and late respiratory depression is the most important potential side effect necessitating long-lasting and close supervision. In the second group, accustomed to opioids, respiratory depression is practically absent if mistakes in dosage and drug associations can be excluded.

In the first group rapid tolerance is seldom seen, in the second group tachyphylaxis can rapidly become a problem.

The other side effects: urinary retention, pruritus, vomiting, nausea, drowsiness may appear for both groups with the same frequency and severity during the initial period of treatment. Differences are rather product, dose or route dependent. Thereafter in cancer patients intensity and severity of side effects become reduced during a period of stabilization. However, at that time mechanical or infection problems may increase.

In cancer patients avoidance of constipation is a more crucial problem than in the surgical patients.

Treatment of side effects:

- *Constipation:*
  Laxative or stool softener every day, e.g. lactulose 1-3 spoons/day
  An ileus can be hidden by ileus-diarrhea. When diarrhea is monitored during chronic opioid therapy, a careful, clinical examination (perhaps with X-ray) has to be done.
- *Nausea:*
  Antiemetic, e.g. domperidone 10 mg x 3/day
- *Urinary retention:*
  For outpatients a trial with 4 x 10 mg phenoxybenzamine can be done (cave hypotension), for inpatients intravenous naloxone can be tried (cave cardiac stimulation).

14.6.2 TECHNICAL PROBLEMS

14.6.2.1 Pain on epidural injection

Pain experienced on epidural injection of the opioid is a common problem with lumbar catheters. The reason for such pain can only be speculated. Possibly the open end of the catheter is situated opposite a nerve root. The injected fluid is pressed against the nerve root, thus inducing pain. The steps that can be taken to overcome the problem are:

- remove the catheter for 1 cm
- decrease the injection volume
- give the injection very slowly (over 10 min)
- precede the opioid injection with 2 ml lignocaine 1%
- if all the steps above fail: try to reposition the catheter
- if this fails, then insert the catheter into the intrathecal space (Cherry et al. 1987 a, b).

14.6.2.2 Fibrous mass

Epidural (not intrathecal) catheters may be complicated by fibrous mass formation as a foreign body reaction within the epidural space. This may lead to displacement of the spinal cord and nesessitate surgical decompression (Rodan et al. 1985; Van Diejen et al. 1987). The catheter material in the above case has been silastic.

14.6.2.3 Infection

The risk of epidural infection due to haematogenous spread, direct extension or cutaneous sources although not frequent is real and may be devastating.

Ventafridda et al. (1987 b) concluded that closed systems have proved to be more suited for long-term treatment without giving any hard data on this conclusion. The incidence of infection (local or spinal) is very different in different reports. It is nearly always concluded that tunnelling or pump implantation prevents infection. However, the available literature presents another picture.

Examples:

- In 20 patients treated either with conventional percutaneous catheters or ports the incidence of infection was higher in the port group (Vainio and Tigerstedt 1988).
- Six from 37 patients treated with a lumbar drug release system (catheter/port) had bacterial meningitis (16%) (Schoeffler et al. 1986).
- With a new model of an exteriorized epidural catheter no infection was recorded in 55 patients treated for 5133 days (Du Pen et al. 1987 c).
- In a number of 10 patients treated with continuous epidural morphine infusion via a tunnelled catheter 1 tunnel infection occurred (Caballero et al. 1986).
- The same occurred in a series of 100 patients in 3 cases (Carl et al. 1984).
- The incidence of meningitis has been higher in series with complete tunnelling of the intrathecal catheter and connection to a port (Blond et al. 1985 c; Madrid et al. 1987) than in a series with a percutaneous epidural catheter (Zenz et al.1988), (Tab. 65).

So, on one hand, it seems that unreflected tunnelling or port implantation is recommended to prevent infection, whereas current data do not demonstrate a consistent confirmation of this recommendation. Indeed critical analysis of most results has put in evidence that the risk of infection is equal for both externalized and internalized systems. On the other hand, patient's comfort and easy nursing, are serious arguments in favour of tunnelling and port implantation.

Diagnosis of catheter related epidural abscess (Du Pen 1988, personal communication):

- pain on injection, not present earlier in therapy
- pain increases during injection and stops after injection
- decreased effectiveness of epidural opioid analgesia
- epidurogram shows location of dye in abscess space
- irrigate and aspirate sample from space for gram stain
- stop use of epidural catheter and convert to intravenous opioid.

Treatment of catheter related infections (Du Pen 1988, personal communication):

- Tunnel infection, distal to the Dacron cuff:
  . systemic broad spectrum antibiotic
  . antibiotic ointment to exit site.
- Tunnel infection, proximal to the Dacron cuff:
  . remove the epidural catheter
  . intravenous broad-spectrum antibiotic
  . specific 10 days I.V. antibiotic when culture date back
  . scan to evaluate epidural space before replacing catheter
  . consider epidural catheter replacement after therapy.
- Epidural infection or abscess:
  . remove catheter and culture
  . scan of epidural space to evaluate extent of abscess
  . 10 days specific agressive I.V. antibiotic treatment
  . scan to reevaluate the epidural space after treatment
  . consider catheter replacement after therapy.

14.6.2.4 Catheter dislodgement or occlusion

In our own patients with percutaneous epidural catheters this complication occurs quite frequently but it requires seldom more than 15 minutes to insert a new catheter or correct the old one by removing for some cm. In patients with completely implanted systems catheter complications sometimes require complete removal and new tunnelling (Madrid et al. 1987, Blond et al. 1985 c; Coombs et al. 1984 a; Krames et al. 1985). In 17 patients treated with completely implantable pumps 4 catheters demonstrated dislodgement or obstruction (Krames et al. 1985).

14.6.2.5 Port failure

Leakage of the portal system may develop and necessitate new implantation (Blond et al. 1985 c; Motsch and Robert 1987 a). In other cases a disconnection between catheter and port is reported (Vainio and Tigerstedt 1988). In a series of 50 patients in 5 cases (10%) the ports required removal. Surprisingly, one patient was successfully treated with oral opioids after removal of the port (Cherry et al. 1985 a).

14.6.2.6 Pump failure

In four cases, from nine implanted programmable pumps, pump failure occurred, two requiring replacement (Penn et al. 1984). In another series of 9 patients with chronic intraspinal baclofen treatment pump malfunction gave rise to two incidents of massive overdose requiring intubation (Penn and Kroin 1987).

14.6.3 Dose escalation and tolerance

Rapid dose escalation is frequently observed after mistakes in treatment. In many cases diagnosis of tolerance is done on an erratic interpretation of the phenomenon.

The causes for inadequate pain control with chronically administered spinal opioids for cancer patients and pseudotolerance have been discussed in Chapter 6.4. True drug tolerance and spinal receptor tolerance are common during chronic opioid treatments.

On the other hand some reports of continuous intraspinal opioid analgesia are encouraging in regard to the resulting cancer pain control (80-90% success rates). However, these reports have not always sufficiently documented the duration of useful analgesia and the need for concomitant analgesic therapies. The overall outcome of 14 cancer pain patients implanted with continuous epidural or intrathecal infusion devices was analyzed by Coombs et al. (1984 a). No clear difference was found in pain control requirements between epidural and intrathecal morphine infusion. Comparison with pre-implant opioid requirements revealed equal or reduced opioid use for up to six months of therapy. But there has been a definite trend toward escalation of intraspinal opioids, systemic analgesics and adjunctive procedure after two months. After six months, failure of pain control was the rule with continuous intraspinal opioids. Failure to control pain does not necessarily equate with failure of the intraspinal system. Bolus of intrathecal opioid, local anaesthetics, clonidine, DADL, etc. may help to interrupt a pain crisis. However, this analysis has been made on patients treated with spinal and systemic opioids. The systemic opioids were administered on a p.r.n. basis which is known to induce tolerance very quickly.

If the daily opioid dose becomes excessive it may be useful to assess the response to sympathectomy. In some patients this permits a temporary arrest in the dosage escalation (Coombs 1983 e). However, this fact suggests that spinal morphine was not really indicated in the very beginning. Sympathectomy or neurolytic blocks should be considered before resorting to spinal opioids (Zenz 1984 c, 1985 b).

With continuous infusion techniques tolerance phenomena are expected to be slower in their appearance than following repeated opioid bolus treatment.

According to the experience of many authors, the opioid doses necessary may remain relatively low over several weeks: 8 mg/d during 2 to 3 months (Coombs et al. 1984 a; Reig et al. 1986). But the same has been shown for the bolus technique, too (Eriksson et al. 1982; Zenz et al. 1985 a). On the other hand, with continuous infusion, in some cases doses increased very rapidly. A dose increase from 15 mg to 150 mg of morphine within two months of therapy with continuous intrathecal infusion was reported by Greenberg et al. (1982).

Samuelsson et al. have re-examined the problem of dose escalation in some patients treated with epidural opioids. Two patients demonstrated decreased CSF morphine concentrations in spite of increasing epidural doses. The authors concluded that impaired drug diffusion from the epidural to the intrathecal space was responsible for this "tolerance" (Samuelsson et al. 1987).

Boersma et al. (1988) reported successful results in 35 cancer patients using ED sufentanil in continuous infusion: loading dose 50 μg/70 kg + continuous infusion 10-25 μg/h (total 350 μg/24h), with a tunnelled catheter, a port A Cath implant and a Deltec portable pump. The plasma concentration of sufentanil was 0.1-0.2 ng/ml. Tolerance development was absent.

14.7 Multicenter survey

14.7.1 Epidural administration

a) During 2 years the data of the Danish epidural opiate study group (26 anaesthesiological departments) were collected. Epidural catheter treatment was applied to 711 patients, for a mean duration of 49 days (3-292). The treatment was effective in 65%, fair in 14%, inadequate in 21%. Morphine was used in 97%, buprenorphine in 3% of the cases. The daily doses, were 13.50 mg morphine initially, 32.5 mg terminally and 1.35 mg buprenorphine initially and 1.75 mg terminally. Side effects were: nausea 21%, vomiting 24%, pruritus 6.8%, constipation 16%, pain on injection 24%, urinary retention 24%, respiratory depression 1.6% (Andersen HB and Eriksen 1984).

b) Personal data from Zenz covering the observations collected during 5 years are summarized in Tab. 66 a.

c) The global results and the frequency of the most serious problems reported in 24 important studies or personal communications on epidural opioid analgesia for chronic cancer pain treatment with morphine are summarized in Tab. 66 b, c, d.

The results are compared with another survey collecting the results of intra-

Table 66a. A survey of the results of a five years period of treatment of severe cancer pain with epidural opioid analgesia.

1 - PATIENTS	
- number of patients	n = 163
- age	57 ± 13 years
- sex	female = 100, male = 63
- ambulatory patients	79
- bedridden patients	84
2 - OPIOID USED: MORPHINE	
- mean bolus dose	6.20 ± 3.82 mg (1 - 60)
- mean dose/day	16.91 ± 22.10 mg (2 - 290)
- mean duration of analgesia	11.20 ± 6.1 h (1 - 93)
after one bolus injection	
BUPRENORPHINE	
- mean bolus dose	0.33 ± 0.10 mg (0.10 - 1.8)
- mean dose/day	0.91 ± 0.58 mg (0.15 - 7.2)
- mean duration of analgesia	9.70 ± 5.4 h (1 - 72)
after one bolus injection	
3 - POSITION OF EPIDURAL CATHETER	n = 282
- lumbar	234
- thoracic	45
- sacral	2
- cervical	1
4 - SIDE EFFECTS (%)	
- vomiting }	13.9
- nausea }	
- pruritus	0.7
- urinary retention	3.3
- severe constipation	2.6
(all patients treated with laxatives)	
- respiratory depression	0
5 - CATHETER COMPLICATIONS (n)	
- obstruction	11
- leakage	16
- involuntarily removed	30
- kinking	5
- removed for therapeutic reasons	36
- local infection	21
- spinal infection	2
6 - DURATION OF CATHETER TREATMENT	
- mean duration of catheter	41 ± 53 days (1 - 501)
- mean duration of treatment	72 ± 88 days (1 - 700)
- total	11 736 days

1 - 50 days: n = 89	206 days: n = 1	267 days: n = 1
51 - 100 days: n = 37	218 days: n = 1	339 days: n = 1
101 - 150 days: n = 15	222 days: n = 2	348 days: n = 1
151 - 200 days: n = 11	224 days: n = 1	378 days: n = 1
	250 days: n = 1	700 days: n = 1

(Zenz 1988)

thecal opioid analgesia treatments. For simplification, only severe respiratory depression, infection, equipment problems, and tolerance are taken into account.

However, it is evident that also other side effects (constipation, urinary retention, etc.) may be important.

d) An interesting model of comparing data from different reports with different techniques has been presented by Du Pen et al. (1987 a). They have related the complications with catheters to the total of treatment days. From the presented data it is obvious that by no means tunnelling or port implantation can prevent from catheter problems or from local or spinal infection.

By this method the problems encountered with a simple percutaneous catheter system (Zenz 1988) may be compared with those observed with the use of tunnelling, ports or pump techniques in Tab. 66. (Andersen et al. 1986 b; Blond et al. 1985; Du Pen et al. 1987 a; Krames et al. 1985; Malone et al. 1985; Motsch and Robert 1987 a; Vainio and Tigerstedt 1988).

The data indicate that neither infection is dependent on the applied technique nor that the use of implanted ports can prevent from catheter problems and infection risk.

e) A Swedish multicentre survey reports on 750 patients treated with epidural opioids for chronic malignant or non-malignant pain. The longest duration of treatment has been 450 days.The study concludes that long term spinal opioid treatment is fully accepted in Sweden. One of the main problems, tachyphylaxis, is not completely clear to be due to pain increase or a real tolerance. Respiratory depression has not been observed, and the reported technical problems are manageable. (Arnér et al. 1988).

It must be underlined that none of these studies are done in comparable conditions and it is beyond any question to compare them with each other. Nevertheless, the present data collected from these publications, covering > 2000 patients indicate clearly the following points:

- Overall results with epidural opioid analgesia in chronic cancer pain treatment are good and even excellent in a high percentage of cases.
- In the majority of the cases superficial infections, respiratory depression or severe tolerance rarely occur.
- If superficial infections occur, they respond well on antibacterial treatment. In addition to withdrawal of the implanted catheters, ports or pumps may be necessary in a high number of the cases.

However, these surveys bring in evidence that epidural opioid analgesia treat-

Table 66b. Prospective survey on the use of the epidural morphine analgesia in cancer pain.

Authors	Date	Pain clinic	Number of patients
Adriaensen *	1986	Leuven	21
Andersen HB and Eriksen	1984	Kopenhagen	711
Batier	1986	Montpellier	158
Bayer-Berger and Arnér	1985	Lausanne	26
Caputi et al.	1983	Ancona	43
Carl et al.	1986	Esbjerg	150
Cherry et al.	1986	Adelaide	50
Coombs et al.	1984 a	Hanover	8
Crawford and Ravio	1986	Esjberg	94
Du Pen *	1988	Seattle	213
Esteve et al.	1986	Paris	21
Farcot et al.	1984	Strasbourg	292
Kiegel et al.	1986	Aix-en-Provence	15
Kong et al.	1986	Montpellier	165
Krames	1985	San Francisco	6
Malone et al.	1985	Reno	15
Michon et al.	1985	Suresnes	44
Müller et al.	1986 c	Gießen	40
Mulder *	1986	Rotterdam	304
Niv et al.	1986	Tel-Aviv	134
Nobili et al.	1985	Milano	28
Penn et al.	1984	Chicago	10
Roquefeuil *	1986 b	Montpellier	1675
Vainio and Tigerstedt	1988	Helsinki	20
Vedrenne and Esteve	1984	Paris	44
Yablonski-Peretz et al.	1985	Jerusalem	80
Zenz *	1988	Bochum	163
27 authors			4530 cases

* = personal communication

ment applied to patients no longer responding to classical treatments, offers the best solution:

- A high success rate can be obtained with acceptable side effects that becomes relatively low after a period of adaptation.
- Most worrying are tolerance problems and technical problems due to the infusion equipment.

Table 66c. Prospective survey on the use of the intrathecal morphine analgesia in cancer pain.

Authors	Date	Pain clinic	Number of patients
Adriaensen *	1986	Leuven	12
	1988	Antwerpen	5
Blond et al.	1985	Lille	126
Coombs et al.	1984 a	Hanover	6
Gestin	1986	Montpellier	175
Krames et al.	1985	San Fransisco	11
Laugner et al.	1986	Strasbourg	41
Lazorthes et al.	1985 c	Toulouse	52
Motsch and Robert	1987	Homburg	14
Muller *	1986	Strasbourg	63
Müller et al.	1988 a	Gießen	23
Obbens et al.	1987	Houston	20
Penn and Paice	1985 c	Chicago	26
Penn et al.	1984	Chicago	10
Ranchere et al.	1986 b	Lyon	305
Rodriquez-Hernandez	1986	Tenerife	40
Wang WK	1985	Yale	46
16 authors			975 cases

* = personal communication.

Conclusions on epidural opioid treatment for cancer pain

Epidural opioid analgesia has, in an important way, extended the possibilities of providing relief for cancer pain, depending on the severity, prognosis, failure with previous treatment, tolerance, etc. A progressive escalation in the complexity of the epidural opioid analgesia treatment can be scheduled (Tab. 62, Fig.85). Epidural opioid administration by means of implanted injection ports or pumps provides for cancer patients with intractable pain an important therapeutic progress. Not only hospitalization can be significantly reduced, but such a treatment makes it possible for the patient to be at home surrounded by his or her family in a more pleasant environment. This plays a very important psychological role in the patient's general conditions.

Table 66d. Prospective survey on the use of the spinal morphine analgesia in cancer pain, global results of 24 investigators using the epidural route and 14 using the intrathecal route.

		Epidural	Intrathecal
Investigators		27	16
Number of patients (N)		4530	975
Duration of study (y)		2 - 5	1 - 7
Bolus dose (mg/70 kg)		2 - 5	0.2 - 2
Efficient dose of morphine (mg/d)			
• at the start	x̄	7 (1 - 30)	2 (0.25 - 20)
• at the end	x̄	17 (5 - 60)	8 (1 - 56)
Number of injections / day	x̄	1 (1 - 4)	1 (1 - 4)
Duration of treatment (day)	x̄	100 (1 - 700)	91 (3 - 579)
Efficacy			
• excellent or good	x̄	78 (45 - 98)	84 (52 - 100)
• poor	x̄	22 (2 - 55)	16 (0 - 19)
Side effects (%) *			
• pain on injection	x̄	21 (0 - 27)	0 (0)
• severe resp. depression	x̄	1 (0 - 18)	0.6 (0 - 4)
• pruritus	x̄	16 (1 - 68)	21 (0 - 30)
• urinary retention	x̄	12 (0 - 24)	22 (0 - 53)
• nausea, vomiting	x̄	18 (7 - 22)	25 (0 - 44)
• drowsiness	x̄	7 (2 - 16)	27 (0 - 68)
• headache	x̄		15 (0 - 22)
• euphoria, dysphoria	x̄	8 (0 - 30)	8 (0 - 14)
• tolerance moderate **	x̄	90 (12 - 100)	42 (11 - 100)
severe	x̄	10 (0 - 14)	1 (0 - 3)
• infection superficial	x̄	4 (0 - 9)	8 (0 - 10)
severe	x̄	1 (0 - 7)	1.5 (0 - 10)
Technical problems			
• catheter, pulled out	x̄	10 (0 - 19)	
rupture	x̄	3 (0 - 11)	
leakage	x̄	6 (0 - 14)	↕
obstruction	x̄	2 (0 - 5)	
withdrawal	x̄	10 (0 - 38)	
reposition	x̄	20 (0 - 28)	
total		51 %	21 %

* = often only at the start of treatment, ** = tolerance or pain increase ?

Table 67. Comparative results with intrathecal and intracerebroventricular analgesia using morphine for severe cancer pain treatment.

	IT	IC
Duration of treatment (d)	102 (3 - 579)	63 (3 - 132)
Number of patients Age of patients (y)	n = 126 58 ± 13	n = 55 49 ± 9
Morphine: (mg) • start of treatment • end of treatment	2.9 ± 1.8 3.3 ± 1.6	0.50 ± 0.15 0.66 ± 0.33
Duration of analgesia for 1 injection (h) • start of treatment • end of treatment	52 ± 17 37 ± 17	33.6 ± 18.2 27.0 ± 11.1
Results (%) • excellent • good • poor	67 25 8	76 20 4
Side effects (%) * • nausea, vomiting • headache • pruritus • urinary retention • euphoria • hallucinations • respiratory depression • infection • tolerance ⎮ moderate ⎮ severe	44 10 29 10 2 0 0 3.17 62.70 0	25 11 18 3.5 0 4 0
Technical complications (%)	4.76	

* mostly at the start of treatment.
(Adapted from Blond et al. 1986; Meynadier et al. 1986 b).

14.7.2 INTRATHECAL ADMINISTRATION

The principal data collected, based on 14 important clinical studies on the use of intrathecal morphine for chronic cancer pain treatment, are summarized in Tab. 66 c, d.
It is not possible to make a valid comparison of those studies because they are performed in very different technical conditions. Nevertheless, regarding the reported results it can be stated that also the use of intrathecal morphine for treatment of chronic oncologic pain provides good and even excellent pain relief in a high number of patients. Side effects and technical failures, however, are relatively high during the first phase of treatment. Growing experience with the equipment and high quality of the nursing care will surely improve the results.

The Tab. 66 d summarizes the results and the frequency of the problems reported in the most important studies on intrathecal opioid analgesia for chronic cancer pain treatment with morphine.

For the sake of simplification we will only consider the most serious problems, such as severe respiratory depression, infection, technical hazards, and tolerance, outweighing them against the global results. Notwithstanding the fact that it is impossible to find in those papers all the information necessary for comparison, the following statements about those 662 treatment observations can be made:
- Overall results are good and even excellent in most cases
- Respiratory depression exceptionally occurs but is always due to errors in dose or technique.
- The use of catheter tunnelling and ports may contribute to higher patient comfort, easier nursing and better treatment acceptance.
- Notwithstanding the use of ports and tunnelled catheters, infection problems are still present.
- Technical problems, although minor in most cases are frequent (21%).
- Tolerance is manifest but develops mostly only at the end of several weeks.

Finally, a trial can be made to compare the intrathecal results with the epidural opioid analgesia results and the intracerebroventricular opioid analgesia results (Tab. 66 d, 67). The results are highly satisfying with all 3 treatment methods. However, in respect of the presented data, side effects and technical problems are more severe and frequent after intrathecal opioid analgesia than after epidural opioid analgesia.

Conclusions

In chronic cancer pain, good pain relief may be obtained in many cases and for a long period with classical methods. However, if these methods are exhausted, epidural or intrathecal and perhaps, later, intracisternal or intracerebroventricular opioids may change the quality of life of many patients.

The right selection of delivery device and injection technique for each individual case, a well-controlled test period with the selected material and clear and extended nursing instructions for patient and family are the main keys of successful treatment.

14.8 Intracisternal opioids

The intracisternal route was initially used for investigations on drug diffusion through the CSF after epidural administration (Usubiaga et al. 1964). Secondly, this route was used to assess the analgesic response in patients suffering from chronic intractable pain prior to initiating intracerebroventricular opioid therapy. Finally, the method producing by itself satisfying results the intracisternal route was proposed as a new regional opioid analgesia technique (Fig. 87 a, b, c).

A low dose of morphine bolus (0.25-0.5 mg) in 1 ml volume was injected into the cisterna magna. With the patient aware and in a sitting position, the cisterna magna was entered medially with a 22 gauge spinal needle between C1 and the skull, with the bevel oriented downward. The needle was carefully advanced (4-6 cm) while aspirating with a syringe. Once there was evidence of free flow of CSF confirming penetration in the cisterna magna, the patient was placed in a lateral decubitus position.

The method was applied in 58 patients and obtained pain relief in a majority of cases within 6 to 20 minutes after injection. Analgesia was obtained without production of serious side effects and lasted 3 to 26 hours (Madrid et al. 1987). Poor to fair pain relief was mostly seen in patients with deafferentation pain. The morphine treatment produced, 30 to 60 min after injection, very high opioid concentrations in the cisterna magna (3500 ng/ml), but these concentrations were significantly different in patients reporting good quality of pain relief versus in those with poor analgesia (Madrid et al. 1987).

The same technique was used in 29 patients not as a test treatment prior intracerebroventricular catheter placement, but as full treatment in cancer patients with intractable pain, irrespective of the anatomical location of pain. Implantation was performed under local anaesthesia.

After penetration of the cisterna magna a silastic catheter was gently threaded down (2-3 cm). A reservoir (Neurone® AMD Rirmed Inc.) filled with saline was then implanted subcutaneousely on the shoulder and connected to the tunnelled catheter. To avoid CSF leakage at the puncture site tissue adhesive (Histoacry ®) was used. Pain relief was obtained with morphine injected once a day in the reservoir. Complete analgesia was obtained in all cases with initial doses of 2 .2

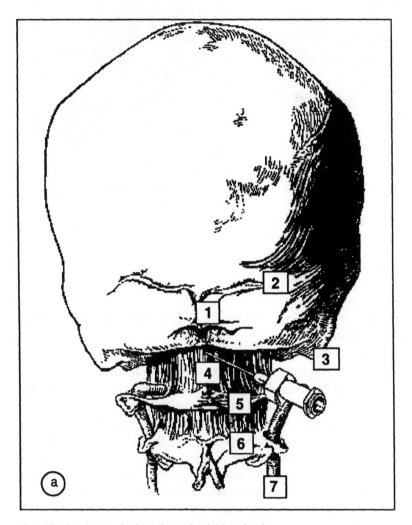

Fig. 87a. Landmarks for intracisternal opioid analgesia.

1. external occipital protuberance
2. superior nuchal line
3. mastoid process
4. atlanto-occipital membrane
5. atlas
6. axis
7. vertebral artery

(Adapted from Schoeffler et al. 1987 b)

400

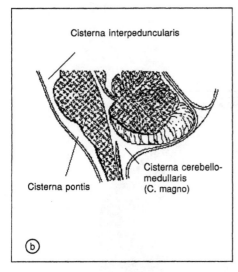
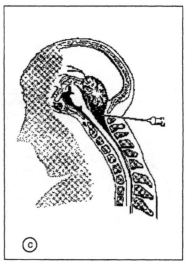

Fig. 87b,c.

b) The cisterna at the base of the brain.

c) Puncture of the cerebellomedullary cisterna.

(Adapted from Chrubasik 1985; Schoeffler et al. 1987 b)

mg/d (1-3) and mean final doses of 5.6 mg/d (2-15), for a mean duration of 74 days (2-413) of treatment.

There were no technical problems during implantation.

Respiratory depression was not observed, transient somnolence and urinary retention was seen in 14% of the cases. Six patients developed infection of the implanted reservoir responding well to antibiotic treatment. Tolerance developed slowly leading to an increase of doses (Schoeffler et al. 1987 a, b).

The wide distribution of opiate receptor sites in the middle brain and pons (aqueductal grey matter, nucleus raphe magnus, trigeminal and vagal nuclei) suggest that opioids injected in the cisterna magna act by influencing more areas concerned with processing nociceptive stimuli than those reached after spinal opioid injections performed at lower levels.

The interesting report of Schoeffler indicates that intracisternal opioid treatment can be sucessful irresponsive of the anatomical location of pain. The results with intracisternal opioid analgesia are comparable to those obtained with intracerebroventricular opioid treatment (see Section 14.9). However, the technique is easier to perform, the large volume of the cisterna magna facilitates the introduction of the catheter and it can be anticipated that acceptance by the patients will be higher. Neuropsychic effects are perhaps rarer than those observed after intracerebroventricular opioid treatment.

Proposed criteria for patient selection

- oral or parenteral opioids ineffective or associated with pronounced side effects
- pain located mainly in the upper body
- palliative treatment ineffective or not possible (surgery or radiotherapy)
- absence of cerebral metastasis
- informed consent

(Landmarks for injection see Fig. 87 a).

In summary: intracisternal opioid analgesia via an implanted device may offer a hopeful, safe, and easy to perform alternative in the management of terminal cancer pain.

14.9 Intracerebroventricular opioids

The discovery of opioid receptors in the region surrounding the fourth ventricle stimulated some workers to investigate the administration of opioids by the intra-cerebroventricular route. Morphine 20 µg/kg and buprenorphine 0.2 µg/kg, have been used in this context (Fig. 88 a, b, c).

Pioneers for investigation in animals with this method were Blancquaert et al. (1982); Colpaert et al. (1978); Freye and Gupta (1979); Freye and Arndt (1980 b); Freye and Hartung (1981); Laubie et al. (1979) and Pascaud et al. (1980).

Many clinicians, promoters of the method, have by now acquired an extensive and positive experience in this new field.

Nevertheless, the use of the intracerebroventricular route is not completely anodyne but provides a method of secondary resort, in cases where the epidural intrathecal or intracisternal administration of the opioid is not active enough for a sufficiently long period (Batier et al. 1983).

The intracerebroventricular injection of small doses of morphine results in the more selective activation of the µ-receptors which are widely distributed in the CNS. In particular, they are especially concentrated in areas involved in the modulation of pain, such as the limbic system, the thalamus, the locus coeruleus, the periaqueductal grey and the median raphe nuclei.

In this way, the central pain receptors are affected without the undue side effects produced by activation of the peripheral receptors as observed following the usual routes of opioid administration. Intracerebroventricular morphine treatment avoids or reduces some peripheral effects produced by conventional morphine treatment.

These effects include the following:

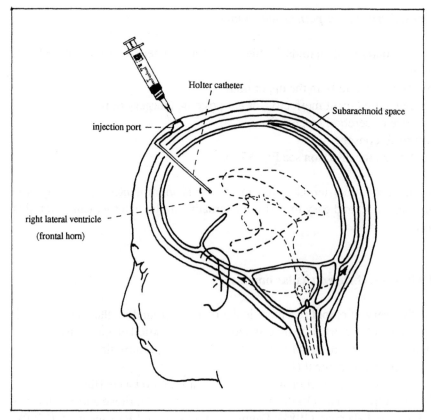

Fig. 88a. Schematic representation of an IC opioid administration.
(Adapted from Macintosh 1985)

- histamine liberation
- first pass effect
- hepatic glycuronoconjugation and enzymatic induction
- problems of blood brain barrier crossing
- effects on the gastric intestinal and urinary tract.

The opioid is delivered with virtually no spillover into the systemic circulation as near as possible to the important supraspinal sites for pain control, with multiple μ-receptors located in the periventricular structures, so that minimal doses have a maximal potency with minimal side effects.

The IC administration of 0.3 mg morphine sulfate produced satisfactory control of intractable pain without any change in other sensory modalities. In addition IC morphine caused a reduction in rectal temperature due to cutaneous vasodilatation and sweating. Metabolism or respiratory rate was not changed, however, blood levels of glucose, prolactin and growth hormone showed a transient elevation for 1-3 hours (Su et al. 1987).

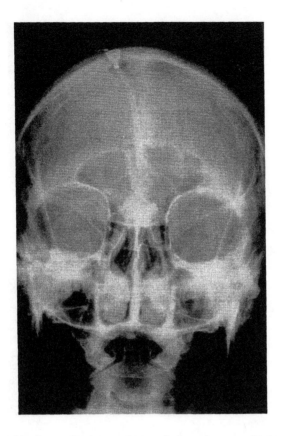

Fig. 88b. Radiographic picture of an intracerebroventricular catheter + an implanted subcutaneous injection port; front view

(Blond et al. 1985 d)

14.9.1 INDICATIONS AND CONTRA-INDICATIONS

The intracerebroventricular administration of an opioid is a reliable method to achieve pain relief in selected cancer patients with severe chronic pain when the maximum tolerated dose of systemic or spinal opioids has become insufficient to control the pain (Obbens et al. 1987).

The following rules can be adopted for patient selection:

- a limited life expectancy (< 6 months)
- severe diffuse neoplastic pain
- rostrally located cancer pain of the head, neck, upper limb region

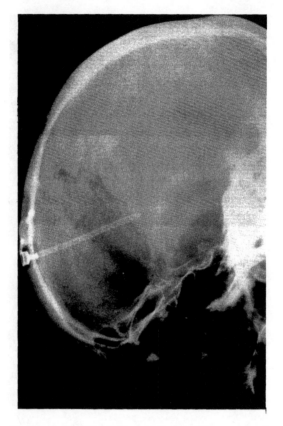

Fig. 88c. Radiographic picture of an intracerebroventricular catheter + an implanted subcutaneous injection port; profile view

(Blond et al. 1985 d)

- pain of multifocal or bilateral in location
- diffuse metastatic pain or disseminated malignancies: prostate, breast, haematologic cancer, bone metastases particularly
- intractable pain resistant to systemic opioids
- difficulties with or failure of epidural or intrathecal opioids
- conventional neuroablative procedures no longer effective or not indicated.

Contra-indications

Contra-indications are identical to those observed for spinal opioids:

Table 68. IT or IC implantation devices in cancer patients: indications and contra-indications.

INDICATIONS	
IT or IC:	- Severe primary cancer pain - Patients who have failed conventional methods of pain control - Patients with a life expectancy > 3 months - Good response to a testdose injection (for at least 6 hours)
IT:	- Median and bilateral cancer located in the lower part of the body

IC:	- Cancer located in the upper part of the body
	- Diffuse cervicofacial pain
	- Pain with bilateral,
	      multifocal or
	      diffuse localization
	- Anatomical difficulties or
	- Failure of IT implantation

CONTRA-INDICATIONS	
IT or IC:	- Allergy to morphine - Abnormal sensitivity to opioids - Coagulopathy - Sepsis - Local skin infection - Deafferentation pain

(Adapted from Blond et al. 1986 d; Coombs 1985 a)

- sepsis
- coagulation disorders
- allergy to opioids
- intracranial pathology (hypertension, infection e.g.) (Tab. 68).

14.9.2 TECHNIQUE

The intracerebroventricular administration of an opioid can be performed by three methods:

a) An implantation of a subcutaneous reservoir

The subcutaneous reservoir is located in the frontal scalp (Heyer Schulte type,

MPAP Cordis, Ommaya, AHS). Fig. 88 gives a schematic representation of the procedure.

b) An auto-administration device consisting of:

- an externally worn unidirectionally metered Hakin valve, connected with a Terumo plastic bag (Roquefeuil et al. 1982).
- a tunnelled catheter
- a Holter catheter in the ventricle.

c) A fully implanted pump

The first method is economic, and is the most frequently used, notwithstanding the increased responsibility created for the nursing staff and the risk of infection.
The second method is economic and avoids the daily nursing constraints and the risk of infection due to multiple injections. The bag contains a morphine reserve sufficient for two months. The external manual compression effected by the patient, produces a metered injection of the opioid solution. The system carries the risk of drug abuse and voluntary or involuntary overdose.

The third method imposes the least constraint upon the nursing staff and leads to the lowest risk of infection. However, it requires a high financial investment.

Implantation technique of an intracerebroventricular reservoir (Ommaya, Heyer Schulte, A.H.S.)

Before implanting the reservoir, it is recommended that a computed tomography of the brain would be performed in order to determine the position of the cerebral ventricles.
    The technique is very simple and without severe risks but must be performed by the neurosurgeon under strictly aseptic conditions.

Operating room procedure:

- local anaesthesia of the shaved scalp
- drilling of a trepan hole anteriorly, in the right frontal bone
- opening and coagulation of the dura mater
- puncture of the right lateral ventricle
- a catheter is implanted through the trepan hole
- insertion of the catheter into the frontal horn of the right lateral ventricle

- tunnelling of the catheter
- subcutaneous emplacement of the small reservoir under the shaved scalp
- connection of reservoir and ventricle drain by a right-angled catheter fixed under the scalp.

The operation lasts about 30 min. The reservoir forms a little bulge under the scalp.

The catheter may also be tunnelled and connected to the reservoir (2 ml) implanted at supraclavicular level or connected to an external collecting bag by means of a subcutaneous tube coming out of the skin at the superior anterior part of the thorax (Roquefeuil et al. 1983).

The catheter and the reservoir may also be connected to an externally worn, battery-powered, infusion pump for continuous intracerebroventricular infusion (e.g. Act-A pump 1000).

This pump is charged every 20-30 days with a 75 ml disposable fluid reservoir containing preservative free sterile morphine sulfate. With such a device the patient is virtually free for several days from the hospital setting for his pain treatment (Lobato et al. 1987).

The catheter may also be connected to a subclavicular implanted Secor Cordis pump filled up with 10 mg morphine dissolved in a 10 ml NaCl solution. The pump is then connected with an Ommaya reservoir implanted in the mastoid region. Self-administration of the opioid is without problems with this pump device (Lutze et al. 1987).

Doses

After aspiration of a few drops of CSF, a test dose of 0.25 mg morphine can be injected without any risk.

Morphine HCl, in a 1% solution containing 10 mg/ml, is ideal.

The effective dose and the frequency of the injections must first be determined individually, and in some cases during hospitalization in an intensive care unit.

In many cases 0.5 mg morphine /48h is sufficient. After 3-4 days of hospitalization the patient can go home. The subsequent necessary reinjections can be given by a general practitioner or by a nurse. Doses can be increased gradually to 3-5 mg /day.

The supervision of the treatment is maintained by the hospital staff. Using an infusion, the morphine doses may be somewhat lower. With the Secor pump the doses daily used in 19 patients by Lutze et al. (1987) were:

- initial dose between 0.2 mg (0.1 x 2) and 0.6 mg (0.2 x 3)
- chronic or terminal phase between 0.3 mg (0.1 x 3) and 0.8 mg (0.2 x 4).

With the Act-A pump, the daily doses used in 50 patients by Lobato et al. (1987) were:

- initial dose between 0.25 mg and 0.50 mg
- chronic phase between 0.5 mg and 2 mg.

10 min after the morphine administration, the onset of pain relief is observed and analgesia becomes maximal at the end of 30 min. A feeling of well-being and a slight euphoria may become manifest. In the majority of cases, only at the beginning of treatment, do dizziness and nausea appear after 2 hours and at the 3rd hour. After the injection a drowsiness may be noted which lasts for some hours.

The duration of analgesia after each injection is variable but often persists for more than 2 days.

14.9.3 EFFECTS

- Analgesia is very rapid (2-10 min).
- Analgesia is very potent and long-lasting (20-72h).
- The total opioid consumption is reduced (1-2 mg morphine/day, less than 1 mg/ day in some cases or 0.035 mg of buprenorphine).
- Mild euphoria is frequent.
- Development of tolerance and dependence is very slight.
- Side effects , e.g. respiratory depression, are rare and generally disappear after 2-3 injections.

14.9.4 REINJECTION AND DAILY NURSING

The reinjections are to be given generally once daily at home on an outpatient basis. This can be performed by the attendant physician , by a nurse, or in some cases by the family of the patient.

Persons responsible for home treatment were taught the injection technique. The following nursing recommendations should be carried out:

- smooth shaving of the skin
- ideally double desinfection of the scalp with an iodine-alcohol solution and sterile wound dressings
- preparation of the morphine in a 1-2 ml insulin syringe
- puncture of the reservoir, which is held between two fingers, perpendicular to the skin with a hypodermic needle attached to an insulin syringe

- transfixation of the tankwall, bringing about a change in resistance
- retrieval of the CSF by means of a test aspiration
- extremely slow injection of the required morphine after aspiration of a few drops of the CSF
- option of a skin bath with povidone-iodine after the injection
- termination of the reinjection session with the sterile wound dressing
- patient's relatives are given single charts to record the morphine doses delivered
- patients are reviewed periodically and at these occasions quality of analgesia, vital signs and neurological functions are evaluated.
  Regular cytobacteriological analysis of the CSF is advisable.

14.9.5 SIDE EFFECTS AND COMPLICATIONS

Mild respiratory depression
Bradypnea without necessity of special treatment is frequent and transient respiratory acidosis can be observed.

Severe respiratory depression
Severe respiratory depression has not been observed in the series of Blond et al. (1985 a); Lefebvre et al. (1985); Thiebaut et al. (1985); but was observed in four cases of overdose (Garcia March et al. 1986; Lazorthes 1988 b; Lenzi et al. 1985; Nurchi 1984).

Respiratory depression was also observed in 7 out of 197 patients (3.5%): three patients developed this complication 4, 8 and 9 hours, respectively, after receiving the first morphine dose 0.25-0.50-1 mg (Lobato et al. 1987).

"Medic alert bracelets"
Although the risk of fatal respiratory depression after repeated injections is very low, rapid morphine escalation or a dosage error may precipitate a respiratory depression crisis. Patients should have a naloxone kit at their disposal for treatment. "Medic alert bracelets" must be made available to all patients to alert the emergency physician to reverse depression.

In case of overdose, 1 ampoule (0.4 mg) of naloxone is injected directly into the tank and another injection is given intramuscularly. After this treatment, the patient wakes up very quickly, but the naloxone injection must sometimes be repeated.

Reservoir infection
This complication is very rare if all injections are performed under sterile conditions, 2% in the 197 patients reviewed by Lobato et al. (1987). However,

it cannot be completely excluded and it is characterized by fever, shivering and positive bacteriological analysis of the CSF.

In a series of 55 patients 3 cases of local infection and 2 cases of purulent meningitis were reported. Recovery occurred after direct intracerebroventricular administration of antibiotics (Lazorthes, in press). One from 20 patients treated with intraventricular morphine developed meningitis (Obbens et al. 1987). In most cases, the infection can be rapidly managed by antibiotics. The reservoir must be removed and implanted on the other side of the scalp, when antibiotic therapy alone is not sufficient. In most cases, for security reasons, reservoir replacement should be performed.

Tolerance

The initial doses of 0.25 mg morphine achieves excellent analgesia in 93 to 100% of the patients and average duration of pain relief ranges around 24h at the beginning of treatment (Blond et al. 1986).

Patients usually report decreased anxiety, a feeling of overall well-being and resume normal sleep patterns, appetite and activity within the first days of treatment.

After one or two weeks development of tolerance may appear. This has practically not been observed by Blond et al. (1985 a, b) but it is noted by other investigators (Lobato et al. 1985; Thiebaut et al. 1985; San Emetrio and Izquierdo 1985; Roquefeuil 1986 a, b). The decrease in analgesic duration can then be compensated by increasing the frequency of the injections or the dosage of the opioid. As a rule tolerance is not a real problem.

In many cases after 2-3 doses, increases in the prolonged phase without need for further dose escalation, may occur. Tolerance never has required withdrawal of treatment (Lobato et al. 1986).

Other side effects
- Transient confusional hallucination syndrome is a specific side effect of this particular injection site.
- Euphoria and somnolence are frequent.
- Miosis or mydriasis are rarely seen.
- Dizziness, nausea and vomiting generally appear in the beginning of treatment.
- Tachycardia and bradycardia are rare.
- Constipation, nystagmus, pruritus, urinary retention give no problems and are observed far less than after other opiate treatments.

Technical complications

The following technical complications have sometimes been encountered:

- dislodgement of the reservoir
- dislocation of the catheter
- leak at the injection port (Blond et al. 1988).

14.9.6 RESULTS

After an inquiry in 14 university clinics we have gathered results in more than 360 patients (Tab. 69 a, b).

Blond et al. (1986 a, b), and Thiebaut et al. (1985) alone, have treated more than 100 cancer patients with intracerebroventricular morphine in two medical centres during the last two years (Tab. 69 a).

IC morphine produced in 79 patients a long-lasting analgesia (3 hours at the beginning of treatment and 28 hours at the end) with a very low daily morphine consumption (Blond et al. 1989).

In every case, the decision to go ahead with this treatment is to be taken after the failure of other treatments, in consultation with the patient, the family and the family practitioner.

It soon became clear that in cancer patients, the intracerebroventricular morphine treatment produced by far the most complete and most long-lasting pain relief with the lowest quantity of morphine.

Comparative results for intracerebroventricular opioid analgesia and intrathecal opioid analgesia are summarized in Tab. 67- 69. The best results were obtained in cancer patients with head and neck pain, which was the case in 76% of the 55 patients treated by Blond (Blond et al. 1985 a).

Other results:

- Thirty-eight patients suffering from cervicofacial pain were treated with doses between 0.5 mg and 2 mg of morphine with a Cordis unidose reservoir implanted subcutaneously in the epicranium. Patients were followed up for a period of 4 to 274 days. Only in two patients pain relief was poor, in all other 36 cases pain was relieved effectively. Side effects observed were somnolence, constipation, nausea and pruritus. In one patient respiratory depression developed after an overdose but could promptly be reversed by naloxone (Lenzi et al. 1985). However, this report gives the impression that some patients were included in this study without a clear indication for such an invasive method. Seventeen patients were pretreated only by minor analgesics. In those cases a trial with oral opioids should have been the first step.
- Another study from Italy reports on 6 patients with cancer pain treated by intracerebroventricular morphine with doses between 2 and 4 mg (Nurchi 1984). Pain relief lasted between 36 and 48 hours. One respiratory depression

Table 69a. Comparative results with intracerebroventricular treatment with morphine in six medical centres.

	Blond, Meynadier (Lille)	Lazorthes (Toulouse)	Lenzi (Brescia)
Number of patients	n = 79	n = 55	n = 38
Follow up (days)	1 450	1 275	
Total morphine dose (mg/70 kg)			
• start of treatment	0.45 ± 0.15	0.30 (0.1 - 1)	
• end of treatment	0.61 ± 0.35	0.70 (0.1 - 20)	
Efficient morphine dose IC (mg/70 kg)			
• start of treatment	0.50		0.50
• end of treatment	0.66		1.07
Duration of analgesia after 1 injection (h)			
• start of treatment	36 ± 17		24 - 48
• end of treatment	28 ± 12		12 - 24
Number of reinjections (d)	1 - 3		1
Duration of treatment (d)	65 (3 - 225)	110 (12 - 230)	5 - 292
Number of patients under treatment (%)			
• duration < 1 month			32
• duration 1 - 2 months			34
• duration > 2 months			34
Efficacy (%)			
• excellent	75		63.5
• good	20	94	31.0
• poor	5	6	5.5
Side effects (%) *	minimal	minimal **	
• nausea, vomiting	25	25	
• pruritus	11	4	
• euphoria	18	6	
• confusion	3.5	1	
• infection (meningitis)	6	?	
Tendency towards tolerance			
• stable dose (%)	55		50
• weak dose increase (%)	33		33
• high dose increase (%)	12	2	12

* Merely at the beginning of the treatment, ** 1 case of resp. depression excepted.
(Blond et al. 1988; Lazorthes and Verdié 1988 a; Lazorthes 1988 b; Lenzi et al. 1985)

occurred after inadvertent injection of 4 mg of morphine but was reversed by 0.8 mg of naloxone.

- Fifty terminal cancer patients were treated by injection of morphine (0.25-2 mg /day in the initial phase and 0.25-16 mg/day in the chronic phase) into the lateral cerebral ventricle via an Ommaya reservoir. Pain relief with a

Table 69b. Comparative results with intracerebroventricular treatment with morphine in six medical centres.

	Lobato (Madrid)	Roquefeuil (Montpellier)	Thiebaut (Strasbourg)
Number of patients	n = 61	n = 17	n = 40
Follow up (days)			
Total morphine dose (mg/70 kg)			
• start of treatment			
• end of treatment			
Efficient morphine dose IC (mg/70 kg)			
• start of treatment	0.85	0.50	0.12 - 2
• end of treatment	2.41	1.05	0.12 - 15
Duration of analgesia after 1 injection (h)			
• start of treatment	12 - 52	24	
• end of treatment	-	12	
Number of reinjections (d)	1 - 3	1 - 2	1 - 2
Duration of treatment (d)	14 - 120	8 - 210	4 - 230
Number of patients under treatment (%)			
• duration < 1 month	30		12
• duration 1 - 2 months	47		9
• duration > 2 months	23		11
Efficacy (%)			
• excellent	81	80	71
• good	16		18
• poor	-		9.4
Side effects (%) *	minimal	minimal	minimal
• nausea, vomiting			
• pruritus			
• euphoria			
• confusion			
• infection (meningitis)			
Tendency towards tolerance			
• stable dose (%)	53		37
• weak dose increase (%)	36		25
• high dose increase (%)	11		-

* Merely at the beginning of the treatment
(Lobato et al. 1983, 1986, Roquefeuil at al. 1984 a, Roquefeuil 1986 a, b, Thiébaut et al. 1985)

favorable behavioural response was obtained without interference with other sensory modalities.

Physical changes or side effects severe enough for the patient to discontinue the therapy were not noted. The treatment was safely performed on an outpatient basis (Lobato et al. 1983, 1987).

- The same technique, as reported by Roquefeuil et al. (1984 a), provided 100% success.

- Continuous intracerebroventricular morphine infusion for treatment of intractable cancer pain gave constant pain relief with mean hourly morphine rates between 0.02 and 0.015 mg. This dose was maintained up to more than 10 months after a pump implantation. Respiratory disturbances were not observed (Weigel et al. 1985 a) .

- The results of the studies of Lobato et al. (1983); Lenzi et al. (1985) with intracerebroventricular opioid analgesia, correspond very well with the series published by Blond et al. (1988); Lazorthes (1988 b); Roquefeuil et al. (1984 a, 1986 a, b); Thiebaut et al. (1985) Tab. 69). The overall excellent results obtained with the method were higher than 80% in a total number of about 550 patients.

Risk/benefit ratio

The potential risk of intracerebroventricular opioid treatments must be accurately evaluated.

Respiratory depression: risk is minimal in patients accustomed to opioid treatments, but overdose, by accident or drug association, is always possible.

- Infection: the risk is minimal with the use of implanted devices.
- Dependence: The risk exists, but for cancer patients it is generally secondary.

With correct application of the technique the risks are largely compensated by the real advantages.

14.10 Current care and nursing problems during regional opioid analgesia

For safe and successful application of spinal or intracerebroventricular opioids for cancer pain, special training of the medical staff is needed.

Accurate and complete written prescriptions are to be given to the nurses and to all the medical doctors involved in the treatment plan.

We can warmly recommend the nurse care plan conceived by Leib and Hurtig (1985) and written up by Paice (1986),(Tab. 70 a, b, c, d, e).

For the family and for the patient the use of a pain diary may be useful.

Home care

Once the patient has been discharged from the hospital, the general practitioner receives all the necessary informations allowing him to take over the responsibility for further treatment supervision. The injections can be done by a nurse and

Table 70a. Complications and nursing care problems during treatment of chronic pain with epidural opioids.

POTENTIAL PROBLEMS	NURSING INTERVENTION	RATIONALE
1 - <u>Inadequate analgesia</u> related to: - Pharmacokinetics, insufficient dose. - Catheter malposition kinking breakage slippage migration.	1. Monitor and evaluate on analgesic effect; use alternative nursing measures to assist with pain relief, e.g. positioning imagery, distraction, communicate sensitivity to patient's pain by handling gently.	1. ED opioids may vary in time of onset, patient may require assistance in dealing with interim pain.
	2. Check equipment for obvious breaks, knots, etc.; also check for leakage at dressing site.	2. May be alerted to equipment malfunction.
	3. Supplemental analgesics LA or opioid may be necessary to administer: a) LA: monitor vital signs, urinary output; assess fluid volume status. b) Supplemental opioids: (intravenous, intramuscular or epidural) monitor respiratory status closely.	3. Give LA in the event that the initial analgesia is inadequate; this reduces the risk of adverse cumulative effect. a) Awareness of risks and complications of the LA analgesia, e.g. hypotension, urinary retention. b) Respiratory depression unpredictable because of plasma / CSF interactions.
	4 . Aspirate catheter gently before giving any ordered ED injection; if blood or CSF present, stop injection.	4. Presence of blood or CSF in catheter indicative for intravascular or intrathecal placement of catheter.

in some cases by the patient himself. Weekly or two weekly controls in the hospital may be necessary.

Tab. 70 to 73 give examples of printed instructions that nurses, doctors and patients receive for information on regional opioid analgesia therapy.

Conclusions

It can be concluded that the potential risks of intracerebroventricular opioid analgesia, which is an altogether exceptional method, are real, but that these must be weighted against the very considerable advantages.

Table 70b. Complications and nursing care problems during treatment of chronic pain with epidural opioids (continued).

POTENTIAL PROBLEMS	NURSING INTERVENTION	RATIONALE
	5. Injection should not be forced. If difficult, reposition patient with spine slightly flexed. If no improvement: catheter may need to be replaced. If catheter removed, check to ensure that it is intact.	5. Flexion of the spine increases intervertebral spaces, thus decreasing compression.
2 - Inadvertent dural puncture related to: - needle puncture during catheter placement or - catheter migration	1. Recognize signs of intrathecal puncture: a) Aspiration of clear colourless fluid (CSF) in the ED catheter: stop injection b) Development of spinal headache (continuous, throbbing, occipital pain, mostly in upright position).	1. a) Physician may convert ED into IT analgesia before removing the catheter. b) Leakage of CSF through the dural puncture site ➤ decrease in CSF pressure ➤ traction on sensitive meningeal and vascular tissues.
	2 . If spinal headache: a) Increase fluid intake. b) Keep patient flat 12 to 24h. Then ambulate slowly. c) ED autologous blood patch . d) Alternatively ED infusion 200 ml of saline per day. e) Oral dihydroergotamine.	2. a) Replaces CSF fluid. b) Allows stabilization of intracranial pressure. c) Occludes dural puncture site by clot formation. d) Increases ED pressure. e) Symptomatic therapy of vasospastic headache.
	3. Anticipate removal or replacement of ED catheter.	

Table 70c. Complications and nursing care problems during treatment of chronic pain with epidural opioids (continued).

POTENTIAL PROBLEMS	NURSING INTERVENTION	RATIONALE
3 - Catheter shearing related to: - Inadvertent break in catheter.	1. Prevention is best.	1. Removal is a physician's function.
	2. Do not use force in removing the catheter, have patient in flexed spine position.	2. Flexion opens the intervertebral spaces, thus releasing the catheter from vertebral compression.
	3. Reassure patient if catheter does shear.	3. Catheter is non-toxic and non-allergic. Surgical removal is advisable only if neurologic sequela develop.
4 - Intravascular placement related to: - Epidural catheter migration.	1. Recognize signs of possible intravascular placement: a) Aspiration of blood in the ED catheter, stop injection. b) Sudden onset of adverse effects, nausea, hypotension, etc. soon after ED opioid is administered.	1. a) Physicians must reposition or replace catheter. Aspiration of blood may indicate a traumatic tap into the ED space. b) Placement of the ED catheter in an ED vein could possibly shunt high concentrations of opioids to the brain.
	2. If patient experiences hypotension: a) Apply oxygen. b) If not contra-indicated, increase IV fluids. c) Increase supervision if >20 % drop in blood pressure.	
	3. Anticipate removal or replacement of ED catheter.	

Table 70d. Complications and nursing care problems during treatment of chronic pain with epidural opioids (continued).

POTENTIAL PROBLEMS	NURSING INTERVENTION	RATIONALE
5 - Paraesthesiae palsies and paralyses related to: - Contact of catheter with neural tissues. - Administration of drugs or solutions toxic to spinal cord tissues. - Spinal cord compression.	1. Monitor neurologic and vital signs.	1. Perhaps catheter is to be removed for 1 cm.
	2. Increase supervision if any unexpected signs and symptoms of neurologic dysfunction arise (e.g. numbness, tingling, sensations in lower limbs, bowel or bladder incontinence or lumbar pain).	2. Sensory and motor deficits are expected outcomes of ED analgesia with LA. These may occur if patient has pressure existing CNS disease or if an infection process or cord compression develops, but these are rare.
	3. Reassure the patient if symptoms cause anxiety.	3. Paraesthesiae are commonly due to inadvertent contact of catheter to neural tissues. These symptoms are generally peripheral and transient. The risk of permanent impairment is remote.
	4. a) Keep syringes with ED medication separate from other medications.	4. a) Prevent inadvertent administration of drugs or solutions toxic to spinal cord tissues may be introduced into the spinal canal.
	b) Verify ED drug and dose with another practitioner before administration.	b) Does not decrease individual responsibility.
	c) Do not use alcohol or other disinfectants to clean catheter injection, port, connections, filter or tapes.	c) Small particles may be introduced into the spinal canal.

Table 70e. Complications and nursing care problems during treatment of chronic pain with epidural opioids (continued and end).

POTENTIAL PROBLEMS	NURSING INTERVENTION	RATIONALE
6 - <u>Infection</u> related to: - Failure in maintaining aseptic conditions	1. Strict aseptic technique is mandatory for preparation, administration of solutions and in maintaining sterility of insertion site, ED catheter and infusion lines.	
	2. Ensure all connection and dressing secure.	
	3. To maintain in-line sterility: Cover catheter injection ports, Luer Lock stopcock, connection, rubber tip with sterile dressing.	
	4. Assess for signs of infectious process. Monitor temperature and neurologic signs.	
	5. Prophylactically on all puncture sites: povidone-iodine unguent	

(Adapted from Leib and Hurtig 1985)

Table 71. For the family doctor: information on epidural opioid treatment.

The epidural opioid analgesia is a new method of pain therapy in cases of severe (mostly malignant) pain.

A low dose of opioids is injected through the epidural catheter into the neighbourhood of the spinal cord. At the dorsal horn, the opioids act by binding to certain opioid receptors. Due this local action the analgesic effect is long-lasting (8-10 hours) without affecting the motor force or the skin sensibility. Side effects are seldom, but may be observed:

- nausea and vomiting
- pruritus
- urinary retention
- constipation
- respiratory depression

Severe side effects are treated by intravenous injection of:

- naloxone 0.4 to 0.8 mg

Respiratory depression has never been observed in cancer patients, when treatment was performed according to this information.

The tip of the epidural catheter is situated in fibrous tissue of the epidural space outside the dura mater.

The injection port of the catheter is connected to a bacterial filter and closed by a stopcock. The bacterial filter has to be changed every other day. Careful asepsis has to be given to all injections. Sometimes, the injection necessitates a certain pressure due to the small catheter lumen.

Please inject slowly and carefully to avoid pain on the nerve roots.

The puncture site has to be covered again every other day by povidone-iodine unguent. Your patient might take a whole body bath every other day.

Concomitant analgesic or sedative therapy should only be performed in contact with the pain clinic to avoid respiratory depression.

Don't worry to contact us, if you have some questions or suggestions.

Stamp   Signature

Table 72. Information for the family doctor on current treatment.

Prescription sheet

Name of the patient:
Born:
Address:
Tel. number:

Your patient is under pain therapy with epidural opioids.

The treatment started ....

Into the epidural catheter has to be injected:

.... mg ....dissolved in .... ml NaCl 0.9 %

This mixture has to be injected .... times per day at certain hours:

....

If there are any problems, please call our clinic for help:

Telephone:

At night or at the weekend please call the hospital ....
and contact the anaesthesist on duty.

Stamp   Signature

Table 73a. For the patients information on epidural opioids.

INFORMATION ON EPIDURAL OPIOIDS

The method you are treated with is a very new one. It is called:

"epidural opioid analgesia"

That means that the pain-killing effect is induced by opioids (e.g. morphine)
injected into the epidural space. That is a small space just in the neighbourhood of the
spinal cord. Into this space a small plastic catheter has been introduced. Through the
catheter at given hours a certain amount of a morphine-like drug has to be injected. In
some cases you might do the injection yourself, in other cases, home nurses or the
family doctor will help you. After the injection, it takes some 30 minutes and you will
feel freedom from pain.
This analgesic effect will last for 8 to 12 hours.

The treatment with epidural opioids only influences your pain perception.
Movements or the normal sensitivity of your skin are not affected.

Don't worry that you are being treated by morphine-like drugs. This therapy can easily
be continued over months and years without concern of dependence.

Table 73b. For the patients' information on pain therapy.

Information on your pain therapy

Name	Date of birth	Address

Your chronic pain is treated by the following dose of analgesic into the epidural catheter:

.... mg .... dissolved in .... ml saline solution.

Of this mixture injections have to be performed .... times per day at

given hours ....

The injections into the catheter have to be performed under sterile conditions. At the end of the catheter, there is a bacterial filter, where all the injections have to pass through. The injection might necessitate some pressure. Please, inject slowly and continuously. The bacterial filter has to be changed every other day.
You can also take a whole body bath every day. The bacterial filter should not be dipped into the water. After the bath the cover can easily be removed and replaced. It is highly important, that povidone-iodine unguent is applied to the puncture site every time you change the cover.
The treatment with opioids given into the epidural space influences only the pain perception. The analgesic effect begins about 30 min. after the injection and continues for some 8 to 12 hours.
Other pain killers as tablets or drops might only be given after consultation of your doctor. Side effects are normally seldom.
But there might be some as e.g.:

> Nausea and vomiting
> Difficulties in micturition
> Constipation
> Sleepiness

If there are side effects, please call the pain clinic.
The telephone number is .... (on week days)
At night or at the weekends, please call hospital
....
They will connect you with the anaesthesist on duty. He will help you.

      Stamp   Signature

15. Chronic non-malignant pain

The analgesia obtained with epidural opioid infusion is very helpful for pain control in cancer patients, but the results are far less satisfactory for patients with non-cancer related chronic pain (Harbaugh 1983). This is generally the case if social and psychological factors (anxiety, opioid abuse, insecurity, etc.) play a greater role in pain perception than ongoing tissue injury.

Common characteristics:

- aetiology is very different
- deafferentation, psychological components, drug abuse are frequent
- response to opioids is poor, full relief is rather an exception.

Opioid therapy can only be the treatment of the last choice. It may only be proposed if all other alternatives have failed to help. In such cases treatment is to be started with classical oral or parenteral opioids. Spinal opioids come only at the end of the treatment ladder.

A recent survey from Sweden indicates clearly that non-malignant pain is not a good indication for spinal opioids. From 19 patients only 2 patients had long-lasting pain relief from this method. One patient had a sacral chordoma and the other one a phantom limb pain. All others were presenting ineffectiveness after longer follow-up (Arnér et al. 1988).

The same conclusion was drawn by Murphy et al. (1987). They treated 6 patients with non-malignant pain of different origin with intraspinal opioids and had to remove the catheter in half of the cases due to failure to obtain sufficient analgesia.

15.1 Treatment with epidural opioids

Special precautions

Before locoregional opioid treatment:
- drug abuse must be under control
- a preliminary trial period for response and dose evaluation is necessary.

During locoregional opioid treatment:
- treatment is completed by physical and psychological methods
- only low opioid doses should be used, equivalents of maximum 20 mg of morphine per day (Boureau 1988).

Different questionable indications

Causalgia
Deafferentation pain, is only slightly or not at all relieved by epidural opioid analgesia, side effects and dysphoric effects are frequent (Muller 1985 a).

Persistent postamputation stump and phantom limb pain responded favourably but temporarily to IT fentanyl. IV fentanyl was unable to reproduce this effect. Neuroaxial fentanyl apparently produced this effect by an important segmental pain modulating action (Jacobson et al. 1989).

There is evidence in man that deafferentation pain can be relieved by epidural clonidine (Glynn et al. 1986, 1987 b).

Dramatic improvement of causalgia is also reported by Coventry and Gordon (1989) after ED administration of clonidine 150 µg in 5 ml of normal saline solution.

Neuropathic pain, sympathetic reflex dystrophy
Analgesia is poor or transient and side effects are severe (Farcot et al. 1981). A combined therapy with epidural administration of local anaesthetics, opioids and clonidine together with neurolytic blocks and sympathectomy has been proposed by Magora et al. (1986 a) and Coombs et al. (1985). However, this combination seems to be a kind of polypragmacy, and in most cases there might be minor invasive techniques with the same effectiveness.

Spinal spasticity in multiple sclerosis
The epidural administration of morphine 3 mg or fentanyl 0.2 mg abolished flexor reflex spasms and reduced markedly muscle tone (Struppler et al. 1983).

Degenerative back pain

Patients with disabling pain due to degenerative changes in the spine conventionally managed with non-steroidal anti-inflammatory agents, were treated with a single epidural administration of diamorphine 2 mg in 4 ml plain bupivcaine 0.25%. No serious side effects were encountered although transient nausea and pruritus occurred in some patients. The procedure was considered safe and useful for the inpatient management of this type of pain. Relief of pain for more than two months was seen in 40% of the 20 patients (Campbell 1983). However, this incidence of pain relief is not far in excess of a placebo action.

In chronic low back pain epidural morphine associated with methylprednisolone produced pain relief lasting 6-12 months in 100% of patients (Cohn et al. 1983). However, more recent data from Dallas et al. (1986) do not support such spectacular results. They are to be considered as unrealistic.

A double-blind cross-over study to match the overenthusiastic results of Cohn et al. was performed in 20 patients and did not support the previous observation but was moderately encouraging. Epidural morphine, associated with a steroid, provided pain relief of post-laminectomy back pain in 65% of the patients. The treatment was more effective than steroids alone and the pain relief lasted from 1 day to 6 weeks. A second administration of morphine and steroids seemed to be more effective if given within 2 weeks after the initial dose (Dallas et al. 1987).

The use of spinal opioids + steroids for low back pain cannot be recommended without serious warnings. The implications of a good response with this simple technique in such a common illness are profound and should be further explored.

Enuresis

Epidural opioid analgesia was used for children presenting an enuresis resistant to conventional treatment (Cardan 1985 b). Morphine given epidurally at doses of 0.25 to 1.5 mg depending on the body weight was used. With this treatment a cure rate of 13% was achieved; 70% of the cases having shown an improvement and failure having been observed in 17%.

However, the side effects of such a treatment are not to be underestimated, hospitalization in an intensive care unit was necessary. Respiratory depression was noted in 8% of the cases, deep sedation in 89%, nausea and pruritus in 86%, and transient urinary retention in 30%.

Hyperreflexia of the sympathetic nervous system

This syndrome was successfully treated with 100 mg epidural pethidine in patients with post-traumatic paraplegia, presenting episodic periods of paroxysmic hypertension due to autonomous nervous system hyperreflexia (Baraka 1985).

Ischaemic pain

According to the opinion of Van den Berg et al. (1981), the use of epidural opioid analgesia for chronic ischaemic pain has no advantages compared to the use of analgesics by oral or parenteral administration. Epidural local anaesthetics that produce significant decrease in the peripheral vascular resistance with an increased perfusion of the extremities are to be preferred whereas only weak changes are induced after epidural opioid analgesia.

Association of an epidural opioid and a local anaesthetic

Morphine 2 mg epidural + lignocaine 1%, was used with success (Layfield et al. 1981). Buprenorphine 0.3 mg associated with bupivacaine 0.5% + epinephrine (questionable in this indication), was administered epidurally for the treatment of chronic vascular pain (Szulc et al. 1984). The association ensured a deep analgesia for 12h in most cases, and even up to 48h in some patients. Such long analgesic periods could not be obtained with local anaesthetics alone.

A significant improvement in the results has been obtained with a sympathetic block potentiated by epidural morphine (Mays et al. 1981 a, b).

Pain produced by direct nerve root irritation is not relieved by epidural opioid analgesia treatment (Palitzsch et al. 1982). However, in such cases, results may be improved by the association of epidural opioid analgesia and locoregional analgesia.

Stones

Severe pain associated with stones and spasms of the bladder can be successfully treated with epidural morphine 3-4 mg per dose (Olshwang et al. 1984). However, again this seems to be a strange indication for spinal opioids.

Other indications

The benefits of the epidural opioid analgesia on chronic non-malignant pain (failed back syndromes, intractable pain from multiple sclerosis, Addison's disease, ischaemic neuritis, scoliosis, hip disease, spinal cord injury) were investigated during a period of two years, in 43 patients. During the first phase of the programme, 1 mg epidural morphine was administered. During the second phase for those patients who had good to excellent relief of pain from the epidural injections, a subcutaneous injection port and tunnelled epidural catheter were implanted. Morphine was injected in repeated bolus through the port. This phase with a duration of several weeks allows for the evaluation of side effects. For those patients having a satisfactory trial with the port, 32 continuous delivery systems were implanted. After 2 years of treatment good to excellent relief of pain was noted in 65% of the patients and only fair or poor relief in 16%. In several patients with unsatisfactory infusion results, supplemental self-administered bolus injections relieved the pain. The total epidural morphine dose per day never exceeded 7 mg. Mechanical problems occurred in 3% of the patients, infection in 3.1%, six pumps were removed. Respiratory depression, severe tolerance or addiction were not seen (Auld et al. 1985).

Auld's results, thus far encouraging for the epidural opioid analgesia treatment of severe chronic non-malignant pain, are clearly different from those obtained by Coombs (1983 b) who concluded that epidural opioid analgesia should not be used for benign pain.

A longer follow-up of similar cases is certainly necessary before definite conclusions can be made.

15.2 Treatment with intrathecal opioids and/or non-opioid drugs

In non-malignant pain there is often a poor response to spinal opioids. This is consistent with the unsatisfactory response to many potentially analgesic approaches in chronic non-malignant pain (Coombs 1983 a, b, c).

Spasticity

Intrathecal morphine:
For the treatment of spastic post-traumatic pain intrathecal morphine 1-2 mg in a 0.5 mg/ml solution injected at level L3-L4 were used. With a single injection, good analgesia lasted 24 to 36h . After a trial period to evaluate the sensitivity of the patient, continuous infusion of intrathecal morphine by a catheter could be initiated. Doses of 2 to 4 mg/24h of intrathecal morphine were sufficient for pain-free active mobility of the patient. Severe side effects were not noted. It was necessary to prolong such a treatment. The doses had also to be progressively increased. Covering one year of continuous treatment a daily dose of 30 mg was reached (Lo and Erickson 1984).

IT morphine decreases the severity of spasticity associated with spinal cord injury (Gall et al. 1988, Erickson 1985, Loubser 1985).

Similar good results with the use of 1-2 mg intrathecal morphine were reported for the treatment of pain and spasticity in neurosurgical patients of a rehabilitation service (Erickson et al. 1985; Lazorthes and Verdié 1988 a). It seems that in addition to a block of afferent pain transmission, the reflex arch contributing to spasticity might also be inhibited by intrathecal opioids. If prolonged control of the spasticity is necessary, pump implantation may be considered (Lazorthes and Verdié 1988 a).

Good results with an intrathecal catheter and an external pump were obtained by Loubser et al. (1986). A bolus dose of 0.5 or 1 mg intrathecal morphine was followed by a continuous infusion starting with an initial rate of 0.5 mg/d. The infusion was continued for a period of 4-5 days after which the catheter was removed. This treatment provided a significant reduction in tonic spasticity without muscle flaccidity. Pain and discomfort were decreased. The continuous administration of intrathecal morphine permitted the use of small opioid amounts, thus minimizing the incidence of side effects.

Intrathecal morphine given at low doses (0.2-0.25 mg) at segmental sacral cord sites produced a profound increase in bladder capacity during 18-24 h in subjects with complete suprasacral spinal cord lesions transforming a low capacity bladder to a moderate capacity bladder. Lack of clinical effectiveness of commonly utilized, systematically administered pharmacologic agents is a current observation in patients with disabling impaired micturition reflexes. In such situations this treatment might be therapeutically advantageous (Hermann et al. 1988).

Intrathecal baclofen

In chronic pain from spinal spasticity caused by multiple sclerosis or by spinal cord contusion, intrathecal opiates reduce pain but have little influence on spasticity. In such cases intrathecal baclofen can be given with good results.

For chronic pain due to spinal spasticity, baclofen may be used in intrathecal doses of 100-150 μg twice daily. In this way, 30-60 min after injection, spinal spasticity is completely inhibited, nociceptive threshold is increased and pre-existing hypersensibility vanishes. The duration of the effect lasts 14-18h. In the mentioned dosage baclofen has no adverse effect on motor power, but in higher doses (300-500 μg), it may elicit side effects such as limb flaccidity, drowsiness and vomiting.

Satisfying results are also obtained with a continuous intrathecal infusion of 3μg/h and additional bolus injections of 75-180 μg twice daily.

Examples:

- In a study on 6 patients with severe spasticity intrathecal baclofen was used at doses between 12 μg and 400 μg daily by programmed infusion via a Medtronic pump. Spasticity was effectively relieved without central side effects over a period of 7 months, spontaneous spasms were eliminated, daily activities were again more easily accomplished (Penn and Kroin 1985 a).

- In a more recent paper Penn and Kroin (1987) reported on a two years' follow-up with intrathecal baclofen for treatment of spinal spasticity. With a gradual dose increase the symptoms could be well controlled. However, two severe drug overdoses occurred due to pump malfunction and took several days to clear up. The two patients presented drowsiness, loss of consciousness and muscle weakness. For safety, both patients were intubated. Nevertheless, the results indicate in certain cases to substitute oral baclofen by the intrathecal route.

- This treatment was also applied with success in post-traumatic spasticities and spasticities secondary to demyelinization and cerebral motor disability by Lazorthes and Verdié (1988 a): six patients received implants: 4 with reservoirs and 2 with a programmable micropump.

- The segmental action of intrathecal baclofen was demonstrated by Dralle et al. (1985). Their clinical examinations on a four year old boy clearly indicated the segmental progression of the action of the intrathecal baclofen by time-related segmental distribution of the antispastic activity.

- In contrast, epidural baclofen, even in high doses of 1.5 mg, had little effect on spinal spasticity and pain, which indicates that the dura mater is a strong barrier for this substance (Müller-Schwefe and Milewski 1985 a).

Baclofen proved to be more efficient than morphine, however, the lack of a specific antagonist limited its applications. Overdose of baclofen may produce loss of consciousness and hypoventilation. Small doses of morphine were much easier to control without causing residual deficiencies in motor function (Lazorthes and Verdié 1988 a).

Conclusions

Real indications for use of spinal opioids in chronic non-malignant pain with the exception made for severe chronic spasticity are according to actual investigations poorly defined. They need further research.

16. Perineural opioid analgesia (PNOA)

After the good analgesic results obtained with the epidural, intrathecal or intra-cerebroventricular adminstration of opioids, some authors have made an attempt to administer opioids by the perineural route, especially for pain treatment of the extremities.

Animal investigations

Investigations in animals by Jurna (1966) and Frazier (1972) showed that morphine, in relatively high doses, depressed action potentials in isolated nerves, suggesting the presence of opiate receptors.

In 1977 it was reported that in cats, morphine when administered intra-arterially, caused changes in the compound action potential of a superficial nerve (Jurna and Grossman 1977).

In man, one mg intravenous morphine affected both spinal cord function as well as afferent volleys in dorsal roots. The presynaptic inhibition caused by morphine was completely reversed by naloxone (Maruyama et al. 1980).

Morphine was said to have caused changes in presynaptic excitability in single cutaneous afferent C- and A-fibres (Carstens et al. 1979).

One study indicated that there exist opiate receptors on primary afferent fibres in the area near the dorsal root ganglia (Field et al. 1980). Rats, made hyperalgic by the injection of prostaglandines, became pain-free after perineural morphine or naloxone injections (Ferreira 1979).

When applying morphine or naloxone topically to the desheated saphenous nerve of rats, both substances showed at high doses (1-2 mg/ml) local anaesthet-ics' properties (Gilly et al. 1985). In a rat model of inflammation, local admini-stration of fentanyl into an inflamed paw, produces a dose related analgesia restricted to the injected area (Joris et al. 1987).

High concentrations of fentanyl and sufentanil exerted a local anaesthetic type action on isolated rabbit nerves (Gissen et al. 1987).

Hassan and Akerman (1989) administering in rats opioids perineurally for infraorbital nerve block, produced localized analgesia with pethidine in doses > 1 mg/kg. The duration of analgesia increased dose dependence. However, localized analgesia was not obtained, with morphine or with fentanyl. It was concluded that pethidine exerted is analgesic effect by a local anaesthetic action and not by the activation of opioid receptors.

Gupta et al. (1989) have performed assays incubating a membrane suspension of homogenized and centrifugated human nerves with DAGO (a potent opioid and μ-receptor agonist), with DSTLE (a δ-receptor agonist) and with EKC (a κ-receptor agonist). They demonstrated binding for all 3 receptor subtypes. The existence of opioid receptors on human peripheral nerves suggests a mechanism of action for opioids administered in peripheral nerve blocks.

Clinical investigations

The first clinical report has been given by Mays et al. (1981 a,1987). In patients with somatic pain 1-6 mg morphine injected in a 0.02% solution, into the perineural space (just as in the case of conventional locoregional techniques) produced pain relief.

 The analgesia was comparable to that obtained by bupivacaine 0.5%. If the patient received morphine and bupivacaine at the same time he experienced the same pain relief but the duration of the effect was longer.

The relationship between the sympatho-adrenergic system and the endorphin or enkephalin receptors was also evidenced by the results of Sprotte (1986). In cases of severe chronic pain related to vascular diseases, he obtained constant and profound pain relief for 2 to 3 days after the infiltration of the sympathetic trunc with only 0.06 mg buprenorphine dissolved in 10 ml saline. In one patient after more than 60 infiltrations the good result remained constant.

Two mg morphine (diluted in 7 ml of normal saline) was injected instead of local anaesthetics, directly around the stellate ganglion in 10 adults with sympathetic pain, 80% obtained substantial relief. Pain relief following admini-stration of morphine was more profound than after the use of local anaesthetics and was achieved without any evidence of sympathetic block. None of the patients presented any systemic opioid effect. After 8 months of treatment, 70% of the patients had no or minimal pain (Mays et al. 1981). The author has no explanation for the results but draws attention to the fact that in recent papers (DiGuilio et al. 1978; Schultzberg et al. 1979) the presence of opiate activity in sympathetic ganglia has been demonstrated. Fine and Ashburn (1988) reported of a patient with postherpetic neuralgia, where stellate ganglion blocks with fentanyl relieved the pain effectively and for a long time. In the same patient intravenous fentanyl had a significantly minor effect. As well, Arias et al. (1989) reported on 2 patients with refractory reflex sympathetic dystrophy, who experienced long-lasting pain relief after sufentanil stellate ganglion injection.

Brachial plexus blocks were applied for surgery of the arm, either using a local anaesthetic alone (lignocaine 1%, or bupivacaine 0.25%), or an association of these local anaesthetics with morphine or buprenorphine. The association of an opioid using a local anaesthetic drug produced a clear-cut prolongation of the analgesic effects (Boogaerts et al. 1983).

The authors demonstrated the peripheral analgesic effects of the opioid with the aid of a percutaneous electrical nerve stimulator. With lignocaine alone the pain level was increased for a maximal duration of 8h. If the association of lignocaine and buprenorphine was used then the analgesic effect was prolonged for more than 24h. The rise of the pain level was clearly an ipsilateral effect indicating that it was not only produced by a systemic action of the opioid. However, it is also possible to explain the observed side effects with this technique in terms of an additional systemic action of the opioid.

By applying morphine and fentanyl directly on the A-β-, A-δ- and C-fibres of the superficial radial nerve in decerebrated cats, neither drug caused any significant change in primary afferent nerve conduction (Yuge et al. 1985 and Kumeta et al. 1985).

In a double-blind investigation, Bullingham et al. (1982, 1983, 1984) reevaluated this pain treatment problem with 2-4 mg morphine at the plexus for postoperative pain treatment in patients after bilateral foot surgery. In contrast to previous authors, the study failed to demonstrate any peripheral effect of the morphine administred by this route.

In another double-blind study the effects of perineural (perifemoral) injection of 5 mg morphine were compared with epidural injection with the same amount of morphine in patients after knee surgery. Better pain relief scores were achieved during treatment with epidural morphine.

The hypothesis of neuro-axonal transport of morphine from the periphery to the spinal cord was not confirmed by the results of this investigation (Dahl et al. 1988).

These investigations, even if they provide contradictory results, have important theoretical and perhaps also practical consequences so that further research in this field is required.

17. Comparative evaluation of the risk/benefit ratio

During the last years there has been very substantial progress in obtaining key pharmacokinetic and pharmacodynamic data to permit rational decisions concerning the safe and effective use of spinal opioid and non-opioid drugs and to decide upon the relative merits of this route of administration, compared with other options for the control of acute and chronic pain (Cousins 1988).

Before a decision can be made to install a regional opioid analgesia treatment, several questions are to be answered and a risk/benefit evaluation, in comparison to the possibilities offered by other analgesia techniques, is to be done.

Which drug, by which route and by which technique, will provide the safest and most effective analgesia with the least side effects for a particular pain situation?

Which drug?

- Morphine versus a lipid soluble opioid.
- Opioid alone versus opioid + local anaesthetic.

Which route and which dose?

- Epidural versus intrathecal route.
- Catheter: percutaneous versus tunnelling.

Which technique?

- Intermittent bolus versus continuous infusion

Which port or pump?

- External portable pump versus implanted pump (Tab. 74).

The right answers will be very different according to an acute or a chronic pain situation to the pain aetiology, to the physio-pathological condition of the patient to previous treatment, to the equipment and to the nursing at our disposal.

Table 74. Which drug by which route and by which technique will provide the safest and the most effective analgesia, with the least effects for a particular situation?

WHICH DRUG ?

    1. Morphine versus a lipophilic opioid
    2. An opioid alone versus an opioid + a local anaesthetic

WHICH ROUTE AND WHICH DOSE ?

    3. Epidural versus intrathecal route
    4. Percutaneous versus tunnelled catheter

WHICH TECHNIQUE ?

    5. Intermittent bolus versus continuous infusion
    6. External portable pump versus implanted pump

Table 75. Differences in morphine effects according to different administration routes.

	ED	IT	IV	IM	PO
ANALGESIA ONSET (min)	20	15	5	15	25
DURATION (h)	8 - 12	10 - 15	4	4	4
PAIN TREATMENT	Acute Chronic	Acute Chronic	Acute	Acute	Chronic
INDICATION	Postop. Polytraum. Delivery Cancer	Postop. Polytraum. Delivery Cancer	Myocard. infarction Postop. Trauma	Postop.	Cancer
CONTRAINDICATION	Coagulation problems	Coagulation problems	Chronic pain	Chronic pain Infarction	Acute pain
DOSE-COEFFICIENT	1 / 3	1 / 20	1	1	3

(Adapted from Zenz 1984 a)

17.1 Epidural opioid analgesia versus peroral, intravenous or intramuscular opioids

Since at present there is an increasing tendency for investigations to be conducted in double-blind fashion, the comparison of results using different techniques of analgesia has become a highly fruitful area of research.

Recently, a substantial number of randomized prospective controlled studies have confirmed the analgesic efficacy of spinal opioids and have documented a relative superiority of analgesia for this route of administration compared with

Table 76. Comparison of results obtained after epidural and intramuscular morphine using a six grade mobilization scale.

Grade	Mobilization	IM morphine + ED saline mean + SEM (min)	ED morphine + IM saline mean + SEM (min)	Statistics
1	Sit up on bedside (feet hanging) with assistance	403 ± 57	312 ± 25	NS
2	Sit up on bedside (feet hanging) without assistance	438 ± 80	359 ± 35	NS
3	Stand with assistance	846 ± 115	619 ± 80	NS
4	Stand without assistance	$1\,359 \pm 218$	880 ± 68	$p < 0.05$
5	Walk with assistance	$1\,941 \pm 258$	$1\,116 \pm 67$	$p < 0.05$
6	Walk freely without assistance	$2\,049 \pm 330$	$1\,153 \pm 66$	$p < 0.05$

Meantime (min) taken from the end of the operation until the patient performed each of the following exercises on encouragement.
NS = not significant.
(Rawal et al. 1984 b)

the use of intravenous, intramuscular or oral opioids (Banning et al. 1986; Bonnet et al. 1984; Brownridge and Frewin 1985; Cohen and Woods 1983; Cullen et al. 1985; El-Baz et al. 1984; Gustafsson et al. 1986; Hasebos et al. 1985; Raj et al. 1985; Rawal et al. 1984; Rechtine et al. 1984; Rosenberg et al. 1984; Shulman et al. 1984; Vella et al. 1985; Writer et al. 1985 e.g.).

However, a clear-cut superiority of epidural opioid analgesia over continuous intravenous opioid analgesia or spinal local anaesthetics for treatment of postoperative pain has not yet been consistently demonstrated (Benhamou et al. 1983).

Comparing the pros and cons of epidural opioid analgesia and intravenous or intramuscular opioid analgesia we can summarize the potential advantages and drawbacks of epidural opioid analgesia for postoperative pain relief (particularly for obese patients and after major surgery) as follows: (Tab. 75, 76, 77)

Advantages:

- Analgesia is more comfortable:
  . there is greater patient mobility
  . drowsiness is not so frequent
  . nausea and vomiting are slightly less frequent
  . intestinal motility is not as disturbed
  . dysphoria is absent
  . hospitalization is generally shorter.
- Analgesia is longer-lasting (Purves et al. 1987).
- Total dose of the opioid is reduced if hydrophilic substances are used (Chovaz and Sandler 1985). The dose reduction is low or non-existent using lipophilic opioids (Van den Hoogen 1987 a; Van den Hoogen and Colpaert 1987 c).
- If the patient is having a spinal anaesthetic then it is easy to give a small dose of an opioid for postoperative analgesia (Glynn et al.1987 b).

Drawbacks:

- Epidural treatment is more difficult to apply.
- Onset of pain relief is slower.
- Results are not as reliable.
- Some side effects are more frequent:
  . pruritus
  . urinary retention.
- Possibility of delayed respiratory depression is higher
  (Rawal and Wattwil 1984 a; Shulman et al. 1983).

Table 77. Comparison of results obtained after epidural and intramuscular morphine. Effects on postoperative gastro-intestinal motility and hospitalization time.

	IM morphine + ED saline mean + SEM	ED morphine + IM saline mean + SEM	Statistics
Postoperative hospitalization time (d)	9.0 ± 0.60	7.1 ± 0.30	$p < 0.05$
Flatus (h)	75.1 ± 3.08	56.7 ± 3.06	$p < 0.05$
Feces (h)	92.7 ± 2.92	68.2 ± 3.51	$p < 0.05$
Postoperative gastric aspirate Day 1 (ml/d) Day 2 (ml/d) Day 3 (ml/d)	211 ± 43.9 192 ± 43.2 243 ± 62.8	227 ± 44.0 351 ± 57.9 422 ± 53.8	NS $p < 0.05$ $p < 0.05$

Mean time from the end of the operation.
(Rawal et al. 1984 b)

The last point can be avoided by a judicious choice of lipophilic opioids and reduced opioid doses (Chovaz and Sandler 1985), but even by doing so a close and prolonged supervision is required.

17.2 Epidural opioids versus intravenous patient controlled analgesia

Comparison of epidural opioids with intravenous PCA was done by Harrison et al. (1988); Rosenberg et al. (1984); Weller et al. (1988). Better analgesic quality for one technique over another was not clearly demonstrated. Patient's satisfaction was comparable, opioid consumption was the same and respiratory rate was

Table 78 a. Comparison of spinal opioid analgesia versus spinal analgesia using local anaesthetics.

	EDOA or ITOA	EDLA or ITLA
1 - Action site	- Substantia gelatinosa of dorsal horn in spinal cord and other sites where opioid receptors are present.	- Nerve roots and long tracts in spinal cord
2 - Type of blockade	- Pre- and postsynaptic inhibition of nerve cell excitation	- Blockade of nerve impulse conduction in axonal membrane
3 - Block modalities	- Selective block of pain conduction	- Pain, motor, sensory, sympathetic fibre block
4 - Pain relief conditions • Peroperative • Postoperative • Labor pain • Post-traumatic pain	- Partial - Good relief - Partial relief - Good relief	- Complete relief possible in all cases
5 - Potential analgesic profile • Comfort • Onset • Duration • Segmental action	- Equal - Slower - Longer - Diffuse	- Equal - More rapid - Shorter - Limited

similar with the two methods. However, in the Harrison study epidural analgesia produced the highest incidence of side effects (the most notable was pruritus).

17.3 Epidural opioids versus epidural anaesthesia with a local anaesthetic

Advantages of the epidural opioid analgesia (Tab.1, 2, 77, 78 a, b):

- Duration of analgesia is longer-lasting.
- Quality of analgesia is better (absence of numbness and motor weakness)
- Mobility, coordination and sensibility is maintained.

Table 78 b. Pros and cons of spinal opioid analgesia versus spinal analgesia using local anaesthetics.

	EDOA or ITOA	EDLA or ITLA
6 - Side effects		
• Cardiovascular system:	- Minor changes	- Hypotension - Bradycardia
Vasoconstriction	- Intact	- Decreased
• Early | respiratory delayed | depression:	- Possible - Possible	- No
• CNS system:		
Sedation	- Possibly marked	- Rare or mild
Convulsions	- Rare	- Possible
Confusion	- Possible	- Rare
Withdrawal	- Rare; possible if rapid dicontinuation of systemic opioids	- No
Nausea, vomiting	- Possible	- Less frequent
Urinary retention	- Possible	- Possible
Pruritus	- Possible	- Absent
Miosis	- Possible	- Absent
Sensory block	- Absent	- Present
Motor block	- Absent	- Present
Sympathetic block	- Absent	- Present
7 - Treatment of side effects:	- Antidote: naloxone	- No antidote - Fluids Ephedrine Sedatives Atropine
8 - Therapeutic ratio	- > 2	< 2
9 - Failure rate	- ?	≈ 10 %

- Postural hypotension is rare.
- Sympathetic block is absent.
- Risk of convulsions, tachycardia, are reduced.
- Safety margin is greater.
- Antidote is available.
- Inadvertent dislodgement of the catheter into the intrathecal space or intravenous injection are not so dangerous.
- The height of the injection level is less important for epidural opioid analgesia.
- Lumbar injections are efficient in most cases.

Drawbacks of epidural anaesthesia with local anaesthetics:

- Regional anaesthesia has a failure rate that approaches 10% depending upon the operator and the technique.
- Significant hypotension may occur (5-55 %) (Brown 1988).
- Prolonged use of local anaesthetics epidurally results in tachyphylaxis.

Drawbacks of epidural opioid analgesia:

- It is difficult to obtain a sufficient depth for surgical anaesthesia with an opioid as sole agent (high doses of pethidine excepted).
- Sympathetic block is suitable after vascular surgery.
- Risk of respiratory depression requires close monitoring.
- Pruritus.

Epidural opioid infusion plus local anaesthetics has been reported to decrease the dose of local anaesthetic required to produce effective analgesia (El Baz et al. 1984) and adverse effects of pain on various organ systems are decreased by the combination (Bonnet et al. 1984; Bromage et al. 1980; Cohen and Woods 1983; Cousins and Bridenbaugh 1986; Cullen et al. 1985; Hjortsø et al.1985, 1986; Logas and El Baz 1987; Raj et al. 1985; Scott DB 1987; Shulman et al. 1984; Yeager et al. 1987).

Associations of low doses of local anaesthetics and opioids were developed in order to minimize the dose of both classes of drugs and presumably to decrease the potential side effects while retaining an efficacious or even increased spinal action (Cousins 1988).

17.4 Epidural opioid versus intrathecal opioid

Unfortunately, there are no comparable data for epidural versus intrathecal placement of catheters. Nevertheless, without any doubt, for postoperative pain treatment, the epidural route is the route of choice for opioid analgesia .

We can summarize the pros and cons of the epidural opioid analgesia compared to intrathecal opioid analgesia techniques as follows (Tab. 78 a, b):

Potential advantages:

- Protective functions of the dura mater are retained.
- Risk of infection is lower.

- Post-spinal headache is avoided.
- Incidence of side effects are lower.

Drawbacks:

- Transfer of drug across the dura mater is different for individual patients.
- Spread in CSF is impossible to control vascular uptake.
- Systemic uptake is greater.
- Analgesia is not as constant in depth and duration.
- Long-term epidural injections may produce epidural fibrosis leading to a loss of efficacy (Müller et al. 1988).

17.5 Advantages and drawbacks of intrathecal opioid analgesia

The intrathecal route is cleaner and requires smaller doses of drug (Glynn et al. 1987 b).

Subarachnoidal administration is not complicated by the simultaneous effect of systemic absorption, which is a co-product of the larger dose which needs to be used for the epidural administration. Systemic absorption, unknown complicating factors as a result of dural transfer and uptake into the extradural fat complicate the dosage of epidural opioids and delay the onset of analgesia (Camporesi and Redick 1983 b).

For the postoperative pain treatment, (Fromme and Gray 1985 a) compared, following thoracic surgery, the results obtained by 0.79 mg (0.5-0.2) of intrathecal morphine with those using 6.2 mg (3-10) epidural morphine. They observed that the analgesia evoked by the two routes of administration, was practically the same, but that the duration of analgesia produced by the intrathecal route was much longer. In this respect, the intrathecal technique, in some cases, can obviate the use of a catheter. Reinjections are less frequently required and the technique itself is simpler than the epidural technique. On the other hand, epidural opioid analgesia may be preferred in other cases, as adaptation of the doses, to the requirement of the patients, is easier.

Intrathecal opioid analgesia provides a more precise and more active technique for pain treatment than epidural opioid analgesia. However, the choice of such treatment being limited by a consideration of the side effects, intrathecal opioid analgesia must be confined to well selected groups of patients.

17.6 Limits and contra-indications of regional opioid analgesia

Without any doubt, spinal opioid analgesia has enlarged and diversified the methods at our disposal in the fight against pain. However, this treatment also has limitations and contra-indications, so that only rational use of this technique can be advised.

Advantages:

- The total drug doses required for analgesia is, compared to other administration routes, reduced.
- The analgesic effects are longer-lasting.
- In some cases, there is a lower incidence of side effects.
  The first two points are only practical advantages whereas the last point is of real clinical interest and importance.

Disadvantages:

- From the technical point of view, a proper application of spinal opioid analgesia requires more skill and time than oral or parenteral treatments.
- The technique requires more intensive care than necessary for systemic injections or oral applications.
- It is difficult to standardize the choice of the product and the doses. The fraction of the injected opioid acting directly on the opioid spinal receptors and the fraction of the injected product acting by systemic route cannot be easily determined.
- Side effects are not always negligible, sometimes they are delayed and extended supervision is necessary.
- The problem of tolerance is perhaps, in the case of postoperative opioids not so acute, but it cannot be completely eliminated.
- The results obtained using spinal opioid analgesia are not always superior to those obtained by other methods.

However, the biggest problems connected with spinal opioid analgesia remain:

- the possibility of delayed respiratory depression
- inadvertent puncture of the dura mater
- infection.

Data available at the present time indicate that the ratio between a minimal effective epidural dose and a dose that will produce side effects is approximately two. Failure to pay due attention to this therapeutic index will result in the administration of inappropriately large doses of spinal opioid in individual patients, so that a predominant spinal action will be lost and any resultant analgesia will be as much determined by brain effects as by spinal effects. This would negate any advantage of the spinal route of administration (Cousins 1988).

18. Future directions in spinal opioid research and conclusions

A broad future is open for further spinal opioid research:

- new and more specific analgesic opioids or non-opioids
- investigation of additional routes of administration
- improvement in administration equipment
- extension of these techniques to children.

We need to know:

- why some patients derive only limited pain relief from spinal opioids
- how to best manage tachyphylaxis to spinal opioids
- whether patients receiving spinal opioids can safely be cared for in a regular nursing ward or whether a special care unit is necessary.

Long-term studies of outcome addressing risk versus benefit are required.

General conclusions

The possibility of effecting in man, a selective pain block by the administration of opioids by the epidural, intrathecal, or intracerebroventricular route is now clearly established.

The demonstration of the existence of different opioid receptors and multiple other non-opioid systems in the spinal cord, modulating pain stimuli, has raised the hope that in the near future other major advances in spinal pain control will become possible. In this connection we can expect a complete or at least partial solution to the ancient problem of opioid tolerance and opioid respiratory depression.

The success of the method depends, above all, on a precise indication and a correct application of the technique. Before a definite statement about these methods can be made, the practitioner interested in these methods must give clear answers to the following questions:

- Is the regional opioid analgesia a good indication for the nature and the severity of the pain that I have to treat?
- If so, which is the opioid of choice? For acute pain preference is to be given to a lipophilic product.
- What doses should be administered? A weak test dose, to start the treatment, reinjection of small doses, or better still, a continuous on-demand infusion of small opioid doses generally offer a satisfactory and adequate solution.
- What is the most suitable route of administration: epidural, intrathecal, intra-cerebroventricular? The epidural route, even if not so precise, in contrast to the others, is associated with only minor side effects.
- To what extent should the opioid be administered? What position should be adopted by the patient after injection?
- Is an association of the opioid with a local anaesthetic advisable?
- If so, with which local anaesthetic, at what dose and without epinephrine if possible?
- What are the possible side effects? They have been widely discussed.
- How can they be prevented? Above all, by careful application of the technique and a sufficient period of supervision.
- How should they be treated? Often by naloxone.
- Finally, is the technical equipment at our disposal adequate and is the nursing staff sufficiently well trained for the effective supervision of the patient?

Spinal opioids are certainly one of the most important steps ahead in the history of acute or chronic pain therapy. This is true in two respects. On the one hand, this method is one of the most effective measures in controlling the pain. On the other hand, with the introduction of spinal opioids the interest in pain therapy started in some cases and increased extraordinarily in other cases. Pain relief for many thousands of patients became better both in quantitative and qualitative respect.

In the last years, perhaps this increasing interest misled pain management to overtreatment in some patients. Regional anaesthetics, oral pharmacotherapy, e.g. with opioids, have still the same function and cannot be substituted by spinal opioids.

What is the function of these newer methods? Regional opioid analgesia is certainly not indicated in those situations where, by non-opioid measures, the pain can successfully be treated. Ischaemic pain, causalgia, headache are strange indications for regional opioids. Obstetric pain still is a questionable indication for the use of spinal opioids alone. Cancer pain without any trial of oral opioids is certainly not an indication for invasive use of catheter and pumps systems.

After ten years of regional opioid analgesia, this method can only hold its place in pain therapy, when proper indications, equipment, drugs and supervision are guaranteed. This book has collected the most actual information on these fields.

We hope it may help to lead the overenthusiasm to a well indicated use of this new valuable method in pain therapy. We hope as well that pain management in some years might become as self-evident as it should be as one of the main duties of medicine. We are still away from this stage but regional opioid analgesia certainly can help on this way.

19. What is regional opioid analgesia?

Administration of opioids by the epidural, intrathecal and intra-cerebroventricular route is a new method for the treatment of severe pain. It has been developed since 1979.

Goal

The introduction of opioids into the organism, as near as possible to their specific receptors, in order to obtain maximum efficacy with minimum quantities of the drug is the rational ground of the procedure.

Administration routes

Among the various routes suitable for the administration of opioids, e.g. the epidural (ED), intrathecal (IT), intracerebroventricular (IC) or perineural (PN) routes, the epidural route is the most popular.

Used drugs

Theoretically, all the pure opioid agonists or agonist-antagonists of the opioid family prepared in preservative-free solution (with the exception of piritramide because of its excessive acidity) can be used. The most commonly administered substances after morphine are buprenorophine, fentanyl, methadone, pethidine. However, alfentanil, hydromorphone, sufentanil and nalbuphine are also of particular interest for these techniques.

Various drug associations may be considered as well. The most fruitful of these being provided by an opioid with local anesthetic but also the association of an opioid with clonidine or midazolam can be justified.

Injection modalities

Administration mode

A single shot injection, repeated as necessary or a loading bolus plus a continuous on-demand infusion are suitable.

Solutions

Glucose, saline, isobaric, hypobaric or hyperbaric solutions can be used and depending on the circumstances, each may have its own indication.

Volumes

2-10 ml of an opioid solution according to the selected injection space.

Injection devices:

- stationary pumps
- external portable pumps
- implantable pumps
- subcutaneous, implantable catheter access ports

They are available from many different manufacturers.

Administration levels

The lumbar level is currently used but also, sacral, thoracic or cisternal administration may be considered.
All these technical modalities must be selected accurately.

Effects

The analgesia obtained by these techniques is, in most cases, more effective and of longer duration than that obtained by the parenteral route.

Side effects

The frequency and severity of these vary according to products, doses, indications and administrative modalities.

They are principally:

- respiratory depression either early or delayed and markedly more frequent with hydrophilic opioids and with the intrathecal route.
- urinary retention
- pruritus
- nausea and vomiting
- drowsiness
- withdrawal syndrome
- tolerance and dependence.

Drug interactions:

- Potentiation and prolongation of the opioid effects are produced by all the central nervous system depressant drugs.
- Antagonism of most side effects and even reduction of analgesia is obtained by naloxone.

Principal indications:

- postoperative pain
- severe acute pain
- cancer pain
- labour pain
- supplement for regional anaesthesia with local anaesthetics

Contra-indications:

- opioid dependence
- coagulation disorders

Drawbacks and limitations

Potential side effects have to be considered on a risk/benefit basis and the possibility of unreliable or unsatisfactory results are to be evaluated.

Conclusions

The new regional administration routes for opioid analgesia have expanded our therapeutic possibilities. The methods have actually gained full credit. If the techniques are used with sufficient caution, care and discrimination, optimal results may be expected.

20. Technical data of equipment for spinal opioid therapy

In many situations the anaesthesiologist will have the task to select and adapt the already existing equipment in his clinic to the special requirements of the patients, the treatment and the financial costs involved in spinal opioid therapy. That is the reason why we have compiled in this chapter an overview of the equipment, mainly on an objective informative basis. The technical data do not provide any commercial promotion, they are certainly incomplete and the authors decline any responsibility for incomplete or inaccurate information.

20.1 Special needles

20.1.1 EPIDURAL NEEDLES

For the choice of an epidural needle the following characteristics can be specified. (Fig. 89, 90, 91).

20.1.1.1 Type of bevel

For single shot administration

- Crawford needle ®: short-bevelled, conic, rounded, blunt point, straight needle.

Gauge:
G 19 1.1 x 76 mm
G 19 1.1 x 88/86 mm
G 18 1.3 x 76/75 mm
G 18 1.3 x 88/86 mm

G 17 1.5 x 76 mm
G 17 1.5 x 88 mm

The variance of outer diameter with the same inner gauge is very high between the different manufacturers, e.g. from 1.3 mm to 1.7 mm for the 16 gauge needle (Kumar and Messahel 1987). There is also a difference on the reference dimensions of nominal diameters for US Standard and standard wire gauge, for the spinal needles, as pointed out by Hoel and Lind (1987).

For catheter use

- Tuohy needle :
side orifice (Huber point).

Gauge:
      G 18 1.3 x 76/80 mm
      G 18 1.3 x 88 mm
      G 18 1.05 x 76 extra thin mm
      G 18 1.05 x 88 extra thin mm

      G 17 1.5 x 76 0/ int 1.2 mm
      G 17 1.5 x 88 0/ int 1.2 mm
      G 16 1.6 x 76/80 mm
      G 16 1.6 x 88 mm
      G 14 2.0 x 93 mm

20.1.1.2 Other specifications

Multiple-use or disposable, centimeter markings, intern metallic or plastic mandrin.

20.1.1.3 Type of the hub

Metallic or plastic, transparent or not, with or without wings, mobile wings or not (a winged needle allows both hands to grasp the needle during insertion into the spinal space).
  - Scott needle = Tuohy type + modified hub
  For current use: Tuohy G 18.

20.1.1.4 Manufacturer

Arrow ®, Braun ®, Medimex ®, Palex ®, Portex ®, Vygon ®, e.g.

20.1.2 INTRATHECAL NEEDLES

20.1.2.1 Type of bevel

- Whitacre needle: pencil point, conic, side orifice.
    Gauge:
        G 22   0.7 x 88 mm
        G 18   1.2 x 38 mm

- Quincke needle: sharp point cutting bevel of medium length.
    Gauge:
        G 29 ** 0.3 x 88 mm
        G 25 ** 0.5 x 88 mm
        G 26 0.45 x 86 mm
        G 22 0.7 x 76 mm
        G 22 0.7 x 88 mm
        _____

        G 20 0.9 x 88 mm
        G 19 1.1 x 88 mm
        G 18 1.2 x 88 mm
- Tuohy needle:
        G 18
        G 22

20.1.2.2 Other specifications

Multi-use or disposable, internal metallic mandrin,
    - Introducer (Fig. 92):
        G 23 (0.6 mm) 30 or 76 mm
        G 20 (0.9 mm) 45 mm
        G 18 (1.2 mm) 38 mm

20.1.2.3 Type of hub

Metallic or plastic, with or without wings, transparent or not.
For current use: single shot: G 25.

20.1.3 OTHER NEEDLES

- Tunnelling needle
- Port needle:
  . Huber needle
     19 G
     20 G
     22 G
     24 G

20.1.4 MANUFACTURERS

Arrow ®, Becton Dickinson ®, Braun ®, Kendall ®, Medimex ®, Palex ®, Portex ®, Vygon ®, e.g.

20.2 Epidural or intrathecal catheters

For the choice of catheter the following characteristics may be specified (Fig. 93, 94, Tab. 79, 80).

20.2.1 TYPE OF DISTAL ENDING

Tip closed with side holes.
Tip open with tip hole (Fig. 93).

20.2.2 TYPE OF PROXIMAL ENDING

Amovible, Luer-Lock connection male or female, barbed, standard connection.
    Special ending (e.g. easy lock silicone connection for connection with catheter access port, pump, filter, non-return valve, stopcock)
    Material (semi-rigid or soft, plastic, vinyl, PVC, nylon, Teflon, polyamide, polyurethane, silicone rubber) (Fig. 94).

20.2.3 OTHER CHARACTERISTICS

- gauge: 16 G, 18 G, 19 G, 28 G
- length: 50 cm, 75 cm, 85 cm, 105 cm
- disposable
- guide wire or not: metallic, nylon
- spring wire or not
- radiopaque or not
- transparent or not

Catheter for current use: 18 G, int 0.45 mm, ext 0.85 mm, passes through a 18 G Tuohy needle.

20.2.4 EPIDURAL AND INTRATHECAL PACKS

Disposable sets are now available (Arrow, Braun, Portex, Vygon etc.), consisting of a plastic tray with small containers, syringes, needles, gauze holder, ampoules, drug solution, etc. All the items are sterilized by gamma radiation. Although expensive, these packs have proved to be very satisfactory (Fig. 95).

20.3 Filters

Filters used for RGOA treatments must have the following properties:

- a low deadspace volume for priming
- a bi-directional support allowing aspiration to check proper catheter placement
- a pore size of 0.20 microns
- an automatic air trap.

For ambulant patients, flat filter models have the advantage that wound dressing becomes easier (Fig. 96, Tab. 81).

20.4 Extension tube for connection between pumps and ports and catheters

The connections between external pump and port or catheter have to cope with 2 problems:

1. They have to be leak-proof and kink-proof.

2. They must have a low priming volume.

The tubings between the pump or the port and between the port and the catheter must have a reduced dead space. A low priming volume of the line ensures a rapid drug response. The use of microtubing sets reducing the dead space to 0.18 ml/min is particularly recommended (Tab. 81).

20.5 Implantable catheter access port

20.5.1 DESCRIPTION

A catheter access port (Tab. 82, Fig. 98 to 102) is composed of the following parts:

- an infusion chamber (port) in medical grade polysulfone, silicone rubber or stainless steel
- a thick self-sealing raised, percutaneously palpable silicone membrane
- an integrated catheter connection fixed to the side of the port body
- a plastic or metallic baseplate (ensuring the needle stop when the membrane is punctured)
- anchor rings for immobilization of the port by suturing to the fasciae.

20.5.2 INJECTION TECHNIQUE INTO A PORT

Use only special 22 G Huber point needles (e.g. Cytocan or Surecan Braun) for injections into the port. Aseptic technique is important to avoid infection, e.g., the skin above the port is carefully disinfected and the required syringes and cannulas are aseptic and disposable.

To perform the puncture, palpate the port between 2 fingers of the left hand. With the right hand holding the needle, pierce the centre of the membrane, until the needle reaches the basal membrane. During the subsequent manipulations it has to be ensured that the position of the needle is not changed so that the silicone membrane is not irritated by movements of the needle. It can be useful to connect an extension tube with a three-way stopcock between the needle and the syringe.

The patency of the catheter system is checked with a sterile saline solution. Before each change of the syringe the three-way stopcock should be closed to maintain a continuous fluid column inside of the port system. Injections are made at moderate pressure (5 ml/min).

After injection the needle is removed and the skin disinfected once more.

20.5.3 INFUSION TECHNIQUE THROUGH A PORT

For starting of an infusion (short-term or long-term infusion) it is recommended to use a 90° needle or a special needle which is connected to an adhesive cap which can be affixed to the skin. Affix a folding compress over the entire visible needle. Attach an extension tube with a three-way stopcock to the needle. To prevent catheter occlusion connect a filter of 0.22 micron.

20.6 Infusion pumps

Spinal administration of opioids demands very accurate infusion control. This can be achieved by volumetric pumps which deliver a given volume of fluid per unit time (ml hourly). The variety of volumetric devices has increased dramatically in the last few years.

20.6.1 CLASSIFICATION OF INFUSION PUMPS

Infusion pumps can be classified in several ways:

a) According the mode of operation:

- linear peristaltic pumps
- rotary peristaltic pumps
- reciprocating piston pumps
- piston actuated diaphragm pumps.

b) According to the fluid containers:

- reservoir pumps
- syringe pumps.

c) According to the energy sources:

- self-powered, by elasticity or gas expansion
- manual
- motor driven.

d) According to the control possibilities by the patient (PCA)

e) According to the weight, the volume and the materials used:

- stationary
- portable
- implantable.

f) According to computerized or telemetric programme and function (Tab. 83).

Important properties of infusion pumps used for spinal opioids are :
- accuracy of infusion rate
- consistency of flow
- safety
- reliability of alarm conditions
- miniaturization and robusticity
- ease of clinical use:
  . setting-up
  . priming
  . change of disposables.

The most important characteristics of infusion pumps are enumerated in Tab. 84.

In Tab. 85-89 these characteristics are used to allow a practical comparison between particular groups of pumps.

The listings are far from complete. They are only based on the information that we have at our disposal at this moment.

The most representative pump models used are represented in Fig. 104-119.

20.6.2 Patient controlled analgesia systems

20.6.2.1 Principles

The patient controlled analgesia (PCA) technique involves the use of machines which allows the patient to self-administer an analgesic drug, in a preset dose, without outside help and according to his needs.

The PCA device consists mostly of three parts (separated from each other or not):

- a pump
- a programmable controller device
- a push button for the patient.

With certain models, the pump may provide a continuous background infusion and at the same time a push button allows the delivery of a supplemental bolus.

In other types of PCA devices the pump is only activated if the patient presses the button in order to receive a dose of drug over a preset time. The concentration of the drug solution, the continuous infusion rate, size, the duration and the repetition of the bolus are programmed, limited and set by the clinician.

The patient controls the amount of analgesic he receives within these limits. After delivering a dose, the machine is refractory to further requests for analgesia over a pre-fixed time. This allows each supplemental bolus to have time to become efficient and helps to prevent overdose.

The drug is administered through a one-way valve to prevent dose accumulation in the spinal tubing.

Early PCA devices were bulky and cumbersome (Fig. 108) but advances in microprocessor technology have allowed the development of more compact apparatus (Fig.110).

The infusion pumps with PCA possibilities are listed in Tab. 85, 86, 87.

20.6.2.2 Example 1: Prominject ® pump

The programmable Prominject infusion pump has 3 modes of operation lodged in 3 separate programme modules, only one of which is active at a time (Fig.109):

a) patient controlled analgesia (PCA)
b) consecutive infusions
c) constant infusion.

The desired mode is selected at the start. Each mode comprises a set of dose parameters:

- drug concentrations
- dose
- lockout period
- time for injection.

The dose settings for a) and b) are presented directly in weight (mg or µg) and time (min) for administration and not in volume and time (ml /hourly) as is useful for a continuous flow administration.

a) Patient controlled analgesia (PCA)

The patient can trigger intermittent injections of fixed bolus doses. Each bolus is then administered over a certain period.

Alternatively, the pump can also deliver a split incremental dose. This is a bolus delivered over 1 min followed by a tail dose infusion for one hour.

It is thus possible to deliver, e.g. 5 µg of sufentanil over 1 min, followed by another 10 µg dose over 1h. In this case the patient demand results in $5 + 5$ µg of sufentanil administered over $1 + 60$ minutes.

Patient control also includes a safety feature for selection of a minimum time interval, during which period the pump will not respond to demands for a new bolus dose.

b) Consecutive infusion

Using this programme the infusion will deliver at two different rates:

- a rapid loading infusion, immediately and automatically followed by:
- a maintenance infusion at a low administration rate.

c) Constant infusion

For infusion at a constant rate, the total volume to be given is preset. The constant rate can be varied from 0.1 to 99.9 ml/hourly.

Note: The programme does not allow the simultaneous use of a continuous low background infusion supplemented, on demand, by a PCA microbolus. However, these advantages are offered by the CADD-PCA ® pump and the Chronomat infusion computer.

20.6.2.3 Example 2: Baxter Travenol Infusor

The Travenol Infusor ® PCA device is a completely disposable system for the patient-controlled delivery of drugs. The system consists of the basic Travenol Infusor and a patient control module ("watch"). The infusor provides the reliable, consistent flow rate into the "watch" and the watch allows access to controlled quantities of the drug.

As required for the therapy, the watch is normally closed but will provide a 0.5 ml bolus of the drug solution when the button or lever is activated by the patient. The constant flow rate of the basic Infusor provides the required lock-out time by refilling the bolus reservoir (in the watch) over a period of 6 minutes. With the Infusor PCA system, the patient can potentially activate the device more frequently than the 6 minutes refill time.

However, since the Infusor refills the bolus reservoir at a minimum time of 6 minutes, the patient can only receive drugs at the same rate of 6 minutes (Fig. 111, 112).

20.7 Monitoring devices

Most useful electronic monitoring devices are those facilitating the early diagnosis of respiratory depression.

Six classes of monitoring devices can be found:

- pupil scanners
- respiratory monitors
- transcutaneous oximeters
- combined transcutaneous O_2/CO_2 monitors
- capnometers
- combined gas analyzers O_2/CO_2.

20.7.1 PUPIL SCANNERS

These devices measure the pupil diameter up to 10 mm under widely variable ambient light conditions (Fig. 120).

Examples:

Pupilscan ® (Fairville Medical Optics Inc.)
- Esilor pupillometer.

20.7.2 RESPIRATORY MONITORS

A simple respiratory monitor with alarm which assesses abdominal and supra-sternal movements (Fig. 121).

Examples:

- Air Shield AS 165 Respiratory Monitor ® (Air Shield)
- Cardiff Respiratory Monitor ® (Graseby)
- Respigraph ® (Nims)
- Respirate apnea alarm
- Respiration and Heart rate monitor ® (Eden)
- Rotomed Respiration ® Monitor (series 8600 TMF) (Rototherm)

- RAG-1200A + ECG (Nihon)
- Apnoea monitor ® (Smad)
- Ventilation monitor ® (Japan Medical Supplies)
- Neonatal Monitor ® (Sorensen and Weel)
- Vitalmon 5010 ® (Kontron).

20.7.3 PULSE OXIMETERS, SaO$_2$

Continuous non-invasive measurement of the oxyhaemoglobin saturation
(SaO$_2$%) with alarms for saturation when SaO$_2$ and/or heart rate fall beyond the
pre-selected limits allows an early detection of hypoxemia.

Examples:

- Accusat® Datascope pulse oximeter
- Bird 4400 portable Pulse Oximeter ® (Bird)
- Biox IVA continuous print-out portable oximeter ® (Ohmeda)
- Biox 3700 Pulse Oximeter ® (Ohmeda)
- In vivo Pulse Oximeter, mod 4500 ® (Invivo Research Lab.)
- Lifestat 1600 Pulse Oximeter ® (Physiocontrol)
- Miniox 100 Pulse Oximeter ® (Catalyst Research)
- N-100 Pulse Oximeter ® (Nellcor) (Fig.122)
- Lifespan 100 Monitor ® (Biochem International)
- Novametrix Pulse Oximeter ® (Novametrix)
- OXI ® Radiometer
- Oxyshuttle Sensor ® (Medics)
- Pulse Oximeter 90501 ® (Spacelab International)
- 501 + Pulse oximeter ® (Criticare Systems Inc).
- Pulsox - 7 ® (Minolta)
- Pulse oximeter R (Sensor Medicis)
- Satlite, Pulse Oximeter ® (Datex)

20.7.4 COMBINED TRANSCUTANEOUS O$_2$/CO$_2$ MONITORS (PTcO$_2$, PTcCO$_2$)

Examples:

- Micro Span Combo ® (Biochem Int Inc)
.- Combi Sensor ® (Kontron)
- Micro Span Combo ® (Biochem Int.)

- Mod 850B ® (Novametrix)
- POET (CSI)
- TCR 3 tc Recorder ® (Radiometer)
- TINA transcutaneous pO_2/pCO_2 monitor ® (Radiometer)

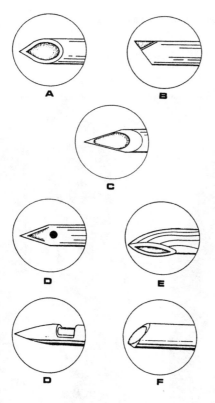

Fig. 89. Spinal needles: A Quincke-Babcock   D Whitacre
　　　　　　　　　　　　　B Pitkin　　　　　　　E Tuohy
　　　　　　　　　　　　　C Green　　　　　　　　F Crawford

470

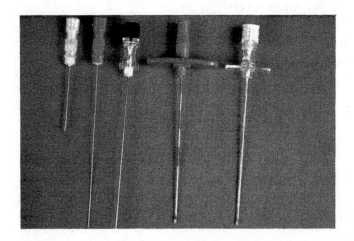

Fig. 90. Various needles used in spinal analgesia.

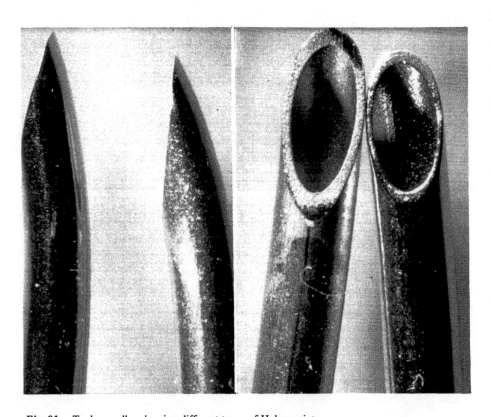

Fig. 91 a. Tuohy needles showing different types of Huber points

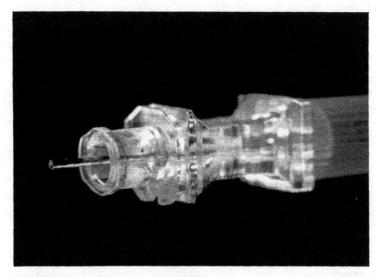

Fig. 91 b. Scott epidural needle. The shaft of this needle protrudes from the hub so that is has an advantage when any obstruction is met to the forward movement of the catheter (Covino and Scott 1985).

472

Table 79. Most frequently used catheters.

Material	Commercial name	Manufacturer
- Nylon	Portex [R]	Portex Inc.
- Polyamide	Perifix [R] Periplant [R]	Braun, Vygon
- Polyethylen	Rilsan [R] PD-Katheter (L) [R]	Ato-Chimie Viggo, Vygon
- Polysiloxampolyurethan	Avothane [R]	
- Polyurethan - Polyvinylchloride (PVC)	Hydrocath [R] Port-A-Kath [R]	Viggo, Vygon Pharmacia
- Silicone rubber	Silastic [R]	A.H.S. Cook, Cordis Infusaid, Micmed, Davol
- Polytetrafluoroethylen compound = teflon	Deseret [R] RACZ [R] Secalon [R]	Sandy Arrow Viggo

Table 80. Microtubing sets.

Microtubing sets	Volume ml	Length cm
- Minimum held-up volume catheter (Markwell-Rand Rocket)	0.16	61
- GO Harvard microbore [R] (Bard)	0.11	60
- Micro volume tubing Travenol [R]	0.19	105

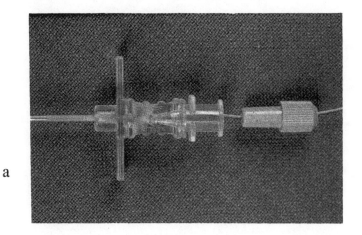

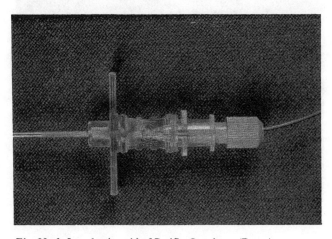

Fig. 92a,b. Introduction aid of Perifix ® catheter (Braun).

474

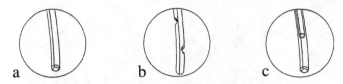

Fig. 93. Epidural catheter tips for chronic treatment (Vygon).

- a) Open tip
- b) Side hole
- c) Open tip + guide wire.

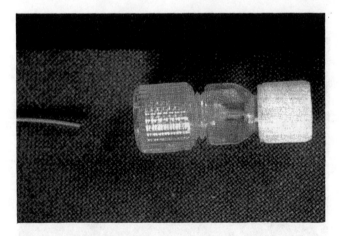

Fig. 94. Catheter adapter (Braun).

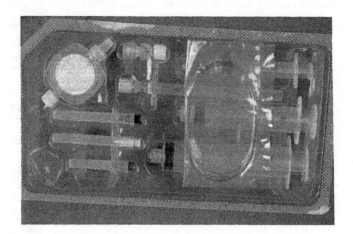

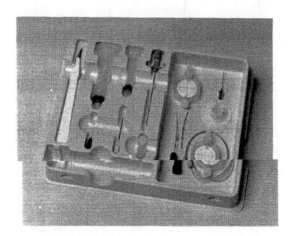

Fig. 95 a,b. Sterile disposable, epidural catheter tray.
a) Braun
b) Portex

Table 81. Comparative properties of different filters used in regional opioid analgesia.

	Cathi-vex SVGS 02505	Millex - OR SLGL 02505	Portex Steril filter	Sterifix Braun
- Transparency:	+	+	+	+ +
- Shape:	round	round	round	round flat
- Deadspace (ml):	0.2	0.2	0.36	
- Filter membrane pore size (μm):	0.22	0.22	0.22	0.2 0.2
- Perfusion pressure limits:	$3\,Kp/cm^2$	$3\,Kp/cm^2$	$5.3\,Kp/cm^2$	$5\,Kp/cm^2$ round $9\,Kp/cm^2$ flat
- Allows fluid aspiration*:	-	+	+	+ +
- Automatic air trap:	+	+	-	
- Dimensions (cm):	3.7 x 2.8	3.8 x 2.8		2.1 x 2.7 round 1.5 x 3.5 flat

* Bi-directional support: allows aspiration to check proper catheter placement.

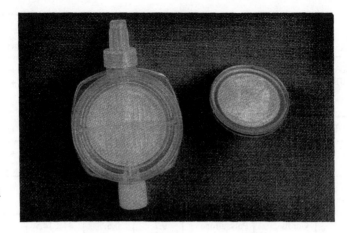

a

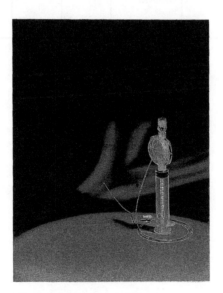

b

Fig. 96. Sterifix filter ® (Braun).
a) The filter
b) Filter catheter and syringe

Table 82a. Catheter injection ports, technical data.

Name model	Manufacturer	Material	Weight dry (g)	Internal Volume (ml)	Dimension (mm)	Connection PD IT IC
CAP 8500 CAP 8501	Medtronic Medtronic	Titanium + Silicone elastomer	9 26	0.07 0.5	38 x 10 50 x 17	+ + + +
Infuse-A-Port	Infusaid	Silicone rubber	14.3	0.2	48 x 16	+ + +
Intraport	Fresenius	Polysulfone silicone	5	0.41	35 x 12.5	+ +
Life Port	Strato Medical					
MPAP multi purpose Access port	Cordis	Polysulfone	9.7	0.6	44 x 14.5	+ +
Ommaya CSF reservoir (Leroy-Hickman)	A H S	Silicone elastomer			15 x 25	+ +

Table 82b. Catheter injection ports, technical data (continued).

Name model	Manufacturer	Material	Weight dry (g)	Internal volume (ml)	Dimension (mm)	Connection PD IT IC
Pain port Sitimplant	Vygon	Silicone	6.8	0.1	10.0 x 35	+ +
			7.5	0.5	12.5 x 35	+ +
			8.1	1.0	15.0 x 35	+ +
Periplant	Braun Melsungen	Polysulfone Silicone	7.4 3.5	0.33 0.1	46 x 10.5 36 x 10.5	+ + + +
Port-A-Cath	Pharmacia	Stainless steel	26	0.5	25 x 13	+ +
Portal PN 550 1874	Pharmacia	Silicone	28	0.4	25.4 x 13.5	+ +
Secor	Cordis	Polysulfon	44	12	65 x 15	+ +
Polysite	LPI	Silicone	7.3		30 x 14.3	+

480

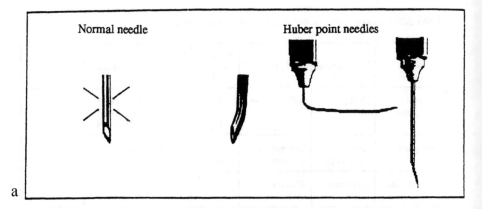

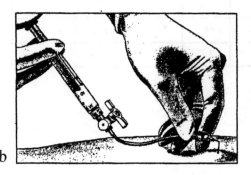

Fig. 97a, b. a) Special 22 g needles with Huber point. The special bevel of the needle avoids damage of the silicone membrane of the port during injection or infusion.

b) Administration of the opioid in a subcutaneous implanted port.

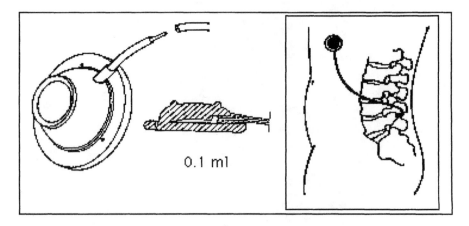

Fig. 98. Painport (Vygon): Complete indwelling system.

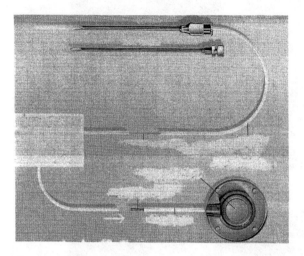

Fig. 99. Intraport Fresenius.

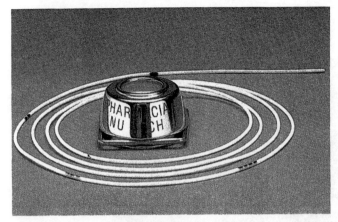

a

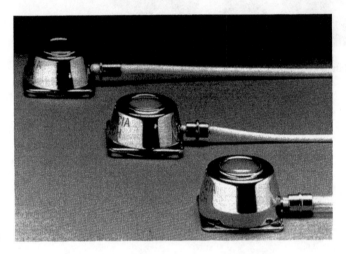

b

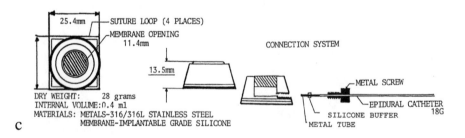

c

25.4mm — SUTURE LOOP (4 PLACES)

MEMBRANE OPENING
11.4mm

CONNECTION SYSTEM

13.5mm

DRY WEIGHT: 28 grams
INTERNAL VOLUME:0.4 ml
MATERIALS: METALS-316/316L STAINLESS STEEL
          MEMBRANE-IMPLANTABLE GRADE SILICONE

METAL SCREW
EPIDURAL CATHETER
                18G
SILICONE BUFFER
METAL TUBE

Fig. 100. Pharmacia port
a) Port and catheter.
b)The port in different sizes.
c) Cross section and connection system.

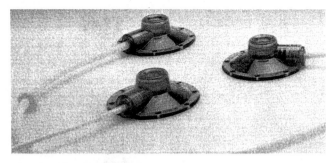

Fig. 101. Infusaid ® port.

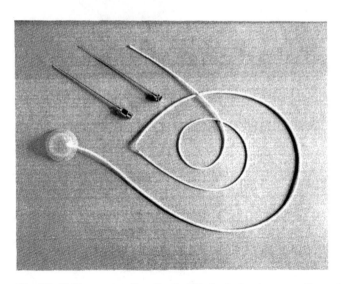

Fig. 102. Unidose access Port Cordis ® and spinal catheter, needles and mandrin.

484

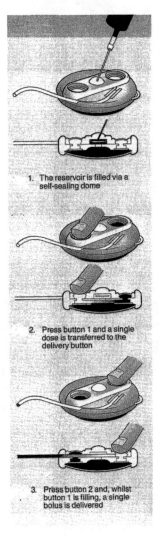

Fig. 103. The Secor ® Cordis device.
Refill and auto-injection system.

Table 83. Classification of infusion pumps used for epidural, intrathecal or intracerebroventricular opioid analgesia.

A - Stationary infusors

1. Stationary syringe infusors
2. Stationary programmable syringe or volumetric infusors

B - Portable infusors

3. Portable manual or self-powered infusors
4. Portable syringe infusors
5. Portable volumetric reservoir infusors

C - Implantable reservoir pumps

6. Implantable pumps with external programming device
7. Implantable pumps with fixed rate

486

Table 84. Characteristics of an infusion pump.

1 - Use:	- Stationary - Portable - Implantable	
2 - Dimensions		
3 - Weight (+battery)		
4 - Principles:	- Volumetric . linear peristaltic	
		. rotary peristaltic
	(not used in RGOA)	. reciprocating piston
	. piston actuating diaphragm pump	
	- Syringe pump	
5 - Reservoir:	- Volume	. 3-60 ml
	- Type	. Syringe (type, disposable, size) . refill cartridge . Plastic pack . elastomeric balloon
	- Refill system	
6 - Catheter microbore		
7 - Basal infusion	- Type	. continuous . pulsatile . programmable, pulse interval start delivery, total hours . bolus: size, duration
	- Rate	. ml/min, h, d
8 - Memory features:	- Total volume infused, digital display - Printer	
9 - Alarms: - Runaway		
	- High pressure occlusion - Air in line - Fluid near empty - Battery low	
10-Power: - Self powered		
	- Manual - Alternative C - Battery	. type . voltage . capacity . rechargeable . recharge interval
11- Accuracy		
12- PCA	- Patient demand signal - Preset dose size - Increments in size - limits: lock-out time, total amount/h	
13- Price		

Table 85. Order of presentation of the infusion pump characteristics as appearing comparatively (from a to i) in the next tables.

Name, model	Manufacturer
1. STATIONARY, SYRINGE INFUSORS	
- Auto Syringe AS 20A	Baxter Travenol
- Auto Syringe 5C	Baxter Travenol
- Dual Syringe I.P. 800	Imed
- Injectomat S	Fresenius
- IVAC 700	IVAC
- Medfusion M 1001	Medfusion Syst. Inc.
- Perfusor Secura	Braun Secura
- Program 1 S.P.	Vial Medical
- PS 2000	Sky Electronics-Habel
- PS A 50	Habel
- PS A 52	Habel
- PS A 55	Habel
- SE 200	Vial Medical
- SE 300	Vial Medical
- SE 400	Vial Medical
- Spritzomat	Vygon
- Terufusion S.P.M.STC 521	Terumo
- Ulis I BM	I.D.F. Medicorep
- Ulis II BM dual	I.D.F. Medicorep
2. STATIONARY PROGRAMMABLE SYRINGE OR VOLUMETRIC INFUSORS	
- Abbott Life Care PCA	Abbott
- Harvard PCA 4000	Bard Medisystem Inc
- Injectomat PCA ** ***	Fresenius
- MS 2000	Graseby
- ODAC PCA	Janssen Scientific Instruments
- Palliator MS 402	Graseby
- PCAS	Graseby
- Cardiff Palliator *	Graseby
- Prodac DAC ** controller + infuser MS 16	Oxford Univ. Clin. Research
- Prominject PCA	Pharmacia
- Leicester micro-palliator ** controller + infuser MS 16	Leicester Infirmary
- PCA infuser model 310	Ivac

* = discontinued   ** = syringe drive part: portable   *** = prototype

Table 86. Infusion pumps: name, model, manufacturer.

Name, model	Manufactures
3. PORTABLE MANUAL OR SELF-POWERED INFUSORS	
- Baxter Travenol Infusor - PCA Infusor	Baxter Travenol Baxter Travenol
- Pen Pump Infusor	Markwell, Rand Rocket
- Perfusor M	Braun
4. PORTABLE SYRINGE INFUSORS	
- Auto Syringe AS 2F - Auto Syringe AS 3B - Auto Syringe AS 6C - Auto Syringe AS 6H pulsastile - Auto Syringe AS 2FH	Baxter Travenol Baxter Travenol Baxter Travenol Baxter Travenol Baxter Travenol
- Harvard mini-Infuser 950 (AF)	Bard
- Microjet bolus 2	Miles-Ames
- MS 16 A - MS 18 - MS 26 (bolus) - MS 27	Baxter Travenol Baxter Travenol Baxter Travenol Baxter Travenol
- Nordisk Infuser	Muirhead
- Perfuser ME	Braun
5. PORTABLE VOLUMETRIC RESERVOIR INFUSORS	
- Act-A-Pump - CADD-1 - CADD-PCA	Pharmacia Pharmacia Deltec Pharmacia Deltec
- Chronomat	Fresenius
- Cormed II	Cormed
- Infumed 200	Medfusion System Inc.
- Promedos El * - Promedos EVI *	Siemens Siemens

* = discontinued   (AF) = programmed for alfentanil only

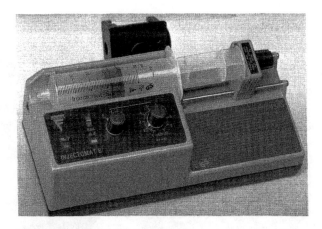

Fig. 104. Injectomat S ® Fresenius.

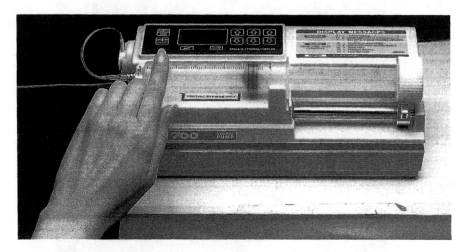

Fig. 105. IVAC 700 ® (IVAC).

490

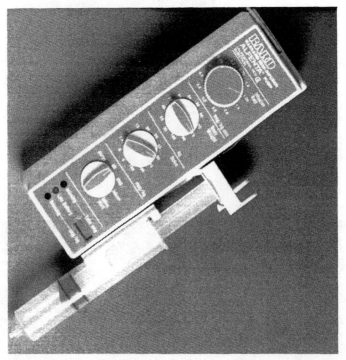

Fig. 106. Harvard Mini-Infuser 950 ® (Bard) for alfentanil infusion only.

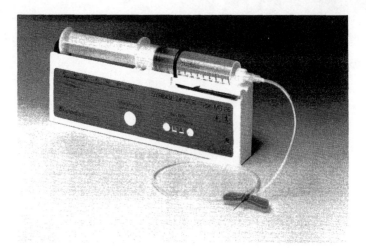

Fig 107. Syringe driver MS 26 (Gaseby Medical).

491

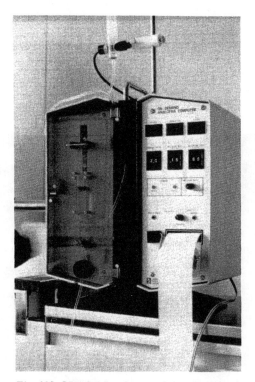

Fig. 108. ODAC PCA (Janssen Scientific Instrument).

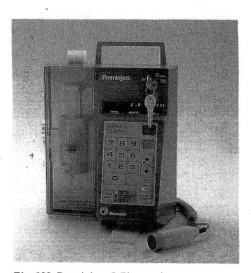

Fig. 109. Prominject ® Pharmacia.

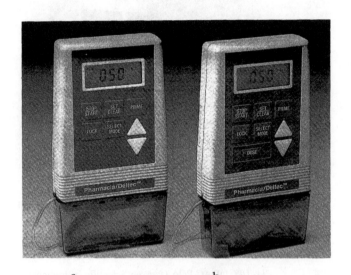

a   b

Fig. 110a,b. Pharmcia Deltec Pumps.
  a) CADD 1 ®
  b) CADD-PCA ®

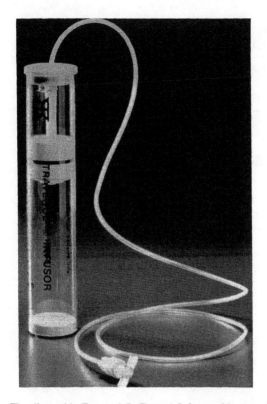

Fig. 111a. The disposable Travenol ® (Baxter) Infusor with a non-kinking tubing and luer lock connection for the ED catheter.

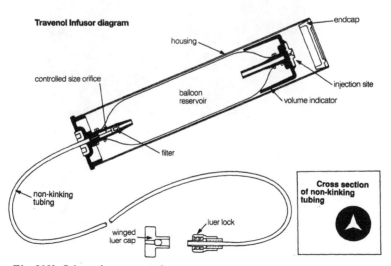

Fig. 111b. Schematic representation.

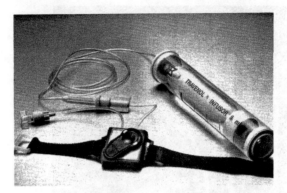

Fig. 112a. The disposable Travenol Infusor ® with programming device.

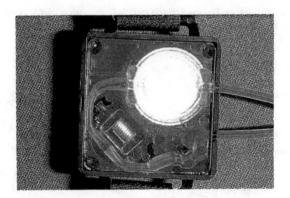

Fig. 112b. The disposable Travenol Infusor®: The programming device.

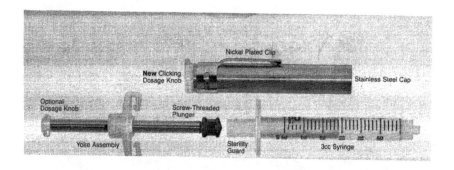

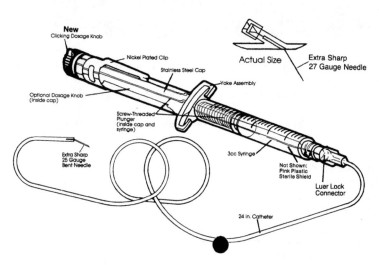

Fig. 113. The Pen Pump Infusor (Rand Rocket, Markwell).

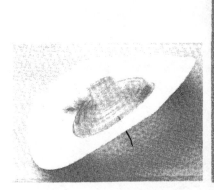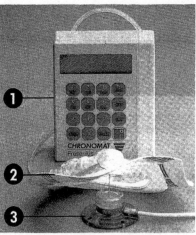

Fig. 114. The Chronomat ® infusion computer (1) with Intraport Stick ® (22 g needle (2) and Spinal Intraport ® (3) Fresenius.

This external pump device for spinal drug infusion consists of the following components:

1) A portable programmable roller pump with a disposable drug reservoir bag of 10 ml. Dimensions: 66,5 x 80,5 x 27,5 mm; weight: 185 g.

The pump provides multiple drug delivery possibilities
-infusion periods from 1 sec to 24 h,
-infusion pause periods from 1 sec to 24 h,
-supplemental bolus from 1 sec to 24 h,
-bolus interval from 1 sec to 24 h,
-program set up for: a) continuous infusion
                 b) pulsatile infusion
                 c) microbolus administration with or without a basic infusion rate.

2) An Intraport Stick with Huber needle and fixation pad for connection between pump and port.

3) An implantable drug port: Intraport with a silicone catheter, guide wire and Tuohy needle.

Table 87a. Implantable pumps (continued): name, model, manufacturer.

Name, model	Manufacturer
6. IMPLANTABLE, PROGRAMMABLE PUMPS	
- DAD Mod 8800	Medtronic
- Pace Setter implantable	Pace Setter, John Hopkins Universitiy
- Promedos IDI *, **	Siemens
- Infusaid M 1000	Infusaid Inc.
7. IMPLANTABLE PUMP, FIXED RATE	
- Infusaid Mod 100 - Infusaid Mod 200 - Infusaid Mod 400 - Infusaid Mod 500	Infusaid Inc., Fresenius Infusaid Inc., Fresenius Infusaid Inc., Fresenius Infusaid Inc., Fresenius
- Secor Cordis	Cordis

Table 87b. Implantable pumps (continued): volumes of reservoir, routes of administration (continued).

Name, model	Volume (ml)	ED	IT	IC
6. IMPLANTABLE, PROGRAMMABLE PUMPS				
- DAD Mod 8800	20	+	+	-
- Pace Setter implantable	15	+	+	-
- Promedos IDI	10	+	+	-
- Infusaid M 1000	22	-	+	+
7. IMPLANTABLE PUMP, FIXED RATE				
- Infusaid Mod 100 - Infusaid Mod 200 - Infusaid Mod 400 - Infusaid Mod 500	47 32 47 22	+	+	+
- Secor Cordis	12	+	+	-

Table 87c. Implantable pumps (continued): PCA possibility.

Name, model	PCA	Background inf.	Programmable bolus
6. IMPLANTABLE, PROGRAMMABLE PUMPS			
- DAD Mod 8800	+	+	+
- Pace Setter implantable	-	-	+
- Promedos IDI	-	-	+
- Infusaid M 1000	+	+	+
7. IMPLANTABLE PUMP, FIXED RATE			
- Infusaid Mod 100 - Infusaid Mod 200 - Infusaid Mod 400 - Infusaid Mod 500	- - - -	- - - -	- - - -
- Secor Cordis	+	-	-

Table 87d. Implantable pumps (continued): weight and dimensions.

Name, model	weight (g)	Dimensions		
		length or diameter (cm)	width (cm)	height (cm)
6. IMPLANTABLE, PROGRAMMABLE PUMPS				
- DAD Mod 8800	175	7.04		2.75
- Pace Setter implantable	200	8.10		2.0
- Promedos IDI	180	8.50	6	2.2
- Infusaid M 1000	272	9.02		2.25
7. IMPLANTABLE PUMP, FIXED RATE				
- Infusaid Mod 100 - Infusaid Mod 200 - Infusaid Mod 400 - Infusaid Mod 500	187 172 208 165	8.70 8.70 8.70 8.70		2.8 2.8 2.8 2.8
- Secor Cordis	45	6.50		1.5

Table 87e. Implantable pumps (continued): basal infusion.

Name, model	Basal cont. infusion
6. IMPLANTABLE, PROGRAMMABLE PUMPS	
- DAD Mod 8800	+
- Pace Setter implantable	+
- Promedos IDI	+
- Infusaid M 1000	+
7. IMPLANTABLE PUMP, FIXED RATE	
- Infusaid Mod 100 - Infusaid Mod 200 - Infusaid Mod 400 - Infusaid Mod 500	+ + + +
- Secor Cordis	-

Table 87f. Implantable pumps (continued): infusion rate and mode.

Name, model	Infusion rate (ml/h)	Infusion mode	Infusion increments (ml/h)
6. IMPLANTABLE, PROGRAMMABLE PUMPS			
- DAD Mod 8800	0.009 - 0.9 0.009 - 1.4	variable	variable
- Pace Setter implantable		variable	2
- Promedos IDI	0.001 - 0.015		variable
- Infusaid M 1000	0.001 - 0.5	variable	variable
7. IMPLANTABLE PUMP, FIXED RATE			
- Infusaid Mod 100 - Infusaid Mod 200 - Infusaid Mod 400 - Infusaid Mod 500	0.04 - 0.25 0.04 - 0.25 0.04 - 0.25 0.04 - 0.25	fixed fixed fixed fixed	- - - -
- Secor Cordis	-	-	-

Table 87g. Implantable pumps (continued): memory features.

Name, model	Memory features			Printer
	Total volume	Total hours	Display num.	
6. IMPLANTABLE, PROGRAMMABLE PUMPS				
- DAD Mod 8800	-	+	+	+
- Pace Setter implantable				-
- Promedos IDI	-	-	-	-
- Infusaid M 1000	+	+	+	+
7. IMPLANTABLE PUMP, FIXED RATE				
- Infusaid Mod 100 - Infusaid Mod 200 - Infusaid Mod 400 - Infusaid Mod 500	- - - -	- - - -	- - - -	- - - -
- Secor Cordis	-	-	-	-

Table 87h. Implantable pumps (continued): alarms.

Name, model	Memory features					
	Audible	Run away	High pressure	Air	Empty fluid	battery
6. IMPLANTABLE, PROGRAMMABLE PUMPS						
- DAD Mod 8800	+	-	-	-	+	+
- Pace Setter implantable	+	-	-	-	+	+
- Promedos IDI	-	-	-	-	-	+
- Infusaid M 1000	+	+	+	-	-	+
7. IMPLANTABLE PUMP, FIXED RATE						
- Infusaid Mod 100 - Infusaid Mod 200 - Infusaid Mod 400 - Infusaid Mod 500	- - - -	- - - -	- - - -	- - - -	- - - -	- - - -
- Secor Cordis	-	-	-	-	-	-

Table 88. Comparison between the Secor implanted multidose port and two implanted pump devices.

	Medtronic system	Infusaid system	Secor (Cordis)
Programmable	yes	no	no
Administration route	ED or IT	ED or IT	IT
Working principle	peristaltic pump	vapor pressure	manual activation
Battery	yes	no	no
Electronic parts	yes	no	no
Dimensions (cm)	7 x 2.7	9 x 3	6.5 x 1.5
Weight (g)	175	200	45
Capacity (ml)	20	50	12
Administration rate	variable 0 - 0.9 ml/h	continuous 0.04 - 0.25 ml/h	on demand bolus 0.1 ml
Preset maximal dose	yes	no	fixed
Possibility to change opioid concentration	yes refill	yes refill	yes refill
Possibility to stop drug delivery	yes	no	yes
Side port access	no	yes	no
Alarm	yes	no	no
Investment	high	high	relatively low

Table 89. Comparison of the properties of different implantable disposable pumps.

	Promedos I D I *	Medtronic system	Infusaid system 400	Pacesetter J. Hopkins **	Infusaid M 1000
Programmable	yes	yes	no	yes	yes
Pump system	peristaltic	peristaltic	vapor pressure	pulsatile solenoid	vapor pressure
Dimensions (cm)	8.5 x 6 x 2.2	7 x 2.7	8.7 x 2.8	8.1 x 2	9.02 x 2.25
Weight (g)	180	175	200	200	272
Capacity (ml)	10	20	47	15	22
Basal flow rate	variable 24 steps	variable 0 - 0.9 ml/h	fixed 4 ml/day	variable 2 ml steps	variable 0.001 - 0.5 ml/h
Supplementary bolus	yes	yes	yes	yes	yes
Adjustability	high	high	limited	high	high
Refill interval	relatively short	relatively short if high doses	longer 3 - 4 weeks	short	variable
Power source	internal battery	internal battery	no battery vapor pressure	internal battery	vapor pressure + battery
Alarm	yes	yes	no	yes	yes
Possibility to stop	yes	yes	no	yes	yes
Auxilliary side port	no	no	yes	no	yes

*Production stopped, ** experimental use only.

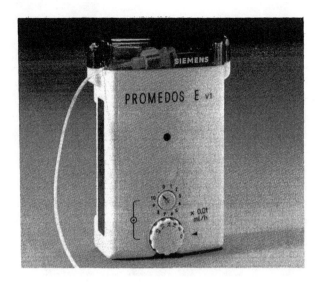

Fig. 115. Promedos E VI (Siemens), discontinued.

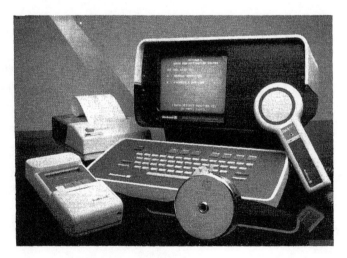

Fig. 116. DAD mod 8800 (Medtronic).
The Medtronic Drug administration System consists of an implantable infusion pump (DAD), a variety of implantable catheters, an implantable catheter access port and a clinician's programmer.

The programmer can (non-invasively) programme the implanted infusion pump to a specific prescription.

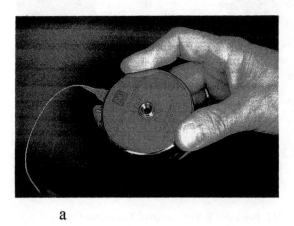

a

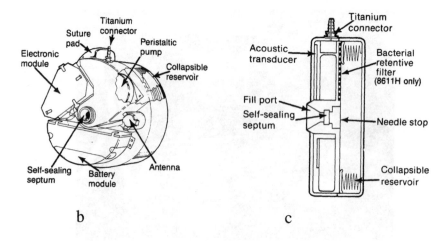

b

c

Fig. 117a,b,c.
The device is programmed to deliver for individual patient needs combined with bolus injection.
a) Medtronic device.
b, c) Cross section of Medtronic administration device.

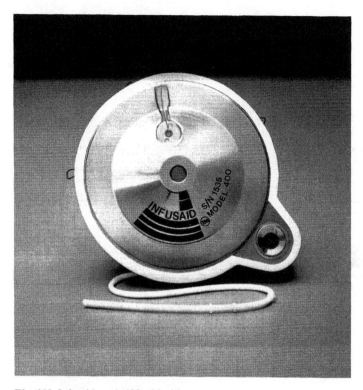

Fig. 118. Infusaid mod. 400 with side port.

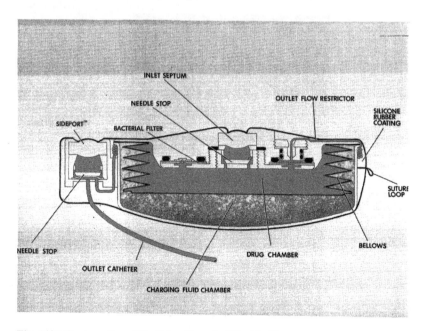

Fig. 119a. Cross section of the Infusaid mod. 400 with side port.

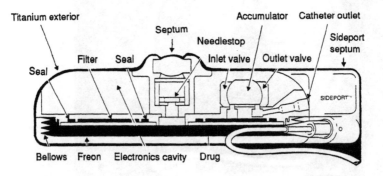

Fig. 119b. Schematic representation of the programmable implantable pump Infusaid M1000.

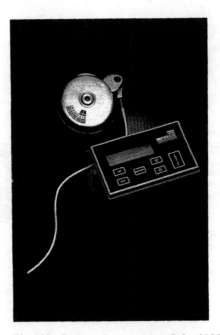

Fig. 119c. Pump and programmer (Infusaid M1000).

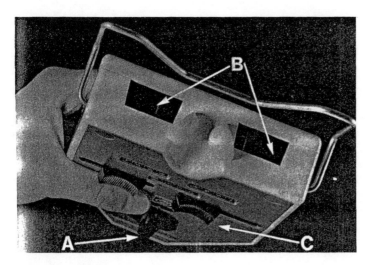

Fig. 120. The Essilor pupillometer.
A) eye of the observer
B) eyes of the subject
C) slide and scale
(Ravnborg et al. 1987)

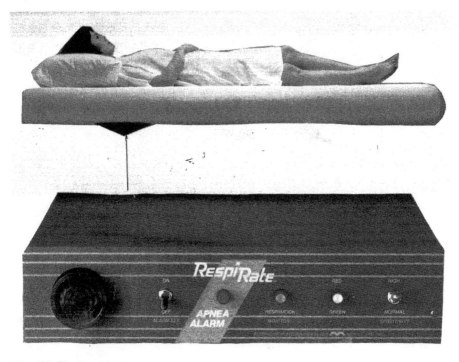

Fig. 121. The Respi-Rate.

508

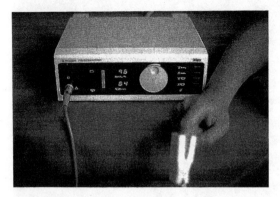

Fig. 122. Pulse Oximeter Nellcor N-100.

Bibliography and references

510

Aantaa R, A Kallio, J Kanto, H Scheinin, M Scheinin. Dexmedetomidine reduces thiopental anesthetic requirements in man. Anesthesiology (Suppl), 1989, 71, 253.

Abboud TK, J Raya, R Noueihed, J Daniel. Intrathecal morphine for relief of labor pain in a parturient with severe pulmonary hypertension. Anesthesiology, 1983, 59, 477.

Abboud TK, SM Shnider, PA Dailey, JA Raya, F Sarkis, NM Grobler, S Sadri, SS Khoo, B De Sousa, CL Baysinger, F Miller. Intrathecal administration of hyperbaric morphine for the relief of pain in labour. Brit J Anaesth, 1984, 56, 1351. (a)

Abboud TK, U Goebelsmann, J Raya, DI Hoffman. Effect of intrathecal morphine during labor on maternal plasma beta-endorphin levels. Amer J Obstet Gynecol, 1984, 149, 709. (b)

Abboud TK, M Moore, J Zhu, K Murakawa, M Minehart, M Longhitano, J Terrasi, ID Klepper, Y Choi, S Kimbal. Epidural butorphanol for the relief of postoperative pain after cesarean section. Anesthesiology, 1986, 65, A397.

Abboud TK, M Moore, J Zhu, K Murakawa, M Minehart, M Longhitano, J Terrasi, ID Klepper, Y Choi, S Kimball, G Chu. Epidural butorphanol or morphine for the relief of post-cesarean section pain: ventilatory responses to carbon dioxide. Anesth Analg, 1987, 66, 887.

Abboud TK. Mini-dose intrathecal morphine for analgesia following cesarean section. Anesthesiology, 1988, 69, 805.

Abboud TK, A Dror, P Mosaad, J Zhu, M Mantilla, F Swart, J Gangolly, P Silao, A Makar, J Moore, H Davis, J Lee. Mini-dose intrathecal morphine for the relief of post-cesarean section pain: safety, efficacy, and ventilatory responses to carbon dioxide. Anesth Analg, 1988, 67, 137.

Abboud TK, A Reyes, M Richardson, A Afrasiabi, L D'Onofrio, M Kalra, J Zhu et al. Epidural morphine or butorphanol augments bupivacaine analgesia during labor. Regional Anesthesia, 1989, 14, 115.

Abboud TK, K Lee, M Chai, J Zhu, A Afrasiabi, M Mantilla, Z Steffens, S Edwards, M Dhillon. Prophylactic oral naltrexone with intrathecal morphine for cesarean section: effects on adverse reactions and analgesia. Anesthesiology (Suppl), 1989, 71, 836.

Abdul-Rasool IH, J Hsieh, DS Ward, B Bloor. The respiratory effects of the alpha-2 agonist, dexmedetomidine in unanesthetized dogs. Anesthesiology (Suppl), 1989, 71, 1092.

Abou Hatem R, P Hendrickx, C Nicaise, M Titeca, I Elfunas. A new totally implantable device for epidural drug delivery. In: W Erdmann, T Oyama, MJ Pernak (Eds.): Pain Clinic I, VNU Science Press, Utrecht, 1985, 293.

Abouleish E, MA Barmada, EM Nemoto, A Tung, P Winter. Acute and chronic effects of intrathecal morphine in monkeys. Brit J Anaesth, 1981, 53, 1027.

Abouleish E, N Rawal, K Fallon, D Hernandez. Combined intrathecal morphine and bupivacaine for cesarean section. Anesthesiology, 1987, 67, A619.

Abouleish E. Apnoea associated with the intrathecal administration of morphine in obstetrics. Brit J Anaesth, 1988, 60, 592. (a)

Abouleish E, N Rawal, K Fallon, D Hernandez. Combined intrathecal morphine and bupivacaine for cesarean section. Anesth Analg, 1988, 67, 370. (b)

Abouleish EI, ES Hanley, SM Palmer. Can epidural fentanyl control autonomic hyperreflexia in a quadriplegic parturient? Anesth Analg, 1989, 68, 523.

Acalovschi I, V Ene, E Lörinczi, F Nicolaus. Saddle block with pethidine for perineal operations. Brit J Anaesth, 1986, 58, 1012. (a)

Acalovschi I, N Secas, F Nicolaus, M Fleseru. Pethidine versus xylocaine as sole intrathecal anaesthetic. VII Eur Congress of Anaesth, 1986, Vienna (Austria), Report, Abstract Nr 648. (b)

Acalovschi I. Herpes simplex after spinal pethidine. Anaesthesia, 1986, 41, 1271. (c)

Ackerman E, J Chrubàsik, M Weinstock, E Wünsch. Effect of intrathecal somatostatin on pain threshold in rats. Schmerz-Pain-Douleur, 1985, 6, 41.

Ackermann WE, MM Juneja. Should epidural fentanyl be given for labor and delivery in a patient with severe pulmonary hypertension. Anaesthesiology, 1988, 69, 284.

Ackerman WE, MM Juneja, GW Colclough, DM Kaczorowski. Epidural fentanyl significantly decreases nausea and vomiting during uterine manipulation in awake patients undergoing cesarean section. Anaesthesiology, 1988, 69 (Suppl), A 679.

Ackerman WE, MM Juneja, DM Kaczorowski, GW Colclough. A comparison of the incidence of pruritus following epidural opioid administration in post cesarean section patients. Regional Anesthesia, 1989, 14 (Suppl), 14.

Ackerman WE, MM Juneja, GW Colclough, DM Kaczorowski. Epidural lipophilic opioids significantly decrease nausea and emesis during uterine manipulation in awake patients undergoing cesarean section. Regional Anesthesia, 1989, 14 (Suppl), 23.

Ackerman WE, MM Juneja, GW Colclough, JM Guiler, DS Guiler. A comparison of epidural fentanyl, buprenorphine and butorphanol for the management of post-cesarean section pain. Anaesthesiology Review, 1989, 16, 37.

Ackerman WE, MM Juneja, DM Kaczorowski, GW Colclough. A comparison of the incidence of pruritus following epidural opioid administration in the parturient. Can J Anaesth, 1989, 36, 388.

Adriaensen H. Personal communication, 1988.

Adu-Gyamfi Y, H Farag, M Naguib. Anaesthesia with continuous thiopentone infusion, epidural morphine and relaxant. J Int Med Res, 1983, 11, 222.

Advokat C. Evidence of place conditioning after chronic intrathecal morphine in rats. Pharmacol Biochem Behav, 1985, 22, 271.

Ahlgren FI, MB Ahlgren. Epidural administration of opiates by a new device. Pain, 1987, 31, 353.

Ahmad S, D Hawes, S Dooley, E Faure, EA Brunner. Intrathecal morphine in a parturient with a single ventricle. Anaesthesiology, 1981, 54, 515.

Ahn NN, D Karambelkar, G Cannelli, TE Rudy. Epidural alfentanil and bupivacaine for analgesia during labor. Anaesthesiology (Suppl), 1989, 71, 845.

Ahuja B. Analgesic effects of intrathecal ketamine in rats. Brit J Anaesth, 1983, 55, 991.

Ahuja B, L Strunin. Ventilatory effects of epidural fentanyl. Can Anaesth Soc J, 1985, 32, S77. (a)

Ahuja BR, L Strunin. Respiratory effects of epidural fentanyl. Changes in end-trial CO2 and respiratory rate following single doses and continuous infusions of epidural fentanyl. Anaesthesia, 1985, 40, 949. (b)

Åkerman B, E Arweström, C Post. Local anesthetics potentiate spinal morphine antinociception. Anaesth Analg, 1988, 67, 943.

Akil H, DJ Mayer, JC Liebeskind. Antagonism of stimulation-produced analgesia by naloxone, a narcotic antagonist. Science, 1976, 191, 961.

Albright G. Epidural morphine, hydromorphone and meperidine for post cesarean - section pain relief, utilizing a respiratory apnea monitor. Anaesthesiology, 1983, 59, A416.

Alexander J, AMS Black. Comparing extradural and i.v. diamorphine and buprenorphine after abdominal surgery. Brit J Anaesth, 1984, 56, 1283P.

Ali MNK, P Conard, M Peterson. A new England survey on the use of epidural opioids for postoperative pain. Anaesthesiology (Suppl), 1989, 71, 705.

Ali NMK. Hyperalgic response in a patient receiving high concentrations of spinal morphine. Anaesthesiology, 1986, 65, 449.

Ali NMK, N Hanna, JS Hoffman. Percutaneous epidural catheterization for intractable pain in terminal cancer patients. Gynecologic oncology, 1989, 32, 22.

Allen PD, A T Walman, DJ Cullen, M Shesky, K Patterson, B Covino. The effects of epidural morphine on post operative analgesia. Anaesthesiology, 1982, 57, A199

Allen PD, T Walman, M Concepcion, M Sheskey, MK Patterson, D Cullen, BG Covino. Epidural

512

morphine provides postoperative pain relief in peripheral vascular and orthopedic surgical patients. Anesth Analg, 1986, 65, 165.

Allinson RR, PE Stach. Intrathecal drug therapy. Drug Intel Clin Pharm, 1978, 12, 347.

Alper MH. Intrathecal morphine: A new method of obstetric analgesia? Anesthesiology, 1979, 51, 378.

Amaki Y, O Nagano, C Sugimoto, K Kobayashi. Trial of double lumen epidural catheter for clinical anesthesia. Anesthesiology, 1982, 57, A181.

Amiot JF, JH Palacci, C Vedrenne, M Pellegrin. Toxicité médullaire de l'acéthyl salycylate de lysine et du chlorhydrate de kétamine administrés par voie intrathécale chez le rat. Ann Fr Anesth Réanim, 1986, 5, 462.

Andelman RJ. Implementing a full-service epidural narcotics programm in a 100-bed community hospital. Regional Anesthesia, 1987, 12, 108.

Andersen HB, A Engquist, BC Jørgensen. Pharmacokinetics of buprenorphine after epidural application. In: Nordic Symposium on Temgesic Meda, Copenhagen, 1981, 84.

Andersen HB, BC Jørgensen, A Engquist. Epidural met-enkephalin (FK 33-824). A dose-effect study. Acta Anaesth Scand, 1982, 26, 69. (a)

Andersen HB, O Benveniste, L Bitsch-Larsen, P Carl, M Crawford, M Djernes, J Eriksen, AM Grell, H Henriksen, E Jansen, H Kaalund- Jørgensen, L Laugesen, C Lønholdt, P Neumann, JE Pedersen, J Wolff. Langtidsbehandling med epidurale opiater. Ugeskr Laeger, 1982, 144, 2633. (b)

Andersen HB. Opiate kinetics after epidural and spinal application. In: JJ Bonica et al. (Eds.): Advances in Pain Research and Therapy, Raven Press, New York, 1983, 477.

Andersen HB, J Eriksen. Paintreatment on long term basis, using extradural opiates. World Congress on Pain, Seattle, 1984.

Andersen HB, J Eriksen, J Kjaergård. Totally implanted access port for epidural injections. Lancet, 1985, 1, 511.

Andersen HB. Mode of action and long term use of spinal opioids II Int Symposium: The Pain Clinic, 1986, Lille (France). (a)

Andersen HB. Experiences in long term treatment with epidural opiates and future trends. In: A Weindl, DW Coombs (Eds.): Proceedings, Int Symposium "Spinal Analgesia": A new approach of cancer pain, Spinger Verlag, 1986. (b)

Andersen HB, J Kjaergård, J Eriksen. Subcutaneously implanted injection system for epidural administration. Acta Anaesth Scand, 1986, 30, 473. (c)

Andersen HB, F Højelse, H Nielsen. Kinetics of ketobemidone in cerebrospinal fluid and plasma after epidural administration. Pain, 1987, S4, S189, 5th World Congress Pain, Hamburg.

Andersen PT. Alopecia areata after epidural morphine. Anesth Analg, 1984, 63, 1142.

Anderson I, WR Thompson, GP Varkey, RL Knill. Lumbar epidural morphine as an effective analgesic following cholecystectomy. Can Anaesth Soc J, 1981, 28, 523.

Anderson P, S Arnér, U Bondesson, L Boréus, P Hartvig. Pharmacokinetics of ketobemidone. In: KM Foley, CE Inturrisi (Eds.): Pain Research and Therapy, Raven Press, New York, 1986, VOL. 8, 171.

Andrews WR, S Stigi, V Jendrek, K Shevde. Intrathecal morphine in cardiac surgical procedures. Can J Anaesth, 1989, 36, S63.

Andrieu G, A Harari, P Viars, K Samii, P Curet, F Richard. Analgésie morphinique péridurale après embolisation artérielle viscérale. La Nouvelle Presse Médicale, 1981, 10, 431.

Andrivet P, JM Ekherian, A Lienhart, R Viars. Bloc moteur induit par la péthidine intrarachidienne. Quantification et comparaison avec la lidocaine. Ann Fr Anesth Réanim, 1987, 6, 419.

Ansuategui M, et al. Cuadro de meningitis en un paciente tratado con morfina epidural (Meningitis nach epiduraler Morphingabe). Rev Esp Anest Reanim, 1983, 30, 60.

Aoki M, LM Kitahata, M Senami, JG Collins. Sufentanil: a drug of choice for spinal opioid analgesia as shown in cats. Anesth Analg, 1985, 64, 190.

Aoki M, M Senami, LM Kitahata, JG Collins. Spinal sufentanil effects on spinal pain-transmission neurons in cats. Anesthesiology, 1986, 64, 225.

Arcario T, J Vartikar, MD Johnson, MJ Lema, S Datta, GW Ostheimer, JS Naulty. Effect of diluent volume on analgesia produced by epidural fentanyl. Anesthesiology, 1987, 67, A441.

Arias LM, RJ Schwartz, R Bartkowski, CM Tom, KL Grossman. Sufentanil stellate ganglion injection in the treatment of refractory reflex sympathetic dystrophy. Regional Anesthesia, 1989, 14, 90.

Arnér S, B Arnér. Differential effects of epidural morphine in the treatment of cancer related-pain. Acta Anaesth Scand, 1985, 29, 32.

Arnér S, N Rawal, LL Gustafsson. Clinical experience of long-term treatment with epidural and intrathecal opioids - a nationwide survey. Acta Anaesth Scand, 1988, 32, 253.

Arroyo JL, L Ponz, F Carrascosa, RP Reiner, L Lecron, MA Nalda. Effects of extradural analgesia with etidocaine and opioids on endocrine function. Brit J Anaesth, 1982, 54, 240P.

Arroyo JL, RP Reiner, JM Rodriguez, C Roux, F Carrascosa, J De Castro. Stimulation de la libération de prostacycline sous anesthésie analgésique. Ann Fr Anesth Réanim, 1983, 2, 133.

Asari H, K Inoue, T Shibata, T Soga. Segmental effect of morphine injected into the epidural space in man. Anesthesiology, 1981, 54, 75.

Atanossoff P, E Alon. Accidental epidural injection of a large dose of morphine. Anaesthesia, 1988, 43, 1056.

Atchison SR, TL Yaksh, P Durant. Cardiovascular and respiratory effects of intrathecal DADL in awake dogs. Anesthesiology, 1984, 61, A219.

Atchison SR, P Durant, TL Yaksh. Cardiorespiratory effects and kinetics of intrathecally injected D-Ala-D-Leu-Enkephalin and morphine in unanesthetized dogs. Anesthesiology, 1986, 65, 609.

Attia J, P Sandouk, C Ecoffey, K Samii. Pharmacokinetics following epidural morphine in children. Anesthesiology, 1985, 63, A469.

Attia J, C Ecoffey, P Sandouk, J Gross, Samii K. Epidural morphine in children: pharmacokinetics and CO_2 sensitivity. Anesthesiology, 1986, 65, 590.

Attig G, G Cierpka, R Lober. Intrathekale Morphinapplikation zur Schmerztherapie nach ausgedehnten gynaekologischen Operationen. ZBL Gynakol, 1985, 107, 738.

Atweh SF, LC Murrin, MJ Kuhar. Presynaptic localization of opiate receptors in the vagal and accessory optic systems: an autoradiographic study. Neuropharmacology, 1978, 17, 65.

Atweh SF, MJ Kuhar. Autoradiographic localization of opiate receptors in rat brain. Brain Res, 1977, 124, 53-67 (I);129, 1-12 (II);134, 393-405 (III)

Auld AW, A Maki-Jokela, DM Murdoch. Intraspinal narcotic analgesia in the treatment of chronic pain. Spine, 1985, 10, 777.

Aun C, D Thomas, LSt John-Jones, MP Colvin, TM Savege, CT Lewis. Intrathecal morphine in cardiac surgery. Eur J Anaesth, 1985, 2, 419.

Auroy P, P Schoeffler, C Maillot, JP Haberer, A Woda. Tolérance intrathécale midazolam. Etude histologique. Ann Fr Anesth Réanim, 1988, 7, 81.

Ausems ME, CC Hug, DR Stanski, AGL Burm. Plasma concentrations of alfentanil required to supplement nitrous oxide anesthesia for general surgery. Anesthesiology, 1986, 65, 362.

Ausman RK, G Caballero. Epidural morphine by continuous infusion in the management of pain in oncology patients. ICRCT 85, Giessen, (W Germany) 1985, August 26-28, Congress report.

Babcock NK, WW Foreward. In: LH Maxson (Ed.): Spinal Anesthesia, Philadelphia, JB Lippincott, 1938.

Babcock NK, P Nance, JW Chapin. Respiratory arrest after intrathecal morphine (letter). JAMA, 1981, 245, 1528.

Bach V, P Carl, O Ravlo, ME Crawford, L Kruse. Extradural droperidol potentiates extradural opioids (letter). Brit J Anaesth, 1985, 57, 238.

Bach V, P Carl, O Ravlo, ME Crawford, M Werner. Potentiation of epidural opioids with epidural droperidol. Anaesthesia, 1986, 41, 1116.

Badaev FI, AA Popov, AL Levit, et al. Postoperative peridural analgesia with morphine, fentanyl and dipidolor. Vestnik Khirurgii Imeni I.I. Grekova, 1984, 132, 104.

Badner NH, AN Sandler, L Leitch, G Koren. Analgesic and respiratory effects of continuous lumbar epidural in post-thoractomy patients. Can J Anaesth, 1989, 36, S69.

Badner NH, AN Sandler, ME Colmenares. Lumbar epidural fentanyl infusions for post-thoracotomy patients. Anesthesiology (Suppl), 1989, 71, 667.

Bagley WP, LJ Rice, LM Broadman. Does pH change contribute to combined epidural narcotic-local anesthetic synergism? Anesthesiology, 1987, 67, A278.

Bahar M, IA Orr, JW Dundee. Central action of spinal opiates. Anesthesiology, 1981, 55, 334. (a)

Bahar M, IA Orr, JW Dundee. Shrinking pupils as a warning of respiratory depression after spinal morphine. Lancet, 1981, I, 893. (b)

Bahar M, M Rosen, MD Vickers. Chronic cannulation of the intradural or extradural space in the rat. Brit J Anaesth, 1984, 56, 405.

Bailey CJ, B Gulczynski, D Racky, K Vehrs. Epidural morphine infusion. Continuous pain relief. AORN J, 1984, 39, 997.

Bailey PW, BE Smith. Continuous epidural infusion of fentanyl for postoperative analgesia. Anaesthesia, 1980, 35, 1002.

Baker BW, S Longmire, MM Jones, J Gallen, QT Palacios, et al. The epidural test dose in obstetrics reconsidered. Anesthesiology, 1987, 67, A625.

Balaban M, P Slinger. Severe hypotension from epidural meperidine in a high-risk patient after thoracotomy. Can J Anaesth, 1989, 36, 450.

Ballantyne JC, AB Loach, DB Carr. Itching after epidural and spinal opiates. Pain, 1988, 33, 149.

Ballantyne JC, AB Loach, DB Carr. The incidence of pruritus after epidural morphine. Anaesthesia, 1989, 44, 863.

Banerjee T, D Koons. Chronic epidural analgesia as a method of relieving chronic intractable pain. Pain (Suppl.), 1981, 1, S124.

Banning AM, JF Schmidt, B Chraemmer-Jørgensen, A Risbo. Comparison of oral controlled release morphine and epidural morphine in the management of postoperative pain. Anesth Analg, 1986, 65, 385.

Bapat AR, NA Kshirsagar, RD Bapat. Aspect of epidural morphine. Lancet, 1979, 2, 584.

Bapat AR, NA Kshirsagar, RD Bapat. Extradural pethidine (letter). Brit J Anaesth, 1980, 52, 637. (a)

Bapat AR, NA Kshirsagar, RD Bapat. Epidural morphine in the treatment of chronic pain. J Postgrad Med, 1980, 26, 242. (b)

Bapat AR, NA Kshirsagar, RB Padmashree, KC Bhagtand, RD Bapat, GB Parulkar. Improvement in peripheral perfusion in peripheral vascular disease cases with epidural morphine. J Postgrad Med, 1980, 26, 246. (c)

Baraka A, R Noueihid, S Hajj. Intrathecal injection of morphine for obstetric analgesia. Anesthesiology, 1981, 54, 136.

Baraka A, M Maktabi, R Noueihid. Epidural meperidine-bupivacaine for obstetric analgesia. Anesth Analg, 1982, 61, 652. (a)

Baraka A. Rostral spread of intrathecal morphine in man. Middle East J Anaesth, 1982, 6, 178. (b)

Baraka A. Epidural meperidine for control of autonomic hyperreflexia in paraplegic parturient. Anesthesiology, 1985, 62, 688.

Bardon T, M Ruckebusch. Changes in 5-Hiaa and 5-HT levels in lumbar CSF following morphine administration to conscious dogs. Neuroci Lett, 1984, 49, 147.

Bardon T, M Ruckebusch.Comparative effects of opiate agonists on proximal and distal colonic motility in dogs. Eur J Pharmacol, 1985, 110, 329.

Barlogie B, L Smith, R Alexanian. Effective treatment of advanced multiple myeloma refractory to alkylating agents. New Engl J of Med, 1984, 310, 1353.

Barré J, G Pfister, C Lelarge, D Debant, J Rendoing. L'analgésie péridurale par étidocaine et fentanyl. Résultats de 635 anesthésies pour prothèses totales de hanches. In: Ars Medici, Bruxelles, Congress Series, 3, II, 1983, 393.

Barré J, D Debant, M Vinsonneau, M Payen, J Rendoing. Essais de prévention des anomalies de distribution. A propos de 1000 anesthésies péridurales pour prothèse de la hanche. Forum Club, AFAR, 9, 1984, Paris.

Barrier G, C Sureau. Effects of anaesthetic and analgesic drugs in labour, fetus and neonate. Clin Obstet Gynaecol, 1982, 9, 351.

Barron DW, Strong JE. Postoperative analgesia in major orthopaedic surgery. Epidural and intrathecal opiates. Anaesthesia, 1981, 36, 937.

Barron DW. Evaluation of antiemetics in association with intrathecal diamorphine. Ann R Coll Surg Engl, 1984, 66, 359. (a)

Barron DW, Strong JE. The safety and efficacy of intrathecal diamorphine. Pain, 1984, 18, 279. (b)

Barron DW, DP O'Toole. Postoperative analgesia following total hip replacement - a comparison between intrathecal diamorphine and methadone. VII Eur Congress of Anaesth, 1986, Vienna (Austria), Report, Abstract 422.

Barros D'Sa AAJ, S Bloom, JH Baron. Direct inhibition of gastric acid by growth hormone releasing hormone in dogs. Lancet, 1975, 1, 886.

Barrow MEH. Postoperative pain control with intrathecal morphine (letter). Anaesthesia, 1981, 36, 825.

Basbaum AI. Cystochemistry of the neural substrate for the processing of noxious information. Symposium on Pain Control, Leuven (Belgium), 1986.

Baskoff JD, RL Watson, SM Muldoon. Respiratory arrest after intrathecal morphine. Anesthesiology Review, 1980, 7, 12.

Bates RFL, GA Buckley, CA McArdle. Comparison of the nociceptive effects of centrally administered calcitonins and calcitonin gene- related peptide. Brit J Pharm, 1983, 80, 518P.

Batier C, P Blanchet, J Benezech, B Roquefeuil. Intéret et problèmes posés par l'administration intraventriculaire de morphine. Commentaires à propos de douze cas. Ann Fr Anesth Réanim, 1983, 2, 233.

Batier C, P Blanchet, J Benezech, B Roquefeuil. Comparaison de l'analgésie morphinique par injections péridurales sous arachnoidiennes et intracérébrales ventriculaires. Cahiers d'Anesth 1985, 33, 43.

Batier C. Point de vue sur la morphinothérapie par voie péridurale dans le douleur cancéreuse. Euromédecine 1986, Montpellier (France) Report, Editel Paris.

Bause H, M Blendl, W Pothmann. Kontinuierliche peridurale Langzeit-Morphinanalgesie bei einem ambulanten Karzinom-Patienten. Regional Anaesthesie, 1984, 33, 86.

Bause H. Erwiderung auf die vorstehenden Bemerkungen von J Chrubasik et al. Regional Anaesthesie, 1985, 8, 41.

Baxter AD, G Kiruluta. Detrusor tone after epidural morphine (letter). Anesth Analg, 1984, 63, 464.

Baxter AD, B Samson, R Doran. Prevention of epidural morphine-induced respiratory depression with intravenous nalbuphine infusion in post-thoracotomy patients. Can J Anaesth, 1989, 36, 503.

Baxter AD, B Samson, S Laganiere, K Hull. Is nalbuphine an effective epidural analgesic? Anesthesiology (Suppl), 1989, 71, 701.

Bayer-Berger MM, S Arnér. Morphine péridurale dans les douleurs cancéreuses rebelles. Moyens

516

et obstacles. Ann Fr Anesth Réanim, 1985, 4, 343.

Bazin JE, V Dissait, CM Monteillard, G Le Bouedéc, JF Trolese, PF Schoeffler. Variations in uterine activity related to epidural fentanyl during labour. Anesthesiology (Suppl), 1989, 71, 849.

Beaumont I, T Deeks. Determination of morphine, diamorphine and their degradation products in pharmaceutical preparation by reversed-phase high-performance liquid chromatography. J Chromatogr, 1982, 238, 520.

Beck H, F Brassow, M Doehn, H Bause, A Dziadzka, J Schulte Am Esch. Epidural catheters of the multi-orifice type: dangers and complications. Acta Anaesth Scand, 1986, 30, 549.

Beeby D, KC McIntosh, M Bailey, DB Welch. Postoperative analgesia for caesarean section using epidural methadone. Anaesthesia, 1984, 39, 61.

Behar M, F Magora, D Olshwang, JT Davidson. Epidural morphine in treatment of pain. Lancet, 1979, 1, 527.

Belcher G, T Smock, HL Fields. Effects of intrathecal ACTH on opiate analgesia in the rat. Brain Res, 1982, 247, 373.

Bell SD, A Levette, GE Larijani. The use of continuous lumbar epidural fentanyl for postoperative pain relief in abdominal aortic aneurysms. Anesthesiology, 1987, 67, A234.

Bell SD. The use of continuois lumbar epidural sufentanil for post operative pain relief in thoracotomies. Regional Anesthesia, 1989, 14 (Suppl), 33.

Bellamy CD, FJ McDonnell, GW Colclough. Postoperative epidural pain management results in shorter hospital stay than iv PCA morphine: a comparison in anterior cruciate ligament repair. Anesthesiology (Suppl), 1989, 71, 686.

Bellanca L, MT Latteri, S Latteri, L Montalbano, C Papa, A Sansone. Plasma and CSF morphine concentrations after i.m. and epidural administration. Pharm Res Comm, 1985, 17, 189.

Bellet M, JL Elghozi, P Meyer, MG Pernollet, H Schmitt. Central cardiovascular effects of narcotic analgesics and enkephalins in rats. Brit J Pharm, 1980, 71, 365.

Benahmed M, P Carde, A Laplanche, J Renaux, J Rouesse, M Spielmann, H Sancho-Garnier. Chimiothérapie en perfusion continue ambulatoire par pompe portable: essai de fiabilité. Bull Cancer (Paris), 1985, 72, 30.

Benedetti C. Intraspinal analgesia: an historical overview. Acta Anaesth Scand, 1987, 31, 17.

Bengtsson M, JB Löftröm, H Merits. Postoperative pain relief with intrathecal morphine after major hip surgery. Regional Anesthesia, 1983, 8, 139.

Bengtsson M, A Bengtsson, L Jorfeldt. Diagnostic epidural opioid blockade in primary fibromyalgia at rest and during exercise. Pain, 1989, 39,171.

Benhamou D, K Samii, Y Noviant. Effect of analgesia on respiratory muscle function after upper abdominal surgery. Acta Anaesth Scand, 1983, 27, 22.

Benlabed M, C Ecoffey, JC Levron, B Flaisler, J Gross. Analgesia and ventilatory response to CO_2 following epdiural sufentanil in children. Anesthesiology, 1987, 67, 948.

Bennett MRD, AP Adams. Postoperative respiratory complications of opiates. Clinics in Anaesthesiology, 1983, 1, 41.

Bentley JB, JH Finley, LR Humphry. Obesity and alfentanil pharmacokinetics. Anesth Analg, 1983, 62, 251.

Berde CB, N Fischel, JP Filardi, CS Coe, HE Grier, SC Bernstein. Caudal epidural morphine analgesia for an infant with advanced neuroblastoma: report of a case. Pain, 1989, 36, 219.

Berg-Seiter S, B Koßmann, W Dick, W Lorenz. Untersuchungen zum Verhalten der Plasmahistaminspiegel nach periduraler Morphinapplikation. Anaesthesist, 1985, 34, 388.

Berkowitz BA, SH Ngai, JC Yang, J Hempstead, S Spector. The disposition of morphine in surgical patients. Clin Pharm Ther, 1975, 17, 629.

Bernard JM, T Lechevalier, M Pinaud, N Passuti. Postoperative analgesia by iv clonidine. Anesthesiology (Suppl), 1989, 71, 154.

Bernatzky G, I Jurna. Intrathecal injection of codeine, buprenorphine, tilidine, tramadol and nefopam depresses the tail-flick response in rats. Eur J Pharm, 1986, 120, 75.

Bernheim J. Améliorer la qualité de (sur)vie des malades cancéreux. Revue Médicale de Liège, 1er Février 1984, 39, 3.

Bernstein J, S Ramanathan, K Ramabadran, H Turndorf. Body temperature changes with epidural and intrathekal morphine. Anesthesiology, 1988, 69 (3A), A688.

Berre J. Relief of pain in intensive care patients. Ressucitation, 1984, 11, 157.

Besson JM, D Le Bars, D Memetrey, C Conseiller. Action de la morphine et des morphinomimétiques sur la transmission du flux nociceptif au niveau spinal. In: Utilisation des Morphinomimétiques en Anesthésie et Réanimation Arnette, Paris, 1974, 125.

Besson JM, D Le Bars, JL Oliveras. L'analgésie morphinique: données neurobiologiques. Ann Anesth Fr, 1978, 19, 343.

Besson JM, MC Wyon Maillard, MC Benois, C Conseiller, K Haman. Effects of phenoperidine on lamina V cells in the cat dorsal horn. J Pharm Exp Ther, 1983, 187, 239.

Besson JM, Y Lazorthes. Spinal opioids and the relief of pain. Symposium Toulouse (France) 1984, Editions INSERM, Paris 1985.

Besson JM. What the brain tells to the spinal cord? Electrophysiological and behavioural approaches. Acta Anaesth Belgica, 1988, 39, 87.

Bibbings J. Epidural analgesia. Nurs Times, 1984, 80, 53.

Biehl DR. Obstetrical anaesthesia update - 1984. Can Anaesth Soc J, 1984, 31, S23.

Bigler D, W Dirkes, R Hansen, J Rosenberg, H Kehlet. Effects of thoracic paravertebral block with bupivacaine versus combined thoracic epidural block with bupivacaine and morphine on pain and pulmonary function after cholecystectomy. Acta Anaesthesiol Scand, 1989, 33, 561.

Bilsback P, G Rolly, O Tampubolon. A double-blind epidural administration of lofentanil, buprenorphine or saline for postoperative pain. 6th Eur Congress of Anaesth, London, 1982. Volume of summaries, p 49.

Bilsback P, G Rolly. A double-blind epidural administration of lofentanil, buprenorphine or saline for postoperative pain. Acta Anaesth Belgica, 1983, 34, 88.

Bilsback P, G Rolly, O Tampubolon. Efficacy of the extradural administration of lofentanil, buprenorphine or saline in the management of postoperative pain. Brit J Anaesth, 1985, 57, 943.

Binsted RJ. Epidural morphine after caesarean section. Anaesth Intens Care, 1983, 11, 130.

Birkhan HJ, B Rosenberg, K Simon, B Moskowitz. Epidural appliziertes Morphium (epidural administration of morphine). Munchen Med Wochenschr, 1982, 124, 634.

Birks RJS, DRG Marsh. Epidural meptazinol. Anaesthesia, 1986, 41, 883.

Blacklock JB, GL Rea, RE Maxwell. Intrathecal morphine during lumbar spine operation for postoperative pain control. Neurosurgery, 1986, 18, 341.

Blackshear P. Implantable drug delivery systems. Scientific American, 1979, 241, 66.

Blaise G, M Jaminet. Postoperative analgesia by epidural injection with morphine. Acta Anaesth Belgica, 1981, 32, 161.

Blaise G, JC McMichan, M Nugent, LH Hollier. Nalbuphine produces side-effects while reversing narcotic-induced respiratory depression. Anesth Analg, 1986, 65, S19.

Blanchard J, EJ Menk, S Ramamurthy, J Hoffman. Subarachnoid & epidural calcitonin for the management of cancer pain. Anesth Analg, 1988, 67, S2, S17.

Blanco J, E Blanco, JM Carceller, A Sarabia, G Solares. Epidural analgesia for post-caesarean pain relief: a comparison between morphine and fentanyl. European J Anaesthesiology, 1987, 4, 365.

Blancquaert JP, RA Lefebvre, JL Willems. Gastric relaxation by intravenous and intracerebroventricular administration of apomorphine, morphine and fentanyl in the conscious dog. Arch Int Pharmacodyn, 1982, 256, 153.

Blanloeil Y, A Levrel, P Michel, D Moreau, A Larichi, A Vairon, M Bourveau. Analgesie post-

518

operative apres oesophagectomie avec thoracotomie: morphine iv continue vs peridurale thoracique au fentanyl + adrenaline. Ann Fr Anesth Réanim, 1987, 6, R26.

Bläss J, H Gerber, K Spelina. Untersuchung über epidurales Morphin. Anaesthesist, 1982, 31, 340.

Blass NH, RB Roberts, K John, K Wiley. The case of errant epidural catheter. Anesthesiology, 1981, 54, 419.

Bledsoe SW, LB Ready. Fentanyl and alfentanil versus morphine for epidural analgesia. Anesthesiology, 1988, 69, 1024.

Blond S, J Meynadier, Th Dupard, M Dubar, M Combelles-Pruvot, JL Christiaens, A Demaille. La neurochirurgie chimique dans le traitement des douleurs cancéreuses: la morphinothérapie intrathécale et la morphinothérapie intra-cérébro-ventriculaire. LARC Medical, 1985, V, 7, 361. (a)

Blond S, J Meynadier, J Chrubasik, Th Dupard, M Dubar, M Combelles-Pruvot, JL Christiaens, A Demaille. Intrathekale und intraventrikuläre Morphin-Analgesie bei Karzinompatienten: Langzeit-Erfahrungen. Schmerz-Pain-Douleur, 1985, 4, 129. (b)

Blond S, M Combelles-Pruvot, J Meynadier. La morphinothérapie intra-cérébro-ventriculaire dans les algies cancéreuses. NPN Médecine, 1985, V, 81, 43. (c)

Blond S, M Dubar, J Meynadier, M Combelle-Pruvot, P Vitrac. Cerebral intraventricular administration of morphine in cancer patients with intractable pain. In: W Erdmann, T Oyama, MJ Pernak (Eds.): Pain Clinic I, VNU Science press, Utrecht, 1985, 77. (e)

Blond S, J Meynadier, M Combelles-Provot, L Vilette, T Dupard, JL Christiaens. Indications et résultats de la morphinothérapie intra-cérébroventriculaire dans les algies cancéreuses: à propos de 55 patients. II Int Symposium: Pain Clinic, 1986, Lille (France).

Blond S, J Meynadier, D Brichard, JD Guieu, JC Willer, D Le Bars. Intra-cerebro-ventricular morphinotherapy (ICVM) (n=79) and study of the supraspinal action of morphine. Pain, 1987, S4, S391.

Blond S, J Meynadier, T Dupard, R Assaker, C Brichard, JL Christiaens, A Demaille. La morphinothérapie intracérébro-ventriculaire: à propos de 79 patients. Neurochirurgie, 1989, 35, 52.

Bloom FE. Neurohumoral transmission of the central nervous system. In: Goodman and Gilmans's (Eds.). The pharmacological basis of therapeutics. MacMillan Publ Co Inc, New York 7th, 1985, 236.

Bloor BC, D Raybould, M Shurtliff, J Gellmann, SW Stead. MPV-1440, an alpha-2 adrengergic agonist with potent anesthetic qualities. Anesthesiology (Suppl), 1988, 69, 614.

Boas RA. Hazards of epidural morphine (letter). Anaesth Intens Care, 1980, 8, 377.

Boas RA, VS Cahill. Epidural buprenorphine compared to other analgesic methods for postoperative pain relief. 4th Int Symposium Düsseldorf (W Germany), june 1983, 22.1.

Boas RA, JW Villiger. Clinical actions of fentanyl and buprenorphine. The significance of receptor binding. Brit J Anaesth, 1985, 57, 192.

Boas RA, JW Villiger. Epidural opioids in postoperative pain treatment. In: HJ Wüst, M Stanton-Hicks (Eds.): Anaesthesiologie und Intensivmedizin, New aspects in regional anesthesia 4. Springer Verlag, Berlin, Heidelberg, New York, 1986, 176, 114.

Bochenek KJ, SN Iovan, EM Brown. Continuous infusion epidural 0.125% bupivacaine/fentanyl and the second stage of labor. Anesth Analg, 1987, 66, S15.

Bodnar RJ, A Kirchgessner, G Nilaver, J Mulhern, EA Zimmerman. Intraventricular capsaicin: alterations in analgesic responsivity without depletion of substance P. Neuroscience, 1982, 7, 631.

Bodnar RJ, DA Simone, JH Kordower, AL Kirchgessner, G Nilaver. Capsaicin treatment and stress-induced analgesia. Pharmacol Biochem Behav, 1983, 18, 65.

Boersma FP. Pain treatment of cancer patients using continuous epidural sufentanil on outpatient basis. Symposium on epidural sufentanil, Brussels, Belgium, 1987.

Boersma FP. Epidural pain treatment in the northern Netherlands. Pain Clinics, 1987, 2, 1.

Boersma FP, AB Buist, J Thie. Epidural pain treatment in the northern Netherlands Organizational and treatment aspects. Acta Anaesth Belgica, 1987, 38, 213.

Boersma FP, H Noorduin, G van den Bussche. Epidural sufentanil for cancer control in outpatients. Annual meeting of the Intern. Society of Regional Anesthesia, Williamsburg, Virginia 1988.

Boersma FP, H Noorduin, G Vanden Bussche. Continuous epidural sufentanil infusion for relief of terminal cancer pain on outpatient basis. Annual Scientific Meeting, 1988.

Boersma FP, H Noorduin, W Pieters, R Woestenborg, J Heykants. Sufentanil concentrations in the spinal cord after long term epidural infusion. Anesthesiology (Suppl), 1989, 71, 706.

Bohannon TW, MD Estes. Evaluation of subarachnoid fentanyl for postoperative analgesia. Anesthesiology, 1987, 67, A237.

Bohus B. Pro-opiocortin fragments and memory function. Symposium: analgesia by peridural and spinal opiates, 1980 Nijmegen (Holland) Congress report, summary 4.

Boico O, F Bonnet, S Rostaing, JF Loriferne, L Quintin, M Ghignone. Epidural clonidine produces postoperative analgesia. Anesthesiology (Suppl), 1988, 69, 388.

Boico O, F Bonnet, S Rostaing, JF Loriferne, P Catoire, K Abhay. Analgesie postoperative induite par la clonidine: comparison de l'administration peridurale et im. Ann Fran Anest Rean, 1989, 8, R205.

Boico O, F Bonnet, PL Darmon, P Catoire, B Rey. Effects of epinephrine and clonidine on pharmacokinetics of spinal bupivacaine. Anesthesiology (Suppl), 1989, 71, 646.

Boldt J, D Kling, G Hempelmann. Hemodynamic and respiratory effects of meptazinol, a new analgetic substance. Acta Anesth Scand, 1987, 31, No 101.

Bonica JJ. Importance of effective pain control. Acta Anaesth Scand (Suppl.), 1987, 31, 1.

Bonnardot JP, M Maillet, JC Colau, F Millot, P Deligne. Maternal and fetal concentrations of morphine after intrathecal administration during labor. Brit J Anaesth, 1982, 54, 487.

Bonnet F, A Harari, M Thibonnier, P Viars. Suppression of antidiuretic hormone hypersecretion during surgery by extradural anaesthesia. Brit J Anaesth, 1982, 54, 29.

Bonnet F, Ch Blery, M Zatan, O Simonet, D Brage, J Gaudy. Effect of epidural morphine on postoperative pulmonary dysfunction. Acta Anaesth Scand, 1984, 28, 147.

Bonnet F, O Boico, S Rostaing, JF Loriferne, L Quintin, M Ghignone. Clonidine for postoperative analgesia: epidural versus im study. Anesthesiology (Suppl), 1988, 69, 395.

Bonnet F, O Boico, S Rostaing, M Saada, JF Loriferne, C Touboul, K Abhay, M Ghignone. Postoperative analgesia with extradural clonidine. Brit J Anaesth, 1989, 63, 465.

Boogaerts J, E Balatoni, N Lafont, L Lecron, J Jacquy, JJ Vanderhaegen. Utilisation des morphiniques dans les blocs nerveux périphériques. In: Ars Medici, Bruxelles, Congress Series 3, I, 1983, 143.

Boogaerts J, L Lecron. Technique et intéret des associations médicamenteuses. In: L Lecron (Ed.): Anésthesie locoregionale, Arnette Paris, 1986, 193.

Booker PD, RG Wilkes, THL Bryson, J Beddard. Clinical experience with epidural morphine.

520

Anaesthesia, 1980, 35, 129. (a)

Booker PD, RG Wilkes, THL Bryson, J Beddard. Obstetric pain relief using epidural morphine. Anaesthesia, 1980, 35, 377. (b)

Bormann von B, B Weidler, R Dennhardt, N Frings, H Lennartz, G Hempelmann. Plasma-ADH-Spiegel als perioperativer Stressparameter (plasma-antidiuretic hormone level as indicator of postoperative stress). Anaesth Intensivther Notfallmed, 1981, 16, 319.

Bormann von B, N Frings, B Weidler, R Dennhardt, G Hempelmann. Postoperative Schmerztherapie durch epidurale Gabe von Fentanyl. Klinikarzt, 1982, 11, 709. (a)

Bormann von B, B Weidler, R Dennhardt, N Frings, G Hempelmann. Plasma-ADH-Spiegel unter kombinierter Neurolept-Analgesie/Peridurale Opiat-Analgesie (variations in vasopressin (ADH) levels during NLA/ epidural opiat analgesia) Regional Anaesthesie, 1982, 5, 7. (b)

Bormann von B, B Weidler, D Kling, G Sturm, HH Scheld, G Hempelmann. Intubationsnarkose (kombinierte Opiatanalgesie) plus modifizierte Periduralanaesthesie und endokrine Stress-Reaktion. Regional Anaesthesie, 1983, 6, 52. (c)

Bormann von B, B Weidler, R Dennhardt, G Hempelmann. Anaesthesieverfahren und postoperative ADH-Sekretion. Anaesthesist, 1983, 32, 177. (a)

Bormann von B, B Weidler, R Dennhardt, G Sturm, HH Scheld, G Hempelmann. Influence of epidural fentanyl on stress-induced elevation of plasma vasopressin (ADH) after surgery. Anesth Analg, 1983, 62, 727. (b)

Börner U, H Müller, M Stoyanov, G Hempelmann. Epidurale Opiatanalgesie. Gewebe und Liquorverträglichkeit der Opiate. Anaesthesist, 1980, 29, 570.

Boskovski N, A Lewinski, J Xuereb, V Mercieca. Caudal epidural morphine for postoperative pain relief (letter). Anaesthesia, 1981, 36, 67.

Boskovski N, A Lewinski. Epidural morphine for the prevention of headhache following dural puncture. Anaesthesia, 1982, 37, 217.

Botney M, HL Fields. Amitriptyline potentiates morphine analgesia by a direct action on the central nervous system. Ann Neurol, 1983, 13, 160.

Boureau F. Ya-t-il une place pour les opiaces dans le douleurs chroniques non-malignes? Schmerz-Pain-Douleur, 1988, 1, 2.

Bourgoin S, D Le Bars, F Artaut, AM Clot, R Boubouton, MC Faurmie-Zaluski, BP Roques, M Hamon, F Cesselin. Effects of ketalorphan and other peptidase inhibitors on the in vitro and in vivo release of methionine-enkephalin - like material from the rat spinal cord. J Pharm Exp Ther, 1986, 238, 360.

Bouvier A, C Lai, Ph Martin, S Francois, JJ Gouedart, P Lunaud, CHG Monod. Etude prospective en double aveugle de l'état neurologique du nouveau-né sous anesthésie épidurale á la bupivacaine seule et á l'association bupivacaine-fentanyl. Rapport foeto-maternel á la naissance. In: Ars Medici, Bruxelles, Congress Series, 3, II, 1983, 383.

Bovill JG, PS Sebel, Cl Blackburn, J Heykants. The pharmacokinetics of alfentanil (R 39209). A new opioid analgesic. Anesthesiology, 1982, 57, 439.

Bovill JG, SP Sebel, TH Stanley. Opioid analgesics in anesthesia, review. Anesthesiology, 1984, 61, 755.

Bowen-Wright RM, T Goroszeniuk. Epidural fentanyl for pain of multiple fractures. Lancet, 1980, 2, 1033.

Bower S. Plasma protein binding of fentanyl. J Pharm Pharmacol, 1981, 33, 507.

Bower S, CJ Hull. Comparative pharmacokinetics of fentanyl and alfentanil. Brit J Anaesth, 1982, 54, 871.

Bray RJ, PA Davies, JA Seviour. The stability of preservative-free morphine in plastic syringes. Anaesthesia, 1986, 41, 294.

Brazenor GA. Long term intrathecal administration of morphine: a comparison of bolus injection via reservoir with continuous infusion by implanted pump. Neurosurgery, 1987, 21, 484.

Brescia FJ. An overview of pain and symptom management in advanced cancer. J of Pain and Symptom Management, 1987, 2, S7.

Breslow MJ, DA Jordan, R Christopherson, B Rosenfeld, CF Miller, DF Haney, C Beattie, RJ Traystman, MC Rogers. Epidural morphine decreases post-operative hypertension by attenuating sympathetic nervous system hyperactivity. Anesthesiology, 1988, 69 (Suppl) A44.

Breslow MJ, DA Jordan, R Christopherson, B Rosenfeld, CF Miller, DF Hanley, C Beattie, RJ Traystman, MC Rogers. Epidural morphine decreases postoperative hypertension by attenuating sympathetic nervous system hyperactivity. J A M A; 1989, 261, 3577.

Bridenbaugh PO, WF Kennedy. Spinal, subarachnoid neural blockade. In: MJ Cousins, PO Bridenbaugh (Eds.): Neuronal blockade. Lippincott, Philadelphia, 1980, 147.

Brizgys RV, SM Shnider. Hyperbaric intrathecal morphine analgesia during labor in patient with Wolff-Parkinson-White syndrome. Obstet Gynecol (Suppl.), 1984, 64, 44S.

Broadman LM, TT Higgings, RS Hannallah, H Desoto, SS Nason. Intraoperative subarachnoid morphine for postoperative pain control following Harrington rod instrumentation in chidren. Can J Anaesth, 1987, 34, S96.

Brock-Utne JG, S Kallichurun, E Mankowitz, RJ Mahary. Intrathecal ketamine with preservative, histological effects on spinal nerve roots of baboons. S Afr Med J, 1982, 440.

Brock-Utne JG, JW Downing, E Mankowitz, J Rubin. Intrathecal ketamine in rats. Brit J Anaesth, 1985, 57, 837.

Brodsky JB, RC Merrell. Epidural administration of morphine postoperatively for morbidly obese patient. West J Med, 1984, 140, 750.

Brodsky JB, MS Shulman, SK Kim. Epidural morphine following abdominoplasty (letter). Plast Reconstr Surg, 1986, 7 125.

Brodsky JB, KM Kretzschmar, JBD Mark. Caudal epidural morphine for post-thoracotomy pain. Anesth Analg, 1988, 67, 409.

Brodsky JB, WG Brose, K Vivenzo. A postoperative pain management service. Anesthesiology, 1989, 70, 719.

Bromage PR, AC Joyal, JC Binney. Local anesthetic drugs. Penetration from the spinal extradural space the neuroaxis. Science, 1963, 140, 392.

Bromage PR. Epidural analgesia, Saunders, Philadelphia, 1978.

Bromage PR, E Camporesi, D Chestnut. Epidural narcotics for postoperative analgesia. Anesth Analg, 1980, 59, 473. (a)

Bromage PR, Camporesi E, Leslie J. Epidural narcotics in volunteers. Sensitivity to pain and to carbon dioxide. Pain, 1980, 9,145. (b)

Bromage PR, Camporesi E, Leslie J. Neurological effects of epidural dilaudid and methadone in volunteers. Anesth Analg, 1980, 59, 531. (c)

Bromage PR. Epidural narcotics for postoperative pain relief: comparison of methadone, hydromorphone and morphine. Symposium: Analgesia by epidural and spinal opiates, Nijmegen (Holland), 1980, Congress, summary 11. (d)

Bromage PR, EM Camporesi, PAC Durant, CH Nielsen. Rostral spread of epidural morphine. Anesthesiology, 1981, 55, A149. (a)

Bromage PR. The price of intraspinal narcotic analgesia. Basic constraints (editorial). Anesth Analg, 1981, 60, 461. (b)

Bromage PR, EM Camporesi, PAC Durant, CH Nielsen. Non respiratory side effects of epidural morphine. Anesth Analg, 1982, 61, 490. (a)

Bromage PR, EM Camporesi, PAC Durant, CH Nielsen. Rostral spread of epidural morphine. Anesthesiology, 1982, 56, 431. (b)

Bromage PR, EM Camporesi, PAC Durant, CH Nielsen. Influence of epinephrine as an adjuvant to morphine. Anesthesiology, 1983, 58, 257. (a)

Bromage PR. Epidural and spinal narcotics. Seminars in Anaesthesia,1983, 2, 75. (b)

522

Bromage PR. Epidural anaesthetics and narcotics. In: PD Wall, R Melzac (Eds.): Textbook of Pain, Churchill Livingstone, Edinburgh 1984, 3B, 558. (a)

Bromage PR. Spinal opiate analgesia: its present role and future in pain relief. Ann Chir Gynaecol, 1984, 73, 183. (b)

Bromage PR. Subdural migration of an epidural catheter. Anesth Analg, 1985, 64, 1029.

Bromage PR, S Al-Faquih, GH Kadiwal, A Tamilrason. Evaluation of bupivacaine and fentanyl epidural analgesia. Anesthesiology, 1987, 67, A226.

Bromage PR. Repeated epdiural anesthesia for extracorporeal shock-wave lithotripsy (ESWL) is not unreliable (letter). Anesth Analg, 1988, 67, 482.

Bromage P. A postoperative pain management service. Anaesthesiology, 1988, 69, 435.

Brooks GZ, Y Donchin, JG Collins, LM Kitahata, SA Jefferson. Epidural morphine does not affect the duration of action of epidural 2-chloro-procaine following caesarean section. Can Anaesth Soc J, 1983, 30, 598.

Brookshire GL, SM Shnider, TK Abboud, DM Kotelko, R Nouiehed, JW Thigpen, SS Khoo, JA Raya, SE Foutz, RV Brizgys RV. Effects of naloxone on the mother and neonate after intrathecal morphine for labor analgesia. Anesthesiology, 1983, 59, A417.

Brose WB, M Powar, SE Cohen. Oxygen saturation in post-cesarean patients using epidural morphine, PCA, or im narcotic analgesia. Anesth Analg, 1988, 67, S24.

Brose WG, SE Cohen. Oxyhemoglobin saturation following cesarean section in patients receiving epidural morphine, PCA, or im meperidine analgesia. Anesthesiology, 1989, 70, 948.

Brown CE, SC Roerig, VT Burger, RB Cody, JM Fujimoto. Analgesic potencies of morphine 3- and 6-sulfates after intracerebroventricular administration in mice: relationship to structural characteristics defined by mass spectrometry and nuclear magnnetic resonance. J Pharm Sci, 1985, 74, 821.

Brown DL. Postoperative analgesia following thoracotomy. Danger of delayed respiratory depression. Chest, 1986, 88, 779.

Brown DL. Risk and outcome in anaesthesia. Lippincott Publications, Philadelphia, 1988.

Brown G, GL Atkinson, SB Standiford. Subdural administration of opioids. Anesthesiology, 1989, 71, 611.

Brown M, P Rein. Securing the epidural catheter. Anesthesiology, 1985, 62, 373.

Brownridge P. Epidural pethidine (letter). Anaesth Intens Care, 1981, 9, 401.

Brownridge P. Epidural and intrathecal opiates for postoperative pain relief. Anaesthesia, 1983, 38, 74. (a)

Brownridge P, J Wrobel, J Watt-Smith. Respiratory depression following accidental subarachnoid pethidine. Anaesth Intens Care, 1983, 11, 237. (b)

Brownridge P. Another misplaced epidural catheter. Anaesth Intens Care, 1984, 12, 369.

Brownridge P, DB Frewin. A comparative study of techniques of postoperative analgesia following caesarean section and lower abdominal surgery. Anaesth Intens Care, 1985, 13, 123.

Brückner JB (ED). Schmerzbehandlung. Epidurale Opiatanalgesie. In: Anaesthesiologie u Intensivmedizin, 1982, 153.

Bruera E, R Fox, S Chadwick, C Brenneis, N MacDonald. Changing pattern in the treatment of pain and other symptoms in advanced cancer patients. J of Pain and Symptom Management, 1987, 2, 139.

Bryant RM, MB Tyers. Antinociceptive actions of morphine and buprenorphine given intrathecally in conscious rats (proceedings). Brit J Pharm, 1979, 66, 472P.

Bryant RM, JE Olley, MB Tyers. Antinociceptive actions of morphine and buprenorphine given intrathecally in the conscious rat. Brit J Pharm, 1983, 78, 659.

Buchwald H, TD Rhode. Implantable drug infusion devices. Surgical rounds, 1984, 16.

Budd K. Update publication. Pain, London, 1982.

Budd K, PM Brown, PJ Robson. The treatment of chronic pain by the use of meptazinol administered into the epidural space. Postgrad Med J (Suppl.), 1983, 59, 68.

Budd K. Clinical use of opioid antagonists, In clinical Anaesthesiology, 1987, 1, 4, 993.

Budiamal LR, CL Muetterties, JL Seltzer, J Jacoby, WH Vogel. Beta endorphin in pregnant women at term. Anesthesiology, 1981, 55, A322.

Bullingham RES, HJ McQuay, RA Moore. Unexpectedly high plasma fentanyl levels after epidural use. Lancet, 1980, 1, 1361. (a)

Bullingham RES, HJ McQuay, RA Moore, MRD Bennett. Buprenorphine kinetics. Clin Pharmaceut Ther, 1980, 28, 667. (b)

Bullingham RES, HJ McQuay, RA Moore. Extradural and intrathecal narcotics. In: RS Atkinson, C Langton Hewer (Eds.): Rec Adv Anaesth Analg, Churchill Livingstone, 1982, 14, 141.

Bullingham RES, G O'Sullivan , H McQuay, P Poppleton, M Rolfe, P Evans, A Moore. Perineural injection of morphine fails to relieve postoperative pain in humans. Anesth Analg, 1983, 62, 164.

Bullingham RES, HJ McQuay, RA Moore. Studies on the peripheral action of opioids in postoperative pain in man. Acta Anaesth Belgica (Suppl.), 1984, 35, S285.

Bundsen P, LE Peterson, U Selstam. Pain relief during delivery and evaluation of conventional methods. Acta Obstet Gynecol Scand, 1982, 61, 289.

Bunodiére M, N Colbert, J Renaud. Sédation des douleurs cancéreuses par injection péridurale quotidienne de morphine grace á un accès sous cutané implanté. Ann Fr Anesth Réanim, 1984, 3, 129.

Bunodiére M, S Havel. L'analgésie par morphine péridurale: injection par les trou sacrés. VII Eur Congress of Anaesth, 1986, Vienna (Austria), Report, Abstract 425.

Burton RJ, SW Krechel, MA Helikson. Intrathecal morphine for post thoracotomy pain relief in children. Anesth Analg, 1989, 68 (Suppl), S 44.

Busch EH, PM Stedman. Epidural morphine for postoperative pain on medical - surgical ward - a clinical review. Anesthesiology, 1987, 67, 101.

Bussières JS, L Thibault, JP Weber, LA Ferron, A McClish. Epidural fentanyl: description of a closed infusion system and study of the stability of fentanyl solution in this system. Regionalanesthesia, 1989, 14 (Suppl), 30.

Caballero GA, RK Ausman, J Himes. Epidural morphine by continuous infusion with an external pump for pain management in oncology patients. Amer Surg, 1986, 52, 402.

Cabo Franch JL, JL Marti Viano. Anestesia intradural con tetracaina y fentanyl. XV Congreso Nacional de anestesiologia y reanimacion, 1981, Valencia, Abstract 068.

Cahill J, D Murphy, D O'Brien, J Mulhall, G Fitzpatrick. Epidural buprenorphine for pain relief after major abdominal surgery. Anaesthesia, 1983, 38, 760.

Cahill J, G Fitzpatrick, J Holohan, M Cody. Epidural morphine for post-operative analgesia: experience with ten cases. Ir J Med Sci, 1984, 153, 247.

Calvey TN. Side effect problems of μ and k agonists in clinical use. In: Update in Opioids p 803. Baillieres Clinical Anaesthesiology, 1987, 1, 4.

Calvillo O, JL Henry, RS Neuman. Effects of morphine and naloxone on dorsal horn neurons in cats. Can J Physiol and Pharmacol, 1974, 52, 1207.

Calvillo O, M Ghigone. Presynaptic effects of clonidine on unmyelinated afferent fibers in the spinal cord of the rats. Neurosci Lett, 1986, 64, 335.

Camara PB, ADM de Salinas, RG Guasch, FC Rivera, MA Nalda-Felipe. Epidural fentanyl with etidocaine or bupivacaine compared in hip surgery. Rev Esp Anest Reanim, 1984, 31, 144.

Camarata PJ, TL Yaksh. Characterization of the spinal adrenergic receptors mediating the spinal effects produced by the microinjection of morphine into the periaqueductal gray. Brain Res, 1985, 336, 133.

Campailla A. Fixation of extradural catheters (letter). Brit J Anaesth, 1985, 57, 1043.

Campbell WI. Epidural opiates and degenerative back pain. Ulster Med J, 1983, 52, 161.

Campbell C. Epidural opioids - the preferred route of administration. Anesth Analg, 1989, 68, 710.

Camporesi EM, CH Nielsen, PR Bromage, PA Durant. Ventilatory CO_2 sensitivity after intravenous and epidural morphine in volunteers. Anesth Analg, 1983, 62, 633. (a)

Camporesi EM, LF Redick. Clinical aspects of spinal narcotics: postoperative managements and obstetrical pain. Clinics in Anaesth, 1983, 1, 57. (b)

Camu F, C Verborgh, D Van de Auwera, E Van Droogenbroeck. Pharmacokinetics and analgesic effects of epidural sufentanil administration for postoperative pain relief. Acta Anaesth Scand (Suppl.), 1985, 29, N° 133.

Candeletti S, S Ferri. Clinical use of subarachnoid neuropeptides: an experimental contribution. Anesth Analg, 1989, 69, 416.

Capogna G, D Celleno, P McGammon, G Richardson, RL Kennedy. Neonatal neurobehavioral following maternal administration of epidural fentanyl during labor. Anesthesiology, 1987, 67, A461.

Capogna G, D Celleno, V Tagariello, C Loffreda-Mancinelli. Intrathecal buprenorphine for postoperative analgesia in the elderly patient. Anaesthesia, 1988, 43, 128.

Caputi CA, G Busca, A Fogliardi, F Giugliano. Evaluation of tolerance in long-term treatment of cancer pain with epidural morphine. Int J Clin Pharm Ther Tox, 1983, 21, 587.

Cardan E. Herpes simplex after spinal morphine (letter). Anaesthesia, 1984, 39, 1031.

Cardan E. Intrathecal frusemide (letter). Anaesthesia, 1985, 40, 1025. (a)

Cardan E. Spinal morphine in enuresis. Brit J Anaesth, 1985, 57, 354. (b)

Carl P, ME Crawford, J Wolff. A comparison between buprenorphine and morphinechloride administered epidurally in treatment of postoperative pain. In: N Valentin, M Crawford, CR Volquardsen (Eds.): Nordic Symposium on Temgesic, Meda, Copenhagen, 1981, 90.

Carl P, ME Crawford, O Ravlo. Fixation of extradural catheters by means of subcutaneous tissue tunnelling. Brit J Anaesth, 1984, 56, 1369.

Carl P, ME Crawford, O Ravlo, V Bach. Longterm treatment with epidural opioids. A retrospective study comprising 150 patients treated with morphine. Anaesthesia, 1986, 41, 32.

Carli P, C Ecoffey, J Chrubasik, M Benlabed, JB Gross, K Samii. Spread of analgesia and ventilatory responses to CO_2 following epidural somatostatin. Anesthesiology, 1986, 65, A216.

Carmichael FJ, SH Rolbin, EM Hew. Epidural morphine for analgesia after caesarean section. Can Anaesth Soc J, 1982, 29, 359.

Carp H, MD Johnson, AM Bader, S Datta, GW Ostheimer. Continuous epidural infusion of alfentanil and bupivacaine for labor and delivery. Anesthesiology, 1988, 69, 3A (Suppl), A687.

Carrasco MS, LM Torres, F Requena, ML Martin, R Garcia de Sola. Acción analgésica del midazolam administrado intraduralmente en el perro. Rev Esp Anest Reanim, 1985, 32, 96.

Carrie LES. Epidural fentanyl in labour. Anaesthesia, 1980, 35, 1129.

Carrie LES, GM O'Sullivan, R Seegobin. Epidural fentanyl in labour. Anaesthesia, 1981, 36, 965.

Carstens E, L Turloch, W Zieglgansberger, M Zimmerman. Presynaptic excitability changes induced by morphine on single cutaneous afferent C and A fibers. Pflugers Arch, 1979, 379, 143.

Carton EG, N McDonald, JR McCarthy. Intrathecal morphne in labour - efficacy and side effects. I J M S, 1987, 158, 323.

Castillo R, I Kissin, EL Bradley. Selective kappa opioid agonist for spinal analgesia without the risk of respiratory depression. Anesth Analg, 1986, 65, 350. (a)

Castillo RA, I Kissin, EL Bradley. Opioid agonist for spinal analgesia without risk of respiratory depression. Anesth Analg, 1986, 65, S28. (b)

Castro MI, JC Eisenach. Pharmacokinetics and dynamics of intravenous, intrathecal and epidural clonidine in sheep. Anesthesiology, 1989, 71, 418.

Casy AF. The structure of narcotic analgesic drugs. In: DH Clouet (Ed.): Narcotic drugs,

Biochemical Pharmacology, Plenum Press, New York, 1971, 1.

Catalano RB. Pharmacology of analgesic agents used to treat cancer pain. Sem Oncol Nurs, 1985, 1, 126.

Caute B, B Monsarrat, C Gounardères, JC Verdie, Y Lazorthes, J Cros, R Bastide. CSF morphine levels after lumbar intrathecal administration of isobaric and hyperbaric solutions for cancer pain. Pain, 1988, 32, 141.

Celleno D, G Capogna. Epidural fentanyl plus bupivacaine 0.125 per cent for labour: analgesic effects. Can J Anaesth, 1988, 35, 375.

Celleno D, G Capogna. Spinal buprenorphine for postoperative analgesia after caesarean section. Acta Anaesth Scand, 1989, 33, 236.

Cervero F. Modulación medular y supramedular de la información nociceptiva: base neurofisiologica del alivio de por los opiáceos intrathecales. Dolor, 1986, 1, 65.

Ceserani R, U Colombo, VR Olgiati, A Pecile. Calcitonin and prostaglandin system. Life Sci, 1979, 25, 1851.

Chabal C, L Jacobson, J Little. Effects of intrathecal fentanyl and lidocaine on somatosensory-evoked potentials, the H-reflex, and clinical responses. Anesth Analg, 1988, 67, 509.

Chabal C, L Jacobson, J Little. Intrathecal fentanyl depresses nociceptive flexion reflexes in patients with chronic pain. Anesthesiology, 1989, 70, 226.

Chadwick HS, LB Ready. Comparison of intrathecal and epidural morphine sulphate for postcesarean section analgesia. Regional Anesthesia, 1987, 12, 40.

Chadwick HS, LB Ready. Intrathecal and epidural morphine sulfate for postcesarean analgesia - a clinical comparison. Anesthesiology, 1988, 68, 925.

Chamberlain DP, MN Bodily, GL Olssen, DH Ramsey. Comparison of lumbar versus thoracic epidural fentanyl for post-thoracotomy analgesia using patient-controlled dosage. Regionalanesthesia, 1989, 14 (Suppl), 26.

Chambers WA, CJ Sinclair, DB Scott. Extradural morphine for pain after surgery. Brit J Anaesth, 1981, 53, 921.

Chambers WA, A Mowbray, J Wilson. Extradural morphine for the relief of pain following caesarean section. Brit J Anaesth, 1983, 55, 1201.

Chang HM, CB Berde, GG Holz, GF Steward, RM Kream. Sufentanil, morphine, met-enkephalin, and kappa-agonist (U-50,488H) inhibit substance P release from primary sensory neurons: a model for presynaptic spinal opioid actions. Anesthesiology, 1989, 70, 672.

Chapman CR. New directions in the understanding and management of pain. Soc Sci Med, 1984, 19, 1261.

Chauvin M, K Samii, JM Schermann, P Sandouk, R Bourdon, P Viars. Plasma concentration of morphine after i.m., extradural and intrathecal administration. Brit J Anaesth, 1981, 53, 911. (a)

Chauvin M, K Samii, JM Schermann, P Sandouk, R Bourdon, P Viars. Plasma morphine concentration after intrathecal administration of low doses of morphine. Brit J Anaesth, 1981, 53, 1065. (b)

Chauvin M, K Samii, JM Schermann, Sandouk P, R Bourdon, P Viars. Plasma pharmacokinetics of morphine after i.m., extradural and intrathecal administration. Brit J Anaesth, 1982, 54, 843. (a)

Chauvin M, A Lienart, P Viars. Traitement de la douleur postopératoire. Comparaisons cliniques et pharmacologiques des différents morphiniques administrés par voie péridurale et intrathécale. In: Ars Medici, Bruxelles, 1982, Congress Series, 3, I, 193. (b)

Chauvin M, J Salbaing, D Perrin, JC Levron, P Viars. Comparison between intramuscular and

526

epidural administration of alfentanil for pain relief and plasma kinetics. Anesthesiology, 1983, 59, A197.

Chauvin M, J Salbaing, D Perrin, JC Levron, P Viars. Clinical assessment and plasma pharmacokinetics associated with intramuscular or extradural alfentanil. Brit J Anaesth, 1985, 57, 886. (a)

Chauvin M. Study of analgesia, side effects and pharmacokinetics after epidural administration of two single doses of alfentanil. Report, Janssen Pharmaceutica, 1985. (b)

Chauvin M. New opiates. II Int Symposium: The Pain Clinic, 1986, Lille (France). In: P Scherpereel, J Meynadier, S Blond (Eds.): Pain Clinic II, VNU Science Press, Utrecht, 1987, 109.

Chauvin M. Facteurs déterminants la diffusion des substances administrées par voie péridurale. VII Eur Congress of Anaesth, 1986, Vienna (Austria), Report, Abst 288.

Chauvin M. Modalités particulières d'utilition de la morphine péridurale et intrathécale, choix du morphinique. J.E.P.U. Paris, 1988, Ed. Arnette, Paris.

Chayen MS, V Rudick, A Borvine. Pain control with epidural injection of morphine. Anesthesiology, 1980, 53, 338.

Cheng EY, RF Koebert, M Hopwood, KA Stommel, D Roerhig, J Kay. Continuous epidural sufentanil infusion for postoperative analgesia. Anesthesiology, 1987, 67, A233.

Cheng EY, KA Stommel. Respiratory monitoring for postoperative patients receiving epidural opioids. Anesth Analg, 1988, 67, S28.

Cheng EY, J May. Nalbuphine reversal of respiratory depression after epidural sufentanil. Crit Care Med, 1989, 17 (4), 378.

Cherry DA, GK Gourlay, MJ Cousins, BJ Gannon. A technique for the insertion of an implantable portal system for the long-term epidural administration of opioids in the treatment of cancer. Anaesth Intens Care, 1985, 13, 145. (a)

Cherry DA, GK Gourlay, MM Lachlan, MJ Cousins. Diagnostic epidural opioid blockade and chronic pain: preliminary report. Pain, 1985, 21, 143. (b)

Cherry DA, GK Gourlay, MJ Cousins. Epidural mass associated with lack of efficacy and epidural morphine and undetectable CSF morphine concentrations. Pain, 1986, 25, 69.

Cherry DA. Drug delivery systems for epidural administration of opioids. Acta Anaesth Scand, 1987, 31, 54. (a)

Cherry DA. Epidural administration of morphine. II Int Symposium: Pain Clinic, 1986, Lille (France). In: Ph Scherpereel, J Meynadier, S Blond (Eds.): Pain Clinic II, VNU Science Press, Utrecht, 1987, 311. (b)

Cherry DA, GK Gourlay, JL Plummer, PJ Armstrong, MJ Cousins. Cephalad migration of pethidine and morphine following lumbar epidural administration in patient with cancer pain. Pain, 1987, S4, S69. (c)

Cherry DA. Use of opioids by implanted systems and self administration. In: Update in Opioids. Baillieres Clinical Anaesthesiology, 1987, 1, 4, 955. (d)

Chester WL, A Schubert, D Brandon, MA Pudimat, CW Pray. Intrathecal morphine: perioperative hemodynamic effects. Anesthesiology, 1987, 67, A267.

Chestnut DH, WW Choi, TJ Isbell. Epidural hydromorphone for postcesarean analgesia. Anesthesiology, 1985, 63, A355.

Chestnut DH, WW Choi, TJ Isbell. Epidural hydromorphone for postcesarean analgesia. Obstet Gynecol, 1986, 68, 65.

Chestnut DH, CL Owen, LG Ostman, JN Bates, WW Choi. Continuous infusion epidural analgesia during labor: a randomized, double-blind comparison of 0.0625 % Buipivacaine/0.0002 % Fentanyl versus 0.125 % Bupivacaine. Anesthesiology, 1987, 67, A443.

Chestnut DH, CL Owen, JN Bates, LG Ostman, WW Choi, MW Geiger. Continuous infusion epidural analgesia during labor: a randomized, double-blind comparison of 0.0625% bupivacaine/0.0002% fentanyl versus 0.125% bupivacaine. Anesthesiology, 1988, 68, 754.

Chestnut DH, KL Pollack, LJ Laszewski, JN Bates, NW Choi. Continuous epidural infusion of bupivacaine-fentanyl during the second stage of labor. Anesthesiology (Suppl), 1989, 71, 841.

Child CS, L Kaufman. Effect of intrathecal diamorphine on the adrenocortical, hyperglycaemic and cardiovascular responses to major colonic surgery. Brit J Anaesth, 1985, 57, 389.

Chiu L, P Chan, K Tse. Epidural morphine (letter). Can Anaesth Soc J, 1982, 29, 79.

Choi HJ, KK Tremper, R Scruggs, RV Asrani, BF Cullen. Continuous transcutaneous PCO2 monitoring during epidural morphine analgesia. Crit Care Med, 1985, 13, 584.

Choi HJ, MS Little, RA Fujita, SZ Garber, KK Tremper. Pulse oximetry for monitoring during ward analgesia: epidural morphine versus parenteral narcotics. Anesthesiology, 1986, 65, A371.

Chovaz PM, AN Sandler. Respiratory effects following epidural and systemic morphine in post-thoracotomy patients. Can Anaesth Soc J, 1985, 32, S87.

Chraemmer-Jørgensen B, HB Andersen, A Engquist. CSF and plasma morphine after epidural and intrathecal application (letter). Anesthesiology, 1981, 55, 714 .

Christensen FR. Epidural morphine at home in terminal patients. Lancet, 1982, 1, 47. (a)

Christensen FR, LW Andersen. Adverse reaction to extradural buprenorphine (letter). Brit J Anaesth, 1982, 54, 476. (b)

Christensen P, MR Brandt. Extradural morphine and Stokes-Adams attacks (letter). Brit J Anaesth, 1982, 54, 363. (a)

Christensen P, MR Brandt, J Rem, H Kehlet. Influence of the extradural morphine on the adrenocortical and hyperglycemic response to surgery. Brit J Anaesth, 1982, 54, 23. (b)

Christensen V. Respiratory depression after extradural morphine (letter). Brit J Anaesth, 1980, 52, 841.

Chrubasik J. Programmierte Medikamentendosierung zur postoperativen Schmerzbehandlung. Deut Med Wochenschr, 1983, 108, 1297.

Chrubasik J. Epidural, on demand, low dose morphine infusion for postoperative pain. Lancet, 1984, 1, 107. (a)

Chrubasik J. Individuelle postoperative Schmerzbehandlung durch klein, extern tragbare, programmierbare Morphinpumpe. Anaesth Intensiv Notfallmed, 1984, 19, 30. (b)

Chrubasik J. Low-dose epidural morphine by infusion pump. Lancet, 1984, 1, 738. (c)

Chrubasik J, KL Scholler, K Wiemers, K Weigel, G Friedrich. Low-dose infusion of morphine prevents respiratory depression. Lancet, 1984, 1, 793. (d)

Chrubasik J. Individuelle Schmerzbehandlung durch kontinuierliche, peridurale, bedarfsgesteuerte Morphininfusion. Elektromedica, 1984, 52, 123. (e)

Chrubasik J. Externally worn morphine infusion devices in treatment of intractable cancer pain. Proceedings: "New Aspects in Chemotherapy", Symposium, Freiburg (W Germany), May 26, 1984. (f)

Chrubasik J, J Meynadier, S Blond, P Scherpereel, E Ackerman, M Weinstock, K Bonat, H Cramer, E Wünsch. Somatostatin, a potent analgesic. Lancet, 1984, 2, 1208. (g)

Chrubasik J, W Vogel, G Friedrich. Morphinkonzentrationen im Serum unter bedarfsgesteuerter periduraler Morphininfusion. Anaesth Intensiv Notfallmed, 1984, 19, 231. (h)

Chrubasik J. On-demand epidural morphine infusion (letter). Anaesth Intens Care, 1984, 12, 272. (i)

Chrubasik J. The analgesic potency of epidural buprenorphine. In: W Erdman, T Oyama, MJ Pernak (Eds.): Pain Clinic I, VNU, Science Press, Utrecht, 1985, 299. (a)

Chrubasik J. Externe Morphinpumpen in der Behandlung unerträglicher Krebsschmerzen. Symposium: new aspects in chemotherapy, Freiburg, 26 may 1985. (b)

Chrubasik J. Spinal infusion of opioids and somatostatin in treatment of pain. Schmerz-Pain-Douleur, 1985, 6, 120. (c)

528

Chrubasik J. Zur spinalen Infusion von Opiaten und Somatostatin (spinal infusion of opiates and somatostatin). Fresenius foundation, 6370 Oberursel, FRG, 1985. (d)

Chrubasik J. Somastostatin, eine Übersicht. Anaesth Intensiv Notfallmed, 1985, 20, 165. (e)

Chrubasik J, G Friedrich, W Vogel. Morphinmetabolismus bei Intensivpatienten unter bedarfsgesteuerter periduraler Morphininfusion zur postoperativen Schmerzbehandlung. Schweiz Med Wochenschr, 1985, 115, 197. (f)

Chrubasik J, J Meynadier, Ph Scherpereel, F Magora, JT Davidson, S Wünsch. Erste Untersuchungen zur intraoperativen Anwendung spinal applizierten Somatostatins. Anaesth Intensiv Notfallmed, 1985, 20, 139. (g)

Chrubasik J, J Meynadier, P Scherpereel, E Wünsch. Somatostatin for anaesthesia. ISA Newsletter, 1985, 22, 6. (h)

Chrubasik J, J Meynadier, P Scherpereel, F Magora, JT Davidson, E Wünsch. Somatostatin für die Anaesthesie. Anaesthesist, 1985, 34, 322. (i)

Chrubasik J, J Meynadier, Ph Scherpereel, E Wünsch. The effect of epidural somatostatin on postoperative pain. Anesth Analg, 1985, 64, 1085. (j)

Chrubasik J, J Meynadier, Ph Scherpereel. Somatostatin versus morphine in epidural treatment after major abdominal operations. Anesthesiology, 1985, 63, A237. (k)

Chrubasik J, KL Scholler, H Cramer, E Wünsch. Epidurales Somatostatin und seine Durchgängigkeit. Anaesthesist, 1985, 34, 322. (l)

Chrubasik J, KL Scholler, K Wiemers, G Friedrich, K Weigel, H Roth, G Berg. Zum Einfluss des Volumens periduraler Morphinbolusinjektionen auf die Morphinkonzentration in der Zisterna magna des Hundes. Anaesthesist, 1985, 34, 304. (m)

Chrubasik J, KL Scholler, J Bammert. Epidural morphine injection and cisternal cerebromedullary CSF bioavailability of morphine in dogs. In: W Erdmann, T Oyama, MJ Pernak (Eds.): Pain Clinic I, VNU Science Press, Utrecht, 1985, 47. (n)

Chrubasik J, W Vogel, J Waninger. Die analgetische Potenz von epiduralem Buprenorphin. Anaesthesist, 1985, 34, 322. (o)

Chrubasik J, B Volk, U Wetterauer, H Trötschler. Externe Opiat-Dosiergeräte bei unerträglichen Krebsschmerzen. Z Allg Med, 1985, 61, 17. (p)

Chrubasik J, K Wiemers. Kein analgetischer Wirkungsverlust durch peridurale "Low Volume" Morphingabe. Anaesth Intensiv Notfallmed, 1985, 20, 19. (q)

Chrubasik J, K Wiemers. Continuous plus on demand epidural infusion of morphine for postoperative pain relief by means of a small externally worn infusion device. Anesthesiology, 1985, 62, 263. (r)

Chrubasik J, K Weigel, G Friedrich. Ergänzende Information zur Anwendung extern tragbarer Dosiergeräte in der Behandlung unerträglicher Krebsschmerzen. Regional Anaesthesie, 1985, 8, 39. (s)

Chrubasik J, K Wiemers, Epidural long-term infusion of morphine for relief of cancer pain. In: W Erdmann, T Oyama, MJ Pernak (Eds.): Pain Clinic I, Science Press, Utrecht, 1985, 301. (t)

Chrubasik J, A Kapsch, K Bonath, K Gerlach, H Cramer, KL Scholler, E Wünsch. Zur Durapermeabilität peridural applizierten Somatostatins. Schmerz, 1985, 1, 13. (u)

Chrubasik J, B Volk, J Meynadier, G Berg, E Wünsch. Observations in dogs receiving chronic spinal Somatostatin and Calcitonin. Schmerz-Pain-Doleur, 1986, 1, 10. (a)

Chrubasik J, KJ Falke, M Zindler, P Vitrac, S Blond, P Scherpereel. Epidural salmon infusion in long-term treatment of cancer pain. VII Eur Congress of Anaesth, 1986, Vienna (Austria), Report, Abst 221. (b)

Chrubasik J. Clinical use of new peptides in pain relief. In: II Int Symposium: Pain Clinic, 1986, Lille (France). In: Ph Scherpereel, J Meynadier, S Blond (Eds.): Pain Clinic II, VNU Science Press, Utrecht, 1987, 123. (a)

Chrubasik J, H Wüst, J Schulte-Mönting, K Thon, M Zindler. Analgesic potency of postoperative epidural fentanyl and alfentanyl. Anesthesiology, 1987, 67, A236. (b)

Chrubasik J, L Warth, H Wüst, M Zindler. Analgesic potency of epidural tramadol after abdominal surgery. Pain, 1987, S4, S154. (c)

Chrubasik J, L Warth, H Wüst, H Bretschneider, J Schulte-Mönting, HD Röher, M Zindler. Untersuchung zur analgetischen Wirksamkeit peridural applizierten Tramadols bei der Behandlung von Schmerzen nach abdominalchirurgischen Eingriffen. Schmerz-Pain-Douleur, 1988, 9, 12. (a)

Chrubasik J, H Wüst, J Schulte-Monting, K Thon, M Zindler. Relative analgesic potency of epidural fentanyl, alfentanil and morphine in treatment of postoperative pain. Anesthesiology, 1988, 68, 929. (b)

Chrubasik J, F Magora. Spinal administration of somatostatin in animals and humans. Anesthesiology, 1988, 69, 808.

Chrubasik J. Bemerkungen zur Arbeit von G. Steiner et al.: Wirkungen und Nebenwirkungen von Somatostatin. Anaesthesist, 1989, 38, 46.

Chrubasik J. Analgetische Wirkung von Somatostatin. Münch Med Wschr, 1989, 131, 199.

Chubra-Smith NM, RP Grand, LC Jenkins. Perioperative transcutaneous oxygen monitoring in thoracic anaesthesia. Can Anaesth Soc J, 1986, 33, 745.

Clark RSJ. The hyperglycemic response to different types of surgery and anaesthesia. Brit J Anaesth, 1970, 42, 45.

Clarke IMC. Narcotics in the treatment of non malignant chronic pain. In: Update in opioids, Baillières Clinical Anaesthesiology, London 1987. Anesthesiology, 1987, 1, 4, 905.

Clergue F, C Montembault, O Despierres, F Ghesquiere, A Harari, P Viars. Respiratory effects of intrathecal morphine after upper abdominal surgery. Anesthesiology, 1984, 61, 677.

Coates G. Management of cancer pain. A practical approach. Med J Aust, 1985, 142, 30.

Cobb CA, BN French, KA Smith. Intrathecal morphine for pelvic and sacral pain caused by cancer. Surg Neurol, 1984, 22, 63.

Cohen AM, WC Wood, M Bamberg, A Risaliti, C Poletti. Continuous canine epidural morphine analgesia with an implanted drug infusion pump. J Surg Res, 1982, 32, 32.

Cohen AT. A computer-controlled syringe driver for use during anaesthesia. Brit J Anaesth, 1986, 58, 670.

Cohen DE, JJ Downes, RC Rapheley. What difference does pulse oximetry make? Anesthesiology, 1988, 68, 181.

Cohen SE, WA Woods. The role of epidural morphine in the postcesarean patient: efficacy and effects on bonding. Anesthesiology, 1983, 58, 500. (a)

Cohen SE, AJ Rothblatt, GA Albright. Early respiratory depression with epidural narcotic and intravenous droperidol. Anesthesiology, 1983, 59, 559. (b)

Cohen SE, S Tan, GA Albright, J Halpern. Epidural fentanyl/bupivacaine for labor analgesia: effect of varying dosages. Anesthesiology, 1986, 65, A368.

Cohen SE, S Tau, GA Albright, J Halpern. Epidural fentanyl/bupivacaine mixtures for obstetric analgesia. Anesthesiology, 1987, 67, 403.

Cohen SE, S Tan, PF White. Sufentanil analgesia following cesarean section: epidural versus intravenous administration. Anesthesiology, 1988, 68, 129.

Cohen SE, LL Subak, WG Brose, J Halpern. Analgesia following cesarean section: comparison of five opioid techniques. Anesthesiology (Suppl), 1989, 71, 832.

Cohn ML, M Cohn. Barrel rotation induced by somatostatin in the non lesioned rat. Brain Res., 1975, 96, 138.

Cohn ML, CT Huntington, S Byrd, DJ Wooten, C Kochman, M Cohn. Computed tomographic and electromyographic evaluation of epidural treatment for chronic low back pain. Anesthesiology,

530

1983, 59, A194.

Collier CB. Epidural morphine (letter). Anaesthesia, 1981, 36, 67.

Collier Cl. Epinephrine and epidural narcotics (letter). Anesthesiology, 1984, 60, 168.

Collins JG, M Matsumoto, LM Kitahata, O Yuge, A Tanaka. Do pharmacokinetic parameters derived from systemic administration adequately describe spinal drug actions? Anesthesiology, 1983, 59, A381.

Colpaert FC. Can chronic pain be suppressed despite suported tolerance to narcotic analgesia? Life Sci, 1979, 24, 1201.

Colpaert FC, CJE Niemegeers, PAJ Janssen, JM Van Ree. Narcotic cueing properties of intraventricularly administered sufentanil, fentanyl, morphine and met-enkephalin. Eur J Pharmacol, 1978, 47, 115.

Colpaert FC. Acute toxicity of epidurally administered sufentanil citrate (R 33800) in rats. Janssen Preclinical Reseach Report, 1984.

Colpaert FC, JE Leysen, M Michiels, R van den Hoogen. Epidural and intravenous sufentanil in the rat: analgesia, opiate receptor, and drug concentrations in plasma and brain. Anesthesiology, 1986, 65, 41.

Cookson RF. Analgesic plasma concentrations. Brit J Anaesth, 1980, 52, 959.

Cookson RF, CJE Niemegeers, S Van den Bussche. The development of alfentanil. Brit J Anaesth, 1983, 55, S157.

Coombs DW, RL Saunders, MS Gaylor, MG Pageau, MG Leith, C Schaiberger. Continuous epidural analgesia via implanted morphine reservoir (letter). Lancet, 1981, 2, 425. (a)

Coombs DW, RL Saunders, CL Schaiberger, G Pageau. Epidural narcotic infusion pump I: implant (method / flow rates). Anesthesiology, 1981, 57, A152. (b)

Coombs DW, RL Saunders, M Gaylor, MG Pageau. Epidural narcotic infusion reservoir. Implantation technique and efficacy. Anesthesiology, 1982, 56, 469. (a)

Coombs DW, DR Danielson, MG Pageau, Rippe E. Epidurally administered morphine for postcesarean analgesia. Surg Gynecol Obstet, 1982, 154, 385. (b)

Coombs DW, RL Saunders, MG Pageau. Continuous intraspinal narcotic analgesia, technical aspects of an implantable infusion system. Regional Anesthesia, 1982, 7, 110. (c)

Coombs DW, MG Pageau, RL Saunders, WT Mroz. Intraspinal narcotic tolerance: preliminary experience with continuous bupivacaine HCl infusion via implanted infusion device. Int J Artificial Organs, 1982, 5, 379. (d)

Coombs DW. Pharmacokinetics. Intraspinal narcotic analgesia for acute and chronic pain. Palm Springs, USA, 1983, Symposium report. (a)

Coombs DW. New approaches to chronic pain therapy. Intraspinal narcotic analgesia for acute and chronic pain. Palm Springs, USA, 1983, Symposium report. (b)

Coombs DW. Mechanism of epidural lidocaine reversal of tachyphylaxis to epidural morphine analgesia. Anesthesiology, 1983, 59, 486. (c)

Coombs DW, RL Saunders, MS Gaylor, AR Block, T Colton, R Harbaugh, MG Pageau, W Mroz. Relief of continuous chronic pain by intraspinal narcotics infusion via an implanted reservoir. JAMA, 1983, 250, 2336. (d).

Coombs DW. The patient with the pump: long term management considerations. Intraspinal narcotic analgesia for acute and chronic pain. Palm Springs, USA, 1983, Symposium report. (e)

Coombs DW, RL Saunders, WT Mroz, MG Pageau. Complications of continuous intraspinal narcotic analgesia (letter). Can Anaesth Soc J, 1983, 30, 315. (f)

Coombs DW, LH Maurer, RL Saunders, M Glayor. Outcomes and complications of continuous intraspinal narcotic analgesia for cancer pain control. J Clin Oncology, 1984, 2, 1414. (a)

Coombs DW, C Allen, FA Meier, JD Franklin. Chronic intraspinal clonidine in sheep. Regional Anesthesia, 1984, 9, 47. (b)

Coombs DW, RL Saunders, D Lachance, S Savage, TS Ragnarsson, LE Jensen. Intrathecal morphine tolerance: Use of intrathecal clonidine, DADLE and intraventricular morphine. Anesthesiology, 1985, 62, 358. (a)

Coombs DW. Potential hazards of transcatheter serial epidural phenol neurolysis. Anesth Analg, 1985, 64, 1205. (b)

Coombs DW, RL Saunders, S Savage, L Jensen, C Murphy. Chronic intrathecal clonidine and narcotic tolerance. Can Anaesth Soc J, 1985, 32, S63. (c)

Coombs DW, RL Saunders, C Allen, J Fratkin, LH Maurer. Chronic intrathecal clonidine analgesia for intractable cancer pain. Schmerz-Pain-Douleur, 1985, 6, 115. (d)

Coombs DW, JD Fratkin, FA Meier, DW Nierenberg, RL Saunders. Neuropathologic lesions and CSF morphine concentrations during chronic continuous intraspinal morphine infusion. A clinical and post-mortem study. Pain, 1985, 22, 337. (e)

Coombs DW. New approches to chronic pain therapy. Seminars in Anesthesia, 1985, 4, 287. (f)

Coombs DW. Management of chronic pain by epidural and intrathecal opioids: newer drugs and delivery systems. Int Anesth Clin, 1986, 24, 59. (a)

Coombs DW, RL Saunders, JD Fratkin, LE Jensen, CA Murphy. Continuous intrathecal hydromorphone and clonidine for intractable cancer pain. J Neurosurg, 1986, 64, 890. (b)

Coombs DW. Continuous intraspinal morphine analgesia for relief of cancer pain: A current review. Inovasions, Intermedics Publ, Norwood, 1986. (c)

Coombs DW, JD Fratkin. Neurotoxicology of spinal agents. Anesthesiology, 1987, 66, 724. (a)

Coombs DW, LB Jensen, C Murphy. Microdose intrathecal clonidine and morphine for postoperative analgesia. Anesthesiology, 1987, 67, A238. (b)

Coombs DW, Rl Saunders, H Maurer, LE Jensen, C Murphy. Continuous intraspinal narcotics for cancer pain in cervicothoracic dermatomes. Regional Anesthesia, 1987, 12, 26. (c)

Cooper GM, NW Goodman, C Prys-Roberts, L Jacobson, G Douglas. Ventilatory effects of extradural diamorphine. Brit J Anaesth, 1982, 54, 239P.

Copel JA, D Harrison, R Whittemore, JC Hobbins. Intrathecal morphine analgesia for vaginal delivery in a woman with a single ventricle. J Reprod Med, 1986, 31, 274.

Corke CF, RG Wheatley. Respiratory depression complicating epidural diamorphine. Two case reports of administration after dural puncture. Anaesthesia, 1985, 40, 1203.

Corsen G, JG Reves, TH Stanley. Intravenous anesthesia and analgesia. Publ. Lea and Febiger, Philadelphia, 1988.

Cousin MT, T Hentz, P Levron, D Pathier. Le fentanyl par voie péridurale en obstétrique. Effets maternels et foetaux et taux plasmatiques. Ann Fr Anesth Réanim, 1983, 2, 201.

Cousins MJ, LE Mather, CJ Glynn, PR Wilson, Graham JR. Selective spinal analgesia (pethidine). Lancet, 1979, 1, 1141. (a)

Cousins MJ, CJ Glynn, PR Wilson, LE Mather, JR Graham. Aspects of epidural morphine (letter). Lancet, 1979, 2, 584. (b)

Cousins MJ et al. Neurolytic lumbar sympathetic blockade: duration of denervation and relief of rest pain. Anaesth Intens Care, 1979, 7, 121. (c)

Cousins MJ, CJ Glynn, PR Glynn, PR Wilson, LE Mather, JR Graham. Epidural morphine (letter). Anaesth Intens Care, 1980, 8, 217. (a)

Cousins MJ, PO Bridenbaugh (Eds.) Neural blockade in clinical anesthesia and management of pain. Lippincott Co., Philadelphia, Toronto, 1980. (b)

Cousins MJ, GD Phillips. Pain, anxiety, sleep. In: ML, Shoemaker, ML Thompson, PR Holbrook, WB Saunders (Eds.): Textbook of critical care, Philadelphia, 1984, 787. (a)

Cousins MJ, LE Mather. Intrathecal and epidural administration of opioids. Anesthesiology, 1984, 61, 276. (b)

Cousins MJ, PO Bridenbaugh. Spinal opioids and pain relief in acute care, in acute pain management. In: MJ Cousins, CD Phillips (Eds.): Acute pain management, Livingstone, 1986, 151. (a)

532

Cousins MJ, GD Phillips. Acute pain management Publ. Churchill Livingstone, NY, 1986. (b)

Cousins MJ, PO Bridenbaugh. Clinical anaesthesia and management of pain. 2nd Edit. Lippincott, Philadelphia, 1987. (a)

Cousins MJ. The spinal route of analgesia for acute and chronic pain. Pain, 1987, S4, S223. (b)

Cousins MJ. Comparative pharmacokinetics of spinal opioids in humans: a step toward determination of relative. Anesthesiology, 1987, 67, 875. (c)

Cousins MJ. The spinal route of analgesia. Acta Anaesth Belgica, 1988, 39, 71.

Cousins MJ. The spinal route of analgesia for acute and chronic pain. In: Dubner R, GF Gebhart, MR Bond (Eds): Proceedings of the Vth World Congress on Pain, Elsevier Science Publishers BV, 1988, 454.

Cousins MJ. The spinal route of analgesia for acute and chronic pain. In: Proceedings of the 5th World Congress on Pain, Dubner R, GF Gebhart, MR Blond (Eds.), 1988, 454-471, Elsevier Science Publishers BV.

Coventry DM, G Todd. Epidural clonidine in lower limb deafferentation pain. Anesth Analg, 1989, 69, 424.

Covino BG, DB Scott. Handbook of epidural anaesthesia and analgesia. Schultz Med Inf, Copenhagen, 1985.

Cowen M, RES Bullingham, GMC Paterson, HJ McQuay, M Turner, MC Allen, A Moore. A controlled comparison of the effects of extradural diamorphine and bupivacaine on plasma glucose and plasma cortisol in postoperative patients. Anesth Analg, 1982, 61, 15.

Cozian A, M Pinaud, JY Lepage, F Lhoste, R Souron. Effects of meperidine spinal anaesthesia on hemodynamics, plasma catecholamines, angiotensin I, aldosterone, and histamine concentrations in elderly men. Anesthesiology, 1986, 64, 815.

Craft JB, H Lim, NH Goldberg, E Landsberger, A Stolte, M Braswell, P Mazel. Epidural sufentanil: maternal and fetal effects in the sheep model. Unpublished report.

Craft JB, JC Bolan, LA Coaldrake, M Mondino, P Mazel, RM Gilman, LK Shokes, WA Woolf. The maternal and fetal cardiovascular effects of epidural morphine in the sheep model. Am J Obstet Gynecol, 1982, 142, 835.

Crawford CP, ME Ravio. Longterm treatment with epidural opioids. Anaesthesia, 1986, 41, 32.

Crawford JS. Experiences with epidural morphine in obstetrics. Anaesthesia, 1981, 36, 207. (a)

Crawford JS. Site of action of intrathecal morphine (letter). Brit Med J, 1980, 281, 1144.

Crawford JS. Intrathecal morphine in obstetrics (letter). Anesthesiology, 1981, 55, 487. (b)

Crawford RD, MS Batra, F Fox. Epidural morphine dose response for postoperative analgesia. Anesthesiology, 1981, 55, A150.

Crawford JS. Epidural morphine (letter). Can Anaesth Soc J, 1982, 5, 286.

Crawford ME, HB Andersen, G Augustenborg, J Bay, O Beck, D Benveniste, LB Larsen, P Carl, M Djernes, J Eriksen, AM Grell, H Henriksen, SH Johansen, HOK Jørgensen, IW Møller, JEP Pedersen, O Ravlo. Pain treatment on outpatient basis utilizing extradural opiates. A Danish multicenter study comprising 105 patients. Pain, 1983, 16, 41.

Cripps TP, CS Goodchild. Intrathecal midazolam and the stress response to upper abdominal surgery. Brit J Anesth, 1986, 58, 1324P.

Crone L, J Conly, C Storgard, A Zbitnew, S Cronk, L Rea, K Greer, E Berenbaum, L Tan, T To. Recurrent herpes simplex virus labialis in parturients receiving epidural morphine. Anesth Analg (Suppl), 1989, 68, 63.

Crone LL, JM Conly, KM Clark, AC Crichlow, GC Wardell, A Zbitnew, LM Rea, SL Cronk, CM Anderson, LK Tan, WL Albritton. Recurrent herpes simplex virus labialis and the use of epidural morphine in obstetric patients. Anesth Analg, 1988, 67, 318.

Crosby G, J Cohen. Local spinal blood flow during spinal analgesia with fentanyl (rat). Anesthesiology, 1984, 61, A224.

Cullen ML, ED Staren, A El-Gan Zouri, WG Logas, AD Ivankovich, SG Economou. Continuous epidural infusion for analgesia after major abdominal operations. A randomized, prospective, double blind study. Surgery, 1985, 98, 717.

Cullen M, AH Altstatt, NJ Kwon, S Benzuly, JS Naulty. Naltrexone reversal of the side effects of epirudal morphine. Anesthesiology, 1988, 69 (3A), A336.

Cunin G, A Serrie, C Thurel, JB Thiebaut. Présentation d'une pompe implantable pour auto-administration séquentielle de morphine par voie intrathécale. II Int Symposium: Pain Clinic, 1986, Lille (France) Abst AP 10.

Cunningham AJ, JA McKenna, DS Skene. Single injection spinal anaesthesia with amethocaine and morphine for transurethral prostatectomy. Brit J Anaesth, 1983, 55, 423.

Cuschieri RJ, CG Morran, JC Howie, CS Mcardle. Postoperative pain and pulmonary complications: comparison of three analgesic regims. Brit J Surg, 1985, 72, 495.

Dagi TF. Low-dose, single inoculation, intraoperative epidural morphine hastens recovery after lumbar spine operation. Neurological Surgery, Surgical Forum, 1984, 35, 496.

Dagi TF, J Chilton, A Caputy, D Won. Long-term, intermittent percutaneous administration of epidural and intrathecal morphine for pain of malignant origin. Amer Surg 1986, 52, 155.

Dahl HD. Peridurale Applikation von Buprenorphin. Regional Anaesthesie, 1984, 7, 56.

Dahl JB, JJ Daugaard, E Kristoffersen, HV Johannsen, JA Dahl. Perineuronal morphine: a comparison with epidural morphine. Anaesthesia, 1988, 43, 463.

Dahlström B. Pharmacokinetics and pharmacodynamics of epidural and intrathecal morphine. Int Anesth Clin, 1986, 24, 29. (a)

Dahlström B, T Hedner, T Mellstrand, G Nordberg, et al. Plasma and cerebrospinal fluid kinetics of morphine. In: KM Foley, et al. (Eds.): Advances in pain research and therapy, vol. 8, Raven press New York, 1986, 37. (b)

Dailey PA, CL Baysinger, G Levinson, SM Shnider. Neurobehavioral testing of the newborn infant. Effects of obstetric anesthesia. Clin Perinatol, 1982, 9, 191.

Dailey PA, GL Brookshire, SM Shnider, TK Abboud, DM Kotelko, R Noueihid, JH Thigpen, SS Khoo, JA Raya, SE Foutz, RV Brizgys, U Göbelsmann, MW Lo. The effects of naloxone associated with the intrathecal use of morphine in labor. Anesth Analg, 1985, 64, 658.

Dailland Ph, JD Lirzin, P Jacquinot, JC Jorrot. Effect of diluting fentanyl on epidural bupivacaine during labor analgesia. Anesthesiolgy, 1988, 69 (3A), A685.

Dallas TL, RL Lin, WH WU, P Wolskee. Epidural morphine and methyl prednisolone for low-back pain. Anesthesiology, 1986, 65, A203.

Dallas TL, RL Lin, WH Wu, P Wolskee. Epidural morphine and methylprednisolone for low-back pain. Anesthesiology, 1987, 67, 408.

Dalmas S. Les effets analgésiques de la somatostatine. Thèse pour le doctorat en médecine (étude expérimentale et clinique). 1986, Université de Lille (France).

Dalmas S, J Meynadier, J Chrubasik, P Scherpereel. Effets de la somatostatine intrathécale sur la sensibilité thermoalgésique du rat. Ann Fr Anesth Réanim (Suppl.), 1987, 6, R35.

Dalmas S, J Meynadier, S Blond, J Chrubasik, P Scherpereel. Substances non morphiniques utilisées en analgésie spinale. Acta of the XXth Int. Meeting of Anaesthesia and Critical care. Ed. Arnette Paris CPU 1988.

Daly MY, AM Woods, CA DiFazio. Continuous naloxone infusion following epidural morphine: a dose-response study. Anesthesiology, 1988, 69 (3A), A683.

Danielson DR, DW Coombs, M Pageau, E Rippe. Epidural morphine for post-cesarean analgesia. Anesthesiology, 1981, 55, A323.

Daugaard JJ, JB Dahl, CB Christensen. Concentrations of morphine in the cerebrospinal fluid after femoral perineural morphine administration. Anesth Analg, 1989, 68, 413.

Davies GK, CL Tolhurst-Cleaver, TL James. CNS depression from intrathecal morphine (letter). Anesthesiology, 1980, 52, 280. (a)

Davies GK, CL Tolhurst-Cleaver, TL James. Respiratory depression after intrathecal narcotics. Anaesthesia, 1980, 35, 1080. (b)

Davies GG, R From. A blinded study using nalbuphine for prevention of pruritus induced by epidural fentanyl. Anesthesiology, 1988, 69, 763.

Davis I. Intrathecal morphine in aortic aneurysm surgery. Anaesthesia, 1987, 42, 491.

De Castro J. Contribution à l'étude de la pharmacologie clinique des analgésiques centraux; analyse de certaines actions du fentanyl utilisé à hautes doses en anesthésie et en réanimation. Thèse d'agrégation, 1972, ULB Bruxelles.

De Castro J, A Van de Water, L Wouters, R Xhonneux, R Reneman. Comparative study of cardiovascular, neurological and metabolic side effects of eight narcoticts in dogs. Acta Anesth Belgica, 1979, 30, 5. (a)

De Castro J. Use of narcotic antagonists in anaesthesia. Brit J Clin Pharm (Suppl.), 1979, 7, 319S. (b)

De Castro J, E D'Inverno, L Lecron, D Levy, E Toppet-Balatoni. Perspectives d'utilisation de morphinoides en anesthésie loco- régionale. Justification - Premiers résultats. Anesth Analg Réanim, 1980, 37, 17. (a)

De Castro J, St Kubicki. Agonistic morphine antagonists and their antidotes in anaesthesia. Symposium, 7th World Congress of Anaesth. Hamburg, Ed AIAREF, 1980, Charleroi. (b)

De Castro J, S Andrieu. Basic principles of general pharmacology and uses of opiate antagonists. In: Agonistic morphine antagonists and their antidotesin anaesthesia, Publ. AIAREF Charleroi, 1980, 11. (c)

De Castro J, C Hörig. Die Pharmakokinetik von Fentanyl und deren Konsequenzen für Atemdepression und Remorphinisierung bei der analgetischen Anaesthesie. Anaesth Intens Med, 1981, 11, 190. (a)

De Castro J, L Lecron. Peridurale Opiatanalgesie. Verschiedene Opiate. Komplikationen und Nebenwirkungen. In: M Zenz et al. (Eds.): Peridurale Opiatanalgesie, Gustav Fischer Verlag, 1981, 103. (b)

De Castro J, S Andrieu, J Boogaerts. Buprenorphine. In: ArsMedici, New Drug Series,1, Kluwer Antwerpen, 1982.

De Castro J. New compounds and new supplements for anaesthesia. In: TH Stanley, WC Petty (Eds.): Anesthesiology: to day and tomorrow. Martinus Nijhoff, Dordrecht, 1985, 49.

De Castro J. Unpublished report 1986. (a)

De Castro J, S Andrieu. Administration de morphiniques par voie loco-régionale. In: L. Lecron: Anesthésie loco-régionale Publ. Arnette Paris 1986. (b)

de la Baume S, JC Schwartz, P Chaillet, H Marcais-Collado, J Costentin Participation of both enkephalinase and aminopeptidase activities in the metabolism of endogenous enkephalins. Neuroscience, 1983, 8, 143.

de la Vega S, H de Sousa. Postoperative analgesia using intrathecal morphine with phenylephrine. Regional Anesthesia, 1987, 12, 91. (a)

de la Vega S, H de Sousa. Dose response of intrathecal morphine for postoperative pain relief. Regional Anesthesia, 1987, 12, 91. (b)

Delander GE, AE Takemori. Spinal antagonism of tolerance and dependence induced by systemically administered morphine. Eur J Pharm, 1983, 94, 35.

Delander GE, PS Portoghese, AE Takemori. Role of spinal mu opioid receptors in the development of morphine tolerance and dependence. J Pharm Exp Ther, 1984, 231, 91.

De Lange S. Stress responses to cardiac surgery, modifying effects of alfentanil and sufentanil anaesthesia. Proefschrift: Rijksuniversiteit, Leiden 1982.

De Lange S, N de Brujn. Alfentanil oxygen anesthesia. Plasma concentrations and clinical effects during variable rate continuous infusion for coronary artery surgery. Brit J Anaesth (Suppl.), 1983, 55, 1835.

Delhaas EM, H Lip, RJ Boskma, JRBJ Brouwers. Low-dose epidural morphine by infusion pump. Lancet, 1984, 1, 690.

Delhaas EM, H Lip, RJ Boskma, JRBJ Brouwers. Longterm epidural morphine by Promedos EV1 infusion pump. In: W Erdmann, T Oyama, MJ Pernak (Eds.): Pain Clinic I, VNU, Science Press, Utrecht, 1985, 317.

Delhaas EM, JRBJ Brouwers, RH Henning. Mini-infusoren voor epidurale/intrathecale opiattoediening bij maligne aandoeningen. Pharmaceutisch Weekblad, 1986, 121, 317.

Dennis GC, R DeWitty. Management of intractable pain in cancer patients by implantable morphine infusion systems. J of the Nat Med Assn, 1987, 79, 939.

Desborough JP, SA Edlin, JM Burrin, SR Bloom, M Morgan, GM Hall. Hormonal and metabolic responses to cholecystectomy: comparison of extradural somatostatin and diamorphine. Brit J Anaesth, 1989, 63, 508.

Desprats R, J Mandry, H Grandjean, B Amar, G Pontonnier, L Lareng. Analgésie péridurale au cours du travail: étude comparative de l'association fentanyl-Marcaine et de la Marcaine seule. J. de Gynécologie, Obstétrique et Biologie de la reproduction, 1983, 12, 901. (b)

Desprats R. Peridural administration of an association bupivacaine - fentanyl: effects on uterine contractibility. ESRA 6th Congress Europ. Soc. Reg Anaesth Report 79, MAPAR, Paris 1987. (a)

Descorp-Declère A, C Bégon, L Brasseur, AM Brunet, JM Vannetzel, JC Boura, L Schwarzenberg, JL Misset, Y Noviant. Interest of medullar analgesia in cancer pain relief. A three years personnal survey of 135 patients. II Int Symposium: Pain Clinic, 1986, Lille (France) Abst IX FP 7. In: Ph Scherpereel, J Meynadier, S Blond (Eds.): Pain Clinic II, VNU Science Press, Utrecht, 1987, 317.

Descorps-Declère A, C Bégon. Site implantable pour injection intrathécale de morphine: Diminution des incidents mécaniques avec un nouveau matériel. Ann Fr Anesth Réanim, 1986, 5, 463.

Devaux C, MC Roussignol, C Oksenhendler, C Winckler. Etude clinique de différents opiacés par voie sousarachnoidienne. Can Anaesth Soc J, 1982, 29, 500. (a)

Devaux C, MC Roussignol, P Deshayes, G Oksenhendler, C Winckler. Side-effects of opiates administered by the subarachnoid route. 6th Eur Congress of Anaesth, London, 1982, Volume of summary, 45. (b)

Devaux C, C Tessier, P Zickler, P Deshayes, G. Oksenhendler, C Winckler. Subarachnoid opiates. A comparative study of morphine, phenoperidine, fentanyl, sufentanyl and buprenorphine. 6th Eur Congress of Anaesth, 1982, London. Volume of summary, 47. (c)

Devaux C, P Zickler, JF Mangez, C Tessier, F Alibert. Pharmcologie clinique des opiacés par voie médullaire. Swiss Med, 1983, 5, 13. (a)

Devaux C, JF Mangez, K Attignon, F Alibert, P Freger, J Godlewski, C Winckler, P Creissard. Etude comparative buprenorphine-morphine par voie intraventriculaire. Ars Medici congress series N°3, 1983, 469. (b)

Devaux C, JF Mangez, F Alibert, P Freger, J Godlewski, C Winckler, P Greissard. Etude comparative buprénorphine - morphine par voie intra-ventriculaire. Ann Franc Anesth Réan, 1983, 2, P193. (c)

Devaux C, P Freger, J Godlewski. Potentiation of opiates administered by the intraventricular route. In: HJ Wüst, M Stanton-Hicks (Eds.): Anaesthesiologie und Intensivmedizin, new aspects in regional anesthesia 4. Springer Verlag, Berlin, Heidelberg, New York, 1986, 176, 122.

Devoghel JC. De petites doses intrathécales d'acétylsalicylate de lysine suppriment la douleur rebelle chez l'homme. Communication 8° réunion interrégionale d'Anesth Réanim et oxyologie Roissy en France, oct 1983. (a)

536

Devoghel JC. Intrathecal lysine acetylsalicylate for pain treatment. Int Med Res, 1983, 11, 90. (b)

Devoghel JC. Small intrathecal doses of lysine-acetylsalicylate relieve intractable pain in man. J Int Med Res, 1983, 11, 90.

Dey PK, W Feldberg. Analgesia produced by morphine when acting from the liquor space. Brit J Pharm, 1976, 58, 383.

Dhiri AK, J Sanford, MG Wyllie. Disposition and pharmacokinetics of meptazinol in the CSF. Brit J Anaesth, 1987, 59, 1140.

DiChiro G, MK Hammock, A Bleyer. Spinal descent of cerebrospinal fluid in man. Neurology, 1976, 26, 1.

DiChiro G. Observations on the circulation of the cerebrospinal fluid. Acta Rad Diagn, 1966, 5, 988.

Dick W, B Kossmann, A Driessen. Studies on blood concentrations after spinal and extradural administration of morphine for the treatment. Brit J Anaesth, 1981, 53, 118.

Dick W, E Traub, RM Möller. Klinische Untersuchungen zur epiduralen Morphinapplikation in der geburtshilflichen Analgesie. Regional Anaesthesie, 1983, 6, 14.

Dickson GR, AJ Sutcliffe. Intrathecal morphine and multiple fractured ribs (letter). Brit J Anaesth, 1986, 58, 1342.

Diesbecq W, A Boel, R Bonneaux. Open pilot trial on the effect of repeated doses of sufentanil epidurally for postoperative pain relief, comparison with morphine. Unpublished Report, Janssen Pharmaceutica 1985.

Diesbecq W. Round table on sufentanil. II Int Symposium: Pain Clinic, 1986, Lille (France).

Dietzel W, L Poloczek, KA Lehmann. Peridurale Analgesie mit Fentanyl in der operativen Intensivtherapie. Anaesth Intensivther Notfallmed, 1982, 17, 38.

DiGuilio AM, HTY Yang, B Lutold, W Fratta, J Houg, E Costa. Characterization of enkephalin-like material extracted from sympathetic ganglia. Neuropharmacology, 1978, 17, 989.

Dirksen R, GMM Nijhuis. Epidural opiate and perioperative analgesia. Acta Anaesth Scand, 1980, 24, 367. (a)

Dirksen R. Results of epidural and spinal endorphinomimetics for surgery and early postoperative pain relief. Symposium: Analgesia by epidural and spinal opiates. Nijmegen 1980, Congress report, summary 12. (b)

Dirksen R, GMM Nijhuis. The relevance of cholinergic transmission at the spinal level to opiate effectiveness. Eur J Pharmacol, 1983, 91, 215.

Dirksen R, GMM Nijhuis, JWM Pinckaers. Selective spinal analgesia: how close to physiological can we get? In: W Erdmann, T Oyama, MJ Pernak (Eds.): Pain Clinic I, NVU, Science Press, Utrecht, 1985, 11.

Dixon R, J Hsiao, W Taaffe, E Hahn, R Tuttle. Nalmefene, radioimmunoassay for a new opioid antagonist. J Pharm Sc, 1984, 73, 1645.

Doblar DD, SM Muldoon, PH Albrecht, J Baskoff, RL Watson. Epidural morphine following epidural local anaesthesia: effect on ventilatory and airway occlusion pressure responses to CO_2. Anesthesiology, 1981, 55, 423.

Dodson ME. A review of methods for relief of postoperative pain. Ann R Coll Surg Engl, 1982, 64, 324.

Doenicke A. Alfentanil. Sertürner Workshops Einbeck. Springer Verlag, Berlin 1986.

Dohi S, N Matsumiya, T Abe. Mechanism of morphine - induced suppression of central nervous system blood flow. No To Shinke, 1983, 35, 1083.

Doi T, I Jurna. Analgesic effect of intrathecal morphine demonstrated in ascending nociceptive activity in the rat spinal cord and in effectiveness of caerulein and cholecystokinin octapeptide. Brain Res, 1982, 234, 399.

Donadoni R, G Rolly, H Noorduin, G Vanden Bussche. Epidural sufentanil for postoperative pain relief. Anaesthesia, 1985, 40, 634.

Donadoni R. Epidural sufentanil administration for pain relief after orthopedic surgery. II Int Symposium: Pain Clinic, 1986, Lille (France). In: Ph Scherpereel, J Meynadier, S Blond, Pain Clinic II, VNU Science Press, Utrecht, 1987, 295. (a)

Donadoni R, G Rolly. Epidural sufentanil versus intramuscular buprenorphine for postoperative analgesia. Anaesthesia, 1987, 42, 1171. (b)

Donadoni R, H Vermeulen, H Noorduin, G Rolly. Intrathecal sufentanil as a supplement to subarachnoid anaesthesia with lignocaine. Brit J Anaesth, 1987, 59, 1523. (c)

Donadoni R, P Capiau. Cardiac arrest after spinal sufentanil: case report. Acta Anaesth Belgica, 1987, 38, 175. (d)

Donchin Y, JT Davidson, F Magora. Epidural morphine for the control of pain after cesarean section. ISR J Med Sci, 1981, 17, 331.

Donnenfeld RM, S Ramanathan, F Parker, L Vargas, H Turndorf. Release of beta-endorphin and antidiuretic hormone by epidural morphine. Anesthesiology, 1987, 67, A446.

Donzelle G, L Bernard, R Deumier, M Lacombe, M Barre, M Lanier, MB Mourtada. Les douleurs oncologiques complexes: essais de traitement par la D-phénylalanine. Anesth Analg Réan, 1981, 38, 655.

Doran R, AD Baxter, B Samson, J Penning, LM Dubé. Prevention of respiratory depression from epidural morphine in post-thoracotomy patients with nalbuphine hydrochloride. Anesthesiology, 1987, 67, A248.

Douard MC, O Marie, F Mourey. Approche nouvelle des cathéters: voies d'abord en général. Encycl Med Chir Cancer, 1985, 50045, 1.

Dougherty TB, CL Baysinger, DJ Gooding. Epidural hydromorphone for postoperative analgesia after delivery by cesarean section. Regional Anesthesia, 1986, 11, 118.

Dougherty TB, CL Baysinger, JC Henenberger. Epidural hydromorphone with and without epinephrine for post-operative analgesia after cesarean delivery. Anesth Analg, 1989, 68, 318.

Douglas MJ, EE Thomas, GH McMorland. Epidemiology of HSV-1 infection in the puerperal population - does epidural morphine cause recrudescence? (abst). Society for obstetric Anesthesia and perinatology, 1986, 125. (a)

Douglas MJ, PLE Ross, GH McMorland. The effect of epinephrine in local anaesthetic on epidural morphine-induced pruritus. Can Anaesth Soc J, 1986, 33, 737. (b)

Douglas MJ, GH McMorland. Possible association herpes simplex type I reactivation with epidural morphine administration. Can J Anaesth, 1987, 34, 426. (a)

Douglas MJ, GH McMorland. A comparison of epidural morphine 3 mg and 5 mg with and without bupivacaine for postoperative analgesia. Can J Anaesth, 1987, 34, 98. (b)

Douglas MJ, GH McMorland, JA Janzen. Influence of bupivacaine as an adjuvant to epidural morphine for analgesia after cesarean section. Anesth Analg, 1988, 67, 1138.

Dover SB. Spinal opioids. Lancet, 1986, 1, 982.

Downing JW, V Williams, R Hascke, D Porte, S Woods, K Fogel, J Horn. Rostral spread of epidural morphine (letter). Anesth Analg, 1984, 63, 375.

Downing R, I Davis, J Black, CWO Windsor. When do patients given intrathecal morphine need postoperative systemic opiates? Ann R Coll Surg Engl, 1985, 67, 251.

Downing R, I Davis, J Black, CWO Windsor. Effect of intrathecal morphine on the adrenocortical and hyperglycaemic responses to upper abdominal surgery. Brit J Anaesth, 1986, 58, 858.

Downing JE, EH Busch, PM Stedman. Epidural morphine delivered by a percutaneous epidural catheter for outpatient treatment of cancer pain. Anesth Analg, 1988, 67, 1159.

Dralle D, H Müller, J Zierski, N Klug. Intrathecal baclofen for spasticity. Lancet, 1985, 2, 1003.

Drasner K, C Bernards, R Ciriales. Intrathecal morphine reduces the minimum alveolar concentration of isoflurane in the rat. Anesthesiology, 1987, 67, A670.

Drasner K, C Bernards, GM Ozanne. Intrathecal morphine reduces the minimum alveolar

538

concentration of halothane in man. Anesth Analg, 1988, 67, S52. (a)

Drasner K, HL Fields. Synergy between the antinociceptive effects of intrathecal clonidine and systemic morphine in the rats. Pain, 1988, 32, 309. (b)

Drasner K, C Bernards, GM Ozanne. Intrathecal morphine reduces the minimum alveolar concentration of halothane in humans Anesthesiology, 1988, 69, 310. (c)

Drasner K, D Ross, N Barbaro, P Weinstein, J Flaherty. A randomized, double-blind, placebo-controlled dose-response study of intrathecal morphine for postoperative pain following lumbar spine surgery. Anesthesiology (Suppl), 1989, 71, 696.

Dray A, R Metsch. Spinal opioid receptors and inhibition of urinary bladder motility in vivo. Neurosci Lett, 1984, 47, 81. (a)

Dray A, R Metsch. Inhibition of urinary bladder contractions by a spinal action of morphine and other opioids. J Pharm Exp Ther, 1984, 231, 254. (b)

Dray A. The rat urinary bladder. A novel preparation for the investigation of central opioid activity in vivo. J Pharm Methods, 1985, 13, 157. (a)

Dray A, L Nunan. Opioid inhibtion of reflex urinary bladder contractions: dissociation of supraspinal and spinal mechanisms. Brain Res, 1985, 337, 142. (b)

Dray A. Epidural opiates and urinary retention: new models provide new insights. Anesthesiology, 1988, 68, 323.

Drenger B, F Magora, S Evron, M Caine. The action of intrathecal morphine and methadone on lower urinary tract in dog. J Urol, 1986, 135, 852.

Drenger B, M Caine, M Sosnovsky, F Magora. Physostigmine and naloxone reverse the effect of intrathecal morphine an the canine urinary bladder. Eur J Anaesth, 1987, 4, 375.

Drenger B, AJ Pikarsky, F Magora. Urodynamic studies after intrathecal fentanyl and buprenor-phine in the dog. Anesthesiology, 1987, 67, A240. (a)

Drenger B, Y Shir, F Magora, JT Davidson. Epidural bupivacaine and methadone analgesia for extracorporeal shock wave lithotripsy. Anesthesiology, 1987, 67, A217. (b)

Drenger B, Y Shir, D Pode, A Shapira, F Magora, JT Davidson. Extradural bupivacaine and methadone for extracorporeal shock-wave lithotripsy. Brit J Anaesth, 1989, 62, 82.

Drenger B, F Magora. Urodynamic studies after intrathecal fentanyl and buprenorphine in the dog. Anesth Analg, 1989, 69, 348.

Driessen A, B Kossmann, W Dick, MR Möller. Untersuchungen zur postoperativen Schmerzthera-pie mit periduralen Morphingaben nach urologischen Operationen. Anaesthesist, 1981, 30, 575.

Drost RH, TI Ionescu, JM van Rossum, RAA Maes. Pharmacokinetics of morphine after epidural administration in man. Arzneim Forsch Drug Res, 1986, 36, 1096.

Duckett JE, MC Donnell, M Zebrowski, M Witte. A comparison of thoracic vs lumbar injections of sufentanil for post-operative analgesia after upper abdominal surgery. Anesthesiology, 1986, 65, A179.

Duckett JE, MC Donnell, M Zebrowski, M Witte. Lumbar versus thoracic continuous epidural sufentanil for postoperative analgesia after upper abdominal surgery. Anesth Analg, 1987, 66, S46.

Dudziak R. Typen der Opiat-Antagonisten. Symposium, Antagonisten in Anaesthesie und Inten-sivemedizin, Dec 1986, Münster (W Germany).

Dufffy BL, MD Read. Epidural pethidine for relief of episiotomy pain. Anaesth Intens Care, 1984, 12, 137.

Duffy BL. Itching as side effect of epidural morphine. Anaesthesia, 1981, 36, 67. (a)

Duffy BL. Experiences with epidural morphine in obstetrics (letter). Anaesthesia, 1981, 36, 822. (b)

Duffy BL. Epidural catheter fixation. Anaesth Intens Care, 1981, 9, 292. (c)

Duffy BL. Epidural opirates (letter). Anaesth Intens Care, 1983, 11, 384.

Duggan AW. Nociception and antinociception: physiological studies in the spinal cord. Clinics in Anaesthesiology, 1985, 3, 17.

Dumas JPh, JL Dupuis, M Suberville, C Chabanier-Poumier, P Colombeau. Analgesie péridurale morphinique continue dans les douleurs rebelles en urologie. Ann Urologie (Paris), 1985, 19, 280.

Duncan JAT. Intrathecal morphine as sole analgesic during labour (letter). Brit Med J, 1980, 20, 515.

Du Pen SL. After epidural narcotics - What next for cancer pain control. Anesth Analg, 1987, 66, S46. (a)

Du Pen SL, D Ramsey, S Chin. Chronic epidural morphine and preservative-induced injury. Anesthesiology, 1987, 67, 987. (b)

Du Pen SL, DG Peterson, A Gogosian, D Ramsey, C Larson, M Omoto. A new permanent exteriorized epidural catheter for narcotic self-administration to control cancer pain. Cancer, 1987, 59, 986. (c)

Du Pen SL. Epidural morphine: guidelines for the clinical management of cancer pain through epidural analgesia. Seattle, Congress, 1988 (personal communication)

Du Pen SL. Reply. Anesthesiology, 1988, 69, 288.

Du Pen SL, DH Ramsey. Diagnosis and treatment of epidural infections - a complication of long-term epidural narcotic administration. Anesthesiology, 1988, 69 (3A), A411.

Du Pen SL, DH Ramsey. Compounding local anaesthetics and narcotics for epidural analgesia in cancer out-patients. Anaesthesiology, 1988, 69 (3A) A405.

Du Pen SL, D Ramsey, S Chin. Chronic epidural morphine and preservative-induced injury. Anesthesiology, 1987, 67, 987.

Durant PAC, TL Yaksh. Distribution in cerebrospinal fluid blood, and lymph of epidurally injected morphine an inulin in dogs. Anesth Analg, 1986, 65, 583. (a)

Durant PAC, TL Yaksh. Epidural injections of bupivacaine, morphine, fentanyl, lofentanil and DADL in chronically implanted rats: a pharmacologic and pathologic study. Anesthesiology, 1986, 64, 43. (b)

Durant PAC, TL Yaksh. Drug effects on urinary bladder tone during spinal morphine-induced inhibition of the micturition reflex in unanesthetized rats. Anesthesiology, 1988, 68, 325.

Durkan WJ, LT Baker, CH Leicht. Postoperative epidural morphine analgesia after 3% 2-chloroprocaine (nesacaine-MPF) or lidocaine epidural anesthesia. Anesthesiology (Suppl), 1989, 71, 834.

D'Athis F, M Macheboeuf, H Thomas, C Robert, G Desch, M Galtier, P Mares, JJ Eledjam. Epidural analgesia with a bupivacaine-fentanyl mixture in obstetrics: comparison of repeated injections and continuous infusion. Can J Anaesth, 1988, 35, 116.

Ebert J, PD Varner. The effective use of epidural morphine sulfate for postoperative orthopedic pain. Anesthesiology, 1980, 53, 257.

Eckstein KL, Z Rogacev, A Vincente-Eckstein, Z Grahova. Prospektiv vergleichende Studie postspinaler Kopfschmerzen bei jungen Patienten (< 51 Jahre). Regional Anaesthesie, 1982, 5, 57.

Ecoffey C, J Attia, K Samii, Fr Kremlin-Bicetre. Analgesia and side effects following epidural morphine in children. Anesthesiology, 1985, 63, A470.

Ecoffey CL. Cancer pain. In: Edimav (Ed.): Congress Report, Montpellier Euromedicine, 1986, 231.

Ecoffey C. Spinal opiates. Schmerz, Pain, Douleur, 1989, 10, 58.

Editorial. Epidural and intrathecal morphine: an old analgesic finds a new use. Inpharma, 1980, Nov., 10. (a)

Editorial. Epidural opiates. Lancet, 1980, I, 962. (b)

540

Editorial. Spinal opiates revisted. Lancet, 1986, I, 655.

Edwards RD, NK Hansel, HT Pruessner, B Barton. Intrathecal morphine for labor pain. Texas Med, 1985, 81, 46.

Edwards WT, RG Burney, D Cappadona, U DeGirolami. Histopathologic changes induced in the epidural space and central neural elements of the guinea pig during chronic epidural morphine administration. Regional Anesthesia, 1985, 10, 45.

Edwards W, U DeGirolami, RG Burney, D Cappadona, R Brickley. Histopatholic changes in the epidural space of the guinea picduring long-term morphine infusion. Regional Anesthesia, 1986, 11, 14.

Ehring E, A Boekstegers. Mophologische-histologische Veränderungen durch kontinuierliche Periduralanalgesie bei einem Karzinom-Patienten. Regional Anaesthesie, 1986, 9, 46.

Eimerl D, D Papir-Kricheli, S Evron, A Carmon. The effects of on pain threshold in rats (letter). Pain, 1983,16, 2, 207. (a)

Eimerl D, D Papir-Kricheli, S Evron, A Carmon. Experimental epidural analgesia: direct effect of morphine at the spinal level In: JJ Bonica, et al. (Eds.): Advances in Pain Research and Therapy, Vol. 5, Raven Press New York, 1983, 487. (b)

Eimerl D, G Uretzky, J Chrubasik, P Magora. Continuous plus on demand epidural infusion of methadone for postoperative pain relief. II Int Symposium: Pain Clinic, 1986, Lille (France), Abst II P6. (a)

Eimerl D, F Magora, Y Shir, J Chrubasik. Patient-controlled analgesia with epidural methadone by means of an external infusion pump. Schmerz-Pain-Douleur, 1986, 4, 156. (b)

Eintraub SJ, JS Naulty. Acute abstinence syndrome after epidural injection of butorphanol. Anesth Analg, 1985, 64, 452.

Eisenach JC, JC Rose, DM Dewan, SC Grice. Intravenous clonidine produces fetal hypoxemia. Anesthesiology, 1987, 67, A 449. (a)

Eisenach JC, JC Rose, DM Dewan, SC Grice. Effects of epidural clonidine in pregnant ewes. Anesthesiology, 1987, 67, A448. (b)

Eisenach JC, S Grice. Epidural clonidine in sheep: hemodynamic and spinal cord blood flow effects. Pain, 1987, S4, S45. (c)

Eisenach JC, SC Grice. Epidural clonidine does not decrease bloodpressure or spinal cord blood flow in awake sheep. Anesthesiology, 1988, 68, 335. (a)

Eisenach JC, SC Grice, DM Dewan. Patient-controlled analgesia following cesarean section: a comparison with epidural and intramuscular narcatics. Anesthesiology, 1988, 68, 444. (b)

Eisenach JC. Demonstrating safety of subarchnoid calcitonin: patients or animals? (letter) Anesth Analg, 1988, 67, 298. (c)

Eisenach JC, SZ Lysak, MI Castro, DM Dewan. Epidural clonidine analgesia: an open-label, dose-ranging study. Anesth Analg (Suppl), 1989, 68, 79.

Eisenach JC, MI Castro, DM Dewan, JC Rose. Epidural clonidine analgesia in obstetrics: sheep studies. Anesthesiology, 1989, 70, 51.

El-Baz NMI, LP Faber, RJ Jensik . Continuous epidural infusion of morphine for treatment of pain after thoracic surgery. Anesth Analg, 1984, 63, 757.

El-Baz NMI, AR Ganzouri, W Gottschalk, AD Ivankovich, LP Faber. Thoracic epidural morphine analgesia for pain relief after thoracic surgery. Anesthesiology, 1982, 57, A205.

El-Baz NMI, MD Goldin. Continuous epidural mophine infusion for pain relief after open heart surgery. Anesthesiology, 1983, 59, A193. (a)

El-Baz NMI, RJ Jensik, LP Faber, AD Ivankovich. Epidural morphine for thoracic anaesthesia during the use of high frequency ventilation. Anesthesiology, 1983, 59, A373. (b)

El-Baz NMI, M Goldin. Continuous epidural infusion of morphine for pain relief after cardiac operations. J Thorac Cardiovasc Surg, 1987, 93, 878.

Ellis DJ, WL Millar, LS Reisner. Comparison of epidural and intravenous fentanyl infusions after cesarean section. Anesthesiology (Suppl), 1989, 71, 1153.

Ellis JS, S Ramamurthy. More problems with the Arrow-Racz epidural catheter (letter). Anesthesiology, 1986, 65, 124.

Elmas C. Thorakale peridurale Opiat-Analgesie. Regional Anaesthesie, 1986, 9, 120.

Engelman e, M Lipszyc, E Gilbart, P van der Linden, B Bellens, A van Romphey, M de Rood. Effects of clonidine on anesthetic drug requirements and hemodynamic response during aortic surgery. Anesthesiology, 1989, 71, 178.

England DW, IJ Davis, AE Timmins, R Downing, CWO Windsor. Gastric emptying: a study to compare the effects of intrathecal morphine and in papaveretum analgesia. Brit J Anaesth, 1987, 59, 1403.

Engquist A, MR Brandt, A Fernandes, H Kehlet. The blocking effect of epidural analgesia on the adrenocortical and hyperglycemic response to surgery. Acta Anaesth Scand, 1977, 21, 330.

Engquist A, J Chraemmer-Jørgensen, B Orgensen. Epidural morphine induced catatonia. Lancet, 1980, 1, 984. (a)

Engquist A, F Fog-Moller, C Christiansen, J Thode, T Vester- Andersen, SN Madsen. Influence of epidural analgesia on the cathecholamine and cyclic AMP responses to surgery. Acta Anaesth Scand, 1980, 24, 17. (b)

Engquist A, BC Jørgensen, HB Andersen. Catatonia after epidural morphine. Acta Anaesth Scand, 1981, 25, 445. (a)

Engquist A . Grundlagen der periduralen Opiate-Analgesie und klinische Erfahrungen. In: M Zenz (Ed.): Peridurale Opiat-Analgesie, Gustav Fischer Verlag, Stuttgart, 1981,1. (b)

Ercan ZS, M Ilhan, RK Tuerker. Alterations by captopril of pain reactions due to thermal stimulations of the mouse foot: interreactions with morphine, naloxone and aprotinin. Eur J Pharm, 1980, 63, 167.

Erickson DL, M Michaelson, JN Lo. Intrathecal morphine for treatment of pain due to malignacy. Pain (Suppl.), 1984, 2, S19.

Erickson DL, JB Blacklock, M Michaelson, KB Sperling, JN Lo. Control of spasticity by implantable continuous flow morphine pump. Neurosurgery, 1985, 16, 215.

Eriksen J, HB Andersen. Paintreatment on long term basis, using extradural opiates. Pain (Suppl.), 1984, 2, S335.

Eriksen S. Particulate contamination in spinal analgesia. Acta Anaesthesiol Scand, 1988, 32, 545.

Eriksson MBE, S Lindahl, JK Nyquist. Experimental cutaneous pain thresholds and tolerance in clinical analgesia with epidural morphine. Acta Anaesth Scand, 1982, 26, 654.

Estafanous FG. Opioids in Anesthesia. Butterworth Publishers, 1984, Boston.

Esteve M, JB Vedrenne, A Guillaume. Traitement ambulatoire des douleurs néoplasiques sus-diaphragmatiques - Injection de morphine par cathéters périduraux dorsaux et cervicaux. II Int Symposium: Pain Clinic, Lille (France), 1986, Abst IX FP 8.

Estok PM, PSA Glass, JS Goldberg, JJ Freiberger, RN Sladen. Use of patient controlled analgesia to compare intravenous to epidual administration of fentanyl in the postoperative patient. Anesthesiology, 1987, 67, A230.

Etches RC, AN Sandler. Analgesic effects of epidural nalbuphine in post-thoractomy patients. Can J Anaesth, 1989, 36 (Suppl), 156.

Etches RC, AN Sandler, M D Daley. Respiratory depression and spinal opioids. Can J Anaesth, 1989, 36, 165.

Evron S, A Samueloff, E Sadovsky, M Berger, F Magora. The effect of phenobenzamine on postoperative urinary complications during extradural morphine analgesia. Eur J Anaesth, 1984, 1, 45. (a)

Evron S, F Magora, E Sadovsky. Prevention of urinary retention with phenoxybenzamine during epidural morphine. Brit Med J, 1984, 288, 190. (b)

Evron S, A Samueloff, A Simon, B Drenger, F Magora. Urinary function during epidural analgesia with methadone and morphine in post cesarean section patients. Pain, 1985, 23, 135.

Faden AI, TP Jacobs. Dynorphin induces partially reversible paraplegia in the rats. Eur J Pharma, 1983, 91, 321.

Falke KJ, J Chrubasik, P Vitrac, S Blond, J Meynadier, M Zindler, Ph Scherpereel. Effectiveness of spinal salmon calcitonin in acute and chronic pain. II Int. Symposium: The Pain Clinic , 1986, Lille (France).

Famewo CE, M Naguib. Meperidine as sole agent for spinal anaesthesia. Can Anaesth Soc J, 1985, 32, S75. (a)

Famewo CE, M Naguib. Spinal anaesthesia with meperidine as the sole agent. Can Anaesth Soc J, 1985, 32, 533. (b)

Fanard L. Epidural sufentanil in caesarean section. Reports of the 5th. international Congress of the Belgien Society of Anaesthesia and Reanimation, Brussels 1988.

Farag H, M Naguib. Caudal morphine for pain relief following anal surgery. Annals of the Royal College of Surgeons of England, 1985, 67, 257.

Farcot JM, B Laugner, A Muller. Intéret des anesthésies épidurales à la morphine dans différents types de douleurs: 492 cas. Anesth Analg Réanim, 1981, 38, 351.

Farcot JM, JB Thiebaut, R Ramboatiana, B Laugner, S Rihaoui, A Muller, F Buchheit. Traitement de la douleur cancéreuse chronique par la morphine au niveau médullaire: y a-t-il une tolérance acquise. La Nouvelle Presse Médicale, 1982, 11, 3063. (a)

Farcot JM, B Laugner, A Muller. Therapeutic and diagnostic uses of morphine epidural in the management of pain. In: TL Yaksh, H Mueller (Eds.): Anaesthesiology and intensive care medicine N°144. Spinal opiate analgesia, experimental and clinical studies, Spinger-Verlag, Berlin, New York, 1982, 40. (b)

Farcot JM, JB Thiebaut, A Muller, J Zwiller, P Basset, MO Revel. Modifications des nucléotides cycliques du LCR induites par des injections de morphine: application à la tolérance. Symposium: Opioides et analgésie médullaire (opiods and spinal analgesia) Toulouse (France) 1984.

Farrar DJ, JL Osborn. The use of bromocriptine in the treatment of the unstable bladder. Brit J Urol, 1976, 48, 235.

Fasano M, HH Waldvogel. Peridural administration of morphine, with or without adrenalin, for postoperative analgesia. Acta Anaesth Belgica, 1982, 33, 195.

Fasmer OB, C Post. Behavioural responses induced by intrathecal injection of 5-Hydroxytryptamine in mice are inhibited by a substance P antagonist, D-Pro2,D-Trp7, 9-Substance P. Neuropharmacology, 1983, 22, 1397.

Fear DW, J Holmes. Epidural morphine. Can Anesth Soc J, 1982, 29, 286.

Fehm HL, KH Voigt, R Lang, KE Beinert, S Raptis, EF Pfeiffer. Somatostatin: a potent inhibitor of ACTH-hypersecretion in adrenal insufficiency. Klin Wochenschr, 1976, 54, 173.

Feith F. Intrathecal morphine administration with a manually operated implantable medication reservoir - Secor. II Int Symposium: The Pain Clinic, 1986, Lille (France), Abst III P 10.

Feldstein GS, SD Waldman, ML Allen. Reversal of apparent tolerance to epidural morphine by epidural methylprednisolone. Anesth Analg, 1987, 66, 264.

Ferreira SF. Site of analgesic action of aspirin-like drugs and opioids. In: Beers RF, EG Basset. (Eds.) Mechanisms of pain and analgesia compounds, Raven Press, New York, 1979, 309.

Ferreira SH. Peripheral analgesia: mechanism of the analgesic action of aspirin-like drugs and opiate antagonists. Brit J Clin Pharm, 1980, 10, S237.

Ferrier C, J Marty, Y Bouffard, JP Haberer, JC Levron, P Duvaldestin. Alfentanil pharmacokinetics in patients with cirrhosis. Anesthesiology, 1985, 62, 480.

Field HL, PC Emson, BK Leigh, RFF Gilgert, LL Iversen. Multiple opiate receptor sites on primary afferent fibers. Nature, 1980, 284, 351.

Fierro G, G Valente, G. Spadaro, F Petruzzi, N DePinto. Analgesia post-operatoria ottenuta mediante iniezione epidurale: valutazione comparativa di morfina e fentanyl. Ann Ital Chir, 1982, 54, 185.

Findler G, D Olshwang, M Hadani. Continuous epidural morphine treatment for intractable pain in terminal cancer patients. Pain, 1982, 14, 311.

Fine PG, MA Ashburn. Effect of stellate ganglion block with fentanyl on postherpetic neuralgia with a sympathetic component. Anesth Analg, 1988, 67, 897.

Fine PG, BD Hare, JC Zahniser. Epidural abscess following epidural catheterization in a chronic pain patient: a diagnostic dilemma. Anesthesiology, 1988, 69, 422.

Finholt DA, JA Stirt, CA DiFazio. Epidural morphine for postoperative analgesia in pediatric patients. Anesth Analg, 1985, 64, 211.

Fink BR. Mechanisms of differential axial blockade in epidural and subarachnoid anesthesia. Anesthesiology, 1989, 70, 851.

Finnegan B, D Moriarty. Opiate sensitivty - a case report. Ir J Med Sci, 1984, 153, 112.

Finster M, HO Morishima, H Pedersen, J Balkon. Meperidine: placental transfer after epidural im or iv injection. Anesthesiology, 1981, 55, A321.

Fiore CE, F Castorina, LS Malatino, C Tamburino. Antalgic activity of calcitonin: effectiveness of the epidural and subarachnoid routes in man. Int J Clin Pharm Res, 1983, 3, 257.

Fischer HBJ, PV Scott. Spinal opiate analgesia and facial pruritus. Anaesthesia, 1982, 37, 777.

Fischer R, T Lubenow, A Liceaga, RJ McCarthy, AD Ivankovich. A comparison of continuous epidural narcotic/local anaesthetic mixtures for postoperative analgesia. Anesth Analg, 1987, 66, S56.

Fischer RL, TR Lubenow, A Liceaga, RJ McCarthy, AD Ivankovich. Comparison of continuous epidural infusion of fentanyl-bupivacaine and morphine-bupivacaine in management of postoperative pain. Anesth Analg, 1988, 67, 559.

Fitzpatrick GF, DC Moriarty. Intrathecal morphine in the management of pain following cardiac surgery. Br J Anaesth, 1988, 60, 639.

Fiume D, M Piccini, M Tamorri. Two years experience of iterative intrathecal morphine for cancer patients. In: JM Besson, Y Lazorthes (Eds.): Spinal opioids and the relief of pain, INSERM, Paris, 1985, 477.

Flacke JW, BC Bloor, WE Flacke, D Wong, S Dazza, SW Stead, H Laks. Reduced narcotic requirement by clonidine with improved hemodynamic and adrenergic stability in patients undergoing coronary bypass surgery. Anesthesiology, 1987, 67, 11.

Flacke JW, WE Flacke, DF McIntee, BC Bloor. Dexmedetomidine: hemodynamic changes in autonomically denervated dogs. Anesthesiology (Suppl), 1989, 71, 495.

Fontanals Dotras J, W Espinosa Soldevilla, R Dubuisson Dumeny, JM Llopart Sulé, J Sainz López, JW Guitiérrez de Simone. Anesthesia locorregional tras la administración de petidina intradural. Rev Esp Anest Rean, 1986, 32, 273.

Fox GS. Epidural morphine for postoperative analgesia. Can J Surgery, 1988, 31, 14.

Fraioli F, A Fabbri, L Gnessi, C Moretti, C Santoro, M Felcici. Subarachnoid calcitonin for intolerable pain. Lancet, 1982, 2, P831.

Frame WT, RH Allison, DD Moir, WS Nimmo. Effect of naloxone on gastric emptying during labour. Brit J Anaesth, 1984, 56, 263.

Francis MD, D Justins, FJM Reynolds. Obstetric pain relief using epidural narcotic agents. Anaesthesia, 1981, 36, 69.

Francis RI, AS Lockhart. Epidural meptazinol (letter). Anaesthesia, 1986, 44, 88.

544

Franetski M, K Prestele, H Kresse. Entwicklungsstand bei programmgesteuerten Insulin-dosiergeräten. Electromedica, 1981, 1, 41.

Franetski M, K Prestele. Insulin delivery devices: what has been achieved, what is feasible, and which medical research is still needed to specify and optimize future devices. In: P Brunetti, et al. (Eds.): Artificial systems for insulin delivery, Raven Press, New York, 1983, 107.

Franetski M. Drug delivery by program or sensor controlled infusion devices. Pharm Res, 1984, 6, 237.

Frankhouser PL. More problems with the Arrow-Racz epidural catheter.Anesthesiology, 1986, 65, 124.

Fratkin J, DW Coombs, RL Saunders, C Allen, LH Maurer. Neuropathologic observations in cancer pain patients receiving chronic spinal analgesics. Schmerz-Pain-Douleur, 1985, 6, 116.

Fratta W, Casu M, A Balestrieri, A Leviselli, G Biggio, GI Fressa. Failure of ketamine to interact with opiate receptors. Eur J Pharmacol, 1980, 61, 389.

Frazier DT, K Murayama, NJ Abbott, T Narahashi. Effects of morphine on internally perfused squid giant axons. Proc Soc Exp Biol Med, 1972, 139, 434.

Frederickson RCA, V Burgus, CE Harrell, JD Edwards. Dual actions of substane P on nociception: possible role of endogenous opioids. Science, 1978, 199, 1359.

Frederickson RCA. Animal and human analgesic studies of metkephamid. In: KM Foley, CE Inturrisi (Eds.): Advances in Pain Research and Therapy, vol 8, Raven Press, New York, 1986, 293.

Freemann AB, L Hicks. Epidural fentanyl as a test dose. Anesth Analg, 1989, 68, 187.

Frenk H, LR Watkins, DJ Mayer. Differential behavioral effects induced by intrathecal microinjec-tion of opiates: comparison of convulsive and cataleptic effects produced by morphine, metha-done and D-Ala2-Methionine-Enkephalinamide. Brain Res, 1984, 299, 31. (b)

Frenk H, BE Stein. Endogenous opioids mediate ecs-induced catalepsy at supraspinal levels. Brain Res, 1984, 303, 109. (a)

Freye E, BN Gupta. A modified technique for the selective perfusion of the fourth cerebral ventricle in conscious dogs. Journal of pharmacological Methods, 1979, 2, 305.

Freye E, BN Gupta. Cardiovascular effects on selective perfusion on the fourth cerebral ventricle in cats with fentanyl, naloxone et methohexital. Indian J of Experimental Biology, 1980, 18, 29. (a)

Freye E, JO Arndt. Perfusion of fentanyl through the fourth cerebral ventricle and its cardiovascular effects in awake and halothane anesthetised dogs. Anaesthesist, 1980, 29, 208. (b)

Freye E, E Hartung. Fentanyl in the fourth cerebral ventricle causes respiratory depression in the anesthetized but not in the awake dog. Acta Anaesth Scand, 1981, 25, 171.

Freye E. Opioid agonists antagonists and mixed narcotic analgesics. Spinger-Verlag, Berlin, 1987.

Friedrich G, J Chrubasik, KL Scholler, P Weigel, H Roth, G Berg, V Renz, P Andreas. Rostral spread of radioactively labelled epidural morphine in dogs. In: W Erdmann, T Oyama, MJ Pernak (Eds.): Pain Clinic I, VNU, Science Press, Utrecht, 1985, 323. (a)

Friedrich G, J Chrubasik, Kl Scholler, K Weigel, HP Rupp. CSF Pharmacokinetics of extradural morphine. Brit J Anaesth, 1985, 57, 936. (b)

Friedrich G, J Chrubasik, Kl Scholler, P Andreas, HP Rupp, K Weigel, H Roth. Peridurale Morphinapplikation: Zum Risiko der Atemdepression. Schmerz, 1985, 1, 10. (c)

Frings N, B von Bormann, H Konder, H Lennartz. Lungenfunktion unter postoperativer periduraler Opiatanalgesie. Zentraleuropäischer Anaesthesiekongress, Berlin, 1981, 321.

Frings N, B von Bormann, H Lennartz. Peridurale Opiatanalgesie. Med Welt, 1982, 33, 163. (a)

Frings N, B von Bormann, U Kroh, H Lennartz. Peridurale Anaesthesie und Analgesieverfahren in der Allgemeinchirurgie. Chirurg, 1982, 53, 184. (b)

Fritz KW, E Lüllwitz, E Kirchner. Die epidurale Anwendung von Buprenorphin. Krankenhausarzt, 1982, 55, 778.

Fromme GA, JR Gray. A comparison of intrathecal and epidural morphine for treatment of post-thoracotomy pain. Anesth Analg, 1985, 64, 214. (a)

Fromme GA, LJ Steidl, DR Danielson. Comparison of lumbar and thoracic epidural morphine for relief of postthoracotomy pain. Anesth Analg, 1985, 64, 454. (b)

Fukushi S. Effects of epidural injection of beta endorphin on endocrine function in man. Jpn J Anesth, 1981, 30, 1112.

Fukushima K, M Nakamura. Postoperative analgesic effect of spinal and epidural morphine with different doses in gynecological surgery. Anesthesiology (Suppl), 1989, 71, 698.

Fukuuchi A, K Yokoyama. Epidural administration of pethidine for the postoperative pain relief (Author's transl). Masui, 1981, 30, 1122.

Furst SR, MB Weinger. Dexmedetomidine, a selective alpha-2 agonist, does not potentiate alfentanil-induced cardiovascular depression in the rat. Anesthesiology (Suppl), 1989, 71, 580.

Fyman P, M Avitable, F Moser, J Reynolds, P Casthely, K Butt, A Kopman. Sufentanil pharmacokinetics in patients undergoing renal transplantation. Anesth Analg, 1987, 66, S62.

Gal RJ, CA DiFazio. Prolonged antagonism of opioid action with intravenous nalmefene in man. Anesthesiology, 1986, 64, 175.

Gall DH, JN Lo, RL Gauthier, DL Erickson, M Michaelson. Intrathecal morphine for the treatment of spasticity. Anesthesiology, 1988, 69 (A3), A353.

Gallon AM. Epidural analgesia for thoracotomy patients. Physiotherapy, 1982, 68, 193.

Garcia-Guasch R, F Campo, P Bello, A Doria, JG Machado, MA Nalda. Extradural fentanyl with etidocaine or bupivacaine compared in hip surgery. 6th Eur congress of Anaesth, London, 1982, Volume of summaries, 360.

Garcia-March G, F Robaina, J Piquer, E Briz, E del Barrio, C Muriel, JL Rodriguez-Hernandez, M Barberá, R Badenes, JA de Vera, JL Barcia- Salorio, J Broseta. Administración intraventricular de morfina en el tratamiento del dolor de origen neoplásico. Estudio cooperativo. Rev Esp Anest Rean, 1986, 33, 68.

Gaumann DM, TL Yaksh. Intrathecal somatostatin in rats: antinociception only in the presence of toxic effects. Anesthesiology, 1988, 68, 733.

Gaumann DM, TL Yaksh, C Post, GL Wilcox, M Rodriguez. Intrathecal somatostatin in cat and mouse studies on pain, motor behavior and histopathology. Anesth Analg, 1989, 68, 623.

Gebert E, J Sarubin. Intrathecal morphine injection for cancer pain. 7th World Congress, Anaesth, Hamburg, 1980. Excerpta Medica, Int Congress Series 533, 458. (a)

Gebert E, J Sarubin, RA Yoeung. Morphin intrathekal, zur Bekämpfung von tumorbedingten und postoperativen Schmerzen. Anaesthesist, 1980, 29, 653. (b)

Gebert E. Überlegungen zu Material und Design der gebräuchlichen Periduralkatheter und zu ihrer Weiterentwicklung. Anaesth und Intensivmed, 1983, 24, 232.

Gebert E, W Grimm, H Nagel, H Scheid. Flüssigkeitsverteilung und Katheterlage im Periduralraum im Rahmen der postoperativen und karzinombedingten Schmerzbekämpfung. Anaesthesist, 1985, 32, 229.

Geerts P. Preservative in fentanyl preparations. Can J Anaesth, 1987, 43, 427.

Gehrmann JE, JR Killam. Assessment of CNS drug activity in rhesus monkeys by analysis of the EEG. Fed Proc, 1976, 35, 2258.

Gennari C, M Montagnani, G Francini, R Nanni, R Civitelli, E Maoili. Rationale dell'uso della calcitonina nelle osteolisi neoplastiche in "Simposio nazionale su calcitonina acquisizioni e prospettive, Venice (Italy) 6-7 March 1981, Abst N°4

Gepts E, L Heytens, F Camu. Pharmacokinetics of placental transfer of intravenous and epidural alfentanil in parturient women. Anesth Analg, 1986, 65, 1155.

Gerber HR. Nebenwirkungen der spinalen Opioidmedikation. Anaesth u. Intensivmed, 1986, 188, 416.

546

Gerber H. Regional anaesthesia. Acta Anaesth Scand (Suppl), 1988, 32,17.

Gerig HJ, F Kern. Postoperative Analgesie mit Morphium epidural nach Hüftoperationen. Anaesthesist, 1982, 31, 87.

Gerig HJ, F Kern. Epidurales Buprenorphin für postoperative Analgesie nach Hüftoperationen. Anaesthesist, 1983, 32, 345.

Germain H, L Frenette, A Néron. Antinociceptive action of clonidine in the epidural space. Pain (Suppl.), 1987, 4, S196.

Germain H, A Néron, A Lomssy. Analgesic effect of epidural clonidine. In: R Dubner, GF Gebhart, MR Blond (Eds.): Proceedings of the 5th World Congress on Pain, Elsevier Science Publishers BV, 1988, 472.

Gessler M, M Rust, R Egbert, W Zieglgänsberger, A Struppler. Segmentale Analgesie bei epiduraler Opiatapplikation. Anaesthesist (Suppl.), 1983, 32, 257.

Gestin Y. Morphinotherapie intrathécale, isobare chez les cancéreux hyperalgiques. In: Ars Medici, Bruxelles, Congress Series 3, II, 1982, 461.

Gestin Y. Morphinothérapie intrathécale ou morphinothérapie péridurale? Que choisir dans le traitement des algies néoplasiques? Méd et Hyg, 1984, 42, 3474.

Gestin Y, GH Safdari, N Pere. Successful paincontrol in neoplastic patients by intrathecal isobaric morphine injections. Int. Symposium Pain Therapy 1985, Rome, abstr. P. 28. (a)

Gestin Y, N Pere, Ch Solassol, P Stapf. Long term subarachnoid administration of morphine. Cahiers d'Anesthésiologie, 1985, 33, 47. (b)

Gestin Y. A propos de 200 abords intrathécaux pour morphinothérpie au long cours à domicile. Euromedecine 1986 Montpellier (France), Abstracts Editel Paris P 158.

Gestin Y. A totally implantable multi-dose pump allowing cancer patients intrathecal access for the self-administration. Anaesthesist, 1987, 36, 377.

Ghignone M, O Calvillo, L Quintin, S Caple, R Kozody. Haemodynamic effects of clonidine injected epidurally in halothane anesthetized dogs. Can J Anaesth, 1987, 34, 46.

Ghignone M, O Calvillo, T Lanier, L Quintin. Comparison of the hemodynamic effect of clonidine administered epidurally (epi) and intravenously (iv). Anesthesiology (Suppl), 1988, 69, 408.

Gibson SJ, JM Polak, SR Bloom, IM Sabate, PM Muldery, MA Ghatei, GP McGregor, JFB Morrison, JS Kelly, RM Evans, MG Rosenfeld. Calcitonin generelated peptide immunoreactivity in the spinal cord of man and of eight other species. J Neurosci, 1984, 4, 3101.

Gieraerts R, A Navalgund , L Vaes et al. Increased incidence of itching and herpes simplex in patients given epidural morphine after cesarean section. Anesth Analg, 1987, 66, 1321.

Gieraerts R, L Vaes, A Navalgund, J Jahr. Recurrent HSVL and the use of epidural morphine in obstetrics. Anesth Analg, 1989, 68, 418.

Gillman MA, FJ Lichtigfeld. Analgesic actions of naloxone suggest the presence of a hyperalgesic opioid system. SAMJ, 1986, 70, 650. (a)

Gillman MA, FJ Lichtigfeld. The hyperalgesic opioid system. S Afr J Sci, 1986, 82, 402. (b)

Gilly H, R Kramer, I Zahorovsky. Lokalanaesthetische Effekte von Morphin und Naloxon. Anaesthesist, 1985, 34, 619.

Gissen AJ, LD Gugino, S Datta, J Miller, BG Covino. Effects of fentanyl and sufentanil on peripheral mammalian nerves. Anesth Analg, 1987, 66, 1272.

Gissen D, LF Wong, M Naroll. Comparison of epidural lidocaine and bupivacaine-fentanyl mixture for extracorporeal shock wave lithotripsy. Regional Anesthesia, 1988, 13, 72.

Gjessing J, PJ Tomlin. Patterns of postoperative pain. A study of the use of continuous epidural analgesia in the postoperative period. Anaesthesia, 1979, 34, 624.

Gjessing J, PJ Tomlin. Postoperative pain control with intrathecal morphine. Anaesthesia, 1981, 36, 268.

Glass DD. Intraspinal morphine in trauma management. Intraspinal narcotic analgesia for acute and chronic pain. Palm Springs, USA, 1983, Symposium report.

Glass P, D Shafron, E Camporesi, J Reves, J Gustafsson, et al. RX77989: a new potent analgesic. Anesthesiology, 1987, 67, A244.

Glass PSA. Respiratory depression following only 0,4 mg of intrathecal morphine. Anesthesiology, 1984, 60, 256.

Glass PSA, B Biagi, S Sischy, E Camporesi. Analgesic action of very low dose intrathecal morphine (0.1 mg) as compared to higher doses (0.2-0.4 mg). Anesthesiology, 1985, 63, A236.

Glass PSA, EM Camporesi, D Shafron, T Quill. Evaluation of pentamorphone in humans: a new potent opiate. Anesth Analg, 1989, 68, 302.

Glenski JA, MA Warner, B Dawson, B Kaufman. Postoperative use of epidurally administered morphine in children and adolescents. Mayo Clin Proc, 1984, 59, 530.

Glynn C, D Dawson, R Sanders. A double-blind comparison between epidural morphine and epidural clonidine in patients with chronic non-cancer pain. Pain, 1988, 34, 123.

Glynn CJ, LE Mather, MJ Cousins, PR Wilson, JR Graham. Spinal narcotics and respiratory depression. Lancet, 1979, 2, 356.

Glynn CJ, LE Mather, MJ Cousins, JR Graham, PR Wilson. Selective spinal analgesia in man following epidural administration of pethidine. Anaesth Intens Care, 1980, 8, 371.

Glynn CJ, LE Mather, MJ Cousins JR Graham, PR Wilson. Peridural meperidine in humans. Analgetic response, pharmacokinetics and transmission into CSF. Anesthesiology, 1981, 55, 520.

Glynn CJ, LE Mather. Clinical pharmacokinetics applied to patients with intractable pain. Studies with pethidine. Pain, 1982, 13, 237.

Glynn CJ, PJ Teddy, MA Jamous, RA Moore. Role of spinal noradrenergic system in transmission of pain in patients with spinal cord injury. Lancet, 1986, 2, 1249.

Glynn CJ. Intrathecal and epidural administration of opiates. In: Update in Opioids. Baillieres Clinical Anaesthesiology, 1987, 1, 4, 915. (a)

Glynn CJ, A Jamous, D Dawson, R Sanders, PJ Teddy, RA Moore. The role of epidural clonidine in the treatment of patients with intractable pain. Pain, 1987, S4, S45. (b)

Gnanadurai TV. Postoperative care (letter). Brit Med J, 1980, 281, 944.

Goldfarb G, ET Ang, B Debaene, S Khon, P Jolis. Effect of clonidine on postoperative shivering in man: a double blind study. Anesthesiology (Suppl), 1989, 71, 650.

Goldman JM, LE Kirson, R Slover. Low-dose intrathecal morphine for postoperative analgesia in patients undergoing transurethral resection of the prostate. Anesth Analg, 1989, 68, S104.

Goldstein A. Opioid peptides (endorphins) in pituary and brain. Science, 1976, 193, 1081.

Gonzalez Navarro A, H Zimman Mansfeld, T Molinero Aparicio MJ Gonzales Hernandez, I Simon Ascarza. Intrathecal opiates for chronic pain in cancer patients. In: JM Besson, Y Lazorthes (Eds.): Spinal opioids and the relief of pain, Basic mechanisms and clinical applications. INSERM, Paris, 1985, 465.

Gonzalez Navarro A, MJ Gonzales Hernandez, H Zimman Mansfeld, T Molinero Aparicio. Epidural administration of calcitonin in pain due to bone metastasis. II Int Symposium: Pain Clinic, 1986, Lille (France), Abst IX FP 1.

Goodchild CS, JM Serrao. Intrathecal midazolam in the rat: evidence for spinally-mediated analgesia. Brit J Anaesth, 1987, 59, 1563.

Goodison R. Epidural narcotics (letter). Anaesth Intens Care, 1983, 2, 389.

Goodman Gilman A, Goodman LS, Gilman A. Goodman and Gilman's. The pharmacological basis of therapeutics. Seventh edition, Macmillan publishing Co., NY, 1985.

Gordh T, U Feuk, K Norlen. Effects of epidural clonidine on spinal cord blood flow and regional and central hemodynamics in pigs. Anesth Analg, 1986, 65, 1312. (a)

548

Gordh T, C Post, Y Olsson. Evaluation of the toxicity of subarachnoid clonidine, guanfacine and a substance P-antagonist on rat spinal cord. Anesth Analg, 1986, 65, 1303. (b)

Gordh T. Epidural clonidine for treatment of postoperative pain after thoracotomy. A double-blind placebo-controlled study. Acta Anaesth Scand, 1988, 32, 702.

Gough JD, AB Williams, RS Vaughan, JF Khalil, EG Butchart. The control of post-thoracotomy pain. A comparative evaluation of thoracic epidural fentanyl infusions and cryo-analgesia. Anaesthesia, 1988, 43, 780.

Gourlay GK, DA Cherry, MJ Cousins. Cephalad migration of morphine in CSF following lumbar epidural administration in patients with cancer pain. Pain, 1985, 23, 317.

Gourlay GK, DA Cherry, JL Plummer, PJ Armstrong, MJ Cousins. The influence of drug polarity on the absorption of opioid drugs intro CSF and subsequent cephalad migration following lumbar epidural administration: application to morphine and pethidine. Pain, 1987, 31, 297.

Gourlay GK, TM Murphy, JL Plummer, SR Kowalski, DA Cherry, MJ Cousins. Pharmacokinetics of fentanyl in lumbar and cervical CSF following lumbar epidural and intravenous administration. Pain, 1989, 38, 253.

Gowan JD, JB Hurtig, RA Fraser, J Kitts, E Torbicki. Lumbar epidural morphine and prophylactic naloxone infusion for post-thoracotomy analgesia. Effects on quality of analgesia and side effects. Anaesth Analg, 1987, 66, S72. (a)

Gowan JD, JB Hurtig, RA Fraser. Epidural bupivacaine at wound closure is a useful adjuvant epidural morphine in the prevention of early post-thoracotomy pain. Can Anaesth Soc J, 1987, 34, 3 (part II), S99. (b)

Gowan JD, JB Hurtig, RA Fraser, E Torbicki, J Kitts. Naloxone infusion after prophylactic epidural morphine: effects on incidence of postoperative side effects and quality of analgesia. Can J Anaesth, 1988, 35, 143.

Grabow L. Schmerzbehandlung durch sub-oder epidurale Opiatapplkation (Pain treatment by sub- or epidural opiate administration). Anaesth Intensivther Notfallmed, 1982, 17, 161. (a)

Grabow L, G Kremer, H Stannigel, P Wesierski. Schmerzbehandlung durch intraoperative epidurale Opiatapplikation bei Eingriffen an der Wirbelsäule. Anaesth Intensivther Notfallmed, 1982, 17, 96. (b)

Grabow L, F Schubert. Karzinompatienten: auch zu Hause ohne Schmerzen. Ärztl Praxis, 1982, 90, P3050. (c)

Grabow L. Opiate und Leitungsanaesthetika epidural in der postoperativen Schmerzbekämpfung. Anaesth und Intensivmed, 1986, 188, 352.

Graham JL, R King, W McCaughey. Postoperative pain relief using epidural morphine. Anaesthesia, 1980, 35, 158.

Grant GJ, S Ramanathan, H Turndorf. Epidural fentanyl reduces isoflurane requirements during thoracotomy. Anesthesiology (Suppl), 1989, 71, 668.

Grant IS. Drowsiness after epidural opioids (letter). Anaesthesia, 1986, 41, 431.

Gray JR, GA Fromme, LE Nauss, JK Wang, DM Ilstrup. Intrathecal morphine for postthoracotomy pain. Anesth Analg, 1986, 65, 873.

Greeley WJ, NP de Bruijn, DP Davis. Pharmacokinetics of sufentanil in pediatric patients. Anesthesiology, 1986, 65, A422.

Greenberg R, EH O'Keefe, MJ Antonaccio. Inhibition of met- enkephalin inactivation by captopril (SQ 14225) in the isolated myenteric plexus-longitudinal muscle strip of guinea-pig ileum. Fed Proc, 1979, 38, 457.

Greenberg HS, J Taren, WD Ensminger, K Doan. Benefit from and tolerance to continuous intrathecal infusion of morphine for intractable cancer pain. J Neurosurg, 1982, 57, 360.

Greenberg HS. Continuous lumbar intrathecal infusion of morphine for intractable cancer pain. Intraspinal narcotic analgesia for acute and chronic pain. Palm Springs, USA, 1983, Symposium report.

549

Greenberg HS. Continuous spinal opioid infusion for intractable pain. In: KM Foley, CI Inturrisi (Eds.): Advances Pain Research and Therapy. Raven Press, Vol 8, 1986, 351.

Greene BA. A 26-gauge lumbar puncture needle: its value in the prophylaxis of headache following spinal analgesia for vaginal delivery. Anesthesiology, 1950, II, 464.

Gregory MA, JG Brock-Utne, S Bux, JW Downing. Morphine concentration in brain and spinal cord after subarachnoid morphine injection in baboons. Anesth Analg, 1985, 64, 929.

Greiner L, L Ulatowksi, P Prohm. Sonographisch gezielte und intraoperative Alkoholblockade der Zöliakalganglien. Ultraschall, 1983, 4, 57.

Grey D. Intrathecal morphine: relief from intractable pain. Can Nurse, 1983, 79, 50.

Gribomont B. Mode d'action comparée des anesthésiques locaux et des opiacés au niveau spinal. In: Ars Medici, Bruxelles, Congress Series 3, I, 1982, 185.

Grice SC, JC Eisenach, DM Dewan, J Weiner. Effect of epinephrine on the duration of analgesia with epidural bupivacaine and fentanyl. Anesthesiology, 1987, 67, A440.

Grice SC, JC Eisenach, DM Dewan. Effect of 2-chloroprocain test dosing on the subsequent duration of labor analgesia with epidural bupivacaine-fentany- epinephrine. Anesthesiology, 1988, 69 (3A), A668.

Grossi P, S Arnér. Effect of epidural morphine on the Hoffman-reflex in man. Acta Anaesth Scand, 1984, 28, 152.

Grum DF, LG Swenson, J Blum. Intrathecal papaverine for thoracic aortic aneurysm resection: a preliminary report. Anesthesiology, 1988, 69 (3A) A894.

Guéneron JP, C Ecoffey, P Carli, D Benhamou, JB Gross, K Samii. Influence of naloxone infusion on respiratory depression following epidural fentanyl. Anesthesiology, 1986, 65, A174.

Guéneron JP, C Ecoffey, P Carli, D Benhamou, JB Gross. Effect of naloxone infusion on analgesia and respiratory depression after epidural fentanyl. Anesth Analg, 1988, 67, 35.

Guerin JM, B Deraison, M Alouini, E Leleu, D Montpellier, M Ossart. Morphinomimétiques et anesthésiques locaux par voie intrarachidienne. Application à la chirurgie urologique. Ann Fr Anesth Réanim 1983, 2, 232.

Gugath M. Schmerzbehandlung durch epidurale Opiatanalgesie. Med Klinik, 1985, 80, 437.

Guillemin R, N Ling, R Burgus. Endorphines, peptides, d'origine hypothalamique et neurohypo- physaire à activité morphinomimétique. Isolement et structure moléculaire de l'alpha endor- phine. CR Acad Sci (D), Paris 1976, 282, 783.

Gundersen RY, R Andersen, G Narverud. Postoperative pain relief with high-dose epidural buprenorphine: a double blind study. Acta Anaesth Scand, 1986, 30, 664.

Gupta B, JHJ Brooks, GA Tejwani, AK Rattan. Narcotic receptors in human peripheral nerves. Anesthesiology (Suppl), 1989, 71, 635.

Gürel A, N Ünal, M Elevli, A Eren. Epidural morphine for postoperative pain relief in anorectal surgery. Anesth Analg, 1986, 65, 499.

Gustafsson LL, B Feychting, C Klingstedt. Late respiratory depression after concomitant use of morphine epidurally and parenterally. Lancet, 1981, 1, 892.

Gustafsson LL, S Ackerman, H Adamson, M Garle, A Rane, B Schildt. Disposition of morphine in cerebrospinal fluid after epidural administration. Lancet, 1982, 1, 796. (a)

Gustafsson LL, S Friberg-Nielsen, M Garle, A Mohall, A Rane, B Schildt, T Symreng. Extradural and parenteral morphine. Kinetics and effects in postoperative pain. A controlled clinical study. Brit J Anaesth, 1982, 54, 1167. (b)

Gustafsson LL, M Garle, J Johannisson, A Rane, J Stenport, P Walson. Regional epidural analgesia: kinetics of pethidine. Acta Anaesth Scand, 1982, 26, 165. (c)

Gustafsson LL, B Schildt, K Jacobsen. Adverse effects of extradural and intrathecal opiates. Report of a nationwide survey in Sweden. Brit J Anaesth, 1982, 54, 479. (d)

Gustafsson LL, AM Grell, M Garle, A Rane, B Schildt. Kinetics of morphine in cerebrospinal fluid after epidural administration. Acta Anaesth Scand, 1984, 28, 535.

Gustafsson LL, C Post, B Edvardsen, CH Ramsey. Distribution of morphine and meperidine after intrathecal administration in rat and mouse. Anesthesiology, 1985, 63, 483.

Gustafsson L, J Johannisson, M Garle. Exradural and parenteral pethidine as analgesia after analgesia after total hip replacement: effects and kinetics. Eur J Clin Pharmacol, 1986, 29, 529. (a)

Gustafsson LL, C Post. The degree of analgesia correlates to spinal morphine concentration after intrathecal administration in rats. Acta Pharm et Toxicol, 1986, 58, 243. (b)

Gustafsson L, Z Wiesenfeld-Hallin. Spinal opioid analgesia: a critical update. Drugs, 1988, 35, 597.

Gustafsson LL, P Hartvig, K Bergström, H Lundqvist, BS Lindberg, B Längström, H Svärd, H Rane, A Tamsen. Distribution of 11-C-labelled morhine and pethidine after spinal administration to rhesus monkey. Acta Anaesth Scand, 1989, 3, 105.

Haag W, E Hartung, E Freye. Erfahrungen mit Buprenorphin als Monoanaesthetikum und in Kombination mit Bupicacain bei periduralen Katheteranaesthesien. III. Internationales Symposium. New Aspects in Regional Anaesthesia. Düsseldorf O4.O7.-05.07. 1982.

Haavik PE. Epidural morphine for analgesia after caeserean section. Can Anaesth Soc J, 1983, 30, 108.

Håkanson E, H Rutberg, L Jorfeldt, J Mårtensson. Effects of the extradural administration of morphine or bupivacaine, on the metabolic response to upper abdominal surgery. Brit J Anaesth, 1985, 57, 394.

Hakanson E, M Bengtsson, H Rutberg, AM Ulrick. Epidural morphine by the thoracic or lumbar routes in cholecystectomy. Effect on postoperative pain and respiratory variables. Anaesth Intens Care, 1989, 17, 166.

Hales P. Pruritus after epidural morphine. Lancet, 1980, 2, 204.

Hall GM, C Youg, A Holdcraft, J Alaghband-Zadeh. Substrate mobilisation during surgery. Anaesthesia, 1978, 33, 924.

Hallworth RE. Epidural narcotic analgesia. J Am Osteopath Assn, 1984, 84, 47.

Hamar O, S Csoemoer, Z Kazy, Z Vigva'ry. Epidural morphine analgesia by means of subcutaneously tunneled catheter in patients with gynecologic cancer. Anesth Analg, 1986, 65, 531.

Hammond JE. Reversal of opioid-associated late-onset respiratory depression by nalbuphine hydrochloride. Lancet, 1984, 2, 1208.

Hammonds W, RS Bramwell, CC Hug, Z Najak, A Critz. A comparison of epidural meperidine and bupivacaine for relief of labor pain. Anesth Analg, 1982, 61, 187.

Hampton WA, NG Lavies, JW Downing, JG Brock-UTne, RT Salisbury, KI Elson. Cisternal cerebrospinal fluid concentrations of morphine following intrathecal and epidural administration in the babbon. Anaesth Intens Care, 1987, 15, 445.

Han JS, CW Xie. Dynorphin: potent analgesic effect in spinal cord of the rat. Life Sci, 1982, 31, 16-17, 1781-4. (a)

Han JS, GX Xie, ZF Zhou, R Folkesson, L Terenius. Enkephalin and beta-endorphin as mediators of electro-acupuncture analgesia in rabbits: an antiserum microinjection study. Adv Biochem Psychopharmacol, 1982, 33, 369. (b)

Han JS, CW Xie. Dynorphin: potent analgesic effect in spinal cord of the rat. Sci Sin (b), 1984, 27, 169. (a)

Han JS, GX Xie. Dynorphin: important mediator for electroacupuncture analgesia in the spinal cord of the rabbit. Pain, 1984, 18, 367. (b)

Han JS, GX Xie, A Goldstein. Analgesia induced by intrathecal injection of dynorphin in the rat. Life Sci, 1984, 34, 1573. (c)

Hanaoka K, S Itoh, T Kugimiya, N Tachibama, H Yamamura. Analgesic effect of buprenorphine on postoperative pain by epidural injection. Journal of the Association of Anaesthesists of Great Britain and Ireland, 6th European Congress of Anaesthesiology, London, Academic Press Grune

& Stratton, London, Toronto, Sydney, New York, San Francisco, 1982.

Hanks GW, RG Twycross, JW Lloyd. Unexpected complication of successful nerve block. Anaesthesia, 1981, 36, 37.

Hanks GW. Pain the physiological antagonist of opioid analgesics. Lancet, 1984, 1, 1477.

Hanson AL, B Hanson, M Matousek. Epidural anasthesia for cesarean section. Acta Obstet Gynecol Scand, 1984, 63, 135.

Harbaugh RE, DW Coombs, RL Saunders, M Gaylor, M Pageau. Implanted continuous epidural morphine infusion system. J Neurosurg, 1982, 56, 803.

Harbaugh RE. Epidural morphine infusion for chronic non-cancer pain. Intraspinal narcotic analgesia for acute and chronic pain. Palm Springs, USA, 1983, Symposium report.

Hardy PAJ, JCD Wells. Pain after spinal intrathecal clonidine. Anaesthesia, 1988, 43, 1026.

Hare BD, DN Franz. Opiate and clonidine receptors on spinal sympathtic neurons inhibit adenylate cyclase to produce neuronal depression. Pain (Suppl.), 1987, 2, 349.

Harfstrand A, M Kalia, K Fuxe, L Kaijer, LF Agnati. Somatostatin- induced apnea: interaction with hypoxia and hypercapnia in rats. Neuroscience letters, 1984, 50, 37.

Harmer M, M Rosen, MD Vickers. Patient-controlled analgesia. Blackwell Scientific Publications, Oxford, 1985.

Harris MNE. Intrathecal morphine and respiratory depression. VII Eur Congress, 1986, Vienna (Austria), Report, Abst. 415.

Harris MM, MD Kahana, TS Park. Intrathecal morphine for postoperative analgesia in children. Anesth Analg, 1989, 68, S116.

Harrison DM, RS Sinatra, L Morgese, JH Chung, ALZ Mandel. Epidural and patient controlled analgesia for postcesarean section pain relief. Anesthesiology, 1986, 65, A364.

Harrison GR. A model of the extradural space and a reappraisal of the extradural space pressure. Brit J Anaesth, 1987, 59, 1177.

Harrison DM, R Sinatra, L Morgese, JH Chung. Epidural narcotic and patient-controlled analgesia for postcesarean section pain relief. Anesthesiology, 1988, 68, 454.

Hårtensson J. Effects of the extradural administration of morphine or bupivacaine, on the metabolic response to upper abdominal surgery. Brit J Anaesth, 1985, 57, 394.

Hartrick CT, CE Pither, U Pai, PP Raj, TA Tomsick. Subdural migration of an epidural catheter. Anesth Analg, 1985, 64, 175.

Hartung HJ, R Klose, W Wiest, H Bauknecht, A Hettenbach. Die Morphin-induzierte Peridural-anaesthesie. Anaesth Intensivther Notfallmed, 1980, 15, 396. (a)

Hartung HJ, W Wiest, R Klose, H Bauknecht, A Hettenbach. Epidurale Morphin-Injektion zur Schmerzbekämfung in der Geburtshilfe. Fortschr Med, 1980, 98, 3. (b)

Hartung HJ, R Klose, M Schäfer, P Berg. Epidurale Buprenorphin- Applikation und CO2-Antwort. VII Eur Congress of Anaesth, 1986, Vienna (Austria), Report, abst 417.

Hartvig P, K Bergström, B Lindberg, PO Lundberg, et al. Regional distribution in the brain of rhesus monkeys of 11 c-opiates measured with emission tomography. In: Foley KM, et al. (Eds.): Adv in Pain Research and Therapy, Raven Press New York, Vol 8, 1986, 73.

Hartvig P, T Gordh, PG Gillberg, J Petterson, I Jansson, C Post. Spinal carbachol analgesia in the rat. Pain (Suppl.), 1987, 4, S197.

Hasenbos M, J van Egmond, M Gielen, JF Crul. Postoperative analgesia by epidural versus intramuscular nicomorphine after thoracotomy. Part I. Acta Anaesthesiol Scand, 1985, 29, 572. (a)

Hasenbos M, J van Egmond, M Gielen, JF Crul. Postoperative analgesia by epidural versus intramuscular nicomorphine after thoracotomy. Part II. Acta Anaesth Scand, 1985, 29, 577. (b)

Hasenbos M, M Simon, J van Egmond, H Folgering, P van Hoorn. Postoperative analgesia by nicomorphine intramuscularly versus high thoracic epidural administration. Acta Anaesth Scand, 1986, 30, 426.

552

Hasenbos M, J van Egmond, M Gielen, JF Crul. Postoperative analgesia by high thoracic epidural versus intramuscular nicomorphine after thoractomy. Part III. Acta Anaesth Scand, 1987, 31, 608.

Hasenbos MA, MJM Gielen, J Bos, E Tielbeek, M Stantan-Hicks, J van Egmond. High thoracic epidural sufentanil for post-thoracotomy pain: influence of epinephrine as an adjuvant - a double blinc study. Anesthesiology, 1988, 69, 1017.

Hassan HG, B Åkerman, CWT Pilcher, H Renck. Antinociceptive effects of localized administration of opioids compared with lidocaine. Regional Anesthesia, 1989, 14, 138.

Hauck W, A Komnos, B Schnapka. Le controle radiologique des cathéters périduraux: une mesure indispensable. II Int Symposium: The Pain Clinic, 1986, Lille (France) Abst II P 2.

Havliecek V, FS Labella, C Pinsky, R Childiaeva. Beta-endorphin induces general anaesthesia by interaction with opiate receptors. Can Anaesth Soc J, 1980, 27, 535.

Heinrich-Roussignol MC. Analgésie médullaire aux opiacés. Thèse pour le Doctorat en médecine, Faculté de médecine de Rouen 1982.

Helmers JH, H Noorduin, AA Adam, J Giezen, L van Leeuwen. Anaesthesia with alfentanil in the geriatric patient. Anaesthesist (Suppl.), 1983, 32, 228.

Helmers JH, van Peer, R Woestenborghs. Alfentanil kinetics in the elderly. Clin Pharm Ther, 1984, 36, 239.

Hempelmann G, H Müller. Morphin und Naloxon. Deut Med Wochenschr, 1981, 106, 411. (a)

Hempelmann G, H Müller (Eds.) Peridurale Opiatanalgesie. Bibliomed, Melsungen, 1981. (b)

Henderson SK, H Cohen. Nalbuphine augmentation of analgesia and reversal of side effects following epidural hydromorphone. Anesthesiology, 1986, 65, 216.

Henderson SK, EB Matthew, H Cohen, M Avram. Epidural hydromorphone: a double-blind comparison with intramuscular hydromorphone for postcesarean section analgesia. Anesthesiology, 1987, 66, 825.

Hendrickx P, R Abou Hatem, C Nicaise. Implantable injection port for epidural opiates self-administration. Acta Anesth Belgica (Suppl.), 1984, 35, 279.

Hennek K, FW Sydow. Die thorakale Periduralanaesthesie zur intra- und postoperativen Analgesie bei Lungenresektionen. Regional Anaesthesie, 1984, 7, 115.

Henry A, J Cheesman, J Sheldon. A trial of the Pen Pump infuser. Practical Diabetes, 1985, 2, 42.

Henry JL. Pharmacological studies on the prolonged depressant effects of baclofen on lumbar dorsal horn units in the cat. Neuropharmacology, 1982, 21, 1085.

Henry M, A Graizon, J Seebacher, D Vauthier, JC Levron, P Viars. Epidural fentanyl with and without epinephrine plasma levels and pain relief. Anesthesiology, 1988, 69 (3A), A391.

Henry M, A Graizon, J Seebacher, D Vauthier, JC Levron, P Viars. Fentanyl adrénaline ou non par voie péridural en obstétrique: dosages plasmatiques et effets analgesiques. Ann Fr Anesth Réan, 1989, 8 R62.

Herman BH, A Goldstein. Antinociception and paralysis induced by intrathecal dynorphin A. Pharm Exp Ther, 1985, 232, 27.

Herman RM, MC Wainberg, PF delGiudice, MK Willscher. The effect of a low dose of intrathecal morphine on impaired micturition reflexes in human subjects with spinal cord lesions. Anesthesiology, 1988, 69, 313.

Herrera-Hoys JO. Surgery under regional analgesia with narcotics as single agents (letter). Anaesthesia, 1983, 38, 509.

Herz A, HJ Teschemacher. Activities and sites of antinociceptive action of morphine like analgesics and kinetics of distribution following intravenous, intracerebral and intraventricular application. Adv Drug Res, 1971, 6, 79.

Herz A, K Albus, J Metys, P Schubert, HJ Teschemacher. On the central sites for the antinociceptive action of morphine and fentanyl. Neuropharmacology, 1970, 98, 539.

Herz A. Biochemie und Pharmakologie des Schmerzgeschehens. Im: Zimmerman, HO Handwerker (Eds.): Schmerz, Springer-Verlag, 1984, p 61.

Herz A. Opioid peptides and opioid receptors: new perspective for an understanding of analgesic actions. VII Eur Congress of Anaesth, 1986, Vienna (Austria), Report, Abst 802. (a)

Herz A. Endogenous opioid and pain. Symposium on Pain Control, Leuven (Belgium), Nov 1986. (b)

Hettenbach H, W Wiest, HJ Hartung. Peridurale Morphin-Analgesie zur Bekämpfung von tumorbedingten Schmerzen bei gynäkologischen Karzinompatientinnen. Geburtsh Frauenheilk, 1984, 44, 503.

Heykants JJP. Janssen-Pharmaceutica Research Laboratory. Unpublished Report.

Heytens L, H Cammu, F Camu. Extradural analgesia during labour using alfentanil. Brit J Anaesth, 1987, 59, 331.

Hilgier M, J Kacki, B Kaminski. Epidural morphine for postoperative pain prevention. 7th World Congress of Anaesth, Hamburg, 1980, Excerpta Medica, Int Congress series 533, p 459.

Hirlekar G. Is itching after caudal epidural morphine dose related? Anaesthesia, 1981, 36, 68.

Hirsh LF, A Thanki, T Nowak. Sudden loss of pain control with morphine pump due to catheter migration. Neurosurgery, 1985, 17, 965.

Hisamitsu T, WC de Groat. The inhibitory effect of opioid peptides and morphine applied intrathecally and intracerebroventricularly on the micturition reflex in the cat. Brain Res, 1984, 298, 51.

Hitchon PW, V Kumar, JC van Gilder. Intrathecal morphine for cancer related. Pain, 1987, S4, S390.

Hjortsø E, T Vester-Andersen, IW Møller, M Lunding. Epidural morphine for postoperative pain relief. Acta Anaesth Scand, 1982, 26, 528.

Hjortsø NC, T Andersen T, F Frøsig, P Neumann, E Rogon, H Kehlet. Failure of epidural analgesia to modify postoperative depressionof delayed hypersensitivity. Acta Anaesth Scand, 1984, 28, 128.

Hjortsø NC, NJ Christensen, T Andersen T, H Kehlet. Effects of the extradural administration of local anaesthetic agents and morphine on the urinary excretion of cortisol, catecholamines and nitrogen following abdominal surgery. Brit J Anaesth, 1985, 57, 400. (a)

Hjortsø NC, P Neumann, F Frøsig, T Andersen, A Lindhard, E Rogon, H Kehlet. A controlled study on the effects of epidural analgesia with local anaesthetics and morphine on morbidity after abdominal surgery. Acta Anaesth Scand, 1985, 29, 790. (b)

Hjortsø NC, C Lund, T Mogensen, D Bigler, H Kehlet. Epidural morphine potentiates pain relief and maintains sensory analgesia during continuous epidural bupivacaine after abdominal surgery. Anesthesiology, 1986, 65, A178. (a)

Hjortsø NC, C Lund, T Mogensen, D Bigler, H Kehlet. Epidural morphine improves pain relief and maintains sensory analgesia during continuous epidural bupivacaine after abdominal surgery. Anesth Analg, 1986, 65, 1033. (b)

Hoekfelt T, L Skirboll, CJ Dalsgaard, et al. Peptide neurons in the spinal cord with special reference to descending systems. In: B Sjoelund, J Bjoiklund (Eds.): Brain Stem Control of Spinal Mechanisms, Elsevier Biomedical Press, Amsterdam, 1982, 89.

Hoel TM, B Lind. Spinal needles, gauge and headache. Brit J Med, 1987, 59, 808.

Hoffman GM, LC Remynse, AJ Casale, C Francis. Caudal morphine analgesia in children: efficacy advantages, and side effects compared to parenteral morphine. Anesthesiology (Suppl), 1989, 71,

554

1019.

Højkjaer-Larsen V, AD Iversen, P Christensen, PK Andersen. Postoperative pain treatment after upper abdominal surgery with epidural morphine at thoracic or lumbar level. Acta Anaesth Scand, 1985, 29, 566.

Højkjaer-Larsen V, P Christensen, MM Brinkløv, F Axelsen. Postoperative pain relief and respiratory performance after thoracotomy: a controlled trial comparing the effect of epidural morphine and subcutaneous nicomorphine. Dan Med Bull, 1986, 33, 161.

Holland AJC, SK Srikantha, JA Tracey. Epidural morphine and postoperative pain relief. Can Anaesth Soc J, 1981, 28, 453.

Holland RB, MW Levitt, LA Whitton, N Shadbolt. Carbon dioxide response after epidural morphine. Anaesthesia, 1982, 37, 753.

Holmberg L, I Odar Cederlof, LOL Heyner, M Ehrnebo. Comparative dispositions of pethidine and norpethidine in old and young patients. Europ J Clin Pharm, 1982, 22, 175.

Horan CT, DG Beeby, JB Brodsky, HA Oberhelman. Segmental effect of lumbar epidural hydromorphone: a case report. Anesthesiology, 1985, 62, 84.

Hord AH. Comparing the efficacy of epidural opiates with that of patient-controlled analgesia. Anesthesiology, 1988, 69, 632.

Hoskin PJ, GW Hanks. Opioid therapy in malignant disease. In: Update in Opioids p 883. Baillieres Clinical Anaesthesiology, 1987, 1, 4.

Hotvedt R, H Refsum. Cardiac effects of thoracic epidural morphine caused by increased vagal activity in the dog. Acta Anaesth Scand, 1986, 30, 76.

Houde RW. Analgesic effectiveness of the narcotic agonists - antagonists. Brit J Clin Pharm, 1979, 7, 297.

Houghton A. Postoperative analgesia in orthopaedic surgery. Anaesthesia, 1982, 37, 471.

Houlton PG, F Reynolds. Epidural diamorphine and fentanyl for postoperative pain. Anaesthesia, 1981, 36, 1144.

Howard EC, GR Murray, TN Calvey, NE Williams. Prolonged release extradural morphine. Ann R Coll Surg Engl, 1985, 67, 8.

Howard RP, LA Milne, NE Williams. Epidural morphine in terminal care. Anaesthesia, 1981, 36, 51.

Huang HJ, T Ishimaru, T Yamabe. Intrathecal morphine for postoperative pain relief. Asia Oceania J Obstet Gynaecol, 1984, 10, 197.

Huckaby T, K Gerard, J Scheidlinger, Johnson, S Datta. Continuous epidural infusion of alfentanil-bupivacaine vs bupivacaine for labor and delivery. Anesthesiology (Suppl), 1989, 71, 847.

Hug CC. Improving analgesic therapy. Anesthesiology, 1980, 53, 441.

Hug CC, S DeLange. Alfentanil pharmacokinetics in patients before and after cardiopulmonary bypass. Anesth Analg, 1983, 62, 266.

Hug CC, Chaffman M. In alfentanil, pharmacology and uses in anaesthesia. ADIS Press, Ed. Camu F, J Spierdyk, Auckland, N. Zealand, 1984, 1. (a)

Hug CC. Pharmacokinetics of new synthetic narcotic analgesics. In: FC Estafanous (Ed.): Opioids in Anesthesia, Butterworth, London, 1984, 50. (b)

Hughes SC. Intraspinal narcotics in obstetrics. Clin Perinatol, 1982, 1, 167.

Hughes SC. Intraspinal narcotics for postoperative pain and obstetrics. Intraspinal narcotic analgesia for acute and chronic pain. Palm Springs, USA, 1983, Symposium report. (a)

Hughes SC. Complications of intraspinal narcotics. Intraspinal narcotic analgesia for acute and chronic pain. Palm Springs, USA, 1983, Symposium report. (b)

Hughes SC. Intraspinal administration of narcotics: a new approach to pain. Western J Medicine, 1984, 140, 440. (a)

Hughes SC, MA Rosen, SM Shnider, TK Abboud, SJ Stefani, M Norton. Maternal and neonatal effects of epidural morphine for labor and delivery. Anesth Analg, 1984, 63, 319. (b)

Hughes SC, RG Wright, D Murphy, P Preston, W Hughes, M Rosen, S Shnider. The effect of pH adjusting 3% 2-chloroprocaine on the quality of postcesarean section analgesia with epidural morphine. Anesthesiology, 1988, 69 (3A), A689.

Hu Gy, FX Zhong, K Tsou. Dissociation of supraspinal and spinal morphine analgesia by reserpine. Eur J Pharm, 1984, 97, 129.

Hui YL, CS Liew. Implanted epidural morphine analgesic therapy for terminal cancer patients. VII Eur Congress of Anaesth, 1986, Vienna (Austria). Report, Abst 429.

Hull JC. The pharmacokinetics of alfentanil in man. Br J Anaesth, 1983, 55, 157S.

Hull JC. The pharmacokinetics and pharmacodynamics of opioids. Mises au point en anesthésie réanimation, MAPAR, Hopital Bicetre, Paris,1986.

Hulman MS, A Sandler, J Brebner. The reversal of epidural morphine induced somnolence with physostigmne. Can Anaesth Soc J, 1984, 31, 678.

Hunt CO, S Datta, M Hauch, GW Ostheimer, L Hertwig, JS Naulty. Perioperative analgesia with subarachnoid fentanyl-bupivacaine. Anesthesiology, 1987, 67, A621.

Hunt CO, JS Naulty, AM Malinow, S Datta, GW Ostheimer. Epidural butorphanol-bupivacaine for analgesia during labor and delivery. Anesth Analg, 1989, 68, 323.

Hunt CO, JS Naulty, AM Bader, MA Hauch, JV Vartikar, S Datta, LM Hertwig, GW Ostheimer. Perioperative analgesia with subarachnoid fentanyl-bupivacaine for cesarean delivery. Anesthesiology, 1989, 71, 535.

Hüsch M, M Zenz. Peridurale Morphin-Analgesie bei Rippenserienbrüchen. In: M Zenz (Eds): Peridurale Opiate-Analgesie, Gustav Fischer Verlag, Stuttgart, 1981, 69.

Husebø S. Behandlund av kreftsmerter med morfin gjennom epiduralkateter. (Treatment of cancer pain with morphine given via epidural catheters). Tidsskr Nor Laegeforen, 1984, 104, 1715.

Husebø S. Treatment of intractable cancer pain with total implantable reservoir. VII Eur Congress, 1986, Vienna (Austria), Report, Abst 426.

Husegaard HC, TK Petersen, L Rybro, BA Schurizek, M Wernberg. Postoperativ smertebehandling med buprenorfin og morfin epiduralt efter hoje laparotomier. (Treatment of postoperative pain with epidural buprenorphine and morhine after high laparotomies). Ugeskr Laeger, 1984, 146, 14.

Husemeyer RP, MC O'Connor, HT Davenport. Aspect of epidural morphine. Lancet, 1979, 2, 583.

Husemeyer RP, Davenport HT. Epidural opiates in pregnancy. Symposium Analgesia by epidural and spinal opiates, Nijmegen (Holland) 1980, Congress Report. (a)

Husemeyer RP, MC O'Connor, HT Davenport. Failure of epidural morphine to relieve pain in labour. Anaesthesia, 1980, 35, 161. (b)

Husemeyer RP, MC O'Connor, HT Davenport. Epidural morphine for analgesia in labour. Anaesthesia, 1980, 35, 420. (c)

Husemeyer RP, HT Davenport, AJ Cummings, JR Rosankiewicz. Comparison of epidural and intramuscular pethidine for analgesia in labour. Brit J Obstet Gynecol, 1981, 88, 711.

Husemeyer RP, AJ Cummings, JR Rosankiewicz, HT Davenport. A study of pethidine kinetics and analgesia in women in labour following intravenous, intramuscular and epidural administration. Brit J Clin Pharm, 1982, 13, 171.

Husted S, JC Djurhuus, HC Husegaard, J Jepsen, J Mortensen. Effects of postoperative extradural morphine on lower urinary tract function. Acta Anaesth Scand, 1985, 29, 183.

Hyde NH, DM Harrison. Intrathecal morphine in a parturient with cyctic fibrosis. Anesth Analg, 1986, 65,1357.

Hylden JL, GL Wilcox. Intrathecal substance P elicits a caudally-directed biting and scratching behavior in mice. Brain Res, 1981, 217, 212.

Hylden JL, GL Wilcox. Intrathecal opioids block a spinal action of substance P in mice: functional importance of both mu- and delta-receptors. Eur J Pharm, 1982, 86, 95.

Hylden JL, GL Wilcox. Pharmacological characterization of substance P-induced nociception in

556

mice: modulation by opioid and noradrenergic agonists at the spinal level. J Pharm Exp Ther, 1983, 226, 398.

Inagaki Y, E Takeyma. Change of analgesic effect of intrathecal buprenorphine combined with local anesthetic used for postoperative pain relief. Masui, 1988, 37 (8), 955.

Ingemar F, H Ahlgren, BE Ahlgren. Epidural administration of opiates by a new device. Pain, 1987, 31, 353.

Inglis S, P Anderson, A Faggella. A comparative study of the respiratory effects of intrathecal butorphanol vs intrathecal morphine in cats. Acta Anaesth Scand (Suppl.), 1985, 29, 83, N° 137.

Inturrisi CE, J G Umans. Meperidine biotransformation and central nervous system toxicity in animal and humans. Advances in Pain Res and Ther, 1986, 8, 143.

Inturrisi CE. Newer methods of opioid drug delivery. Int Ass F Studdy of Pain. Refresher Course on Pain Managment Hamburg, 1987.

Ionescu TI, A van Maris, RHT Taverne, B Smalhout. Differences in the haemodynamic effects of epidural morphine and epidural bupivacaine anaesthesia for abdominal aortic surgery. VII Eur Congress of Anaesth, 1986, Vienna (Austria), Report, Abst 420.

Ionescu TI, RH Drost, JMM Roelofs, EKA Winckers, RHT Taverne, AA van Maris, JM van Rossum. The pharmacokinetics of intradural morphine in major abdominal surgery. Clin Pharmacokinetics, 1988, 14, 178.

Ionescu TI, RH Drost, EKA Winckers, RHT Taverne, JMM Roelofs, JM Van Rossum. Epidural morphine anesthesia for abdominal aortic surgery pharmacokinetics. Regional Anesthesia, 1989, 14, 107.

Ionescu TI, RHT Taverne, P Houweling, ANJ Schouten, G Schimmel, I van der Tweel, A van Dijk. A study of epidural morphine and sufentanil anesthesia for abdominal aortic surgery. Acta Anaest Belg, 1989, 40, 1, 65.

Isaacson IJ, FI Weitz, AJ Berry, GB Knos, DS Venner. Intrathecal morphine's effect on the postoperative course of patients undergoing abdominal aortic surgery. Anesth Analg, 1987, 66, S86.

Islas JA, J Astorga, M Laredo. Epidural ketamine for control of postoperative pain. Anesth Analg, 1985, 64, 1161.

Ivankovich AD, RJ McCarthy. Epidural ketamine for control of postoperative pain: two comments (letter). Anesth Analg, 1986, 65, 989.

Iversen IH. Systematiseret undervisning i epidural smertebehandling. Sygeplejersken, 1985, 85, 24.

Jacobson L. Site of action of intrathecal morphine (letter). Brit Med J, 1980, 281, 870.

Jacobson L, PD Phillips, CJ Hull, ID Conacher. Extradural versus intramuscular diamorphine. A controlled study of analgesic and adverse effects in the postoperative period. Anaesthesia, 1983, 38, 10.

Jacobson LE, EJ Krane, AM Lynn, C Parrot, DC Tyler. Comparison of caudal morphine with caudal bupivacaine and conventional parenteral morphine therapy. Anesthesiology, 1986, 65, A427.

Jacobson L, MS Kokri, AK Pridie. Intrathecal diamorphine: efficiency, duration, optimal dose and side effects. Anesth Analg, 1987, 66, S89.

Jacobson L, C Chabal. Intrathecal morphine: efficacy, duration, optimal dose and side effects. Anesth Analg, 1988, 67, S102.

Jacobson L, C Chabal, MC Brody. A dose-response study of intrathecal morphine: efficaccy, duration, optimal dose and side effects. Anesth Analg, 1988, 67, 1082.

Jacobson I, C Chabal, MC Brody, RJ Ward, RC Ireton. Intrathecal methadone and morphine for postoperativ analgesia: a comparison of the efficacy, duration and side effects. Anesthesiology, 1988, 69 (3A), A352.

Jacobson L, C Chabal, MC Brody. Relief of persistent postamputation stump and phantom limb pain with intrathecal fentanyl. Pain, 1989, 37, 317.

Jacobson L, C Chabal, MC Brody, RJ Ward. Intrathecal methadone 5 mg and morphine 0.5 mg for postoperative analgesia: a comparison of the efficacy, duration and side effects. Anesth Analg, 1989, 68, S132.

Jacobson L, C Chabal, MC Brody, RJ Ward, RC Ireton. Intrathecal methadone and morphine for postoperative analgesia: a comparison of the efficacy, duration and side effects. Anesthesiology, 1989, 70, 742.

Jacobson L, C Chabal, MC Brody, RJ Ward, L Wasse. Intrathecal methadone: a dose-response study and comparison with intrathecal morphine. Anesthesiology (Suppl), 1989, 71, 695.

Jaffe JH, WR Martin. Opioid analgesic and antagonists. In: Goodman and Gilman's (Eds.): The Pharmacological Basis of Therapeutics, 7th edition, McMillan Publishing Co, 1985, 491.

Jaffe S, V Harbicek, H Friesen, V Chernick. Effect of somastostatin and L-glutamate on neurons of the sensorimotor cortex in awake habituated rabbits. Brain Res, 1978, 153, 414.

James CF, CE Banner, PG Hanna, J Rost, D Caton. Comparison of epidural fentanyl via bolus with or without continuous infusion after cesarean section. Anesthesiology, 1988, 69 (3A), A682.

Jamous MA, CW Hand, RA Moore, PJ Teddy, HJ McQuay. Epinephrine reduces systemic absorption of extradural diacetylmorphine. Anesth Analg, 1986, 65, 1290.

Jansen EC, NE Drenck, A Ulrich. Silicone tubing used as fixation of epidural catheters. Anesthesiology, 1987, 66, 694.

Janssen PAJ. A fentanyl family of analgesics, sufentanil, alfentanil and lofentanil. Research report Janssen Pharmaceutica, 1980,

Janssen PAJ. Report Janssen Research News, 1981, 2, 2.

Janssen PAJ. Potent, new analgesic, tailor made, for different purposes. Acta Anaesth Scand, 1982, 26, 262.

Janssen PAJ. The development of new synthetic narcotics. In: FG Estafanous (Ed.): Opioids in Anesthesia, Butterworth, London, 1984, 37.

Janvier G, E Dardel, G. Dugrais, J Pere, A Vallet, S Winnock. Rachianesthésie à la péthidine en chirurgie générale et vasculaire (expérience clinique à propos de 100 cas). Forum Club AFAR, 1984, Paris.

Janvier G, E Dardel, G. Dugrais, J Pere. A Vallet, S Winnock. Rachianesthésie à la péthidine en chirurgie générale et vasculaire. Ann Fr Anesth Réanim, 1985, 4, 445.

Jasinski DR. Assessment of the abuse potentiality of morphine like drugs. In: WR Martin (Ed.): Drug addiction handbook of exp. pharmacology. Springer Verlag Berlin, 1977, 197.

Jasinski DR. Human pharmocology of narcotic antagonists. Brit J Clin Pharm, 1979, 7, S287.

Jasinski DR. Opioid receptors and classifications. In: Nimmo, Smith (Eds.): Opioid agonist antagonist drugs in clinical practice. Current Clin. Practic Series B, Excerpta Medica, Amsterdam, 1984, 24.

Jayais P, F Millot, M Bunodiére. Concentration de morphine dans le liquide céphalo-rachidien aprés administration péridurale de morphine. Nouv Presse Méd, 1982, 11, 3348.

Jayr C, A Mollié, JL Bourgain, J Alarcon, J Masselot, P Lasser, A Denjean, J Truffa-Bachi, M Henry-Amar. Postoperative pulmonary complications: general anesthesia with postoperative parenteral morphine compared with epidural analgesia. Surgery, 1988, 104, 57.

Jensen BH. Caudal block for postoperative pain relief in children after genital operations: a comparison between bupivacaine and morphine. Acta Anaesth Scand, 1981, 25, 373.

Jensen MP, P Karoly S Braver. The measurement of clinical pain intensity: a comparison of six methods. Pain, 1986, 27, 117.

Jensen NH, K Eliasen, SH Johansen. Postoperativ respirations depression after epidural morphine. Ugeskr Laeger, 1985, 147, 1625.

Jensen PJ, P Siem-Jørgensen, TB Nielsen, H Wichmand-Nielsen, E Wintherreich. Epidural morphine by the caudal route for postoperative pain relief. Acta Anaesth Scand, 1982, 26, 511.

Jessell TM. Substance P in nociceptive sensory neurons. Ciba Found Symp, 1982, 91, 225.

Johannessen JN, LR Watkins, SM Carlton, DJ Mayer. Failure of spinal cord serotonin depletion to alter analgesia eliceted from the periaqueductal gray. Brain Res, 1982, 237, 373.

Johnson SM, AW Duggan. Evidence that the opiate receptors of the substantia gelatinosa contribute to the depression, by intravenous morphine, of the spinal transmission of impulses in unmyelinated primary afferents. Brain Research, 1981, 207, 223.

Johnson MD, FB Sevarino, MJ Lema, S Datta, GW Ostheimer, JS Naulty. Effect of epidural sufentanil on temperature regulation in the parturient. Anesthesiology, 1987, 67, A450.

Johnson A, M Bengtsson, JB Löfström, A Rane, A Wahlström. Influence of postoperative naloxone infusion on respiration and pain relief after intrathecal morphine. Regional Anesthesia, 1988, 13, 146.

Johnson MD, FB Sevarino, ML Lema. Cessation of shivering and hypothermia associated with epidural sufentanil. Anesth Analg, 1989, 68, 70.

Johnson C, N Oriol, D Feinstein. Onset of action between bupivacaine 0.5% vs bupivacaine 0.5% plus fentanyl 75 mcg. Anesthesiology (Suppl), 1989, 71, 843.

Johnson MD, MS Brown, P Barresi, CO Hunt, S Datta. The addition of epinephrine to subarachnoid hyperbaric bupivacaine with fentanyl for cesarean delivery. Anesthesiology (Suppl), 1989, 71, 869.

Johnson MD, L Hertwig, PH Vehring, S Datta. Intrathecal fentanyl may reduce the incidence of spinal headache. Anesthesiology (Suppl), 1989, 71, 911.

Johnston JR, W McCaughey. Epidural morphine. A method of managment of multiple fractured ribs. Anaesthesia, 1980, 35, 155.

Jones G, DL Paul, RA Elton, JH McClure. Comparison of bupivacaine and bupivacaine with fentanyl in continuous extradural analgesia during labour. Brit J Anaesth, 1989, 63, 254.

Jones RDM, JG Jones. Intrathecal morphine: naloxone reverses respiratory depression but not analgesia. Brit Med J, 1980, 281, 645.

Jones SEF, JM Beasley, DWR MacFarlane, JM Davis, G Hall-Davies. Intrathecal morphine for postoperative pain relief in children. Brit J Anaesth, 1984, 56, 137.

Jordan GH, NC Babcock, JJ Mocnik, DF Lynch. Pain control following renal infarction/ablation using continuous epidural combined anesthesia/analgesia. J Urol, 1983, 130, 861.

Jørgensen BC, HB Andersen, A Engquist. Epidural low-dose morphine and postoperative pain: a controlled study. 7th World Congress of Anaesth, Hamburg, 1980, Excerpta medica, Int Congress series N° 533, p 456 N° 1017.

Jørgensen BC, HB Andersen, A Engquist. CSF and plasma morphine after epidural and intrathecal application. Anesthesiology, 1981, 55, 714.

Jørgensen BC, HB Andersen, A Engquist. Influence of epidural morphine on postoperative pain, endocrine-metabolic, and renal responses to surgery. A controlled study. Acta Anaesth Scand, 1982, 26, 63.

Joris JL, R Dubner, KM Hargreaves. Opioid analgesia at peripheral sites: a target for opioids released during stress and inflammation? Anesth Analg, 1987, 66, 1277.

Jorrot JC, JD Lirzin, Ph Dailland, P Jacquinot, Ch Conseiller. Association sufentanil-bupivacaine à 0.25% par voie péridurale pour l'analgésie obstétricale. Comparaison avec le fentanyl et un placebo. Ann Fr Anesth Réanim, 1989, 8, 321.

Josten KU. Erfahrungen mit längerliegenden Periduralkathetern - Peridurale Morphine-Analgesie bei Karzinompatienten (letter). Regional Anaesthesie, 1982, 5, 47.

Joyau M, JC Deybach, M Durand, G Parmentier, Y Nordmann. Analgesie péridurale par procaine et fentanyl chez une parturiente atteinte de porphyrie aigue intermittente. Ann Fr Anesth Réanim, 1986, 5, 453.

Jurna I. Dämpfung repetitiver Aktivierungsvorgänge an der spinal Motorik durch Morphin. In: R

Janzen, WD Keidel, A Herz, C Ateichele (Eds.): Schmerz Grundlagen-Pharmakologie-Therapie, Georg Thieme Verlag, 1972, 267.

Jurna I. Inhibition of the reflex of repetitive stimulation on spinal motorneurons of the cat by morphine and pethidine. Neuropharmacol, 1966, 5, 117.

Jurna I, W Grossman. The effect of morphine on mammalian nerve fibers. Eur J Pharm, 1977, 44, 339.

Jurna I. Die pharmakologischen Grundlagen der Spinalanalgesie mit Morphin. Anaesth Intensivmed, 1983, 24, 381.

Jurna I. Cyclic nucleotides and aminophylline produce different effects on nociceptive motor and sensory responses in the rat spinal cord. Naunyn Schmiedebergs Arch Pharmacol, 1984, 327, 23. (a)

Jurna I. Depression of nociceptive sensory activity in the rat spinal cord due to the intrathecal administraion of drugs: effect of diazepam. Neurosurgery, 1984, 15, 917. (b)

Justins DM, F Reynolds. Intraspinal opiates and itching : A new reflex ? Brit Med J, 1982, 284, 1401. (a)

Justins DM, D Francis, PG Houlton, F Reynolds. A controlled trial of extradural fentanyl in labour. Brit J Anaesth, 1982, 54, 409. (b)

Justins DM, C Knott, J Luthman, F Reynolds. Epidural versus intramuscular fentanyl. Analgesia and pharmacokinetics in labour. Anaesthesia, 1983, 38, 937.

Jyu C, JD Lamb. Respiratory depression following epidural morphine. Can Anaesth Soc J, 1985, 32, 99.

Kadieva VS, CH van Hasselt. Low dose intrathecal morphine for caesarean section. Anaesthesia, 1982, 38, 1229.

Kafer ER, JT Brown, GW Ross, JN Ghia. Effect of epidural morphine on respiratory function and hemodynamic stability. Nc Med J, 1982, 43, 207.

Kafer ER, JT Brown, D Scott, JW Findlay, RF Butz, E Teeple, JN Ghia. Biphasic depression of ventilatory responses to CO2 following epidural morphine. Anesthesiology, 1983, 58, 418.

Kaiko RF, S Wallenstein, AG Rogers, PY Grabinski, et al. Clinical analgesic studies and sources of variation in analgesic responses to morphine. In: KM Foley et al. (Eds.): Adv. Pain research and therapy, Vol. 8, Raven Press, New York, 1986, 13.

Kaiser KG, CR Bainton. Treatment of intrathecal morphine overdose by aspiration of cerebrospinal fluid. Anesth Analg, 1987, 66, 475.

Kalia M, K Fuxe, LF Agnati, I Hökfelt, A Härfstrand. Somatostatin froduces apnea and is localized in medullary respiratory nuclei a possible role in apneic syndromes. Brain Res, 1984, 296, 339.

Kalia PK, R Madan, R Saksena, RK Batra, GR Gode. Epidural pentazocine for postoperative pain relief. Anesth Analg, 1983, 62, 949.

Kalso E. Effects of intrathecal morphine, injected with bupivacaine, on pain after orthopaedic surgery. Brit J Anaesth, 1983, 55, 415.

Kanto J, R Erkkola. Obstetric analgesia: pharmacokinetics and its relation to neonatal behavioral and adaptive functions. Biol Res Pregnancy Perinatol, 1984, 5, 23. (a)

Kanto J, R Erkkola. Epidural and intrathecal opiates in obstetrics. Int J Clin Pharm Ther Tox, 1984, 22, 316. (b)

Kanto J, R Erkkola, L Aaltonen, L Äärimaa. Epidural morphine as postoperative analgesia following cesarean section under epidural analgesia. Int J Clin Pharm Ther Tox, 1985, 23, 43.

Kartha RK, S Velamati, L Penas, R Aravapalli. Epidural butorphanol for postoperative analgesia. Anesthesiology, 1987, 67, A235.

Katz J, W Nelson. Intrathecal morphine for postoperative pain relief. Regional Anesthesia, 1981, 6, 1.

Kaufman JJ, NM Semo, WS Koski. Microelectrometric titration measurement of the pka's and

560

partition and drug distribution coefficients of narcotics and narcotic antagonists and their pH and temperature dependence. J Med Chem, 1975, 18, 647.

Kaufman L. Intrathecal heroin. Lancet, 1981, 2, 1341.

Kavuri S, Y Janardhan, FE Fernando, K Shevde, D Eddi. A comparative study of epidural alfentanil and fentanyl for labor pain relief. Anesthesiology (Suppl), 1989, 71, 846.

Kawamura S, S Sakurada, T Sakurada, K Kisara, Y Akutsu, Y Sasaki, K Suzuki. Antinociceptive effect of centrally administered cyclo (n-Methyl-L-Tyr-L-Arg) in the rat. Eur J Pharm, 1983, 93,1.

Kawana Y, H Sato, H Shimada, N Fujita, Y Ueda, A Hayashi, Y Araki. Epidural ketamine for postoperative pain relief after gynecologic operations: a double-blind study and comparison with epidural morphine. Anesth Analg, 1987, 66, 735.

Kawashima Y, N. Uchida, S Kawahira, K Meguro, T Nampo, Y Fujita. A step towards complete pain relief after surgery. 7th World Congress of Anaesth, 1980, Hamburg. Excerta Medica, Congress series 533, 455 N°1016.

Kay B. Extradural buprenorphine (letter). Brit J Anaesth, 1983, 55, 255.

Kay NH. Epidural fentanyl (letter). Anaesthesia, 1984, 39, 498.

Kehlet H, MR Brandt, J Rem. Role of neurogenic stimuli in mediating the endocrine-metabolic response to surgery. J Parent Ent Nutr, 1980, 4, 152.

Kehlet H. The endocrine-metabolic response to postoperative pain. Acta Anaesth Scand (Suppl.), 1982, 74, 173.

Kehlet H, N Hjortsø. Influence of epidural analgesia with local anesthetics and morphine on morbidity after abdominal surgery. In: G. Hossli, P Frey, G Kreienbühl (Eds.): Anaesthesiologie und Intensivmedizin, ZAK Zürich, 1986, 188, 360. (a)

Kehlet H, N Hjortsø. Influence of epidural opiates on postoperative morbidity and endocrine-metabolic changes. In: HJ Wüst, M Stanton-Hicks (Eds.): Anaesthesiologie und Intensivmedizin, new aspects in regional anesthesia 4, Springer Verlag, Berlin, Heidelberg, New York, Tokyo, 1986, 176, 128. (b)

Kehlet H, NC Hjortsø, C Lund, T Mogensen, D Bigler. Effect of morphine on sensory analgesia during continuous epidural bupivacaine. Schmerz-Pain-Douleur, 1987, 3, 95.

Kehrberger E, E Lanz, D Theiss. Morphin epidural-Einfluss auf Ausbreitung und Verlauf einer Periduralanaesthesie mit Bupivacain 0.75%. VII Eur congress, 1986, Vienna (Austria), Report, Abst. 418.

Kendig JJ, MKT Savola, M Maze. Effects of a sedative/analgesic alpha-2 adrenergic agonist, dexmedetomidine, on the spinal cord of newborn rats. Anesthesiology (Suppl), 1989, 71, 581.

Kennedy BM. Intrathecal morphine and multiple fractured ribs (letter). Brit J Anaesth, 1985, 57, 1266.

Keruel S, M Rosello, J Rouire-Rosello, J Bimar. Comparaison de deux méthodes d'analgésie péridurale dans l'accouchement (à propos de 1100 cas). Ann Fr Anesth Réanim, 1983, 2, 3, 120.

Kiegel P, B Garrigues, AP Blanc, MC Blanc, C Arruidarre. Traitement des douleurs cancéreuses par implantation de site d'injection permettant l'administration périmédullaire de chlorhydrate de morphine. II Int Symposium: Pain Clinic, Lille (France) 1986, Abst. III P 4.

Kierkegaard E, P Hole, MM Brinkløv, P Klint. Preliminary experience with epidural buprenorphine. In: Nordic Symposium on Temgesic, Meda, Copenhagen, 1981, 88.

Kim KC, RK Stoelting. Effect of droperidol on the duration of analgesia and development of tolerance to intrathecal morphine. Anesthesiology, 1980, 53, S219.

King FG, AD Baxter, G Mathieson. Tissue reaction of morphine applied to the epidural space of dogs. Can Anaesth Soc J, 1984, 31, 268.

King GH, MS Mok, SN Steen, M Lippmann. Relief of postoperative pain with low doses intrathecal morphine. 6th Europ congress of Anaesth, London, 1982,147po, S123.

King HK, SK Tsai. Delayed respiratory depression following repeated intrathecal low dose morphine. Anaesth Intens Care, 1985, 13, 334.

Kirson LE, JM Goldman, RB Slover. Low-dose intrathecal morphine for postoperative pain control in patients undergoing transurethral resection of the prostate. Anesthesiology, 1989, 71, 192.

Kiss I, G Spellenberg, M Abel. Perioperative Opiatanalgesie. Anaesth Intensivth Notfallmed, 1981, 16, 343.

Kiss I, M Abel. Die Rippenfraktur, eine Indikation für die peridurale Opiatanalgesie. In: JB Brueckner (Ed.): Anaesthesiologie und Intensivmedizin, Schmerzbehandlung, epidurale Opiatanalgesie. Springer Verlag, Berlin, 1982,153, 90.

Kiss I, H Müller. Thorakale peridurale Opiat-Analgesie. Regional Anaesthesie, 1985, 8, 57.

Kiss I. (Ed.) Karzinomschmerzen. In: Anaesthesiologie und Intensivmedizin, Karzinomschmerzen, Springer Verlag, Berlin, 1987, Band 196.

Kitagawa O. Intrathecal administration of eucaine in combination with morphine. Tokyo Iji Shinski, 13 April, 1901.

Kitahata LM, Y Kosaka, A Taub. Lamina specific suppression of dorsal horn unit activity by morphine sulfate. Anesthesiology, 1974, 41, 39.

Kitahata LM, JG Collins. Spinal action of narcotic analgesics. Anesthesiology, 1981, 54, 153.

Kitahata LM, M Aoki, M Senami, JG Collins. Effects of spinal sufentanil. Soc Neurosci, 1984, Abst 10, Part 1, 106. (b)

Kitahata LM, JG Collins. Intrathecal and epidural shortacting narcotics. Estafanous Opioids in Anesthesiology, Butterworth Publishers, London, 1984, 155. (a)

Kitahata LM. Spinal analgesia with morphine and clonidine. Anesth Analg, 1989, 68, 191.

Klein AS, JP Mickle. Epidural morphine for analgesia after selective dorsal rhizotomy - a report of 18 cases. Regionalanesthesia, 1989, 14 (Suppl), 53.

Klepper ID, DL Sherrill, PR Bromage. Analgesic and respiratory effects of epidural sufentanil in volunteers. ASA, 12-16 Oct 1985.

Klepper ID, DL Sherrill, CL Boetger, PR Bromage. Analgesic and respiratory effects of extradural sufentanil in volunteers and the influence of adrenaline as an adjuvant. Brit J Anaesth, 1987, 59, 1147.

Klinck JR, MJ Lindop. Epidural morphine in the elderly. A controlled trial after upper abdominal surgery. Anaesthesia, 1982, 37, 907.

Klockgether T, M Schwarz, U Wüllner, L Turski, K Sonntag. Myorelaxant effect after intrathecal injection of antispastic drugs in rats. Neuroscience Letters, 1989, 97, 221.

Kloss Th, W Junginger. Kombinierte Anwendung von Katheterperiduralanalgesie und Allgemeinanaesthesie für große urologische Eingriffe. Kurzfassung der Referate des 3. Internationalen Symposiums über Anaesthesie-Reanimations - und Intensivbehandlungsprobleme, Zürs/Arlberg 06.02.-13.02.1983, Referat Nr 47.

Knape JTA. Early respiratory depression resistant to naloxone following epidural buprenorphine. Anesthesiology, 1986, 64, 382.

Knell PJ. Site of action of intrathecal morphine (letter). Brit Med J, 1980, 281, 870.

Knill RL, JL Clement, WR Thompson. Epidural morphine causes delayed and prolonged ventilatory depression. Can Anesth Soc J, 1981, 28, 537.

Knill RL, AM Lam, WR Thompson. Epidural morphine and ventilatory depression. Anesthesiology, 1982, 56, 486.

Knill RL. Wresting or resting ventilation. Anesthesiology, 1983, 59, 599.

Knill RL. Cardiac arrests during spinal anesthesia: unexpected?. Anesthesiology, 1988, 69, 629.

Knitza R, H Hepp. Zur analgetischen Wirkung von Morphin und Bupivacain bei periduraler Applikation in der Geburtshilfe. Z Geburtsh Perinatol, 1981, 185, 220.

Knitza R, G Biro, H Hepp. Serummorphinkonzentrationen und Analgesie bei epiduraler oder subcutaner Morphingabe in der Geburtshilfe. Z Geburtsh Perinatol, 1982, 186, 200.

Koch J, JU Nielsen. Rare misplacements of epidural catheters. Anesthesiology, 1986, 65, 556.

562

Koerker DJ, LA Harker, CJ Goodner. Effects of somatostatin on hemostasis in baboons. N Engl J Med, 1975, 293, 476.

Kong D, A Siou, Cl Batier, B Roquefeuil. Mise au point a propos de de 165 péridurales morphiniques. II Int Symposium: Pain Clinic, Lille (France) 1986, Abst.IX FP 5.

Konieczko KM, JG Jones, MP Barrowcliffe, C Jordan, DG Altman. Antagonism of morphine-induced respiratory depression with nalmefene. Brit J Anaesth, 1988, 61, 318.

Konturek SJ, J Tasler, M Cieszkowski, DH Coy, AV Schally. Effects of growth hormone release-inhibiting hormone on gastrin secretion, mucosal blood flow and serum gastrin. Gastroenterology, 1976, 70, 737.

Koontz WL, EH Bishop. Management of the latent phase of labor. Clin Obstet Gynecol, 1982, 25, 1, 111.

Korbon GA, CA DiFazio, JM Verlander, DJ James, SJ Levy, PC Perry, SM Rosenblum. IM naloxone reverse respiratory depression from epidural morphine while preserving analgesia. Anesthesiology, 1983, 59, A218.

Korbon GA, CJ Lander, AD Jenkins, MC Lippert, PO Carey. Neurological complications after epidural anesthesia for extracorporeal shock wave lithotripsy: a review. Anesthesiology, 1987, 67, A228.

Korbon GA. Repeated epdiural anesthesia for extracorporeal shock-wave lithotrypsy is not unreliable. Anesth Analg, 1988, 67, 484.

Korinek AM, M Languille, A Liénart, P Viars. Tous les traitements de la douleur n'ont pas le même effet sur la sécrétion d'ADH. In: Ars Medici, Bruxelles, Congress Series 3, 1982, 227.

Korinek AM, M Languille, F Bonnet, M Thibonnier, P Sasano, A Lienhart, P Viars. Effect of postoperative extradural morphine on ADH secretion. Brit J Anaesth, 1985, 57, 407.

Korsh J, S Ramanathan, F Parker, H Turndorf. Systemic histamine release by epidural morphine. Anesthesiology, 1987, 67, A445.

Kortum K, H Nolte, HJ Kenkmann. Die Geschlechtsabhängigkeit subjektiver Beschwerden nach Spinalanaesthesie. Regional Anaesthesie, 1982, 5, 1.

Kossmann B, E Voelk, D Spilker. Perioperative Glucoseregulation bei Operation eines Aorto-bifemoralen Bypass unter Neuroleptanalgesie im Vergleich zu thorakaler Epiduralanaesthesie. Zentraleuropäischer Anaesthesiekongress, Berlin, 1981, 265.

Kossmann B, ED Spilker, E Voelk, H Heinrich. Thoracic epidural anaesthesia and the haemodynamic changes during operation of an aorto-bifemoral bypass. 6th Eur Congress of Anaesth, London, vol of summaries, 1982, 389.

Kossmann B, W Dick, KH Wollinsky, E Traub, J Harzenetter, MR Möller. Peridurale Morphin Analgesie: Wirkung und Pharmakokinetik. Anaesthesist, 1983, 32, 284.

Kossmann B, W Dick, I Bowdler, FW Ahnefeld, J Harzenetter. The analgesic action and respiratory side effects of epidural morphine. Regional Anesthesia, 1984, 9, 55. (a)

Kossmann B, W Dick, KH Wollinsky, I Bowdler, HH Mehrkens, M Böck, MR Möller. Vergleichende Untersuchungen der Nebenwirkungen von Morphin nach periduraler, spinaler und intravenöser Applikation. Regional Anaesthesie, 1984, 7, 25. (b)

Kosterlitz HW. Possible physiological significance of multiple endogenous opioid agonists. In: RF Beers (Ed.): Mechanisms of pain and analgesic compounds. Raven Press, New York, 1979, 207.

Kotelko DM, PA Dailey, SM Shnider, MA Rosen, SC Hughes, RV Brizgys. Epidural morphine analgesia after cesarean delivery. Obstetrics & Gynecology, 1984, 63, 409.

Kotelko DM, RL Rottman, WC Wright, JJ Stone, RM Rosenblatt, AY Yamashiro. Improved surgical and postcesarean analgesia with epidural fentanyl/morphine combination. Anesthesiology, 1987, 67, A622.

Kotelko DM, RL Rottman, WC Wright, JJ Stone, AY Yamashiro, RM Rosenblatt. Transderm scop® decreases post-cesarean nausea and vomiting in patients receiving epidural morphine. Anesthesiology, 1988, 69 (3A), A666.

Kotob HIM, CW Hand, RA Moore, PJD Evans, J Wells, AP Rubin, HJ McQuay. Intrathecal morphine and heroine in humans: six-hour drug levels in spinal fluid plasma. Anesth Analg, 1986, 65, 718.

Krames ES, A Lyons, P Taylor, J Gershow, T Kenefick, A Glassberg. Continuous infusion of spinally administered narcotics for the relief of pain due to malignant disorders.In Intraspinal narcotic analgesia for acute and chronic pain. Palm Springs, USA, 1983. Symposium report.

Krames ES, J Gershow, A Glassberg, T Kenefick, A Lyons, P Taylor, D Wilkie. Continuous infusion of spinally administered narcotics for the relief of pain due to malignant disorders. Cancer, 1985, 56, 696.

Krames ES, DJ Wilkie, J Gershow. Intrathecal D-Ala2-D-Leu5-enkephalin (DADL) restores analgesia in a patient analgetically tolerant to intrathecal morphine sulfate. Pain, 1986, 24, 205.

Krames ES, DJ Wilkie. Acute and chronic effects of delta-alanine2-delta-leucin5-enkephalin (DADL) in morphine tolerant cancer. Pain, 1987, S4, S68.

Krane EJ, LE Jacobson, AM Lynn, C Parrot, DC Tyler. Caudal morphine for postoperative analgesia in children: a comparison with caudal bupivacaine and iv morphine. Anesth Analg, 1987, 66, 647.

Krane EJ. Delayed respiratory depression in a child after caudal epidural morphine. Anesth Analg, 1988, 67, 79.

Krane EJ, LE Jacobson, DC Tyler. Caudal epidural morphine in children: a comparison of three doses. Anesthesiology, 1988, 69 (3A), A763.

Krane EJ, DC Tyler, LE Jacobson. The dose response of caudal morphine in children. Anesthesiology, 1989, 71, 48.

Krantz T, CB Christensen. Respiratory depression after intrathecal opioids: report of a patient receiving long-term epidural opioid therapy. Anaesthesia, 1987, 42, 168.

Kraynack BJ, L Moore, EF Klein. Hyperbaric intrathecal morphine for parturients with toxemia. In: HJ Wüst, M Stanton-Hicks (Eds.): Anaesthesiologie und Intensivmedizin, new aspects in regional anesthesia 4, Springer Verlag, Berlin, Heidelberg, New York, Tokyo, 1986, 176, 140.

Kroin JS, RJ McCarthy, RD Penn, JM Kerns, AD Ivankovich. The effect of chronic subarachnoid bupivacaine infusion in dogs. Anesthesiology, 1987, 66, 737.

Krynicki J, L Hjelmerus. Kontinuerlig analgetikatillfoersel epiduralt med infusionspump. Swedish Doctors Journal, june, 1985.

Kühn K, J Hausdörfer, KF Rothe. Schmerzbekämpfung mit epiduralen Morphininjektionen. Anaesthesist, 1981, 30, 521.

Kuhnert BR et al. Meperidine disposition in mother and non pregnant females. Clin Pharm Ther, 1980, 27, 486.

Kuhnert BR, PL Linn, PM Kuhnert. Obstetric medication and neonatal behavior. Current controversies. Clin Perinatol, 1985, 12, 423.

Kumar B, FM Messahel. Evaluation of epidural needles. Acta Anaesth Scand, 1987, 31, 96.

Kumeta Y, M Senami, M Aoki, LM Kitahata, JG Collins. Direct opioid application on peripheral nerves does not alter activity of single C polymodal nociceptive fibers. Anesthesiology, 1985, 63, A233.

Kuo RJ. Epidural morphine for post-hemorrhoidectomy analgesia. Dis Colon Rectum, 1984, 27, 529.

Kuraishi Y, M Satoh, Y Harada, A Akaike, T Shibata, H Tagaki. Analgesic action of intrathecal and intracerebral beta-endorphin in rats: comparison with morphine. Eur J Pharmacol, 1980, 67, 143.

Kuraishi Y, N Hirota, Y Sato, Y Hino, M Satoh, H Takagi. Evidence that substance P and somatostatin transmit separate information related to pain in the spinal dorsal horn. Brain Res, 1985, 325, 294. (b)

Kuraishi Y, N Hirota, M Satoh, H Takagi. Antinociceptive effects of intrathecal opioids, noradrenaline and serotonin in rats: mechanical and thermal algesic tests. Brain Res, 1985, 326, 168. (a)

564

Labaille T, K Samii, C Mann, Y Noviant. Fonction respiratoire post-opératoire après analgésie morphinique par voies sous-cutanée et péridurale. La Nouvelle Presse médicale, 1982, 11, 1309.

Lam AM, RL Knill, WR Thompson, JL Clement, GP Varkey, WE Spoerel. Epidural fentanyl does not cause delayed respiratory depression. Can Anaesth Soc J, 1983, 30, 578.

Lamarche Y, R Martin, J Reiher, G Blaise. The sleep apnoea syndrome and epidural morphine. Can Anaesth Soc J, 1986, 33, 231.

Landa L, EM Berg, H Breivik. Epiduralt morfin for vanskelig traktable cancersmerter (epidural morphine for severe cancer pain). Tidsskr Nor Laegeforen, 1984, 104, 1713.

Landais A, N Darthout, BH Kong-Ky, C St-Maurice. Association fentanyl-bupivacaine péridurale pour l'analgésie obstétricale. Cahiers d'Anesthésiologie, 1983, 31, 297.

Lander CJ, CS Hayworth, JC Moscicki, CA DiFazio. Analgesia and ventilatory characteristics of epidural spiradoline - a specific kappa agonist. Anesthesiology, 1987, 67, A243. (a)

Lander CJ, GA Korbon, CR Monk, WP Arnold, AD Jenkins, M Langley, BR Williamson. Epidural anesthesia and extracorporeal shock wave lithotripsy: pathologic effects on the epidural space. Anesthesiology, 1987, 67, A227. (b)

Landon L. An apparent seizure following inadvertent intrathecal morphine. Anesthesiology, 1985, 62, 545.

Lanz E, D Theiss, W Riess, U Sommer. Epidural morphine for postoperative analgesia. A double-blind study. Anesth Analg, 1982, 61, 236.

Lanz E, M Daubländer, M Lipp, D Theiss. 0.5 mg Morphin intrathekal bei Spinalanaesthesie. Regional Anaesthesie, 1984, 7, 79. (a)

Lanz E, G Simko, D Theiss, MH Glocke. Epidural buprenorphine - A double blind study of postoperative analgesia and side effects. Anesth Analg, 1984, 63, 593. (b)

Lanz E, E Kehrberger, D Theiss. Epidural morphine: a clinical double-blind study of dosage. Anesth Analg, 1985, 64, 786.

Lanz E, E Kehrberger, M Wittig, D Theiss. Epidural morphine analgesia: clinical double blind studies of dose and injection volume. Eur J Anaesth, 1986, 3, 60. (a)

Lanz E, F Däubler, D Eissner, KH Brod, D Theiss. Der Einfluß der spinalen Liquordynamik auf die subarachnoidale Ausbreitung rückenmarksnah applizierter Substanzen. Regional Anaesthesie, 1986, 9, 4. (b)

Larsen JJ, O Svendsen, HB Andersen. Microscopic epidural lesions in goats given repeated epidural injections of morphine: use of a modified autopsy prodedure. Acta Pharmacol et Toxicol, 1986, 58, 5.

Larsen VH, AD Iversen, P Christensen, PK Andersen. Postoperative pain treatment after upper abdominal surgery with epidural morphine at thoracic or lumbal. Acta Anaesth Scand, 1985, 29, 566.

Latarjet J, PY Chomel, JB Cognet, MT Corniglion, JP Galoisy-Guibal, R Joly, A Robert, J Meunier. Effets analgésiques postopératoires de la péthidine injectée par voie péridurale. Ann Fr Anesth Réanim, 1985, 4, 27.

Laubie M, H Schmitt, M Vincent. Vagal bradycardia produced by microinjections of morphine-like drugs into the nucleus ambiguus in anaesthetized dogs. Eur J of Pharm, 1979, 59, 287.

Laugner B, A Muller. L'analgésie morphinique. La Nouvelle Presse Médicale, 1982, 32, 2422.

Laugner B, A Muller, JB Thiebaut, JM Farcot. Analgésie par site implantable pour injections intrathécales itératives de morphine. Ann Fr Anesth Réanim, 1985, 4, 511. (a)

Laugner B. Morphinothérapie intrathécale dans la douleur cancéreuse. Info-Systèmes, 1985, 2, 5, 26. (b)

Laugner B, A Muller, G Buliard. Morphinothérapie intrathécale: utilisation d'un reservoir implantable muni d'une valve activable par voie transcutanée. II Int Symposium: Pain Clinic, 1986, Lille (France).

Layfield DJ, RJ Lemberger, BR Hopkinson, GS Makin. Epidural morphine for ischaemic rest pain. Brit Med J, 1981, 282, 697.

Lazorthes Y, Ch Gouardères, JC Verdié, B Montsarrat, R Bastide, L Campan and J Cros. Analgésie par injection intrathécale de morphine. Etude pharmacocinétique et application aux douleurs irréductibles. Neurochirurgie, 1980, 26A, 159.

Lazorthes Y, J Cros, JC Verdié, JC Lagarrigue, R Bastide, S Boetto. Morphine intrarachidienne chronique dans le traitement des douleurs d'origine néoplasique. Médecine et Hygiène, 1982, 40, 86.

Lazorthes Y, J Siegfried, CH Gouaderes, R Bastide, J Cros, JC Verdie. Periventricular gray matter stimulation versus chronic intrathecal morphine in cancer pain. In: JJ Bonica, V Ventafridda (Eds.): Advances in Pain Research and Therapy, Raven press, New York, 1983, 5, 467.

Lazorthes Y. Administration intra-rachidienne continue de morphine. Infu-Systèmes 1984, 1, 6 (1st part); 1, 14 (2nd part); 1, 30 (3th part).

Lazorthes Y, JC Verdié, R Bastide, B Caute, G Clemente. Les systèmes implantables pour administration épidurale et intrathécale chronique d'opioides. In: JM Besson, Y Lazorthes (Eds.): Spinal Opioids and the Relief of pain. Basic Mechanisms and Clinical Applications, INSERM, Paris, 1985, 391. (a)

Lazorthes Y, R Bastide, JC Verdié, ML Clergue, A Lavados, B Caule, J Cros. Chronic spinal administration of opiate : Application in the treatment of intractable cancer pain. In: JM Besson, Y Lazorthes (Eds.): Spinal Opioids and the Relief of Pain. Basic Mechanisms and Clinical Applications, INSERM, Paris, 1985, 437. (b)

Lazorthes Y, JC Verdié, R Bastide, A Lavados, D Descouens. Spinal versus intraventricular chronic opiate administration with implantable drug delivery devices for cancer pain. Presented at the World Society for Stereotactic and Functional Neurosurgery Congress, Toronto, 4th-7th July, 1985. (c)

Lazorthes Y, JC Verdié. Implantable systems for local chronic administration of drug applications in neuropharmacology In: F Pluchino, G Broggi (Eds.): Advanced Technology in Neurosurgery, Springer Verlag Berlin, Heidelberg, 1988, 217. (a)

Lazorthes Y. Intracerebroventricular administration of morphine for control of irreducible cancer pain. Annals NY Ac Sci , 1988, 531,123.

Leavens ME, CS Hill, DA Cech, JB Weyland, JS Weston. Intrathecal and intraventricular morphine for pain in cancer patients: initial study. J Neurosurg, 1982, 56, 241.

Le Bars D, AH Dickenson, JM Besson. Opiate analgesia and descending control systems. In: JJ Bonica, U Lindblom, A Iggo (Eds.): Advances in Pain Research and Therapie, Raven press, New York, 1983, 341.

Lecron L, D Levy, C Quintana, E Toppet. Prospects of the use of medullary injections of morphinoid drugs. Congress Series, Excerpta Medica, 1979, N 490.

Lecron L, E Toppet-Balatoni, J Bogaerts. Essais comparatifs des différentes techniques antalgiques par voie médullaire. Utilisation des morphiniques. Anesth Analg Réan, 1980, 37, 549. (b)

Lecron L, D Levy, E Toppet. Utilisation de la buprenorphine combinée à l'étidocaine en injection péridurale, premiers essais. In: Agonistic morphine antagonists and their antidotes in anaesthesia,7th World Congress of Anesth, Hamburg, Ars Medici, AIAREF, 1980, 104. (c)

Lecron L, D Levy, E Toppet, S Andrieu, J De Castro. Perspectives d'utilisation des morphiniques par voie médullaire. 15th Latin American Congress of Anesth, Guatemala City, 1979. Ars Medici, 1980, 353. (a)

Lecron L. Anesthésie loco-régionale. Arnette Paris Ed. 1986, and 2nd Ed. 1990.

Lee A, D Simpson, A Whitfield, DB Scott. Continuous epidural infusion of bupivacaine and diamorphine for postoperative pain relief after major gynecologic surgery. Regional Anesthesia,

566

1987, 12, 30.

Lee A, D Simpson, A Whitfield, DB Scott. Postoperative analgesia by continuous extradural infusion of bupivacaine and diamorphine. Brit J Anaesth, 1988, 60, 845-850.

Lefebvre JL, Blond S, Christiaens JL, Combelles-Purvot M, Meynadier J. La morphine intra-cérébro-ventriculaire dans le traitement des algies néoplasiques de la sphère. J Fr ORL, 1985, 34, 487.

Leib RA, JB Hurtig. Epidural and intrathecal narcotics for pain management. Heart and Lung, 1985, 14, 164.

Leicht CH, SC Hughes, PA Dailey, SM Shnider, MA Rosen. Epidural morphine sulfate for analgesia after cesarean section: a prospective report of 1000 patients. Anesthesiology, 1986, 65, A366. (a)

Leicht CH, MA Rosen, PA Dailey, SC Hughes, SM Shnider, BW Baker, DB Cheek, DE O'Connor. Evaluation and comparison of epidural sufentanil citrate and morphine sulfate for analgesia after cesarean section. Anesthesiology, 1986, 65, A365. (b)

Leighton GE, RE Rodriguez, RG Hill, J Hughes. κ-Opioid agonists produce antinociception after i.v. and i.c.v. but not intrathecal administration in the rat. Br J Pharmacol, 1988, 93, 553.

Leighton BL, CA DeSimone, MC Norris, B Ben-David. Intrathecal narcotics for labor revisited: fentanyl 25 mcg and morphine 0.25 mg provide rapid, profound analgesia. Anesthesiology, 1988, 69 (3A) A680.

Leighton BL, CA DeSimone, MC Norris, B Ben-David. Intrathecal narcotics for labor revisited: the combination of fentanyl and morphine intrathecally provides rapid onset of profound, prolonged analgesia. Anesth Analg, 1989, 69, 122.

Lema MJ, F Reiestad, JS Naulty, KE Stromstag, S Datta, GW Ostheimer. Epidural alfentanil administration for postoperative pain relief. Regional Anesthesia, 1987, 12, 28.

Lema MJ, F Reiestad. A comparison of epidural alfentanil, morphine and alfentanil-morphine combinations for postoperative analgesia after total hip replacement (THR). Anesthesiology (Suppl), 1989, 71, 702.

Lenzi A, G Galli, M Gandolfini, G Marini. Intraventricular morphine in paraneoplastic painful syndrome of the cervicofacial region: experience in thirty-eight cases. Neurosurgery, 1985, 17, 6.

Lesley-Ann L, J M Conly, K M Clark, A C Crichlow, G C Wardell, A Zbitnew, L M Rea, S L Cronk, C M Anderson, L K Tan, W L Albritton. Recurent herpes simplex virus labialis and the use of epidural morphine in obstetric patients. Anesth Analg, 1988, 67, 318.

Leslie J, E Camporesi, B Urban, P Bromage. Selective epidural analgesia. Lancet, 1979, 2, 150.

Lettre: Spinal opiates revisited. Lancet, 1986, 2, 655.

Leveque C, C Garen, D Pathier, E Mazuir, R Maneglia, et al. Lofentanil dans l'analgésic obstéticale par voie péridurale. Cahier d'anesthésiologie, 1986, 34, 543.

Levron JC, B Flaisler, P Stephen, M Chauvin, P Salbaing, P Viars. Pharmacokinetics of alfentanil following epidural administration in man. Report Janssen Pharmaceutica, 1983.

Levy RA, HK Proudfit. Analgesia produced by microinjection of baclofen and morphine at brainstem sites. Eur J Pharm, 1979, 57, 43.

Levy RA, HK Proudfit, et al. The analgesic action of baclofen. J Pharm Exp Ther, 1977, 202, 437.

Levy RA, BD Goldstein, MM Elyjiw. Analgesia following local injection of dibutyryl cyclic nucleotides at sites in the rat CNS. Eur J Pharm, 1981, 71, 139.

Leykin Y, D Niv, V Rudik, E Geller. Delayed respiratory depression following extradural injection of morphine. Isr J Med Sci, 1985, 21, 855.

Leysen JE, CJE Niemegeers, TH Stanley. In vivo narcotic effects and opiate receptor occupation. 7th World Congress of Anesth, Hamburg, 1980. Excerpta Medica, Congress Series, 533, 287.

Leysen JE, W Gommeren. Sufentanil, a superior ligand for a mu ligand opiate receptor binding properties of regional distribution in rat brain and spinal cord. Eur J Pharm, 1983, 7, 209.

Licina MG, A Schubert, JE Tobin, HF Nicodemus, L Spitzer. Intrathecal morphine does not reduce the mac of halothane in humans: results of a double blind study. Anesthesiology, 1988, 69 (3A), A643.

Lin DM, HM Shapiro, EM Shipko. Comparison of epidural lidocaine and fentanyl on spinal cord metabolism during sensory stimulation. Anesthesiology, 1985, 63, A232.

Lin DM, K Becker, HM Shapiro. Neurologic changes following epidural injection of potassium chloride and diazepam. Anesthesiology, 1986, 65, 210.

Linder S, A Borgeat, J Biollaz. Meniere-like syndrome following epidural morphine analgesia. Anesthesiology, 1989, 71, 782.

Ling N. Solid phase synthesis of porcine alpha-endorphin and gamma-endorphin, two hypotha-lamic-pituitary peptides with opiate activity. Biohemical and Biophysical Research Communications, 1977, 74, 248.

Lingenfelter RW. Hazard of a new epidural catheter. Anesthesiology, 1983, 58, 293.

Liolios A, FH Andersen. Selective spinal analgesia. Lancet, 1979, 2, 357. Lipp M, M Daubländer, E Lanz. Buprenorphin 0.15 mg intrathecal zur postoperativen Analgesie. Eine klinische Dop-pelblindstudie. Anaesthesist, 1987, 36, 233.

Lipman JL, B Blumenkopf. Comparison of subjective and objective analgesic effects of intrave-nous and intrathecal morphine in chronic pain patients by heat beam dolorimetry. Pain, 1989, 39, 249.

Lippmann M, MS Mok. Epidural butorphanol for the relief of postoperative pain. Anesth Analg, 1988, 67, 418.

Lips U, I Pichlmayr. Vergleich der zentralen Wirksamkeit periduraler und systemischer Morphin-gaben an Hand von EEG-Spekralanalysen. Intensivmed Prax, 1981, 4, 51.

Lisander B, O Stenquist. Epidural fentanyl counteracts sympathetic gastric inhibition. Acta Anaesth Scand, 1985, 29, 560.

Lisander B, O Stenquist. Extradural fentanyl and postoperative ileus in cats (letter). Brit J Anaesth, 1981, 53, 1237.

Little MS, JD McNitt, HJ Choi, KK Tremper. A pilot study of low dose epidural sufentanil and bupivacaine for labor anesthesia. Anesthesiology, 1987, 67, A444.

Lobato RD, JL Madrid, LV Fatela, JJ Rivas, E Reig, E Lamas. Intraventricular morphine for control of pain in terminal cancer patients. J Neurosurg, 1983, 59, 627.

Lobato RD, JL Madrid, LV Fatela, JJ Rivas, E Reig, E Lamas. Analgesia elicited by low-dose intraventricular morphine in terminal cancer patients. In: HL Fields et al. (Eds.): Advances in Pain research and Therapy, Vol 9, Raven Press New York 1985, 673.

Lobato RD, JJ Rivas, R Sarabia, JL Madrid, LV Fatela. Intraventricular morphine for intractable cancer pain: a review Euromedecine, 1986, Montpellier, France, abstract, Editel, Paris.

Lobato RD, JL Madrid, LV Fatela, R Sarabia, JJ Rivas, A Gozalo. Intraventricular morphine for intractable cancer pain rationale, methods, clinical results. Acta Anaesth Scand, 1987, 31, 68.

Logas WG, N El-Baz, A El-Ganzouri, M Cullen, E Staren, LP Faber, AD Ivankovich. Continuous thoracic epidural analgesia for postoperative pain relief following thoracotomy: a randomized prospective study. Anesthesiology, 1987, 67, 787.

Lo JN, DL Erickson. Relief of post-spinal trauma spasticity with intrathecal morphine. Anesthesiology, 1984, 61, A220.

Lomessy A, JP Viale, J Motin. Analgésie post-opératoire au fentanyl par voie péridurale. Ann Anesth Fr, 1981, 1, 17.

Lomessy A, C Magnin, JP Viale, J Motin. A comparative study of epidural and intramuscular fentanyl for postoperative pain. 6th Eur Congress of Anaesth, London, 1982, volume of summaries 406.

Lomessy A, C Magnin, JP Viale, J Motin, R Cohen. Clinical advantages of fentanyl given epidurally for postoperative analgesia. Anesthesiology, 1984, 61, 466. London SW. Respiratory depression after single epidural injection of local anesthetic and morphine. Anesth Analg, 1987, 66, 797.

Loomis CW, J Penning, B Milne. A study of the analgesic interaction between intrathecal morphine and subcutaneous nalbuphine in the rat. Anesthesiology, 1989, 71, 704.

Loper KA, LB Ready, BH Dorman. Prohylactic transdermal scopolamine reduces nausea in postoperative patients receiving epidural morphine. Anesthesiology, 1988, 69 (3A), A409.

Loper KA, LB Ready. Epidural morphine after anterior cruciate ligament repair: a comparison with patient-controlled intravenous morphine. Anesth Analg, 1989, 68, 350.

Loper KA, LB Ready, M Nessly, SE Rapp. Epidural morphine provides greater pain relief than patient-controlled intravenous morphine following cholecystectomy. Anesth Analg, 1989, 69, 826.

Loubser PG, M Dimitrijevic, P Sharkey. Control of spasticity with intrathecal morphine. Anesthesiology, 1986, 65, A202.

Louis Ch, E Freye, E Hartung, W Haag. Buprenorphin in der periduralen Leitungsanaesthesie. Anaesth Intensivther Notfallmed, 1982, 17, 341.

Lowenstein E, DM Philbin. Narcotic anaesthesia. Clinics in Anaesthesiology, 1983, 1, 5.

Lubenow TR, RL Fischer, TP Besser, RJ McCarthy, LM Newman, AD Ivankovich. Comparison of continuous epidural infusions of sufentanil-bupivacaine with morphine-bupivacaine. Anesthesiology, 1988, 69 (3A), A397.

Lubenow TR, J Kroin, RJ McCarthy, S Lyon, R Penn, AD Ivankovich. Analgesic evaluation of intrathecal clonidine and tzantidine. Regional Anesthesia (Suppl), 1989, 14, 31.

Lubenow TR, J Wong, RJ McCarthy, AD Ivankovich. Prospective evaluation of continuous epidural narcotic-bupivacaine infusion in 1500 postoperative patients. Regional Anesthesia, 1989, 14 (Suppl), 32.

Lubenow T, J Kroin, R McCarthy, A Ivankovich. Analgesic and hemodynamic evaluation of intrathecal clonidine and tizanidine. Anesthesiology (Suppl), 1989, 71, 648.

Lucke C, B Hoeffken, A Von zur Muehlen. The effect of somatostatin on TSH levels in patients with primary hypothyroidism. J Clin Endocrinol Metab, 1975, 41, 1082.

Lund C, P Selmar, OB Hansen, NC Hjortsø, H Kehlet. Effects of epidural/intrathecal bupivacaine and morphine on somatosensory evoked potentials to dermatomal stimulation. Anesthesiology, 1986, 65, A177.

Lund C, P Selmar, OB Hansen, CM Jensen, H Kehlet. Effect of extradural morphine on somatosensory evoked potentials to dermatomal stimulation. Brit J Anaesth, 1987, 59,1408.

Lund C, OB Hansen, H Kehlet. Effect of epidural clonidine on somatosensory evoked potentials to dermatomal stimulation. Eur J Anaesth, 1989, 6, 207.

Lund C, S Qvitzau, A Greulich, NC Hjortsø, H Kehlet. Comparison of the effect of extradural clonidine with those of morphine on postoperative pain, stress responses, cardiopulmonary function and motor and sensory block. Brit J Anaesth, 1989, 63, 516.

Lundy P, DJ Jones. Depression of spinal NE uptake by ketamine and its isomers. Anesthesiology, 1983, 59, A383.

Lunn JK, FJ Dannemiller, TH Stanley. Cardiovascular responses to clamping of the aorta during epidural and general anesthesia. Anesth Analg (Cleve), 1979, 58, 372.

Lutze M, B Kaden, K Weigel, M Brock. Intraventrikuläre Opiatapplikation mit implantierten Medikamentenpumpen Deut Ärzteblatt, 1987, 84, 1762.

Lysak SZ, JC Eisenach, CE Dobson. Patient controlled epidural analgesia (PCEA) during labor: a comparison of three solutins with continuous epidural infusion (CEI) control. Anesthesiology, 1988, 69 (3A), A690.

MacDonald R, PJ Smith. Extradural morphine and pain relief following episiotomy. Brit J Anaesth,

1984, 56, 1201.

MacEvilly M, C O'Carroll. Hallucinations after epidural buprenorphine. Br Med J, 1989, 298, 928.

Macintosh's R. Lumbar puncture and spinal analgesia. Lee, Atkinson, Watt, 5th ed, Churchill Livingstone, 1985.

Mackersie RC, SR Shackford, DB Hoyt, TG Karagianes. Continuous epidural fentanyl analgesia: ventilatory function improvement with routine use in treatment of blunt chest injury. J Trauma, 1987, 27, 1207.

Macrae DJ, S Munishankrappa, LM Burrow, MK Milne, IS Grant. Double blind comparison of the efficacy of extradural diamorphine, extradural phenoperidine an i.m. diamorphine folloowing caesarean section. Brit J Anaesth, 1987, 59, 354.

Madej TH, L Immelman, S Roth. Extradural and intraperitoneal sufentanil in the rat: analgesia, antagonism and plasma concentrations. Brit J Anaesth, 1987, 59, 932. (a)

Madej TH, L Strunin. Comparison of epidural fentanyl with sufentanil. Anaesthesia, 1987, 42, 1156. (b)

Madej TH, NC Watson, BC Martin. Large dose epidural sufentanil: management of postoperative pain with few side effects. Anaesthesia, 1987, 42, 1204. (c)

Madrazo I, R Franco-Bourlan, V Leon, I Mena. Analgesic effect of intracerebroventricular (ICV) somatostatin-14, arginine vasopression and oxytocin in a patient with terminal cancer. Pain (Suppl), 1987, 4, S142.

Madrid JL, LV Fatela, RD Lobato, CP Alfranca. Intermittent intrathecal morphine by means of an implantable reservoir: survey of 100 cases. VII Eur Congress of Anaesth, 1986, Vienna (Austria), Report, Abst. 428.

Madrid JL, LV Fatela, RD Lobato, A Gozalo. Intrathecal therapy: rationale, technique, clinical results. Acta Anaesth Scand, 1987, 31, 60.

Madsen K, T Ebert, D McDonald, S Eichner, D Stowe. Comparison of epidural lidocaine and epidural narcotics for extracorporeal shock wave lithotripsy. Anesthesiology, 1988, 69 (3A), A403.

Maggi G. Rilievi clinici e terapeutici sull'uso della calcitonina sintetica di salmone nelle sindrome di Sudeck, nel morbo di Paget e nell'osteoporosi migrante. Clin Therap, 1978, 85, 375.

Magora F, Y Donchin, D Olshwang, JG Schenker. Epidural morphine analgesia in second-trimester induced abortion. Am J Obstet Gynecol, 1980, 138, 260. (a)

Magora F, D Olshwang, P Eimerl, J Shorr, R Katzenelson, S Cotev, JT Davidson. Observations on extradural morphine analgesia in various pain conditions. Brit J Anaesth, 1980, 52, 247. (b)

Magora F. Current status of the utilization of opioids by spinal injection. II Int Symposium: The Pain Clinic, 1986, Lille (France). In: Ph Scherpereel, J Meynadier, S Blond (Eds.): Pain Clinic II, VNU Science Press, Utrecht, 1987, 79. (a)

Magora F, Y Shir, S Fields. Prolonged epidural administration of bupivacaine and methadone followed by alcohol sympathectomy with computerized tomography control for the managemants of sympathetic reflex dystrophy. Schmerz-Pain-Douleur, 1986, 2, 83. (b)

Magora F, S Cotev. Future trends in regional spinal opioids. Int Anesth Clinics, 1986, 24, 2, 113. (a)

Magora F, J Chrubasik, D Damm, J Schulte-Mönting, Y Shir. Application of a new method for measurement of plasma methadone levels to the use of epidural methadone for relief of postoperative pain. Anesth Analg, 1987, 6, 1308. (b)

Magora F, Y Shir, et al. Methadone plasma concentrations after patient controlled epidural analgesia. Pain, 1987, S4, S190. (c)

Maione M, C Mazzi, P Nannicini. Puntura durale accidentale durante l'esecuzione di un blocco peridurale con associazione bupivacaina 0,50 % - fentanyl. Minerva anestesiologica, 1983, 49, 325.

Mak M, E Koski. The accuracy of Infusor® in continuous administration of intravenous indomethacin. VII Eur Congress of Anaesth, 1986, Vienna (Austria), Report, Abst 232.

Malick JB, JM Goldstein. Analgesic activity of substance P following intracerebral administration in rats. Life Science, 1978, 23, 835.

Malinow AM, BLK Mokriski, ML Wakefield, WJ McGuinn, DG Martz, JN Desverreaux, MJ Matjasko. Does pH adjustment reverse nesacaine antagonism of postcesarean epidural fentanyl analgesia? Anesth Analg, 1988, 67, S137. (a)

Malinow AM, BLK Mokriski, ML Wakefield, WJ McGuinn, DG Martz, JN Desverreaux, MJ Matjasko. Anesthetic choice affects postcesarean epidural analgesia. Anesth Analg, 1988, 67, S138. (b)

Malinow AM, BLK Mokriski, MK Nomura, MA Kaufman. Effect of epinephrine on intrathecal fentanyl analgesia. Anesthesiology (Suppl), 1989, 71, 704.

Malins AF, NW Goodman, GM Cooper, C Prys-Robert, RN Baird. Ventilatory effects of pre- and postoperative diamorphine. A comparison of extradural with intramuscular administration. Anaesthesia, 1984, 39, 118.

Malone BT, R Beye, J Walker. Management of pain in the terminally ill by administration of epidural narcotics. Cancer, 1985, 55, 438.

Mamo H. La douleur. Masson, Paris, 1982.

Mandaus L, R Blomberg, E Hammar. Long-term epidural morphine analgesia. Acta Anaesth Scand (Suppl.), 1982, 74, 149.

Manders KL. Integrated approach to the management of pain. Indiana Medicine, 1986, December, 1053.

Mankowitz E, JG Brock-Utne, JE Cosnett, R Green-Thompson. Epidural ketamine. A preliminary report. S Afr Med J, 1982, 61, 441.

Manoharan A. Vincristine by infusion for childhood acute immune thromboccytopenia. Lancet, 1986, I, 317.

Marando R, RS Sinatra, ES Fu, JG Collins. Failure of intrathecally administered nalbuphine to suppress visceral pain in pregnant rats. Anesthesiology, 1987, 67, A447.

Marlowe S, R Engstrom, PF White. Epidural patient-controlled analgesia (PCA): an alternative to continuous epidural infusions. Pain, 1989, 37, 97.

Marshall DC, JJ Buccafusco. Supraspinal and spinal mediation of naloxone-induced morphine withdrawal in rats. Brain Res, 1985, 329, 131.

Martin GE, T Naruse. Differences in the pharmacological actions of intrathecally administered neurotensin and morphine. Regul Pept, 1982, 3, 97.

Martin H, L Kocher, S Chere-Croze. Chronic lumbar intrathecal catheterization in the rat with reduced-length spinal compression. Physiol Behav, 1984, 33, 159.

Martin LL, RL Bouchal, DJ Smith. Ketamine inhibits serotonine uptake in vivio. Neuropharmacology, 1982, 21, 113.

Martin LVH. Postoperative analgesia after circumcision in children. Brit J Anaesth, 1982, 54, 1263.

Martin R, J Salbaing, G Blaise, JP Tétrault, L Tétrault. Epidural morphine for postoperative pain relief: a dose-response curve. Anesthesiology, 1982, 56, 423.

Martin R, Y Lamarche, JP Tétrault. Utilisation de morphiniques épiduraux et sous-arachnoidiens. Can Anaesth Soc J, 1983, 30, 666. (a)

Martin R, Y Lamarche, JP Tétrault. Epidural and intrathecal narcotics. Can Anaesth Soc J, 1983, 30, 662. (b)

Martin R, Y Lamarche, JP Tétrault, L Tétrault, LJ Veilleux. Effect of epinephrine addition to epidural morphine in obstetric analgesia. Regional Anesthesia, 1985, 10, 129.

Martin WR, CG Eades, JA Thompson, RE Huppler, PE Gilbert. The effects of morphine and nalorphine-like drugs in the non-dependent and morphine-dependent chronic spinal dog. J Pharm Exp Ther, 1976, 197, 517.

Martin WR. History and development of mixed opioid agonists, partial agonists and antagonists.

Brit J Clin Pharm, 1979, 7, S273.

Martin WR. The pharmacology of opioids. Parmacological reviews, 1983, 35, 283.

Martindale. The Extra Pharmacopoeia. 25th ed. 1982, Pharmaceutical Press London.

Maruyama Y, K Shimoji, H Shimizu, Y Sato, H Kuribayashi, R Kaieda. Effects of morphine on human spinal cord and peripheral nervous activities. Pain, 1980, 8, 63.

Masoud PJ, JT Ohr, CD Green. Transient neurologic changes after epidural morphine. Anesth Analg, 1981, 60, 540.

Masoud PJ, CD Green. Effects of massive overdose of epidural morphine sulphate. Can Anaesth Soc J, 1982, 29, 377.

Mather LE, PJ Meffin. Clinical pharmacokinetics of pethidine. Clin Pharmacokinetics, 1978, 3, 252.

Mather LE, EG Pavlin. Transfer of pethidine to CSF following intravenous administration. Anaesth Intens Care, 1981, 9, 205.

Mather LE. Pharmacokinetic and pharmacodynamic factors influencing the choice dose and route of administration of opiates for acute pain. Clinics in Anesthesiology, 1983, 1, 117. (a)

Mather LE. Clinical pharmacokinetics of fentanyl and its newer derivatives. Clin Pharmacokinetics, 1983, 8, 422. (b)

Mather LE, GD Phillips. Opioids and adjuvants. Principles of use. In: MJ Cousins, GD Phillips (Eds.): Acute pain management, Publ. Churchill Livingstone, New York, 1986, 77.

Mather LE. Opioid Pharmacokinetics in relation to their effects. Anaesth. Intens. Care, 1987, 15, 15.

Mathews E. Epidural morphine (letter). Lancet, 1979, 1, 673.

Mathews ET, LD Abrams. Intrathecal morphine in open heart surgery (letter). Lancet, 1980, 1, 543.

Matsuki A. Nothing new under the sun - a japanese pioneer in the clinical use of intrathecal morphine (letter). Anesthesiology, 1983, 58, 289.

Matsumiya N, S Dohi. Effects of intravenous or subarachnoid morphine on cerebral and spinal cord hemodynamics and antagonism with naloxone in dogs. Anesthesiology, 1983, 59, 175.

Matsumoto M, O Yuge, JG Collins, LM Kitahata, A Tanaka. Does alfentanil have a role to play in spinal opioid analgesia? Anesthesiology, 1983, 59, A380.

Matsumura H, T Sakurada, A Hara, S Sakurada, K Kisara. Characterization of the hyperalgesic effect induced by intrathecal injection of substance P. Neuropharmacology, 1985, 24, 421.

Matsunaga M, K Dan, K Higa, K Yoshida, K Fukushima. Epidural or intravenous buprenorphine for postoperative pain relief. Masui, 1984, 33, 995.

Mattei A, FP Alberico, F Chiumiento, MP Monti, A Sirignano, A Viglietto. Association between hyperbaric bupivacaine and buprenorphine in subarachnoid anesthesia. Abstract 649, 1986, 7th Europ. Congress Anaesth, Verlag Mandrich Wien.

Matthew EB, SK Henderson, MJ Avram, R Glassenberg, H Cohen. Epidural hydromorphone versus epidural morphine for post-cesarean section analgesia. Anesth Analg, 1987, 66, S112.

Matthews NC, G Corser. Epidural fentanyl for shaking in obstetrics. Anaesthesia, 1988, 43, 783.

Maurette P, P Tauzin-Fin- G Vincon, A Brachet-Lierman. Arterial and ventricular CSF pharmacokinetics after intrathecal meperidine in humans. Anesthesiology, 1989, 70, 961.

Max M, CE Inturrisi, P Grabrinski, RF Kaiko, KM Foley. Epidural opiates: plasma and cerebrospinal fluid (CSF) pharmacokinetics of morphine, methadone and beta-endorphin. Pain (Suppl.), 1982, 1, S122.

Max M, C Inturrisi, R Kaiko, P Grabinski, C Li, K Foley. Epidural and intrathecal opiates: cerebrospinal fluid and plasma profiles in patients with chronic cancer pain. Clin Pharm Ther, 1985, 38, 631.

May AE, J Wandless, RH James. Analgesia for circumcision in children. A comparison of caudal bupivacaine and intramuscular buprenorphine. Acta Anaesth Scand, 1982, 26, 331.

May KS, M Schapp, JJ Limfan, WC North. Pain relief after peripheral perineural injection of morphine. Pain (Suppl.), 1981, 1, S120.

Mayer SE. Neurohormonal transmission and the autonomic nervous system. In: Goodman and Gilman's (Eds.): The pharmacological basis of therapeutics. 6th McMillan Publ, New York, 1980, 56.

Mays KS, M Schnapp, JJ Lipman, WC North. Pain relief after peripheral perineural injection of morphine. Pain (Suppl.), 1981, 1, S120. (a)

Mays KS, WC North, M Schnapp. Stellate ganglion "blocks" with morphine in sympathetic type pain. J Neurol, Neurosurg and Psych, 1981, 44, 189. (b)

Mays KS, M Schnapp, WC North. Comparison between morphine and local anesthetic injections of stellate and celiac ganglia in chronic pain syndroms. In: TL Yaksh, H Müller (Eds.): Anaesthesiologie und Intensivmedizin, Spinal opiate analgesia, Springer Verlag, Berlin, Heidelberg, New York, 1982, 144, 121.

Mays KS, JJ Lipman, M Schnapp. Local analgesia without anesthesia using peripheral perineural morphine injections. Anesth Analg, 1987, 66, 417.

McCaughey W, J Graham. The respiratory depression of extradural morphine. Proc. Anaesthetic Research Society London, November 1981.

McCaughey W, JL Graham. The respiratory depression of epidural morphine. Time course and effect of posture. Anaesthesia, 1982, 37, 990.

McClain DA, JCC Hug. Intravenous fentanyl kinetics. Clin Pharm Ther, 1980, 28, 106.

McClure JH, WA Chambers, E Moore, DB Scott. Epidural morphine for postoperative pain. Lancet, 1980, 1, 975.

McCollum JSC, AC McKay, JW Dundee, DP O'Toole. Intradural bupivacaine with diamorphine obtunds the neuroendocrine response to operative stress. Ir J Med. Sci, 1986, 155, 138.

McCoy DD, MG Miller. Epidural morphine in a terminally ill patient. Anesthesiology, 1982, 57, 427.

McDonald AM. Complication of epidural morphine. Anaesth Intens Care, 1980, 8, 490.

McDonald R, PJ Bickford Smith. Extradural morphine and pain relief following episiotomy. Brit J Anaesth, 1984, 56, 1201.

McDonnell TE, RR Bartkowski, FA Borilla, TK Henthorn, JJ Williams. Nonuniformity of alfentanil pharmacokinetics in healthy adults. Anesthesiology, 1982, 57, A236.

McDonogh AJ, BS Cranney. Delayed presentation of an epidural abscess. Anaesth Intens Care, 1984, 12, 364.

McGrady EM, DK Brownhill, AG Davis. Epidural diamorphine and bupivacaine in labour. Anaesthesia, 1989, 44, 400.

McLelland J. The mechanism of morphine-induced urticaria (letter). Arch Dermatol, 1986, 122, 138.

McMorland GH, MJ Douglas. Epidural morphine for postoperative analgesia. Can Anaesth Soc J, 1986, 33, 115.

McQuay HJ, RES Bullingham, PJD Evans, JW Lloyd, RA Moore. Demand analgesia to assess pain relief from epidural opiates. Lancet, 1980, 1, 768.

McQuay HJ, RA Moore, RES Bullingham. Buprenorphine kinetics. In: KM Foley, CE Inturrisi (Eds.): Advances in Pain Reseach and Therapy, vol 8 Raven Press, New York, 1986, 271.

McQuay HJ. Spinal opiates. Brit J Hosp Med, 1987, April, 354.

McQuay HJ, RA Moore. Urinary retention following spinal opiates. Anesthesiology, 1988, 69, 441.

McQuay HJ, AF Sullivan, K Smallman, AH Dickenson. Intrathecal opioids, potency and lipothilicity. Pain, 1989, 36, 111.

Meddens HJM. The influence of different anesthetic techniques on blood loss in prostatectomy patients (Hryntschak's operation). Acta Anaesth Belgica, 1981, 32, 239.

Meert TF, H Noorduin, HR Lu. Epidural sufentanil: a review of pharmacological clinical data. Report of the 5th. international Congress of the Belgien Society of Anaesthesia and Reanimation,

Brunch, 1988.

Meglio M, B Cioni, V d'Annunzio, GF Rossi. Subarachnoid morphine in the treatment of cancer pain. In: JM Besson, Y Lazorthes (Eds.): Spinal opioids and the relief of pain, Basic mechanisms and clinical applications. INSERM, Paris, 1985, 431.

Mehnert JH, TJ Dupont, DH Rose. Intermittent epidural morphine instillation for control of postoperative pain. Amer J Surg, 1983, 146, 145.

Meier FA, DP Perl, WW Pendlebury, DW Coombs, RL Saunders. Continuous infusion of epidural anesthesia and posterior column deterioration. Lancet, 1982, 2, 659. (a)

Meier FA, DW Coombs, RL Saunders, MG Pageau. Pathologic anatomy of constant morphine infusion by intraspinal silastic catheter. Anesthesiology, 1982, 57, A206. (b)

Meisenberg G, WH Simons. Peptides and the blood-brain barrier. Life Sci, 1983, 32, 2611.

Meistelman C, C Saint-Marice, M Lepaul, et al. A comparision of alfentanil pharmacokinetics in children and adults. Anesthesiology, 1987, 66, 13.

Meldrum BS, C Menini, JM Stutzmann, R Naquet. Effects of opiate-like peptides, morphine, and naloxone in the photosensitive baboon, papiopapio. Brain Res, 1979, 170, 333.

Melendez J, V Cirella, T Dodds. Lumbar epidural analgesia post-thoracic surgery. Anesth Analg, 1988, 67, S147.

Mensink FJ, R Kozody, CH Kehler, JG Wade. Dose-response relationship of clonidine in tetracaine spinal anaethesia. Anesthesiology, 1987, 67, 717.

Messahel FM, PJ Tomlin. Narcotic withdrawal syndrome after intrathecal administration of morphine. Brit Med J, 1981, 283, 417.

Meuldermans WEG, RMA Hurkmans, JJP Heykants. Plasma proteinbinding and distribution of fentanyl, sufentanil, alfentanil and lofentanil in blood. Arch Int Pharmacodyn Ther, 1982, 257, 4.

Meuldermans W, R Woestenborgs, H Noorduin, F Camu, A Van Steenberge, J Heykants. Protein-binding of the analgesics alfentanil and sufentanil in maternal and neonatal plasma. Eur J Clin Pharmacol, 1986, 30, 217.

Meunier J. Analgésie péridurale post-opératoire par la péthidine en chirurgie digestive. Ann Fr Anesth Réanim, 1984, 3, 469.

Meyer G, G Quenet, L Ronchi, E Bonnieux, M Martignon. Anesthésie péridurale avec narcose de complément et controle de la ventilation en chirurgie viscérale. Ann Fr Anesth Réanim, 1983, 2, 178.

Meynadier J, M Dubar, S Blond, M Combelles-Pruvot. Traitement des douleurs néoplasiques par la morphine intrathécale et intra-cérébroventriculaire. AIAREF, Tunis, Juin 1984.

Meynadier J, M Dubar, J Chrubasik, S Blond. Intraventricular morphine in the treatment of cancer pain. Schmerz-Pain-Douleur, 1985, 6, 46. (a)

Meynadier J, M Dubar, J Chrubasik, S Blond. Treatment of intractable pain in cancer patients with intrathecal morphine. Schmerz-Pain-Douleur, 1985, 6, 46. (b)

Meynadier J, J Chrubasik, M Dubar, E Wünsch. Intrathecal somatostatine in terminally ill patients. A report of two cases. Pain, 1985, 23, 9. (c)

Meynadier J, M Dubar, S Blond, M Combelle-Pruvot. Intrathecal morphine in treatment of intractable pain in cancer patients. In: W Erdmann, T Oyama, MJ Pernak (Eds.): Pain Clinic I, VNU, Science Press, Utrecht 1985, 87. (d)

Meynadier J, S Blond, C Gros, JM Lecomte, J Chrubasik, JC Schwartz. First clinical demonstration of analgesia induced by co-intra- thecal administration of enkephalinase and aminopeptidase inhibitors. Poster Session, International Symposium on Pain Therapy, Roma, sept. 1985. (e)

Meynadier J, D Lefébvre, J Beaucaire, M Combelles-pruvot, R Assaker, S Blond. Traitement des douleurs rebelles en cancérologie par la morphinothérapie intrathécale: a propos de 126 cas. II Int Symposium: Pain Clinic, 1986, Lille (France). (a)

Meynadier J. Administration de substances non-morphiniques dans le LCR dans le cadre du traitement des douleurs rebelles en cancérologie. Euromédecine 1986, Montpellier (France), La douleur en cancérologie, Editel, Paris, 151. (b)

Meynadier J, C Gros, JM Lecomte, J Chrubasik, JC Schwartz. Analgesic effectiveness of intrathecal inhibitors of enkephalinase and aminopeptidase in man. Anesth Analg, 1987, 66, S117. (a)

Meynadier J, C Gros, JM Lecomte, J Chrubasik, JC Schwartz. Are the enkephalinase and aminopeptidase inhibitors useful in chronic cancer pain treatment. Anaesthesist, 1987, 36, 387. (b)

Meynadier J, S Blond, C Brichard, D Lefebre, J Beaucaire, Th Dupard, R Assaker. Intrathecal morphintherapy (IM) in intractable cancer pain: four years of experience (n=170). Pain, 1987, S4, S391. (c)

Meynadier J, S Dalmas, JM Lecomte, Cl Gros, JCH Schwartz. Patient analgesia effects of inhibitors enkephaline metabolism administered intrathecally to cancer patients. Pain Clinic, 1989, 2, 201.

Michelangeli F, et al. L'association fentanyl - bupivacaine après césarienne. Conv Med, 1984, 3, 121.

Michon F, C Oxeda, M Girard, M Fischler, O Delalande, L Toty, G Vourc'h. Sédation prolongée de douleurs chroniques rebelles. A propos de trois techniques. In: Ars Medici, Congress Series 3, 1983, II, 475.

Michon F, VG des Mesnards, M Girard, M Fischler, G Vourc'h Analgésie péridurale morphinique de longue durée en pathologie néoplasique et vasculaire. Cahiers d' Anesthésiologie, 1985, 33, 39.

Migaly P. The problem of intrathecal ketamine. Brit J Anaesth, 1986, 58, 684.

Mihic DN, E Binkert, FA Hess, J Orucevic, J Turner. Die peridurale Morphingabe zur Behandlung postoperativer Schmerzen. Regional Anaesthesie, 1982, 5, 42.

Millan MJ, C Schmauss, MH Millan, A Herz. Vasopressin and oxytocin in the rat spinal cord: analysis of their role in the control of nociception. Brain Res, 1984, 309, 384.

Millan MJ. Multiple opioid systems and pain. Review article. Pain, 1986, 27, 303.

Miller D, JA Robblee. Perioperative managment of a patient with a malignant pheochromocytoma. Can Anaesth Soc J, 1985, 32, 278.

Miller MT. Epidural morphine in the treatment of tetanus (letter). S Afr Med J, 1983, 63, 31.

Milne B, FW Cervenko, K Jhamandas, M Sutak. Intrathecal clonidine: analgesia and effect on opiate withdrawal in the rat. Anesthesiology, 1985, 62, 34.

Milne RP, HE Williams. Epidural morphine in terminal care. Anaesthesia, 1981, 36, 51.

Milon D, D Bentue-Ferrer, D Noury, JM Reymann, J Sauvage J, H Allain, C Saint-marc, J van den Driessche. Anesthésie péridurale pour césarienne par association bupivacaine-fentanyl. Ann Fr Anesth Réanim, 1983, 2, 273.

Milon D, H Allain, D Noury, G Lavenac, J van den Driessche. Analgésie péridurale au cours du travail: comparison de trois associations bupivacaine -fentanyl et de la bupivacaine seule (a propos de 202 cas). J de Pharm, 1985, 16, 539. (a)

Milon D, H Allain, D Noury, G Lavenac, J van den Driessche. Analgésie péridurale au cours du travail: comparison de trois associations bupivacaine-fentanyl. J de Pharm, 1985, 16, 631. (b)

Milon D, G Lavenac, D Noury, H Allain, J Van Der Driessche, C Saint- Marc. Analgésie péridurale au cours du travail: comparaison de trois associations fentanyl-bupivacaine et de la bupivacaine seule. Ann Fr Anesth Réanim, 1986, 5, 18.

Minnich ME, JG Quirk, RB Clark. Epidural anesthesia for vaginal delivery in a patient with idiopathic hypertrophic subaortic stenosis. Anesthesiology, 1987, 67, 590.

Miralles FS, F Lopez-Soriano, D Perez, F Lopez-Rodriguez, MM Puig. Subarachnoid administration of calcitonin produces postoperative analgesia. Anesthesiology, 1986, 65, A199.

Miralles FS, F Lopez-Soriano, MM Puig, D Perez, F Lopez-Rodriguez. Postoperative analgesia induced by subarachnoid lidocaine plus calcitonin. Anesth Analg, 1987, 66, 615.

Mircea N. Subarachnoid anaesthesia and analgesia with pethidine. IV Int Congress of Anaesth, Bucarest, 1981, abstract 121.

Mircea N, C Constantinescu, C Jianu, G Busu, C Ene, S Daschievici, A Nedelcu, A Leoveanu. L'anesthésie sous-arachnoidienne par la péthidine. Ann Fr Anesth Réanim, 1982, 1, 167.

Mitterschiffthaler G, Ch Huber, A Theiner, IC Fuith. Selection of patients for intrathecal opioid therapy. ESRA 6th Congress Eur Soc Reg Anaesth, Report 119, MAPAR, Paris 1987

Mocavero G. Perineural, epidural and subarachnoid morphine for the relief of chronic pain. Anaesthesia, 1982, 37, 471.

Modig J, A Hjelmstedt, B Sahlstedt, E Maripuu. Comparative influences of epidural and general anaesthesia on deep venous thrombosis and pulmonary embolism after total hip replacement. Acta Chir Scand, 1981, 147, 125. (a)

Modig J, L Paalzow. A comparison of epidural morphine and epidural bupivacaine for postoperative pain relief. Acta Anaesth Scand, 1981, 25, 437. (b)

Modig J, T Borg, L Bagge, T Saldeen. Role of extradural and of general anaesthesia in fibrinolysis and coagulation after total hip replacement. Brit J Anaesth, 1983, 55, 625. (a)

Modig J, T Borg, G Karlstroem, E Maripuu, B Sahlstedt. Thromboembolism after total hip replacement: role of epidural and general anesthesia. Anesth Analg, 1983, 62, 174. (b)

Moine P, C Ecoffey. Bupivacaine caudal block with fentanyl in children. Anesthesiology (Suppl), 1989, 71, 1017.

Moir DD. Pain relief in labour. Brit J Hosp Med, 1977, 17, 226.

Mok MS, SK Tsai. More experience with intrathecal morphine for obstetric analgesia (letter). Anesthesiology, 1981, 55, 481.

Mok MS, SK Tsai. Analgesic effects of ID butorphanol, nalbuphine, meperidine, and fentanyl. 8th World Congress Anaesth, 1984 Manilla, Vol 11, A213. (a)

Mok MS, M Lippmann, JJ Wang, KH Chan, TY Lee. Efficacy of epidural nalbuphine in postoperative pain control. Anesthesiology, 1984, 61, A187. (b)

Mok MS, BW Louie, BF Hwong BF, KH Chan, M Lippmann. Epidural nalbuphine for the relief of pain after thoracic surgery. Anesth Analg, 1985, 64, 258.

Mok MS, SK Tsai, WM Ho, HS Tso, M Lippmann. Efficacy of epidural butorphanol compared to morphine for the relief of postoperative pain. Anesthesiology, 1986, 65, A175.

Mok MS, SP Shuai, C Lee, TY Lee, M Lippmann. Naltrexone pretreatment attenuates side effects of epidural morphine. Anesthesiology (Suppl), 1986, 65, 200.

Mok MS, KH Chan, SK Chung, TY Lee, M Lippman. Evaluation of the analgesic effects of epidural ketamine. Anesth Analg, 1987, 66, S121.

Mok MS, JJ Wang, JH Chan, SE Liu, M Lippmann. Analgesic effect of epidural clonidine and nalbuphine in combined use. Anesthesiology (Suppl), 1988, 69, 398.

Mokriski BLK, AM Malinow, St Amant, MA Kaufman, JA Snell, DA Nagey. Epidural narcotic analgesia for labor and fetal heart rate variability. Anesthesiology (Suppl), 1989, 71, 856.

Moldenhauer CC, CC Hug. Use of narcotic analgesics as anesthetics. Clinics in Anaesthesiology, 1984, 2, 107.

Molke Jensen F, JB Madsen, H Guldager, AA Christensen, HO Eriksen. Respiratory depresssion after epidural morphine in the postoperative period. Influence of posture. Act Anesth Scand, 1984, 6, 600.

Mollenholt P, N Rawal, C Post, I Paulsson. Neurotoxic and motor actions of somatostatin in the rat after intrathecal administration. ESRA, 6th Congress Eur Soc Reg Anaesth, MAPAR, Paris, 1987, Report 115.

Mollenholt P, C Post, N Rawal, J Freedman, T Hökfelt, I Paulsson. Antinociceptive and 'neurotoxic' actions of somatostatin in rat spinal cord after intrathecal administration. Pain, 1988, 32, 95.

576

Møller IW, T Vester-Andersen, A Steentoft, E Hjortsø, M Lunding. Respiratory depression and morphine concentration in serum after epidural and intramuscular administration of morphine. Acta Anesth Scand, 1982, 26, 421.

Møller TW, J Eriksen. Accidental high dose extradural morphine. Brit J Anaesth, 1982, 54, 1237.

Montpellier D, F Lepointe, P Besserve. Anesthésie loco-régionale intraveineuse du membre supérieur par une association lignocaine-fentanyl. Abstract 975, 1986, 7th Europ. Congress Anaesth, Mandrich Verlag, Wien.

Moon RE, FM Clements. Accidental epidural overdose of hydromorphone. Anesthesiology, 1985, 83, 238.

Moonka NK, S Ramanathan, P Khoo, H Turndorf. Does epinephrine modify the action of epidural morphine? Anesthesiology (Suppl), 1989, 71, 905.

Moore A, R Bullingham, H McQuay, M Allen, D Baldwin, A Cole. Spinal fluid kinetics of morphine and heroin. Clin Pharm Ther, 1984, 35, 40.

Moore AK, A Vilderman, W Lubenskyi, J McCans, GS Fox. The effect of age on postoperative pain relief after standardized doses of epidural morphine. Anesth Analg, 1989, 68, S199.

Moore DC, MS Batra. The components of effective test dose prior to epidural block. Anesthesiology, 1981, 55, 693.

Moore RA, RES Bullingham, HJ McQuay, CW Hand, JB Aspel, MC Allen, D Thomas. Dural permeability to narcotics: in vitro determination and application to extradural administration. Brit J Anaesth, 1982, 54, 1117.

Moore RA, RES Bullingham, HJ McQuay, M Allen, D Baldwin, A Cole. Spinal fluid kinetics of morphine and heroin in man. Clin Pharmacol Ther, 1984, 35, 40. (a)

Moore RA, GMC Paterson, RES Bullingham, MC Allen, D Baldwin, HJ McQuay. Controlled comparison of intrathecal cinchocaine with intrathecal cinchocaine and morphine Clinical effects and plasma morphine concentrations. Brit J Anaesth, 1984, 56, 837. (b)

Moore RA, JW Sear, RES Bullingham, HJ McQuay. Morphine kinetics in renal failure. In: KM Foley et al. (Eds.): Adv. in Pain Research and Therapy, Vol 8, Raven Press New York, 1986, 65.

Moore RA, CW Hand, HJ McQuay. Opiate metabolism and excretion. In: Update in Opioids p 829. Baillieres Clinical Anaesthesiology, 1987, 1, 4.

Morgan B, CJ Bulpitt, P Clifton, PL Lewis. Effectiveness of pain relief in labour: survey of 100 mothers. Brit Med J, 1982, 285, 689.

Morgan M. Editorial. Anaesthesia, 1982, 37, 527.

Morgan M. Epidural and intrathecal opioids. Anaesth Intens Care, 1987, 15, 60.

Morgan M. The rational use of intrathecal and extradural opioids. Brit J Anaesth, 1989, 63, 165.

Mori K, T Komatsu, T Tomemori, K Shingu, N Urabe, N Seo, Y Hatono. Pentobarbital-anaesthetized and decerebrate cats reveal different neurophysiological responses in anaesthetic-induced analgesia. Acta Anaesth Scand, 1981, 25, 349.

Mori K, K Shingu. Epidural ketamine does not produce analgesia. Anesthesiology, 1988, 68, 296.

Moricca G. Intrathecal morphine for the control of the pain of myocardial infarction. Anaesthesia, 1981, 36, 68.

Morisot P, JF Dessanges, J Regnard, A Lockhart. Ventilatory response to carbon dioxide during extradural anaesthesia with lignocaine and fentanyl. Brit J Anaesth, 1989, 63, 97.

Morris RW, M Nairn, TA Torda. A comparison of fifteen pulse oximeters. Part 1: a clinical comparison; part II: a test of performance under conditions of poor perfusion. Anaesth Intens Care, 1989, 17, 62.

Moskowitz B, M Bolkier, Y Ginesin, DR Levin, B Rosenberg. Epidural morphine: a new approach to combined anesthesia and analgesia in urological patients. Eur Urol, 1986, 12, 171.

Mota A, P De Antonio, G Huertas, C Márquez, E Torres, R Noval, A Pajuelo LM Torres. Analgesia espinal monodosis en el curso preoperatorio de la hernia discal. Rev Espan Anaest R., 1989, 36 1, 56, 72.

Motsch J. Über die Periduralanalgesie. Anaesth Intensivmed, 1983, 24, 384.

Motsch J. Anesthesiques locaux et morphinques par voie peridurale. Can Anesth, 1984, 32, 43.

Motsch J, B Robert. Spinale Opiat-Analgesie mit implantierbaren Kathetersystemen. Schmerz-Pain-Doleur, 1987, 3, 115. (a)

Motsch J, G Schüder, B Bier. Use of portable pumps for continuous intrathecal narcotics infusion. Anaesthesist, 1987, 36, 377. (b)

Motsch J, W Bleser, AJ Ismaily. Bedeutung der intrathekalen Opiat-Analgesie in der Therapie terminaler Karzinomschmerzen. Anaesth Intensivmed, 1987, 9, 283. (c)

Motsch J, W Bleser, AJ Ismaily, G Schüder. Continuous intrathecal narcotics in treatment of intractable cancer pain using a small portable pump. Acta Anaesth Scand, 1987, 31, No 165. (d)

Motsch J, W Bleser, AJ Ismaily, L Distler. Kontinuierliche intrathekale Opiattherapie mit tragbaren Medikamentenpumpen bei Karzinomschmerzen. Anästh. Intensivther. Notfallmed., 1988, 23, 271.

Mott JM, JH Eisele. A survey of monitoring practices following spinal opiate administration. Anesth Analg, 1986, 65, S105.

Moulin DE, MB Max, RF Kaiko, CE Inturrisi, J Maggard, TL Yaksk, KM Foley. The analgesic efficacy of intrathecal DADL in cancer patients with chronic pain. Pain, 1985, 23, 213.

Moulin DE, CE Inturrisi, KM Foley. Epidural and intrathecal opioids: cerebrospinal fluid and plasma pharmacokinetics in cancer pain patients. In: KM Foley et al. (Eds.): Adv. in Pain Research and Therapy, Vol 8, Raven Press New York, 1986, 369. (a)

Moulin DE, CE Inturrisi, KM Foley. Cerebrospinal fluid pharmacokinetics of intrathecal morphine sulfate and D-Ala2-Leu5-Enkephalin. Ann Neurol, 1986, 20, 218. (b)

Mourisse P, J Geernaert, L Weyne, H Noorduin, G Van den Bussche. Epidural sufentanil and bupivacaine in labour pain, a comparative study. Janssen Clinical Research report, 1985, R 33800/4, april.

Moyer JR. Alfenta ® (alfentanil HCl injection) Publ. Janssen Pharmaceutica, USA

Mulder JH. Prospective multicenter study about morphine infusion for treatment of chronic cancer pain. Nederlandse vereniging ter bestudering van pyn, Rotterdam. 1986, Personnal communication.

Mule SJ. Physiological disposition of narcotic agonists and antagonists. In: DH Clouet (Ed.): Narcotic drugs: Biochemical pharmacology. New York, Plenum Press, 1971, 99.

Muller A, B Laugner, JM Farcot, M Singer, P Gauthier-Lafaye, R Gandar. Hypoalgésie obstétricale par injection péridurale de morphine. Anesth Analg Réanim, 1981, 38, 35.

Muller A, A Straja, JP Dupeyron, D Franckhauser, E Dumeny. Postoperative hypoalgesia by epidural morphine after abdominal surgery. In: TL Yaksh, H Mueller (Eds.): Anaesthesiology and intensive care medicine N°144. Spinal opiate analgesia, experimental and clinical studies. Spinger-Verlag, Berlin, New York, 1982, 62.

Muller A. Administration périmédullaire de morphiniques. In: P Gauthier-Lafaye (Ed.): Précis d'anesthésie loco-régionale, Masson, Paris 1985, 248. (a)

Muller A, B Laugner, P Diemonsch. Intrathecal opiates: a new implantable reservoir with transcutaneously operated valve. Poster, Sertürner Symposium, Einbeck, 1985. (c)

Muller A, B Laugner. Implantable injection port for intrathecal morphine administration. Poster, Sertürner Symposium, Einbeck 1985 (b)

Muller A, B Laugner. Site d'injection pour morphinothérapie intrathécale lombaire. II Int Symposium: Pain Clinic, 1986, Lille (France).

Müller H, M Stoyanov, U Börner, V Lüben, G Hempelmann. Peridurale Opiatinfusion bei Karzinomschmerz: Implantationstechnik und individuelle Füllung der Pumpe. In: Gh. Sehhati-Chafai (Eds.): Schmerzdiagnostik und Therapie, 141.

Müller H, U Börner, G Hempelmann. Clinical use of epidural opiate analgesia. 7th world Congress of Anaesth, Hamburg, 1980, Excerpta Medica, Int Congress Series N° 533, abstract 825. (a)

578

Müller H, U Börner, M Stoyanov, G Hempelmann. Intraoperative peridurale Opiatanalgesie. Anaesthesist, 1980, 29, 656. (b)

Müller H, U Börner, M Stoyanov, L Gleumes, G Hempelmann. Peridurale Opiatapplikation bei malignombedingten chronischen Schmerzen. Anaesth Intensivther Notfallmed, 1981, 16, 251. (a)

Müller H, A Brähler, M Stoyanov, U Börner, G Hempelmann. Peridurales Morphin als Adjuvans der geburtshilflichen Periduralanaesthesie (Epidural morphine as an adjunct to epidural anaesthesia). Regional Anaesthesie, 1981, 4, 42. (b)

Müller H, W Vogelsberger, K Aigner, HF Herget, G Hempelmann. Kontinuierliche peridurale Opiatapplikation mit einer implantierten Pumpe. Regional Anaesthesie, 1983, 6, 47. (a)

Müller H, J Biscoping, H. Gips, H Schelp, G Hempelmann. Buprenorphin-Konzentrationen in Serum und Liquor: Beziehung zu blutgasanalytischen Veränderungen bei verschiedenen Applikationswegen. Vortrag Internationales Sertürner Symposium "Schmerz, Schmerzforschung und Therapie", Göttingen, 15.-18.06.1983.(b)

Müller H, K Aigner, I Worm, M Lobisch, A Brähler, G Hempelmann. Langzeit-Erfahrungen mit der kontinuierlichen periduralen Opiatanalgesie mittels implantierter Pumpe. Anaesthesist, 1984, 33, 433.

Müller H, J Biscoping, H Gips, F Tilkes, P Strunz, G Hempelmann. Hygienische Verhältnisse und Stabilität der Medikamente bei periduraler Langzeit-Infusion mit implantierten oder externen Pumpen. Anaesthesist, 1985, 34, 247. (a)

Müller H, K Aigner, H Gerlach, I Worm, G Hempelmann. Continuous epidural opiate analgesia via internal or external pumps in chronic pain of malignant origin. In: W Erdmann, T Oyama, MJ Pernak (Eds.): Pain Clinic I, VNU, Science Press, Utrecht, 1985, 327. (b)

Müller H, H Gerlach, J Boldt, P Hild, KU Oehler, G Hempelmann. Local medication of spinal spasticity. Schmerz-Pain-Douleur, 1985, 6, 123. (c)

Müller H, U Börner, H Gips, V Lüben, G Hempelmann. Continuous epidural opiate infusion in cancer pain. Schmerz-Pain-Douleur, 1985, 3, 117. (d)

Müller H, K Aigner, K Schwemmle, G Hempelmann. Implantation of pump or port for epidural opiate analgesia in cancer pain. ICRCT 85, Giessen, FRG, August 26-28, 1985. (e)

Müller H, O Otto, P Marck, G Hempelmann. Continuous epidural opiate in malignant pain. ICRCT 85, Giessen FRG, August 26-28, 1985. (f)

Müller H, K Aigner, J Zierski. Behandlung von Tumorschmerz mit Pumpsystem zur rückenmarknahen Opiatapplikation. Deut Ärzteblatt, 1985, 35, 2475. (g)

Müller H, K Aigner, J Biscoping, I Worm, G Hempelmann. Continuous epidural opiate infusion in malignant pain. Life Support Systems, 1985, 3, 182. (h)

Müller H, HW Pia. Pumpen in der Pharmakotherapie. Deut Ärzteblatt, 1985, 35, 2486. (i)

Müller H, U Börner, J Zierski, G Hempelmann. Intrathecal baclofen in tetanus (letter). Lancet, 1986, 1, 317. (a)

Müller H, J Zierski, H Gerlag. Intrathekales Baclofen bei Tetanus. VII Eur Congress, 1986, Vienna (Austria), report, Abst 314. (b)

Müller H, H Gips, W Krumholz, J Zierski, V Lüben, G Hempelmann. Phamakokinetik der kontinuierlichen periduralen Morphininfusion. Anaesthesist, 1986, 35, 672. (c)

Müller H, et al. Intractecal baclofen in tetanus. Lancet, 1986, 1, 317. (d)

Müller H, W Vogelsberger, K Aigner, I Gerlach, G Hempelmann. Epidural opiate analgesia via implantable, continuous low-flow pump for cancer pain. In: HJ Wüst, M Stanton-Hicks (Eds.): Anaesthesiologie und Intensivmedizin, new aspects in regional anesthesia 4, Springer Verlag, Berlin, Heidelberg, New York, Tokyo, 1986, 176, 149. (e)

Müller H. Personnal communication 1986 (f)

Müller H, U Börner, J Zierski, G Hempelmann. Intrathecal baclofen for treatment of tetanus-induced spasticity. Anesthesiology, 1987, 66, 76.

Müller H, V Lüben, J Zierski, G Hempelmann. Long term spinal opiate treatment. Acta Anaesth Belgica, 1988b, 39, 82.

Müller H, Ch Schnorr, J Zierski, G Hempelmann. Rückenmarksnahe Medikamenteninfusion bei Schmerzen durch maligne Tumoren oder Spastizität. Med Welt, 1988a, 39, 829.

Müller-Schwefe G, P Milewski. Effects of intrathecal baclofen on spinal spasticity in man. Int Symposium, Spinalanalgesia, Munich, april 1985, abstracts. (a)

Müller-Schwefe G, W Frey, S Müller-Schwefe, P Milewski. Ambulant continuous epidural opiate-analgesia using an external portable infusion pump. In: W Erdmann, T Oyama, MJ Pernak (Eds.): Pain Clinic I, VNU, Science Press, Utrecht, 1985, 335. (b)

Murata K, I Nakagawa, Y Kumeta, LM Kitahata, JG Collins. Intrathecal clonidine suppresses noxiously evoked activity of spinal wide dynamic range neurons in cats. Anesth Analg, 1989, 69, 185.

Murchison DJ, FM Davis, JM Gibbs, EJ Maycock. Epidural buprenorphine (letter). Anaesth Intensive Care, 1984, 12, 179.

Murphy DF, P MacGrath, M Stritch. Postoperative analgesia in hip surgery. A controlled comparison of epidural buprenorphine with intramuscular morphine. Anaesthesia, 1984, 39, 181. (a)

Murphy DF, M MacEvilly. Pain relief with epidural buprenorphine after spinal fusion: a comparison with intramuscular morphine. Acta Anaesth Scand, 1984, 28, 144. (b)

Murphy DF, J Cahill, G Fitzpatrick, M MacEvilly. Epidural buprenorphine for postoperative pain relief. Anesth Analg, 1985, 64, 456.

Murphy TM. Intraspinal narcotics for chronic pain: abstract in: Recent advances in intraspinal pain therapy. Vicenza, Sept, 1985, 15.

Murphy TM, S Hinds, D Cherry. Intraspinal narcotics: non-malignant pain. Acta Anaesth Scand, 1987, 31, 75.

Murray K. Prevention of urinary retention with phenoxybenzamine during epidural morphine (letter). Brit Med J, 1984, 288, 645.

Nabil MK, N Hanna, JS Hoffman. Percutaneous epidural catherization for intractable pain in terminal cancer patients. Gynecologic Oncology, 1989, 32, 22.

Naguib M, Y Adu-Gyamfi, GH Absood, H Farag, HK Gyasi. Epidural ketamine for postoperative surgery. Can Anaesth Soc J, 1986, 33, 16. (a)

Naguib M, CE Famewo, A Absood. Pharmacokinetics of meperidine in spinal anaesthesia. Can Anaesth Soc J, 1986, 33, 162. (b)

Naguib M. Epidural ketamine for postoperative analgesia. Anaesth Analg, 1988, 67, 798.

Naito H. Pharmacokinetics of intravenous and epidural buprenorphine analgesia. Masui, 1988, 37 (19), 1180.

Nakagawa I, LM Kitahata, K Murata, K Omote, JG Collins. Spinal mechanism of clonidine analgesia and its synergism with morphine. Anesth Analg, 1988, 67, S157.

Nakazawa T, M Ikeda, T Kaneko, K Yamatsu. Analgesic effects of dynorphin-a and morphine in mice. Peptides (Fayetteville), 1985, 6, 75.

Nalda MA, F Campo, I Burzaco. First administration of epidural fentanyl in obstetric analgesia. 7th world congress of anaesthesiology, Hamburg,1980, Excerpta Medica, Int Congress Series 533, 324.

Nalda MA, F Campo, I Burzaco. Obstetric analgesia with fentanyl administered by the extradural route. Brit J Anaesth, 1981, 53, 113P.

Nalda MA, F Campo, I Burzaco. Obstetric analgesia with fentanyl-bupivacaine by the extradural route. Brit J Anaesth, 1982, 54, 250P.

Nalda MA, JL Gonzalez. Pharmacokinetics of epidural clonidine. Eur J Anaesth, 1986, 3, 60. (a)

Nalda MA, JL Gonzalez. Postoperative pain relief with the synergistic interaction of epidural

580

clonidine and morphine. VI Eur Congress, 1986, Vienna (Austria), Report, Abst 421. (b)

Nanninga JB, F Frost, R Penn. Effect of intrathecal baclofen on bladder and sphincter function. J Urology, 1989,142,101.

Naulty JS, M Johnson, GA Burger, S Datta S, JB Weiss, J Morrison, GW Ostheimer. Epidural fentanyl for postcesarean delivery pain management. Anesthesiology, 1983, 59, A415.

Naulty JS, S Weintraub, J McMahon, GW Ostheimer, C Hunt, R Chantigian. Epidural butorphanol for postcesarean delivery pain management. Anesthesiology, 1984, 61, A415.

Naulty JS, S Datta, GW Ostheimer, MD Johnson, GA Burger. Epidural fentanyl for postcaesarean delivery pain managment. Anesthesiology, 1985, 63, 694.

Naulty JS. Intraspinal Narcotics. Clinics in Anaesthesiology, 1986, 4, 145. (a)

Naulty JS, L Hertwig, CO Hunt, B Hartwell, S Datta, GW Ostheimer, BG Covino. Duration of analgesia of epidural fentanyl following cesarean delivery - effects of local anesthetics drug selection. Anesthesiology, 1986, 65, A180. (b)

Naulty JS, A Malinow, CO Hunt, J Hausheer, S Datta, MJ Lema, GW Ostheimer. Epidural butorphanol-bupivacaine for analgesia during labor and delivery. Anesthesiology, 1986, 65, A369. (c)

Naulty JS, FB Sevarino, MJ Lema, CO Hunt, S Datta, GW Ostheimer. Epidural sufentanil for postcesarean delivery pain management. Anesthesiology, 1986, 65, A396. (d)

Naulty JS, P Labove, S Datta, CO Hunt, GW Ostmeier. Epidural butorphanol/fentanyl for postcesarean delivery analgesia. Anesthesiology, 1987, 67, A463.

Naulty JS, W Bergen, D Zurowski, R Ross, W Grubb. Effect of diluent volume on analgesia produced by epidural sufentanil. Anesthesiology (Suppl), 1989, 71, 700.

Naulty JS, R Ross, W Bergen. Epidural sufentanil-bupivacaine for analgesia during labor and delivery. Anesthesiology (Suppl), 1989, 71, 842.

Nauman CP Rundtischgespräch. Anaesth Intensivmed, 1986, 188, 364.

Navarro GH, MJ Gonzalez, H Zimman Mansfeld, T Molinaro Apricio. Epidural administration of calcitonin in pain due to bone metastasis. II Int Symposium: Pain Clinic, 1986, Lille (France).

Negre I, JP Gueneron, C Ecoffey, J Levron, K Samii. CO2 sensitivity after epidural fentanyl. Anesthesiology, 1985, 63, A507.

Negre I, JP Gueneron, C Ecoffey, C Penon, JB Gross, JC Levron, K Samii. Ventilatory response to carbon dioxide after intramuscular and epidural fentanyl. Anesth Analg, 1987, 66, 707.

Neil A, L Terenius. Receptor mechanisms for nociception. Int Anesth Clin, 1986, 24, 1.

Nelson TW, JK Lilly, JD Baker, JA Ackerly. Prophylactic versus prn naloxone for the treatment of pruritus secondary to epidural morphine. Regional Anesthesia, 1987, 12, 38.

Nelson W, J Katz. Intrathecal morphine for postoperative pain relief. Anesthesiology, 1980, 53, S218.

Netter FH. Nervous System I, Ciba collection of med illustration. Ciba Pharmaceutical Cie Ed, 1977. Neurochir. 1989, 35, 52-57.

Ngai SH, BA Berkowitz, JC Young, J Hempstead, S Spector. Pharmacokinetics of naloxone in rats and men. Anesthesiology, 1976, 44, 398.

Nicaise C, R Abou Hatem, P Hendrickx. Ambulatory use of epidural morphine in cancer patients. Proceedings: 2nd European Conference on Clinical Oncology and Cancer Nursing, Amsterdam, Holland, November 2-5, 1983, 216 (Abstract).

Nicosia F, E Pelliccia, P Dell'Amico, R Troinai, M Lombardi, I Spinelli, A Sicari, M Gianfranchi. Cordotomia cervicale percutanea e morfina spinale da serbatoio sottocutaneo nella strategia contro il dolore da cancro (Percutaneous cervical chordotomy and spinal morphine from a subcutaneous reserve in the management of cancer pain. Minerva Anestsiol, 1983, 49, 663.

Nicosia F, A Albani, M Lombardi, A Tagliagambe. Tolleranza alla buprenorfina per via peridurale nel dolore da cancro. Min Anest, 1984, 50, 669.

Nielsen CH, EM Camporesi, PR Bromage, EM Bukowski, PAC Durant. CO2 sensitivity after epidural and i.v. morphine. Anesthesiology, 1981, 55, A372.

Nielsen TH, HC Husegaard, J Joensen. Tunnelleret epiduralkateter og infektion. (Tunnelled epidural catheter and infection). Ugeskr Laeger, 1985, 147, 1548.

Nimmo WS, G Smith. Opioid agonist/antagonist drugs in clinical practice. Excerpta Medica, Amsterdam, 1984.

Nimmo WS, JG Todd. Fentanyl by constant rate i.v. infusion for postoperative analgesia. Brit J Anaesth, 1985, 57, 250.

Nisho Y, RS Sinatra, LM Kitahata, JG Collins. Spinal cord distribution of 3H-morphine after intrathecal administration: relationship to analgesia. Anesth Analg, 1989, 69, 323.

Niv D, V Rudick, MS Chayen, MP David. Variations in the effect of epidural morphine in gynecological and obstetric patients. Acta Obstet Gynecol Scand, 1983, 62, 455.

Niv D, V Rudick, A Golan, MS Chayen. Augmentation of bupivacaine analgesia in labor by epidural morphine. Obstet Gynecol, 1986, 67, 206.

NN Spinal opiates revisited. Lancet, 1986, I, 655.

NN Epidural morphine (letter). Can Anaesth Soc J, 1982, 29, 286.

Nobili C, A Ambrosino, S Formenti, V Izzo, L Piva, A Svergnini, M Tiengo. Home treatment of terminal cancer pain by epidural morphine. Pain (Suppl), 1984, 2, 335.

Noisser H, P Fuchs, S Wajsberg, H-J Ebell, K Peter. Postoperative pain epidural versus i.v. applications of buprenorphine. Abstracts, Int Symposium, Spinal Analgesia, Munich, April 1985.

Nordberg G, T Hedner, T Mellstrand, B Dahlström. Pharmacokinetic aspects of epidural morphine analgesia. Anesthesiology, 1983, 58, 545.

Nordberg G, T Hedner, T Mellstrand, B Dahlström. Pharmacokinetic aspects on intrathecal morphine analgesia. Anesthesiology, 1984, 60, 448. (a)

Nordberg G. Pharmacokinetic aspects of spinal morphine analgesia. Acta Anaesth Scand, 1984, 28, 1. (b)

Nordberg G, T Hedner, T Mellstrand, L Borg. Pharmacokinetics of epidural morphine in man. Eur J Clin Pharm, 1984, 26, 233. (c)

Nordberg G. Epidural versus intrathecal route of opioid administration. Int Anesth Clin, 1986, 24, 93. (a)

Nordberg G, T Mellstrand, L Borg, T Hedner. Extradural morphine: influence of adrenaline admixture. Brit J Anaesth, 1986, 58, 598. (b)

Nordberg G. Intraspinal opioid analgesia, pharmacokinetics aspects. II Int Symposium, Pain Clinic, Lille, France, June 1986. (c)

Nordberg G, V Hansdottir, L Kvist, T Mallstrand, T Hedner. Pharmacokinetic aspects on the epidural site of morphine administration. VII Eur Congress, 1986 Vienna (Austria), Report Abst. 416. (d)

Normandale JP, C Schmulian, JL Paterson, J Burrin, M Morgan, GM Hall. Epidural diamorphine and the metabolic response to upper abdominal surgery. Anaesthesia, 1985, 40, 748.

Norris FM. Remote effects of cancer on the spinal cord. In: PJ Vinken, GW Bruijn (Eds.): Handbook of Clinical Neurology, 1975, Elsevier, 669.

Norris MC, BL Leighton, CA DeSimone. Naltrexone and subarachnoid morphine following cesarean section. Anesthesiology (Suppl), 1989, 71, 873.

Notcutt WG. Patient-controlled analgesia: the need for caution. Anaesthesia, 1989, 44, 268.

Noueihed R, P Durant, TL Yaksh. Studies on the effects of intrathecal sufentanil, fentanyl, and alfentanil in rats and cats. Anesthesiology, 1984, 61, A218.

Novick D M, M J Kreek, A M Fanizza. Methadone disposition in patients with chronic liver disease. Clinical Pharmacology and Therapeutics, 1981, 30, 353.

Nurchi G. Use of intraventricular and intrathecal morphine in intractable pain associated with

582

cancer. Neurosurgery, 1984, 15, 801.

Nybbel-Lindahl G, C Carlsson, I Ingemarsson, M Westgren, L Paalzow. Maternal and fetal concentrations of morphine after epidural administration during labor. Am J Obstet Gynecol, 1981, 139, 20.

Nyska M, B Klin, Y Shapira, B Drenger, F Magora, GC Robin. Epidual methadone for preoperative analgesia in patients with proximal femoral fractures. Brit Med J, 1986, 293, 1347.

Obbens EAMT, C Statton Hill, ME Leavens, SR Ruthenbeck, F Otis. Clinical note: intravenricular morphine administration for control of chronic pain. Pain, 1987, 28, 61.

Oberoi GS, N Yaubihi. Postoperative epidural morphine analgesia in Papua New Guinea. Anesth Intens Care, 1989, 17, 332.

Ochi G, M Oda, K Kamimura, Y Kuba, A Ishiguro, A Fujii, T Sato. Narcotic dependency in patients with cancer pain treated with epidural morphine). Masui, 1983, 32, 758.

Ochi G, M Oda K Kamimura, Y Kuba, A Ishiguro, A Fujii, T Sato. Narcotic dependency in droperidol mixture for postoperative analgesia. Masui, 1985, 34, 330.

Oden RV. Etiology of pain and altered consciousness following epidural injection of morphine. Anesthesiology, 1988, 69, 287.

Odoom JA, IL Sih. Respiratory depression after intrathecal morphine. Anesth Analg, 1982, 61, 70.

Offermeier J, JM von Rooyen. Opioid drugs and their receptors: a summary of the present state of knowledge. S Afr Med J, 1984, 66, 299.

Ogawa GS. Comment on intrathecal morphine (letter). Drug Intel Clin Pharm, 1984, 18, 531.

Olshwang D, A Shapiro, S Perlberg, F Magora. The effect of epidural morphine on ureteral colic and spasm of the bladder. Pain, 1984, 18, 97.

Onofrio BM, TL Yaksh, PG Arnold. Continuous low dose intrathecal morphine administration in the treatment of chronic pain of malignant origin. Mayo Clin Proc, 1981, 56, 516.

Onofrio BM, TL Yaksh. Intrathecal delta-receptor ligand produces analgesia in man. Lancet, 1983, 1, 1386. (a)

Onofrio BM. Intraspinal narcotic analgesia for acute and chronic pain. Palm Springs, USA, 1983, Symposium report. (b)

Onofrio BM. Treatment of chronic pain of malignant origin with intrathecal opiates. Clin Neurosurg, 1983, 31, 304. (c)

Organowski S, PG Duncan. Clinical differences in spinal opioid efficacy. Can J Anaesth, 1989, 36, 448.

Orr IA, JW Dundee, C McBride. Preservative free epidural morphine denatures in a plastic syringe. Anaesthesia, 1982, 37, 352.

Orwin JM. Buprenorphine pharmacological aspects in man. In: Harcus et al. (Eds.): Pain-new perspectives in measurement, Churchill, 1977, 141.

Ossipov MH, GF Gebhart. Light pentobarbital anesthesia diminishes the antinociceptive potency of morphine administered intracranially but not intrathecally in the rat. Eur J Pharm, 1984, 97, 137.

Ossipov MH, L J Suarez, TC Spaulding. A comparison of the antinociceptive and behavioral effects of intrathecally administered opiates, a alpha2-adrenergic agonists, and local anesthetics in mice and rats. Anesth Analg, 1988, 67, 616.

Ossipov MH, LJ Suarez, TC Spaulding. Antinociceptive interactions between alpha-2-adrenergic and opiate agonists at the spinal level in rodents. Anesth Analg, 1989, 68, 194.

Östman LPö, CL Owen, JN Bates, FL Scamman, K Davis. Oxygen saturation in patients the night after cesarean section during epidural morphine analgesia. Anesthesiology, 1988, 69 (3A), A691.

Otteni JC, C Jeanpierre, T Pottecher. Spinal block with lignocaine and fentanyl for Ender nailing in the elderly. Brit J Anaesth, 1982, 54, 238P.

Oyama T, A Matsuki, T Taneichi, N Ling, R Guillemin. Beta-endorphin in obstetric analgesia. Am

J Obstet Gynecol, 1980, 13, 613. (a)

Oyama T, T Jin, R Yamaya. Profound analgesic effects of beta-endorphin in man. Lancet, 1980, 1, 122. (b)

Oyama T. Endocrinology and the anaesthesist. N°11 series, Monographs in Anaesthesiology, Elsevier Science, Amsterdam, 1980. (c)

Oyama T, S Fukuski, T Jin. Epidural beta-endorphin in treatment of pain. Can Anaesth Soc J, 1982, 29, 24.

Oyama T, T Jin, T Murakawa. Analgesic effect of continuous intrathecal beta-endorphin in cancer patients. In: W Erdmann, T Oyama, MJ Pernak (Eds.): Pain Clinic I, VNU, Science press, Utrecht, 1985, 93.

Oyama T, T Murakawa, S Baba, H Nagao. Analgesic effect of continuous infusion versus single epidural narcotic administration. II Int Symposium: The Pain Clinic II, 1986, Lille (France). In: Ph Scherpeerel, J Meynadier, S Blond (Eds.): Pain Clinic II, VNU Science Press, Utrecht,1987, 313. (a)

Oyama T, T Murakawa, S Baba, H Nagao. Continuous vs. bolus epidural morphine. Acta Anaesth Scand, 1987, 31, 77. (b)

O'Connor M, A Escarpa, C Prys-Roberts. Ventilatory depression during and after infusion of alfentanil in man. Brit J Anaesth, 1983, 55, 217S.

O'Neill P, C Knickenberg, S Bogahalanda, AE Booth. Use of intrathecal morphine for postoperative pain relief following lumbar spine surgery. J Neurosurg, 1985, 63, 413.

Paech MJ. Epidural pethidine or fentanyl during caesarean section: a double-blind comparison. Anaesth Intens Care, 1989, 17, 157.

Pageau MG, DW Coombs. New analgesic therapy relieves cancer pain without oversedation. Nursing, 1985, 15, 47.

Paice JA. Intrathecal morphine sulfate for intractable pain. J Neurosurg Nurs, 1984, 16, 237.

Paice JA. Intrathecal morphine infusion for intractable cancer pain: a new use for implanted pumps. Oncology nursing Forum, 1986, 13, 41.

Palacios QT, MM Jones, J Tessem, J Adenwala, S Longmire, Th Joyce. Comparison of epidural butorphanol and morphine for analgesia after cesarean section. Anesth Analg, 1987, 66, S133.

Palitzsch J, I Becker, S Roth, K Pochodzaj. Epidurale and intrathekale Anwendung von Morphium zur postoperativen Schmerzausschaltung. Anaesth Reanim, 1981, 6, 204.

Palitzsch J. Spinale Opiatanalgesie. Ztschr f Aertzl Fortb, 1982, 76, 581.

Palme M. Morphin intrathekal zur Bekämpfung von tumorbedingten und postoperativen Schmerzen. Anaesthesist, 1981, 30, 530.

Pandit SK, RB Powell, B Crider, ID McLaren, T Rutter. Epidural fentanyl: a simple and novel approach to anesthetic management for extracorporeal shockwave lithotripsy. Anesthesiology, 1987, 67, A 225.

Pandit SK, RB Powell, B Crider, ID McLaren, T Rutter. Epidural fentanyl is not effective for analgesia for extracorporeal lithotripsy (ESWL). Anesthesiology, 1988, 68, 176.

Pant KK, S Gurtu, JN Sinha, KK Tangri, KP Bhargava. Spinal site of antiarrhythmic action of morphine and pethidine in normal and spinal cord transected dogs. J Auton Pharm, 1984, 4, 11.

Parker EO, GL Brookshire, SJ Bartel, RG Menard, ED Culverhouse, LC Ault. Effects of epinephrine on epidural fentanyl, sufentanil and hydromorphone for postoperative analgesia. Anesthesiology, 1985, 63, A235.

Parker EO. Epidural narcotic use for outpatient pain treatment. Anesth Analg, 1989, 69, 408.

Parker F, K Ramabadran, S Ramanathan, H Turndorf. Pharmacokinetics of epidural morphine in obstetrical patients. Anesth Analg, 1988, 67, S162.

Parker GA, DA Fell, JA Young. Intrathecal morphine for cancer pain control. JOSMA, 1987, 80, 849.

584

Parker RK, N Berberich, DL Helfer, PF White. Use of epidural-PCA versus iv-PCA after obstetrical anesthesia. Anesthesiology (Suppl), 1989, 71, 872.

Parkinson SK, TV Whalen, CT Porter, SL Little. The use of continuous epidural morphine infusions in small children: a report of two cases. Regional Anesthesia, 1989, 14, 152.

Partridge BL, D Phil, J Katz. Epidural opioids do not affect skin capillary blood flow. Anesthesiology, 1988, 69 (3A), A386.

Pascaud XB, MG Genton, G Remond, M Vincent. Antral to colonic motility responses to intracerebroventricular administration of D-ALA-2-Enkephalinamide beta-endorphin, methionine, enkephalin, and fentanyl in anesthetized rats. In: J Christensen (Ed.): Gastrointestinal motility, Raven Press, New York,1980, 459.

Pasqualucci V, G Moricca, P Solinas. Intrathecal morphine for the control of the pain of myocardial infarction (letter). Anaesthesia, 1981, 36, 68.

Pasqualucci V, Solinas P. Intrathecal morphine in the treatment of acute myocardial infarction pain. G Ital Cardiol, 1982, 12, 278.

Pasqualucci V, C Tantucci, F Paoletti, ML Dottorini, G Bifarini, R Belfiori, MB Berioli, V Grassi, CA Sorbini. Buprenorphine vs. morphine via the epidural route: a controlled comparative clinical study of respiratory effects and analgesic activity. Pain, 1987, 29, 273.

Patel D, Y Janardhan, B Merai, J Robalino, K Shevde. Intrathecal meperidine in endoscopic urologic procedures: a comparative study with a local anesthetic. Regional-Anesthesia, 1989, 14 (Suppl), 49.

Patel, YC, K Rao, S Reichlin. Somatostatin in human cerebrospinal fluid. New Engl J Med, 1977, 296, 529.

Paterson GMC, HJ McQuay, RES Bullingham, RA Moore. Intradural morphine and diamorphine. Anaesthesia, 1984, 39, 113.

Patt R, V Potenza, E White. Epidural sufentanil as the sole anesthetic for extracorporeal shock wave lithotripsy. Anesth Analg, 1989, 69 S221.

Paulus DA, WL Paul, ES Munson. Neurologic depression after intrathecal morphine. Anesthesiology, 1981, 54, 517.

Payne KA. Epidural and intramuscular pethidine - a pharmacokinetic study. S Afr Med J, 1983, 63, 193. (a)

Payne KA. Epidural versus i.m. pethidine in postoperative pain relief. S Afr Med J, 1983, 83, 196. (b)

Payne R, KM Foley. Advances in the management of cancer pain. Cancer Treat Rep, 1984, 68, 173.

Payne R, CE Inturrisi. CSF Distribution of morphine, methadone and sucrose infusion after IT injection. Life Sci, 1985, 37, 1137.

Payne R, K Foley, C Inturrisi. Cerebrospinal fluid pharmacokinetis of opioids in a sheep model. In: Foley et al. (Eds.): Adv. in Pain Research and Therpy, Vol. 8, Raven Press New York, 1986, 385.

Payne R. CSF distribution of opioids in animals and man. Acta Anaesth Scand, 1987, Suppl 85, 31, 38. (a)

Payne R. Anatomy, physiology, and neuropharmacology of cancer pain. Medical Clinics of North America, 1987, 71, 153. (b)

Payne R. Role of epidural and intrathecal narcotics and peptides in the management of cancer pain. Medical Clinics of North America, 1987, 71, 313. (c)

Payne R, D Pignotti, O Ilercil, CE Inturrisi. CSF distribution of opioids after intracerebroventricular and lumbar intrathecal administration in the sheep. Pain, 1987, S4, S188. (d)

Peat SJ, P Bras, MH Hanna. A double-blind comparison of epidural ketamine and diamorphine for postoperative analgesia. Anaesthesia, 1989, 44, 555.

Pedersen J, MR Madsen. Metastic carcinoma in the extradural space (letter). Brit J Anaesth, 1985,

57, 935.

Peets JM, C Power, B Pomeranz. Long latency spinal cord dorsum potential; suppression by intrathecal morphine and enkephalin analog. Brain Res, 1984, 304, 279.

Pellerin M, D Boule, A Abergel, M Starkman, J Palacci, JF Amiot, N Colbert, D Mechali, P Babinet, F Hardy, R Hamer. Intérèt de l'injection intrarachidienne d'acétylsalicylate de lysine dans le taitement de la douleur chronique rebelle des cancéreux: à propos de 28 cas. II Int Symposium: Pain Clinic, 1986, Lille (France) Abstract IX FP 3.

Pelligrino DA, RD Peterson, SK Henderson, RF Albrecht. Relationship of cisternal CSF morphine levels to changes in ventilation during i.v. or fourth cerebroventricular infusions of morphine sulfate in the awake dog. Anesthesiology, 1987, 67, A553.

Pelligrino DA, RD Peterson, RF Albrecht. Cisternal CSF morphine levels and ventilatory depression following epidural administration of morphine sulfate in the awake dog. Anesth Analg, 1988, 67, S167.

Pelligrino DA, RD Peterson, SK Henderson, RF Albrecht. Comparative ventilatory effects of intravenous versus fourth cerebroventricular infusions of morphine sulfate in the unanesthestized dog. Anesthesiology, 1989, 71, 250.

Peng ATC, SM Shulman, LS Blancato, F Cutrone, K Nyunt. Epidural ketamine improves epidural lidocaine anesthesia during cesarean section: a double blind study. Anesthesiology, 1987, 67, A624.

Penn PR, JS Kroin. Intrathecal baclofen alleviates spinal cord spasticity. Lancet, 1984, I, 1078.

Penn RD, JA Paice, W Gottschalk, AD Ivankovich. Cancer pain relief using chronic morphine infusion. Early experience with a programmable implanted drug pump. J Neurosurg, 1984, 61, 302.

Penn RD, JS Kroin. Continuous intrathecal Baclofen for severe spasticity. Lancet, 1985, 2, 125. (a)

Penn RD. Drug pumps for treatment of neurologic diseases and pain. Neurol Clinics, 1985, 3, 439. (b)

Penn RD, JA Paice. Treatment of cancer pain by chronic intraspinal drug infusion. In: JM Besson, Y Lazorthes (Eds.): Spinal opioids and the relief of pain, Basic mechanisms and clinical applications. INSERM, Paris, 1985, 417. (c)

Penn RD, JS Kroin. Long-term intrathecal baclofen infusion for treatment of spasticity. J Neurosurg, 1987, 66, 181.

Penn RD, JA Paice. Chronic intrathecal morphine for intractable pain. J Neurosurg, 1987, 67, 182.

Penn RD, SM Savoy, D Corcos, M Latash, G Gottlieb, B Parke, JS Kroin. Intrathecal baclofen for severe spinal spasticity. N Engl J Med, 1989, 320, 1517.

Penning JP, B Samson, A Baxter. Nalbuphine reverses epidural morphine induced respiratory depression. Anesth Analg, 1986, 65, S119.

Penning JP, B Samson, AD Baxter. Reversal of epidural morphine-induced respiratory depression and pruritus with nalbuphine. Can J Anaesth, 1988, 35, 599.

Penon C, I Negre, C Ecoffey, JB Gross, K Samii. Analgesia and ventilatory control after intramuscular and epidural alfentanil. Anesthesiology, 1986, 65, A173.

Penon C, I Negre, C Ecoffey, JB Gross, JC Levron, K Samii. Analgesia and ventilatory response to carbon dioxide after intramuscular and epidural alfentanil. Anesth Analg, 1988, 67, 313.

Penon C, C Ecoffey. Effets respiratoires de la clonidine administrée par voie péridurale. Ann Fr Anesth Réanim, 1989, 8, R211.

Penon C, C Ecoffey, SE Cohen. Ventilatory effects of epidural clonidine. Anesthesiology (Suppl), 1989, 71, 649.

Percutaneous epidural catheterization for intractable pain in terminal cancer patients. Gynecologic oncology, 1989, 32, 22.

Peréz-Saad H, J Bures. Cortical spreading depression blocks naloxone- induced escape behaviour in morphine pretreated mice. Pharmacol Biochem Behav, 1983, 18, 145.

Perriss BW. Epidural opiates in labour. Lancet, 1979, 2, 422.

Perriss BW. Epidural pethidine in labour. A study of dose requirements. Anaesthesia, 1980, 35, 380. (a)

Perriss BW. Intrathecal morphine (letter). Anesthesiology, 1980, 53, 82. (b)

Perriss BW, AF Malins. Intrathecal morphine in labour (letter). Brit J Anaesth, 1980, 52, 515. (c)

Perriss BW, AF Malins. Pain relief in labour using epidural pethidine with adrenaline. Anaesthesia, 1981, 36, 631.

Perrot G, A Muller, B Laugner. Surdosage accidentel en morphine intrarachidienne. Traitement par naloxone i.v. seule. Ann Fr Anesth Réanim, 1983, 2, 412.

Pert CB, S Snyder. Opiate receptors: démonstration in nervous tissue. Sience, 1973, 179, 1011.

Perún J, J Vinas, LI Loncan, JE Ajuria. Analgesia morfinica intrathecal en pacientes concerosos. Utilidad del reservorio de morfina. Rev Espanola Anest Réanim, 1987, 34, 38.

Petersen TK, SE Husted, L Rybro, BA Schurizek, M Wernberg. Urinary retention during i.m. and extradural morphine analgesia. Brit J Anaesth, 1982, 54, 1175.

Petit J, G Coulombe, G Oksenhendler, D Lapert, C Winckler. Analgésie péridurale morphinique après chirurgie thoraco- abdominale. Intérêt chez l'insuffisant respiratoire chronique. Ann Fr Anesth Réanim, 1983, 2, 191. (a)

Petit J, G Coulombe, G Oksenhendler, D Lapert, C Winckler. Contribution de l'analgésie péridurale morphinique au traitement des traumatismes du thorax. Ann Fr Anesth Réanim. 1983, 2, 192. (b)

Petit J, G Oksenhendler, ML Eustache, M Dechmani, C Winckler. Analgésie péridurale par la morphine et par la buprenorphine après chirurgie thoracique, étude controlée, randomisée en double aveugle. II Int Symposium: Pain Clinic, 1986, Lille (france) Abst. IX FP 4.

Petit J, D Comar, G Oksenhendler, C Winckler. Analgésie péridurale par la morphine et par la buprénorphine après chirurgie thoracique étude controlée, randomisée, en double aveugle. Ann Fr Anesth Réanim, 1987, 6 , R91, 30th Congres SFAR.

Petit J, D Comar, B Pigot, ML Eustache, G Oksenhendler, C Winckler. Analgésie péridurale après chirurgie thoracique: morphine versus buprénorphine. Ann Fr Anesth Réanim, 1988, 7, 464.

Petit J, G Oksenhendler, G Colas, T Danays, A Leroy, C Winckler. Analgésie péridurale postopératoire à la clonidine. Ann Fr Anesth Rean, 1989, 8, R203.

Petit J, G Oksenhendler, G Colas, T Danays, A Leroy, C Winckler. Pharmacokinetics and effects of epidural clonidine in acute postoperative pain. Regional Anesthesia, 1989, 14 (Suppl), 43.

Petit J, G Oksenhendler, G Colas, A Leroy, C Winckler. Comparison of the effects of morphine, clonidine and a combination of morphine and clonidine administered epidurally for postoperative analgesia. Anesthesiology (Suppl), 1989, 71, 647.

Petry T, U Cloez, JP Pertek, M Heck, J Augure. Depression respiratoire après injection intrathécale de morphine: intérêt de naloxone in situ. Ann Fr Anesth Réanim, 1985, 4, 424.

Pfeifer BL, HL Sernaker, UM Ter Horst. Pain scores and ventilatory and circulatory sequelae of epidural morphine in cancer patients with and without prior narcotic therapy. Anesth Analg, 1988, 67, 838.

Pfeifer BL, HL Sernaker, UM Ter Horst, SW Porges. Crosstolerance between systemic and epidural morphine in cancer patients. Pain, 1989, 39,181.

Pflug AE, JJ Bonica. Physiopathology and control of postoperative pain. Arch Surg, 1977, 112, 773.

Pflug AE, MJ Lindop, TM Murphy, GM Aasheim, HA Beck. Early reversal of postoperative hypoxemia. Anesth Analg (Cleve), 1976, 55, 822.

Phan C, I Azar, IP Osborn, Lobo, E Lear. The quality of epidural morphine analgesia following cesarean delivery as affected by the volume of the injectant. Anesthesiology, 1987, 67, A285.

Phan CQ, I Azar, IP Osborn, OR Salter, E Lear. The quality of epidural morphine analgesia following epidural anesthesia with choloroprocaine or choloroprocaine mixed with epinephrine for cesarean delivery. Anesth Analg, 1988, 67, S171. (a)

Phan CQ, I Azar, IP Osborn, OR Salter, E Lear. The quality of epidural morphine analgesia following epidural anesthesia with lidocaine or chlorophrocaine for cesarean delivery. Anesth Analg, 1988, 67, S172. (b)

Phan CQ, EA Machernis, N Zung, I Azar, E Lear. The quality of epidural morphine-fentanyl analgesia following epidural anesthesia with 2-chloroprocaine. Anesthesiology (Suppl), 1989, 71, 835.

Philbin DM, CH Coggins. Plasma ADH levels in cardiac surgical patients during morphine and halothane anaesthesia. Anesthesiology, 1978, 49, 95.

Phillips DM, RA Moore, RES Bullingham, MC Allen, D Baldwin, A Fisher, JW Lloyd, HJ McQuay. Plama morphine concentrations and clinical effects after thoracic extradural morphine or diamorphine. Brit J Anaesth, 1984, 56, 829.

Phillips GH. Epidural sufentanil in labor. Anesth Analg, 1987, 66, S140. (a)

Phillips GH. Combined epidural sufentanil and bupivacaine for labor analgesia. Regional Anesthesia, 1987, 12, 165. (b)

Phillips GH. Combined epidural sufentanil and bupivacaine for labor analgesia. Regional Anesthesia, 1987, 12, 112. (c)

Phillips GH. Continuous infusion epidural analgesia in labor: the effect of adding sufentanil to 0.125 % bupivacaine. Anesth Analg, 1988, 67, S173. (a)

Phillips GH. Continuous infusion epidural analgesia in labor: the effect of adding sufentanil to 0.125 % bupivacaine. Anesth Analg, 1988, 67, 462. (b)

Phillips GH. Epidural sufentanil/bupivacaine combinations for analgesia during labor: effect of varying sufentanil doses. Anesthesiology, 1988, 67, 835. (c)

Pickerodt VWA, HJ Geiger. Die Häufigkeit von Anastomoseninsuffizienzen nach Dickdarmresektionen unter kombinierter Peridural - Allgemeinanaesthesie. Anaesthesist (Suppl.), 1983, 32, 247.

Piepenbrock S, M Zenz, G Otten. Peridurale Opiat-Analgesie in der postoperativen Phase. In: M Zenz (Ed.): Peridurale Opiat-Analgesie. Gustav Fischer Verlag, Stuttgart, 1981, 47. (a)

Piepenbrock S. Medikamentöse Therapie akuter Schmerzzustände. Munchen Med Wochenschr, 1981, 123, 1526. (b)

Piepenbrock S, M Zenz, GW Sybrecht, G Otten. Peridurale Morphin - Analgesie. II Atemdepression. Regional-Anaesthesie, 1981, 4, 32. (c)

Piepenbrock S. Peridurale Opiat-Analgesie: Grenzen der Methode. Anaesth Intensivmed, 1982, 153, 39.

Pierrot M, M Blaise, A Dupuy, S Hugon, M Cupa. Analgésie péridurale à dose élevée de fentanyl: échec de la méthode pour la kinésithérapie post-opératoire précoce avec chirurgie du genou. Can Anaesth Soc J, 1982, 29, 587.

Pigot B, J Petit, ML Eustache, G Oksenhendler, C Winckler. Influence de la naloxone intraveineuse sur les effets secondaires et l'analgésie après injection péridurale de fentanyl. Ann Fr Anesth Réanim, 1987, 6, 434.

Pitkin GP. Controllable spinal anesthesia. J Med Soc N J, 1927, 24, 425.

Piva L, V Costali, A Severgnini, B Pagnoni, A Calmi, C Nobili, M Tiengo. Somatosensory evoked potentials in postoperative analgesia with fentanyl. 6th Eur Congress of Anaesth, London, 1982, volume of summaries, p 502.

Planner R, RW Cowie, AS Babarczy. Continuous epidural morphine analgesia after radical operations upon the pelvis. Surg Gyn Obst, 1988, 166, 229.

Plewe G, G Nölken, J Schrezenmeir, H Kasper, U Krause, J Beyer. Side effects of somatostatin analogue SMS 201-995 in the treatment of acromegaly over 12 months. Somatostatin Symposium Washington, 1986 (Abstract) II-16.

Poletti CE, AM Cohen, DP Todd, RG Ojemann, WH Sweet, NT Zervas. Cancer pain relieved by long term epidural morphine with permanent indwelling systems for self-administration. J Neurosurg, 1981, 55, 581.

Pomonis SP. Overdose of intrathecal morphine. Anaesthesia, 1986, 41, 670.

Ponz L, F Carrascosa, R Perez-Reiner, JC Franco, JL Arroyo, L Lecron. Adrenocortical function under epidural analgesia: etidocaine with buprenorphine or fentanyl. 6th Eur Congress of Anaesth, London, 1982, volume of summaries, p 346. (a)

Ponz L, F Carrascosa, JM Bermudez de Castro, JL Arroyo, L Lecron. Pituitary function under epidural analgesia: etidocaine with buprenorphine or fentanyl. 6th Eur Congress on Anaesth, London 1982, volume of summaries, p 345. (b)

Porreca F, TF Burks. The spinal cord as a site of opioid effects on gastrointestinal transit in the mouse. J Pharm Exp Ther, 1983, 227, 22.

Porreca F, A Dray. Motilin acts within the CNS to inhibit urinary bladder contractions. Life Sci, 1984, 34, 2577. (a)

Porreca F, HI Mosberg, R Hurst, VJ Hruby, TF Burks. Roles of mu, delta and kappa opioid receptors in spinal and supraspinal mediation of gastrointestinal transit effects and hot-plate analgesia in the mouse. J Pharm Exp Ther, 1984, 230, 341. (b)

Portenoy RK, KM Foley. Chronic use of opioid analgesics in non-malignant pain: report of 38 cases. Pain, 1986, 25, 171.

Post C, J Freedman. A new method for studying the drugs in spinal cord after intrathecal injection. Acta Pharm Toxicol, 1984, 54, 253.

Post C, T Archer, T Gordh. Spinal alpha-adrenergic mechanisms for analgesia. Schmerz-Pain-Douleur, 1987, 3, 107. (a)

Post C, T Gordh, BG Minor, T Archer, J Freedman. Antinociceptive effects of spinal cord tissue concentrations after intrathecal injection of guanfacine or clonidine into rats. Anesth Analg, 1987, 66, 317. (b)

Poupard P, JJ Eledjam, C Peguret, G Draussin, F D'Athis. Effet comparatifs de la prilocaine et de l'association prilocaine- fentanyl en rachianesthésie. Forum Club AFAR, 1984, Paris.

Powell GM, RB Steinberg. Epidural sufentanil alone for analgesia for labor and delivery. Anesth Analg, 1989, 68, S226.

Pozzi E, M Caravatti. Chimiothérapie en perfusion continue chez des patients traités ambulatoirement. SAKK-Bulletin, 1985, 5, 9.

Presper JH, J Denion. Epidural morphine for control of postoperative laminectomy pain. Spine, 1988, 13, 124.

Prestele K, H Funke, R Möschl, E Reif, M Franetzki. Development of remotely controlled implantable devices for programmed insulin infusion. Life Support Systems, 1983, 1, 23.

Preston P, M Rosen, D Daniels, B Glosten, S Shnider, B Ross, P Dailey, S Hughes. Epidural fentanyl with lidocaine for cesarean section. Anesthesiology, 1987, 67, A442.

Preston PG, MA Rosen, SC Hughes, B Glosten, BK Ross, D Daniels, SM Shnider, PA Dailey. Epidural anesthesia with fentanyl and lidocaine for cesarean section: maternal effects and neonatal outcome. Anesthesiology, 1988, 68, 938.

Price DD, A von der Gruer, J Miller, A Rafi, C Price. Potentiation of systemic morphine analgesia in humans by proglunide, a cholecystokinine antagonist. Anesth Analgesia, 1985, 64, 801.

Prior FN, A Thyle. Epidural morphine (letter). Anaesthesia, 1981, 36, 535.

Prithvi P, P Raj. Postoperative analgesia. In: Langloys (Eds.): 6.Congress Eur Soc Loco-Reg Anaesth, MAPAR Bicetze Paris, 1987, 157.

Proudfit HK, DL Hammond. Alteration in nociceptive threshold and morphine - induced analgesia produced by intrathecally administered amine antagonists. Brain Res, 1981, 218, 393.

Przewlocki B, L Stala, W Lason, R Przewlocki. The effect of various opiate receptor agonists on the seizure threshold in the rat. Is dynorphin an endogenous anticonvulsant? Life Sci, 1983, 33, 595. (a)

Przewlocki B, L Stala, M Greczek, GT Sheraman, B Przewlocka, A Herz. Analgesic effects of mu-, delta- and kappa-opiate agonists and, in particular, dynorphin at the spinal level. Life Sci, 1983, 33, 649. (b)

Puig Riera de Conias MM. Analgesia producida por administracion subarachnoidea y epidural de opioides: lugar y mecanismos de accio. Rev Espaniola Anest Rean, 1986, 33, 1.

Purves PG, SJ Sperring, V Dykes, TD Stanley. Improved postoperative analgesia: epidural versus patient controlled i.v. morphine. Anesth Analg, 1987, 66, S143.

Pybus DA, TA Torda. Dose-effect relationships of extradural morphine. Brit J Anaesth, 1982, 54, 1259.

Pybus DA, BE D'Bras, G Goulding, H Liberman, TA Torda. Postoperative analgesia for hemorrhoid surgery. Anaesth Intens Care, 1983, 11, 27.

Pybus DA, T Torda. Opiates and sexual function. Nature, 1984, 310, 636.

Quintin L, C Roux, I Macquin, F Bonnet, M Ghignone. Clonidine blunts the endocrine and circulatory surge during recovery of aortic surgery. Anesthesiology (Suppl), 1989, 71, 155.

Racz GB, M Sabonghy, J Gintautas, WM Kline. Intractable pain therapy using a new epidural catheter. JAMA, 1982, 248, 579.

Racz GB, J Gintautas, G Fabian. Technical Advance: A New Epidural Catheter. Persistent Pain Vol 5, Grune & Stratton, 1985, chap. 12, 268.

Racz GB, RF Haynsworth, S Lipton. Experiences with an improved epidural catheter. In: The Pain Clinic, VNU Science Press, 1986, 1,1, 21.

Ragot P, P Crozat, P Tauzin-Fin, JM Fonrouge, M Sabathie. Blocage de la motilité par la péthidine intra-rachidienne. (Blockade of movement by pethidine (letter). Presse Med, 1983,12, 2258.

Ragot P, P Tauzin-Fin, Ph Crozat, A Brachet-Liermain, Ph Ballanger, M Sabathié. Comparaison de la péthidine et de la prilocaine en rachianesthésie pour 100 interventions urologiques. Agressologie, 1984, 25, 29. (a)

Ragot P, P Tauzin-Fin, Ph Crozat, A Brachet-Liermain, Ph Ballanger, M Sabathié. Relation entre la dépression respiratoire, l'analgésie post-opératoire et les concentrations sanguines après rachianesthésie la péthidine. Forum Club AFAR, 1984, Paris. (b)

Ragot, P, P Tauzin-Fin, P Crozat, JM Fonrouge, M Sabathié. Péthidine intrathécale. Comparaison avec un anesthésique local. Ann Fr Anesth Réanim, 1984, 3, 143. (c)

Raj PP, D Knarr, E Vigdorth, R Gregg, D Denson, CN Hopson. Comparative study of continuous epidural pethidine infusion versus systemic analgesics for postoperative pain relief. Anesthesiology, 1985, 63, A238.

Raj PP. Anesthetic techniques for chronic pain management. Refresher Course ASA, New Orleans, 1989, 136.

Ramanathan S, R Horn, F Parker, H Turndorf. Naloxone infusion is ineffective in preventing the side effects of epidural morphine in postcesarean section patients. Anesthesiology, 1986, 65, A367.

Ranchere JY, P Rebattu, D Coullioud. Problems met in the diagnosis and management of bacterial meiningitis developed from an intrathecal developed. Semaine des Hopitaux, 1986, 62, 1015. (a)

Ranchere JY, R Lombard, C Lupo. Morphinothérapie IT ambulatoire chez le sujet cancéreux. II Int Symposium, 1986, Lille (France), Abstr.IX p70. (b)

Rane A, J Säwe, B Dahlström, L Paalzow, L Kager. Pharmacological treatment of cancer pain with special reference to the oral use of morphine. Acta Anaesth Scand, 1982, 74, 97.

Rankin APN, REH Comber. Management of fifty cases of chest injury with a regimen of epidural

590

bupivacaine and morphine. Anaesth Intensive Care, 1984, 12, 311.

Rao U, IT Campbell, DM Catley, JR Sutherst. Epidural meptazinol for pain relief after lower abdominal surgery. Anaesthesia, 1985, 40, 754.

Rao U, IT Campbell, JR Sutherst, DM Catley. Epidural meptazinol. Anaesthesia, 1987, 42, 218.

Rauch R, D Knarr, D Denson, P Raj. Comparison of the efficacy of the epidural morphine given intermittent injestion or continuous infusion for the management of postoperative pain. Anesthesiology, 1985, 65, A201.

Rauck RL, JC Eisenach, CA Buzzanell. Epidural clonidine for intractable cancer pain management. Anesthesiology (Suppl), 1989, 71, 1151.

Ravalia A, PN Robinson. Respiratory depression and spinal opioids. Can J Anaesth, 1989, 36, 728.

Ravat F, R Dorne, JP Baechle, A Beaulaton, B Lenoir, P Leroy, B Palmier. Epidural ketamine or morphine for postoperative analgesia. Anesthesiology, 1987, 66, 819. (a)

Ravat F, R Dorne, P Leroy, JP Baechle, B Palmier, A Beaulaton, B Lenovi. Epidural ketamine or morphine for postoperative analgesia. ESRA 6th Congress Eur Soc Reg Anaesth, Publ. MAPAR Paris 1987, report 91. (b)

Ravidran R, W Albrecht, M McKay. Apparent intravascular migration of epidural catheter. Anesth Analg, 1979, 58, 252.

Ravnborg M, FM Jensen, NH Jensen, IK Hold. Pupillary diameter and ventilatory CO2 sensitivity after epidural morphine and buprenorphine in volunteers. Anesth Analg, 1987, 66, 847.

Rawal N, UH Sjöstrand, B Dahlström. Postoperative pain relief by epidural morphine. Anesth Analg, 1981, 60, 726. (a)

Rawal N, K Möllefors, K Axelsson, G Lingårdh, B Widman. Naloxone reversal of urinary retention after epidural morphine. Lancet, 1981, 2, 1411. (b)

Rawal N, UH Sjöstrand, B Dahlström, PA Nydahl, J Östelius. Epidural morphine for postoperative pain relief: A comparative study with intramuscular narcotic and intercostal nerve bloc. Anesth Analg, 1982, 61, 93.

Rawal N, K Möllefors, K Axelsson, G Lingårdh, B Widman. An experimental study of urodynamic effects of epidural morphine and of naloxone reversal. Anesth Analg, 1983, 62, 641. (a)

Rawal N, K Möllefors, M Wattwil, K Axelsson, G Lindgårdh. Experimental studies of urodynamic and respiratory changes following epidural morphine. 4th Int Symposium Düsseldorf, June, 1983. (b)

Rawal N, M Wattwil. Respiratory depression following epidural morphine. An experimental and clinical study. Anesth Analg, 1984, 63, 8. (a)

Rawal N, U Sjöstrand, E Christoffersson, B Dahlström, A Avill, H Rydman. Comparison of intramuscular and epidural morphine for postoperative analgesia in the grossly obese. Influence on postoperative ambulation and pulmonary function. Anesth Analg, 1984, 63, 583. (b)

Rawal N, B Dahlström, CE Inturrisi, B Tandon, U Schött, U Sjöstrand, M Wennhager. Prevention of complications of epidural morphine analgesia by low dose naloxone infusion. Acta Anaesth Scand, 1985, 29, N° 135. (a)

Rawal N, U Schött, B Tandom B,U Sjöstrand, M Wennhager. Influence of i.v. naloxone infusion on analgesia and untoward effects of epidural morphine. Anesth Analg, 1985, 64, 270. (b)

Rawal N. Spinal opioids, non-nociceptive effects and their clinical applications. Schmerz-Pain-Douleur, 1985, 3, 119. (c)

Rawal N, B Tandon. Epidural and intrathecal morphine in intensive care units. Intens Care Med, 1985, 11, 129. (d)

Rawal N, U Schött, B Tandon, U Sjöstrand, M Wennhager. Influence of i.v. naloxone infusion on analgesia and respiratory depression following epidural morphine. Anesth Analg, 1985, 64, 194. (e)

Rawal N, U Schött, B Dahlström, CE Inturrisi, B Tandon, U Sjöstrand, M Wennhager. Influence of naloxone infusion on analgesia and respiratory depression following epidural morphine.

Anesthesiology, 1986, 64, 194. (a)

Rawal N. Non-nociceptive effects of intraspinal opioids and their clinical applications. Int Anesth Clin, 1986, 24, 75. (b)

Rawal N. Round table on sufentanil. II Int Symposium, 1986, Lille (France). (c)

Rawal N, K Möllefors, M Wattwil, K Axelsson, G Lingårdh, B Widman. Experimental studies of urodynamic and respiratory changes following epidural morphine. In: HJ Wüst, M Stanton-Hicks (Eds.): Anaesthesiologie und Intensivmedizin, new aspects in regional anaesthesia 4, Springer Verlag, Berlin, Heidelberg, New York, Tokyo, 1986, 176, 135. (d)

Rawal N, UH Sjöstrand. Clinical application of epidural and intrathecal for pain management. Int Anesth Clin, 1986, 24, 43. (e)

Rawal N, S Arnér, LL Gustafsson, R Allvin. Present state of extradural and intrathecal opioid analgesia in Sweden. Brit J Anaesth, 1987, 59, 791.

Ray CD, R Bagley. Indwelling epidural morphine for control of postlumbar spinal surgery pain. Neurosurgery, 1983, 13, 388.

Raybould D, BC Bloor, DF McIntee, JW Flacke, WE Flacke. Reduction of anesthetic requirements and cardiovascular effects of BHT 920, a selective alpha-2 adrenergic agonist. Anesthesiology (Suppl), 1988, 69, 600.

Ready LB. Age alters effective dose of epidural morphine following abdominal hysterectomy. Pain, 1987, S4, S71.

Ready LB, R Oden, HS Chadwick, C Benedetti, GA Rooke, R Caplan, LM Wild. Development of an anesthesiology-based postoperative pain management service. Anesthesiology, 1988, 68, 100.

Ready LB, HS Chadwick. Reply. Anesthesiology, 1988, 69, 436.

Reay BA, AJ Semple, WA Macrae, MacKenzie, IS Grant. Low-dose intrathecal diamorphine analgesia following major orthopaedic surgery. Brit J Anaesth, 1989, 62, 248.

Rechtine GR, CM Reinert, NH Bohlman. The use of epidural morphine to decrease postoperative pain in patients undergoing lumbar laminectomy. J Bone Joint Surg, 1984, 66, 113.

Redding TW, EJ Coy. The disappearance distribution and excretion of 125 J-labeled Thyrosine-1-growth hormone release inhibiting factor (125J-Tyr-1-GIF) in mice, rats and man. 56th Meeting Amer Endocrino Soc Atlanta, June 12-14, 1974, Abst 198.

Reddy Sv, J Maderdrut, TL Yaksh. Spinal cord pharmacology of adrenergic agonist-mediated antinociception. J Pharm Exp Ther, 1980, 213, 525.

Regan JW, VA Doze, K Daniel, M Maze. Is dexmedetomidine's anesthetic action dependent of isoreceptor selectivity? Anesthesiology (Suppl), 1989, 71, 579.

Reig E, E Patino, ML Franco, MC del Cano, F Avello. Ambulant continuous extradural morphine analgesia using an external portable infusion pump. VII Eur Congress of Anaesth, 1986, Vienna (Austria), Report, Abst 427.

Reigle TG. Increased brain norepinephrine metabolism correlated with analgesia produced by the periaqueductal gray injection of opiates. Brain Res, 1985, 338, 155.

Rein P, W Brothers, K Eakins, K Cooper, WC Dunwiddie. Respiratory depressant effects of epidural butorphanol. Anesthesiology, 1985, 63, A247.

Reitz J, JJ McKichan, L Hoffer, J Kryc, MB Howie. Reduced plasma clearance of alfentanil associated with prolonged mayor abdominal surgery. Anesth Analg, 1984, 63, 265.

Reiz S, M Westberg. Side effects of epidural morphine. Lancet, 1980, 2, 203.

Reiz S, J Ahlin, B Ahrenfeld, M Andersson, S Andersson. Epidural morphine for postoperative pain relief. Acta Anaesth Scand, 1981, 25, 111. (a)

Reiz S, S Haeggmark, M Ostman. Invasive analysis of non-invasive indicators of myocardial work and ischaemia during anaesthesia soon after myocardial infarction. Acta Anaesth Scand, 1981, 25, 303. (b)

Reiz S. Epidural morphine for the treatment of pain after multiple rib fractures, a double blind comparison with bupivacaine. In: JB Brueckner (Eds.): Schmerzbehandlung, Epidurale Opiat-

592

analgesie. Springer Verlag Berlin, Heidelberg, New York, 1982, 31.

Renaud B, JF Brichant, F Clergue, M Chauvin, JC Levron, P Viars. Administration péridurale continue de fentanyl: effets ventilatoires et pharmacocinétique. Ann Franc D'Anesth et Réanim, 1985, 4, 87A. (a)

Renaud B, JF Brichant, F Clergue, M Chauvin, JC Levron, P Viars. Continuous epidural fentanyl: ventilatory effects and plasma kinetics. Anesthesiology, 1985, 63, A234. (b)

Renaud B, JF Brichant, F Clergue, M Chauvin, JC Levron, P Viars. Ventilatory effects of continuous epidural infusion of fentanyl. Anesth Analg, 1988, 67, 971.

Renkl F, M Dittmann. Reduktion des postspinalen Kopfschmerzes nach Benutzung von Spinalnadeln 29 G versus 26 G - ein prospektiver Vergleich. Anaesthesist, 1984, 33, 452.

Reny-Palasse V, R Rips. Antinociceptive activity of TRH metabolites in the mouse. Pain, 1987, 30, 259.

Revill SI, JO Robinson, M Rosen, MIJ Hogg. The reliability of a linear analogue for evaluating pain. Anaesthesia, 1976, 31, 1191.

Rexed B. The cytoarchitectonic organisation of the spinal cord in the cat. J Comp Neurology, 1952, 96, 415.

Rexed M, V Havlicek, L Leybin, FS Labella, H Friesen. Opiate-like naloxone reversible actions of somatostatin given intra cerebrally. Can J Physiol Pharmacol, 1978, 56, 227.

Reynolds F. Epidural narcotics (letter). Anesth Analg, 1981, 60, 123.

Reynolds F. Pharmacology of intraspinal opiates (letter). Anaesthesia, 1982, 37, 499.

Reynolds F, PA Roberts, M Pollay, PH Stratemeier. Quantitative anatomy of the thoracolumbar epidural space. Neurosurgery, 1985, 17, 905.

Reynolds F. Plasma transfer of opioids. in Update in Opioids p 859.Baillieres Clinical Anaesthesiology, 1987, 1, 4.

Reynolds F, G O'Sullivan. Epidural fentanyl and perineal pain in labour. Anaesthesia, 1989, 44, 341.

Reynolds F Epidural fentanyl and plasma fentanyl concentrations Anaesthesia, 1989, 44, 864

Reynolds F. Extradural opioids in labour. Brit J Anaesth, 1989, 63, 251.

Rezek M, V Havlizek, L Leybin, FS LaBella, H Friesen. Opiate-like naloxone reversible actions of somatostatin given intracerebrally. Can J Physiol Pharmacol, 1978, 56, 227.

Richter HP, K Schmidt. Neurochirurgische Behandlungsmöglichkeiten maligner Schmerzen. (Neurosurgical treatment possibilies in malignant pain). Chirurg, 1983, 54, 789.

Rico RC, GH Hobika, AM Avellanosa, RJ Trudnowski, J Rempel, CR West. Use of intrathecal and epidural morphine for pain relief in patients with malignant diseases: a preliminary report. J Med, 1982, 13, 223.

Riegler R, A Pernetzky. Festsitzender Epiduralkatheter durch Schlinge und Knoten. Regional Anaesthesie, 1983, 6, 19.

Riegler R, AF Hammerle, GA Albright, J Neumark. Der RACZ - Epiduralkatheter. Regional Anaesthesie, 1984, 7, 109.

Rigoli M. In: M Tiengo, M Cousins (Eds.): Pharmacological basis of Anesthesiology. Raven Press, New York, 1983. (a)

Rigoli M. Epidural analgesia with benzodiazepines. Progress Anesth, 1983, 3, 69. (b)

Rippe ES, JJ Kresel, DW Coombs, WT Mroz, CR Smith. Effect of morphine sulfate concentration on flow rate in an implantable reservoir. Amer J Hosp Pharm, 1984, 41, 496.

Rippe ES, JJ Kresel. Preparation of morphine sulfate solutions for intraspinal administration. Amer J Hosp Pharm, 1986, 43, 1420.

Riss PA, C Bieglmayer. Obstetric analgesia and immunoreactive endorphin peptides in maternal plasma during labor. Gynecol Obstet Invest, 1984, 17, 127.

Ritchel WA. Pharmakinetic aspects of analgesics. Meth Find Exptl Clin Pharmacol, 1982, 417.

Robertson K, MJ Douglas, GH McMorland. Epidural fentanyl with and without epinephrine for postcesarean section analgesia. Can Anaesth Soc J, 1985, 32, 502.

Robinson RJS, S Lenis, M Elliot. Accidental epidural narcotic overdose (letter). Can Anaesth Soc J, 1984, 31, 594.

Robinson RJS, IR Metcalf. Hypertension after epidural meperidine. Can Anaesth Soc J, 1985, 32, 658.

Robinson RJS, S Brister, E Jones, M Quigly. Epidural meperidine analgesia after cardiac surgery. Can Anaesth Soc J, 1986, 33, 550.

Robinson DE, CH Leicht. Epidural analgesia with low-dose bupivacaine and fentanyl for labor and delivery in a parturient with severe pulmonary hypertension. Anesthesiology, 1988, 68, 285.

Robson JA, JB Brodski. Latent dural puncture after lumbar epidural block. Anesth Analg, 1977, 56, 725.

Rocco AG, E Fran, AF Kaul, SJ Lipson, JP Gallo. Epidural steroids, epidural morphine and epidural steroids combined with morphine in the treatment of post-laminiectomy syndrome. Pain, 1989, 36, 297.

Rodan BA, FL Cohen, WJ Bean, SN Martyak. Fibrous mass complicating epidural morphine infusion. Neurosurgery, 1985, 16, 68.

Rodriguez Hernandez JL, F Robaina Padron, J A de Vera Reyes. Administracion intratecal lumbar de morfina en el tratamiento del dolor del cancer avanzado. Rev Esp Anest Rean, 1986, 33, 253.

Rodriguez J, TK Abboud, A Reyes, M Payne, J Zhu, Z Steffens, A Afrasiabi. Continuous infusion epidural analgesia during labor: a randomized, double-blind comparison of 0.0625% bupivacaine/0.002% butorphanol versus 0.125% bupivacaine. Anesthesiology (Suppl), 1989, 71, 840.

Roerig SC, SM O'Brien, JM Fujimoto, GL Wilcox. Tolerance to morphine analgesia: decrease multiplicative interaction between spinal and supraspinal sites. Brain Res, 1984, 308, 360.

Rolly G, P Bilsback, O Tampubolon. Epidural administration of buprenorphine, lofentanil and saline in the treatment of postoperative pain. Royal Soc Med Int Congress Series, 1984, 65, 125.

Román de Jesús JC, JA Aldrete, RA Castillo, D Hursh. Uso del butorfanol en analgesia peridural: comunicación preliminar. Revista Espanola d Anesthesiologia, 1988, 35, 26.

Romijn JA, JJ van Lieshout, DN Velis. Reversible coma due to intrathecal baclofen. Lancet, 1986, II, 696.

Rondomanska M. Postoperative epidural anesthesia and analgesia with buprenorphine. In: Agonistic morphine-antagonists and their antidotes in anaesthesia, De Castro J, St. Kubicki (Eds.) Rep. 7th World Congress of anaesthesiologists Hamburg, Ed AIAREF, 1980, 105.

Ropiquet S, J Petit, G Oksenhendler, C Winckler. Syndrome de servrage lors d'une administration péridurale de morphine après interruption d'un traitement par la clonidine. Ann Fr Anesth Réanim, 1984, 3, 380.

Roquefeuil B, P Blanchet, C Batier, J Benezech. Analgésie morphinique par voie ventriculaire. A propos de quatre cas dont un avec autoadministration. Ann Fr Anesth Réanim, 1982, 1, 649.

Roquefeuil B, J Benezech, C Batier, P Blanchet, C Gros. Intérêt de l'analgésie morphinique par voie ventriculaire dans les algies rebelles néoplasiques. Neurochirurgie, 1983, 29, 135.

Roquefeuil B, P Blanchet, Cl Batier, J Benezech. Intérrêt de l'analgésie morphinique par voie ventriculaire cérébrale dans les algies rebelles néoplasiques. A propos de 17 cas dont 5 par autoadministration. Journées Int. Franco-Magrébiennes d'Anesthésie réanimation, Tunis, 1984. (a)

Roquefeuil B, J Benezech, P Blanchet, C Batier, Ph Frèrebeau, C Gros. Intraventricular administration of morphine in patients with neoplastic intractable pain. Surg Neurol, 1984, 21, 155. (b)

Roquefeuil B. Analgésie morphinique par voie ventriculaire à propos de 17 cas. Euromedecine

594

1986, Montpellier, France, abstracts, Editel Paris. (a)

Roquefeuil B. Results with EDOA and ICOA. Personnal communication 1986 (b)

Roques BP, MC Fournie-Zaluski, G Gacel, P Chaillet, JM Zajac, G Waksman, R Bouboutou et al. Enkephalin degrading enzymes inhibitors and selective agonists for mu or delta receptors: new ways in analgesia. INSERM, 1984, 127, 87.

Rosen K, D Rosen, E Bank. Caudal morphine for postoperative pain control in children undergoing cardiac procedures. Anesthesiology, 1987, 67, A510.

Rosen KR, DA Rosen. Caudal epidural morphine for control of pain following open heart surgery in children. Anesthesiology, 1989, 70, 418.

Rosen MA, SC Hughes, SM Shnider, TK Abboud, M Norton, PA Dailey, JD Curtis. Epidural morphine for relief of postoperative pain after cesarean delivery. Anesth Analg, 1983, 62, 666.

Rosen MA, PA Dailey, SC Hughes, CH Leicht, SM Shnider, CE Jackson, W Baker, D Cheek, D O'Connor. Epidural sufentanil for postoperative analgesia after cesarean section. Anesthesiology, 1988, 68, 448.

Rosenberg PH, A Heino, B Scheinin. A Comparison of intramuscular analgesia, intercostal block, epidural morphine and on demand i.v.- fentanyl in the control of pain after upper abdominal surgery. Acta Anaesth Scand, 1984, 28, 603.

Rosenfeld MG, Mermod JJ, SG Amara, LW Swanson. Production of a novel neuropeptide encoded by calcitonin gene via tissue specific RNA processing. Nature, 1983, 304, 128.

Rosow C. Agonist-antagonist opioids: theory and clinical practice. Can J Anaesth, 1989, 36, S5.

Rosow CE, J Moss, DM Philbin, JJ Savarese. Histamine release during morphine and fentanyl anesthesia. Anesthesiology, 1982, 56, 93.

Rosow CE. New synthetic opioid analgesics. In: G Smith, BG Covino (Eds.): Acute Pain, Butterworths, London, 1985, 68.

Rosseel PMJ, WGM Van den Broek, EC Boer, O Prakash. A comparison between epidural sufentanil and morphine for analgesia after thoracic surgery. ESRA 6th Congress Eur Soc Reg Anaesth, Ed. MAPAR Paris 1987, report 88. (a)

Rosseel PMJ, WGM van den Broek, EC Boer, O Prakash. Epidural sufentanil for intra- and postoperative analgesia in thoracic surgery: a comparative study with intravenous sufentanil. Acta Anaesth Scand, 1988, 32, 193. (b)

Rossignoli L, AM Alcione, L Rossignoli, AM Alcione, et al. Clonidina associata a morphina nella analgesia epidurale a lungo termine. Algos, 1985, 2, 235.

Rossignon MD, D Khayat, R Guesde, JJ Rouby, CL Jacquillat, P Viars. Intravenous anesthesia using fentanyl and benzodiazepine decreases functional activity of polymorphonuclear leukocytes in man. Anesthesiology, 1988, 69 (3A), A595.

Rostaing S, F Bonnet, O Boico, JF Loriferne, P Catoire, K Abhay. Analgésie postopératoire induite par la clonidine péridurale. Ann Fr Anest Réan, 1989, 8, R204.

Roston CE, RP Grant, WB Woodhurst. Postoperative epidural morphine in lumbar spinal surgery. Anesthesiology, 1984, 61, A221.

Rotar VI, YA Feldman, AI Levitsky, PG Zaishlyor. Prolonged postoperative analgesia in elderly urologic patients. Urologia I nefrologia, 1983, 2, 58.

Roure P, N Jean, AC Leclerg, N Cabanel, JC Levron, et al. Pharmacokinetics of alfentanil in children undergoing surgery. Brit J Anaesth, 1987, 59, 1437.

Rubin J, E Mankowitz, JG Brock-Utne, JW Downing. Ketamine and postoperative pain. S Afr Med J, 1983, 63, 443.

Rucci FS, P Migliori, M Cardamone, A Simonelli, S Spaniani. Fentanyl and bupivacaine mixtures for epidural blockade. Minerva Anestesiologica, 1984, 50, 383.

Rucci FS, M Cardmone, P Migliori. Fentanyl and bupivacaine mixtures for extradural blockade. Brit J Anaesth, 1985, 57, 275.

Ruckebusch Y, JP Ferre, C Du. In vivo modulation of intestinal motility and sites of opioid effects in the rat. Regul Pept, 1984, 9, 109.

Rukavina Z, M Aksamija, D Bakranin. Intrathecal morphine for postoperative pain relief. VII Eur Congress of Anaesth, Vienna, Austria, 1986, Abstract 423.

Ruppert M, U Jost, G Putz, M Hirschauer. Buprenorphin (Temgesic) peridural zur operativen Schmerzbekämpfung, Ein Jahres-Studie. Anaesthesist, 1982, 3 Suppl., 516.

Russell B, TL Yaksh. Antagonism by phenoxybenzamine and pentazocine of the antinociceptive effects of morphine in the spinal cord. Neuropharmacology, 1981, 20, 575.

Russell RD, KJ Chang. delta and mu receptor activation: a stratagem for limiting opioid tolerance. Pain, 1989, 36, 381.

Rutberg H, E Håkanson, B Anderberg, L Jorfeldt, J Mårtensson, B Schildt. Effects of the extradural administration of morphine or bupivacaine, on the endocrine response to upper abdominal surgery. Brit J Anaesth, 1984, 56, 233.

Rutgers MJ, PJ Roos. Bacteriological complications of self administered epidural morphine in patients with cancer. Brit Med J, 1986, 292, 992.

Rutter DV, DG Skewes, M Morgan. Extradural opioids for postoperative analgesia. A double blind comparison of pethidine, fentanyl and morphine. Brit J Anaesth, 1981, 53, 915.

Ryan DW. Anaesthesia for cystectomy. A comparison of two anaesthetic techniques. Anaesthesia, 1982, 37, 554.

Rybro L, BA Schurizek, TK Petersen, M Wernberg. Postoperative analgesia and lung function: a comparison of intramuscular with epidural morphine. Acta Anaesth Scand, 1982, 26, 514.

Sagnard P, F Ravat, H Counioux, J Motin. La péthidine en péridurale administrée par injection intermittente ou par infusion continue pour l'analgésie postopératoire. Ann Fr Anesth Réanim, 1987, 6, R27.

Saissy JM, N Drissi-Kamili, A Nouredine, H Mabrouk. Contribution à l'étude de l'analgésie post-opératoire à la kétamine par voie péridurale. Conv Méd, 1984, 3, 399. (a)

Saissy JM. Expérience de la péthidine par voie sous- arachnoidienne en anesthésie. La Nouvelle Presse Médicale, 1984, 13, 2149. (b)

Sale JP, GV Goresky, G Koren, L Strunin. Pharmacokinetics of alfentanil in children. Anesth Analg, 1986, 65, S129.

Salvetti B, J Debout, F Lesoin, R Krivosic-Horber, G Cacheux. Anesthésie péridurale pour la chirurgie du rachis. Ann Fr Anesth Réanim, 1983, 2, 188.

Samaryutel I, I Kolesnikov, G Nikolajev, K Zilmer. Suppression of neuroendocrine stress reaction in oncologic surgery with epidural ketamine and morphine. VII Eur Congress, 1986, Vienna (Austria), Report, Abst 419.

Samii K, J Feret, A Harari, P Viars. Selective spinal analgesia (letter). Lancet, 1979, 1, 1142.

Samii K, M Chauvin M, P Viars. Postoperative spinal analgesia with morphine. Brit J Anaesth, 1981, 53, 817.

Samii K. Les morphiniques par voie rachidienne. Rapport. 29ème Congrès Nat. Soc Fr d'Anesth, Lille (France), 1983, 126.

Samii K. The postoperative use of spinal opioids.. I Int Symposium, 1986, Lille (France).

Samii K. Postoperative epidural opioids. Schmerz-Pain-Douleur, 1987, 3, 101.

Samuelsson H, G Nordberg, T Hedner, J Lindqvist. CSF and plasma morphine concentrations in cancer patients during chronic epidural morphine therapy relation to pain. Pain, 1987, 30, 303.

San Emetrio F, JM Izquierdo. Aportaciones al tratamiento del dolor mediante derivados opiaceos administrados por via intraventricular cerebral y su utilidad an el enfermo canceroso. Thesis Universidad de Valladolid, Spain 1985.

Sandler AN, P Chovaz. Respiratory depression following epidural morphine: a clinical study. Can Anaesth Soc J, 1986, 33, 542.

Sandu L, CO Mungiu, C Ionescu, C Constandache, M Molotiu, A Ianas. Clinical and experimental

596

data in connection with conduction anaesthesia and analgesia with pethidine. IV Int Congress of Anaesth, Bucarest (Roumania), 1981, Abst B55, 153.

Sanford TJ. A review of sufentanil. Seminars in Anesthesia, 1988, 7, 127.

Sangarlangkarn S, V Klaewtanong, P Jonglerttrakool. Meperidine as a spinal anesthetic agent: a comparison with lidocaine-glucose. Anesth Analg, 1987, 66, 235.

Saroynok J, MI Sweency, ID White. Classification of adenosine receptors mediating anti-nocicepton in the rat spinal cord. Brit J Pharma, 1986, 88, 923.

Sarrion J, JM Palanca, JM Aguilar, V Chulia. Analgésie post-opératoire avec chlorhydrate de morphine péridural versus noramidopérinométansulfonate de magnésium intravéneux dans la chirurgie abdominale haute. II Int Symposium: Pain Clinic, 1986, Lille (France), Abst VIII FP 8. (a)

Sarrion J, JM Palanca, JM Aguilar, V Chulia. Analgesia post- operatoria con cloruro morfico epidural en cirugia abdominal alta. Rev Espanola Anest Rean, 1986, 33, 435. (b)

Sarubin J, E Gebert. Schmerzbekämfung mit Morphin intrathekal oder peridural? Fortschr Med, 1983, 101, 122.

Saunders RL, DW Coombs. Dartmouth-Hitchcock Medical Center experience with continuous intraspinal narcotic analgesia. In: Schmidek, Sweet (Eds.): Operative Neurosurgical Techniques, Grune and Stratton, New York, 1983, 2, 1211.

Savola MKT, MB MacIver, VA Doze. Interaction of dexmedetomidine, an alpha-2-adrenoceptor agonist, with isoflurane in rat hippocampal cal neurons. Anesthesiology (Suppl), 1989, 71, 597.

Savolaine ER, JB Pandya, SH Greenblatt, SR Conover. Anatomy of the human lumbar epidural space: new insights using CT-epidurography. Anesthesiology, 1988, 68, 217.

Sawynok J, SM Moochhala, DJ Pillay. Substance P, injected intrathecally, antagonizes the spinal antinociceptive effect of morphine, baclofen and noradrenaline. Neuropharmacology, 1984, 23, 741.

Schauss C, TL Yaksh. In vivo studies on spinal opiates. J Pharm Exp Ther, 1983, 228, 1.

Schaz K, G Stock, W Simon, et al. Enkephalin effects on blood pressure, heart rate, and baroreceptor reflexe. Hypertension, 1980, 2, 395.

Scheinin B, PH Rosenberg. Effect of prophylactic epidural morphine or bupivacaine on postoperative pain after upper abdominal surgery. Acta Anaesth Scand, 1982, 26, 474.

Scheinin B, R Orko, PH Rosenberg. Absorption of epidural morphine. Anaesthesia, 1986, 41, 1257.

Scheinin B, R Asantila, R Orko. The effect of bupivacaine and morphine on pain and bowel function after colonic surgery. Acta Anaesth Scand, 1987, 31, 161.

Schildt B, M Bengtsson, S Friberg, Nelsen, A Mohall, A Rane, T Symreng. Relief of postoperative pain by morphine in the epidural space. A controlled clinical study. Acta Anaesth Scand, 1982, 74, 151.

Schlesinger TS, DJ Miletich. Epidural fentanyl and lidocaine during cesarean section: maternal efficacy and neonatal safety using impedance monitoring. Anesthesiology, 1988, 69 (3A), A649.

Schmauss C, C Doherty, TL Yaksh. The analgetic effects of an intrathecally administered partial opiate agonist, nalbuphine hydrochloride. Eur J Pharm, 1982, 86, 1, 1.

Schmauss C, TL Yaksh, Y Shimohigashi, G Harty, T Jensen, D Robbard. Differential association of spinal mu, delta and kappa opioid receptors with cutaneous thermal and visceral chemical nococeptive stimuli in the rat. Life Sci, 1983, 33, 653.

Schmauss C, TL Yaksh. In vivo studies on spinal opiate receptor sites mediating antinociception. II. Pharmacological profiles suggesting a differential association of mu, delta and kappa receptors with visceral chemical and cutaneous thermal stimuli in the rat. J Pharm Exp Ther, 1984, 228, 1.

Schmauss C, TL Yaksh. Differential association of spinal opiate receptors with various nociceptive inputs. Schmerz-Pain-Douleur, 1985, 6, 112. (a)

Schmauss C, Y Shimohigashi, TS Jensen, D Rodbard, TL Yaksh. Studies on spinal opiate receptor pharmacologa. III Analgetic effects of enkephalin dimers as measured by cutaneous-thermal and visceral-chemical evoked responses. Brain Res, 1985, 337, 209. (b)

Schmidek HH, SG Cutler. Epidural morphine for control of pain after spinal surgery: a preliminary report. Neurosurgery, 1983, 13, 37.

Schmidt JF, AM Banning, B Chraemmer-Jørgensen, A Risbo. Comparison beetwen oral sustained release morphine and epidural morphine given at fixed schedule, in the control of postoperative pain. Acta Anaesth Scand, 1985, 29, N°132. (a)

Schmidt JF, B Chraemer-Jørgensen, JE Pedersen, A Risbo. Postoperative pain relief with naloxone. Severe respiratory depression and pain after high dose of buprenorphine. Anaesthesia, 1985, 40, 583. (b)

Schmidt K, PH Althoff, F Lacey, H Prestele, AG Harris, C Rosak, K Schoeffling. Analgesic effect of the somatostatin-analogue SMS 201-995 in acromegalic patients - a double blind study. Int. Somatostatin Symposium, Washington, 1986, Abstr. II-17.

Schneider I, M Diltoer. Continuous epidural infusion of ketamine during labour (letter). Can J Anaesth, 1987, 34, 657.

Schoeffler P, E Pichard, R Ramboatiana, D Joyon, JP Haberer. Bacterial meningitis due to infection of a lumbar drug release system in patients with cancer pain. Pain, 1986, 25, 75.

Schoeffler P, JP Haberer, CM Monteillard. Morphine injections in cisterna magna for intractable pain in cancer patients. Report: ASA annual meeting Atlanta GA 1987. (a)

Schoeffler PF, JP Haberer, CM Monteillard, E Bouetard. Morphine injections in cistern magna for intractable pain in cancer patients. Anesthesiology, 1987, 67, A246. (b)

Schroeder KA, JA Taren, HS Greenberg, P Layton. Continuous intrathecal morphine for cancer pain: preliminary report of a method for case selection. Surgical Forum, 1984, 35, 498.

Schubert P, H Teschemacher, GW Kreutzberg, A Herz. Intracerebral distribution pattern of radioactive morphine and morhine-like drugs after intraventricular and intrathecal injection. Histochemie, 1970, 22, 277.

Schubert A, MG Licina, PJ Lineberry, JE Tobin, GS Bacon. The effect of intrathecal morphine on lower extremity somatosensory evoked potentials in man. Anesthesiology, 1988, 69 (3A), A350.

Schultzberg M, T Hokfelt, L Terenius, et al. Enkephalin immuno-reactive nerve fibres and cell bodies in sympathetic ganglia of the guinea-pig and rat. Neuroscience, 1979, 4, 249.

Schüttler J, H Schwilden, H Stoeckel. Pharmacokinetics as applied to total intravenous anaesthesia. Anaesthesia (Suppl.), 1983, 38, 56.

Schwartz JC. Metabolism of enkephalins and the in activating neuropeptidase concept. Tr Neurosci, 1983, 6, 45.

Schwartz JC, S de la Beaume, ML Bouthenet, G Giros, C Gros, C Llorens-Cortes, H Pollard, N Sales, B Solhonne, J Costentin, JM Lecomte. Neuropeptidases responsables de l'inactivation des enkephalinases et pharmacologie de leurs inhibiteurs. J Pharm Paris (Suppl.), 1986, 17, 104.

Schwarz T. Prolonged regional analgesia with morphine-epidurally. RN, 1982, 45, 32.

Schwieger I, Z Gamulin, PM Suter. Lung function during anesthesia and respiratory insufficiency in the postoperative period: physiological and clinical implications. Acta Anaesthesiol Scand, 1989, 33, 527.

Sciandra G, D Bono, M Coaloa, G Garelli, L Piazza, AM Viglietti. Studio comparativo tra buprenorfina e morfina nel controllo del dolore nell'immediato postoperatorio per via peridurale. Minerva Anesth, 1984, 50, 607.

Scott DB, J McClure. Selective epidural analgesia. Lancet, 1979, 1, 1410.

Scott DB, CM Sinclair. Advances in regional anaesthesia and analgesia. Clin Obstet Gynaecol, 1982, 9, 273.

Scott DM. Acute pain management. In: Cousins MJ, PO Bridenbaugh (Eds.) Neural blockade in clinical anesthesia and management of pain, 2nd., J.B. Lippincott, Philadelphia, 1987, 861.

Scott H, H Cohen. Nalbuphine augmentation of analgesia and reversal of side effects following epidural hydromorphone. Anesthesiology, 1986, 65, 216.

598

Scott J, EC Huskisson. Graphic representation of pain. Pain, 1976, 2, 175.

Scott JF. Pain treatment in a palliative unit or team of a university hospital. Act Anaesth Scand (Suppl.), 1982, 26, 119.

Scott NB, T Mogensen, D Bigler, C Lund, H Kehlet. Continuous thoracic extradural 0.5 % bupivacaine with or without morphine: effect on quality of blockade, lung function and the surgical stress response. Brit J Anaesth, 1989, 62, 253.

Scott PV, FE Bowen, P Cartwright, BC Rao, D Deely, HG Wotherspoon, IMA Sumrein. Intrathecal morphine as sole analgesic during labour. Brit Med J, 1980, 281, 351.

Scott PV, HB Fischer. Instraspinal opiates and itching: A new reflex? Brit Med J, 1982, 284, 1015.

Sebel PS, C Aun, J Fiolet J, K Noonan, TM Savege, MP Colvin. Endocrinological effects of intrathecal morphine. Eur J Anaesth, 1985, 2, 291.

Seebacher J, P Galli Douani, M Henri, G Andrieu, P Viars. Analgésie péridurale en obstétrique. In: Ars Medici, Congress Series, 3, vol II, 1983, 329.

Seeling W, KH Altemeyer, M Butters, HL Fehm, U Loos, R Mayer, M Nabjinsky, JE Schmitz. Glukose, ACTH, Kortisol, T4, T3 und RT3 im Plasma nach Cholecystektomie. Vergleichende Untersuchungen zwischen kontinuierlicher Periduralanaesthesie und Neuroleptanalgesie. Regional Anaesthesie, 1984, 7, 1. (a)

Seeling W, P Lotz, M Schroeder. Untersuchungen zur postoperativen Lungenfunktion nach abdominalen Eingriffen. Vergleich zwischen kontinuierlicher, segmentaler, thorakaler Periduralanaesthesie und i.m. injiziertem Piritramid. Anaesthesist, 1984, 33, 408. (b)

Seeling W, FW Ahnefeld, G Rosenberg, H Heinrich, D Spilker. Aortofemoraler Bifurkationsbypass-Der Einfluß des Anaesthesieverfahrens (NLA, thorakale kontinuierliche Katheterananaesthesie) auf Kreislauf, Atmung und Stoffwechsel. Anaesthesist, 1985, 34, 217.

Seemann H. Schmerzdokumentation für den ambulanten Patienten. In: M Zimmermann, HO Handwerker (Eds.): Schmerz, Springer-Verlag, Berlin, 1984, 249.

Segal IS, RG Vickery, JK Walton, VA Doze, M Maze. Dexmedetomidine diminishes halothane anesthetic requirements in rats through a postsynaptic alpha-2 adrenergic receptor. Anesthesiology, 1988, 69, 818.

Semple AJ, DJ Macrae, S Munishankarappa, LM Burrow, MK Milne, IS Grant. Effect of the addition of adrenaline to extradural diamorphine analgesia after caesarean section. Brit J Anaesth, 1988, 60, 632.

Serrao JM, CS Goodchild. Intrathecal midazolam in the rat. Evidence for spinally-mediated analgesia. Brit J Anaesth, 1987, 59, 124P.

Serrao JM, SC Stubbs, CS Goodchild. Intrathecal midazolam and fentanyl in the rat: evidence different spinal antinociceptive effects. Anesthesiology, 1989, 70, 780.

Serrie A, G Cunin, C Thurel, JB Thiebaut, P Sandouk, JM Schermann. Etude pharmacocinétique de la morphine administrée par voie intra- ventriculaire, étude préliminaire de 10 cas. II Int Symposium, Pain Clinic, Lille, France 1986, Abstract III P 7.

Serrie A, P Sandouk, G Cunin, JM Scherrmann, C Thurel, G Lot, E Echter. Ventricular versus lumbar CSF morphine concentration and pain assessment following intraventricular administration. Pain, 1987, S4, S191.

Servergnini A, L Piva, C Carabellese, R Rossi, M Zanetta. Fentanyl versus bupivacaine in the analgesic treatment of obstructive arteriopathies. 6th Eur Congress of Anaesth, London, 1982, volume of summaries, 318.

Sevarino FB, MD Johnson, MJ Lema, S Datta, GW Ostheimer, JS Naulty. The effect of epidural sufentanil on shivering and body temperature in the parturient. Anesth Analg, 1989, 68, 530.

Sevarino FB, C McFarlane, V Takla, A Fischer, R Sinatra. The effect of epidural fentanyl on postcesarean delivery analgesic requirements as administered by PCA. Anesthesiology (Suppl), 1989, 71, 871.

Shafer A, PF White, V Coe, DR Stanski. Use of pharmacokinetic variables to determine infusion regimens. Anesthesiology, 1983, 59, A244.

Shafer A, ML Sung, PF White. Differences in pharmacokinetics contribute to postoperative respiratory depression after an alfentanil infusion. Anesthesiology, 1985, 63, A283.

Shafer A, ML Sung, PF White. Pharmacokinetics and pharmacodynamics of alfentanil infusions during general anesthesia. Anesth Analg, 1986, 10, 1021. (a)

Shafer A, PF White, V Coe, DR Stanski. Use of pharmacokinetic variables to determine infusion segments. Anesth Analg, 1986, 65,1021. (b)

Shah M W, D T Jones, M Rosen. Patient demand postoperative analgesia with buprenorphine. Brit J Anaesth, 1986, 58, 508.

Shanker KB, NV Plakar, R Nishkala. Paraplegia following epidural toassium chloride. Anaesthesia, 1985, 40, 45.

Shapiro LA, S Hoffman, R Jedeikin, R Kaplan. Single-injection epidudral anesthesia with bupivacaine and morphine for prostatectomy. Anesth Analg, 1981, 60, 818.

Shapiro LA, RJ Jedeikin, D Shalev, S Hoffman. Epidural morphine analgesia in children. Anesthesiology, 1984, 61, 210.

Sharnick S, GJ Grant, S Ramanathan, H Turndorf. Pharmacokinetics of intrathecal bupivacaine and morphine with and without epinephrine for cesarean section. Anesth Analg (Suppl), 1989, 68, 254.

Shetter AG, MN Hadley, E Wilkinson. Administration of intraspinal morphine sulfate for the treatment of intractable cancer pain. Neurosurgery, 1986, 18, 740.

Shipton EA. Epidural fentanyl in the management of severe pain (letter). S Afr Med J, 1984, 65, 193. (a)

Shipton EA, JM Steyn, FO Müller, HKL Hundt. Preliminary pharmacokinetic profile of the epidural absorption of fentanyl. IRCS Medical Science, 1984, 12, 75. (b)

Shipton EA. Pruritus - a side effect of epidural fentanyl for postoperative analgesia. Sa Meditse Tydskrif, 1984, 66, 61. (c)

Shipton EA, JM Hugo, FO Müller. Epidural fentanyl in the management of postoperative pain. S Afr Med J, 1986, 70, 325.

Shnider SM. Epidural and subarachnoidal opiates in obstetrics, basic considerations. Annual Refresher Course Lectures, ASA San Fransisco, 1985, 165, 1.

Shnider SM. Epidural and subarachnoid opiates in obstetrics. Refresher Course ASA, New Orleans 1989, 235.

Shohami E, S Evron. Intrathecal morphine induces myoclonic seizures in the rat. Acta Pharm Tox, 1985, 56, 50.

Shulman MS, J Brebner, A Sandler. The effect of epidural morphine on postoperative pain relief and pulmonary function in thoracotomy patients. Anesthesiology, 1983, 59, A192.

Shulman MS, A Sandler, J Brebner. The reversal of epidural morphine induced somnolence with physostigmine. Can Anaesth Soc J, 1984, 31, 678. (a)

Shulman MS, AN Sandler, JW Bradley, PS Young, J Brebner. Postthoracotomy pain and pulmonary function following epidural and systemic morphine. Anesthesiology, 1984, 61, 569. (b)

Shulman MS, G Wakerlin, L Yamaguchi, JB Brodsky. Experience with epidural hydromorphone for post-thoracotomy pain relief. Anesth Analg, 1987, 66, 1331. (a)

Shulman MS. Epidural butamben for the treatment of metastatic cancer pain. Anesthesiology, 1987, 67, A245. (b)

Sicuteri F, A Panconesi, PL Del Bianco, G Franchi, B Anselmi. Venospastic activity of somatostatin in vivo in man: naloxone reversible tachyphylaxis. Int J Clin Pharm Res, 1984, 3, 253.

600

Sidi A, JT Davidson, M Bahar, D Olshwang. Spinal narcotics and central nervous system depression. Anaesthesia, 1981, 36, 1044.

Siegfried J, A Kühner, V Sturm. Neurosurgical treatment of cancer pain. Recent Results Cancer Res, 1984, 89, 148.

Siegismund K, M Beutner, C Fiedler. Postoperative Analgesie durch peridurale Piritramidapplikation (Postoperative analgesia by peridural piritramide application). Zbl Gynakol, 1982, 104, 615.

Silbert BS, GC Dixon, R Kluger, J Berg. Epidural opioids as anaeshesia for extracorporeal shock wave lithotripsy in two patients with cardiac disease. Can J Anaesth, 1988, 35, 624.

Silbert BS, R Kluger, AC Meads, K Stasytis. Double-blind trial comparing epidural lignocaine with epidural fentanyl for anaesthesia during extracorporeal shock wave lithotripsy. Anaesth Intens Care, 1989, 17, 9.

Simionescu R. Respiratory depression after epidural and intrathecal narcotics (letter). Anaesthesia, 1982, 37, 600.

Simon EJ, JM Hiller, I Edelman. Opiate receptors: specific binding of the potent narcotic analgesic tritium labelled etorphine to rat brain homogenate. National Academy of Science. Proccedings, USA, 1973, 70, 1947.

Simoneau G, A Vivien, R Sertenne, F Kustlinger, K Samii, Y Noviant, P Duroux. Diaphragmatic dysfunction after upper abdominal surgery: effect of analgesia. Am Rev Disease (sous presse), 1984.

Simpson KH, TH Madej, JM McDowell, R MacDonald, G Lyons. Comparison of extradural buprenorphine and extradural morphine after caesarean section. Brit J Anaesth, 1988, 60, 627.

Sjöström S, A Tamsen, P Hartvig. Patient-controlled analgesia with epidural opiates. In: M Harmer, M Rosen, MD Vickers (Eds.): Patient-controlled Analgesia, Blackwell Scientific Publ. Oxford, 1985, 156.

Sjöström S, P Harvig, P Persson, A Tamsen. Pharmacokinetics of epidural morphine and meperidine in humans. Anesthesiology, 1987, 67, 877. (a)

Sjöström S, A Tamsen, MP Persson, P Harvig. Pharmacokinetics of intrathecal morphine and meperidine in humans. Anesthesiology, 1987, 67, 889. (b)

Sjöström S, D Hartvig, A Tamsen. Patient-controlled analgesia with extradural morphine or pethidine. Brit J Anaesth, 1988, 60, 358.

Skerman JH, A Gupta A, MA Jacobs. Continuous infusions of epidural fentanyl for postoperative pain relief following cesarean section. Soc Obst Anest Perinat, 1985, 1, 95. (a)

Skerman JH, BA Thompson, MT Goldstein, MA Jacobs, A Gupta, NH Blass. Combined continuous epidural fentanyl and bupivacaine in labor: a randomised study. Anesthesiology, 1985, 63, A450. (b)

Skjöldebrand A, M Garle, L Gustafsson, H Johansson, NO Lunell, A Rane. Analgesia during labour with pethidine epidurally. Acta Anaesth Scand (Suppl.), 1982, 74, 74. (a)

Skjöldebrand A, M Garle, LL Gustafsson, H Johansson, NO Lunell, A Rane. Extradural pethidine with and without adrenaline during labour: wide variation in effect. Brit J Anaesth, 1982, 54, 415. (b)

Skoeld M, L Gillberg, O Ohlsson. Pain relief in myocardial infarction after continuous epidural morphine analgesia (letter). N Engl J Med, 1985, 312, 650.

Slater EM, GL Zeitlin, MG Edwards. Experience with epidural morphine for postsurgical pain in a community setting. Anesthesiology Rev, 1985, 12, 37.

Slattery PJ, RA Boas. Newer methods of delivery of opiates for relief of pain. Drugs, 1985, 30, 539.

Slavic-Svircev V, G Heidrich, RF Kaiko, BF Rusby. Ibuprofen in the treatment of postoperative pain. Amer J Med, 1984, 77, 84.

Smith G, BG Covino. Acute Pain. Butterworths, 1985.

Smith G. Management of postoperative pain. Can J Anaesth, 1989, 36, S1.

Snyder S. Opioid receptors in brain. New Engl Med J, 1977, 3, 266.

Solanki DR. Epidural fentanyl for relief of lower extremity tourniquet pain in orthopaedic surgery. Anesth Analg, 1987, 66, S161.

Solomon RE, GR Gebhart. Intrathecal clonidine and morphine in rats: antinociceptive tolerance and cross-tolerance and effects on blood pressure. Pain, 1987, S4, S41.

Soni N, M Russell. Delayed onset spinal after epidrual analgesia. Anaesthesia, 1982, 37, 74.

Sosis M. Spinal opiates revisited. Lancet, 1986, 1, 655.

Sosnowski M, TL Yaksh. Role of spinal adenosine receptors in modulating the hyperesthesia produced by spinal glycine receptor antagonism. Anesth Analg, 1989, 69, 587.

Sosnowski M, TL Yaksh. Symmetric tolerance after continuous spinal infusion of mu agonists in rats. Anesthesioloy (Suppl), 1989, 71, 621.

Sosnowski M, CW Stevens, TL Yaksh. Assessment of the role of A1/A2 adenosine receptor mediating the purine antinociception: motor and autonomic function in the rat spinal cord. J Pharmacol Exp Ther, 1989, 250, 915.

Spampinato S, S Candeletti, E Cavicchini, P Romualdi, E Speroni, S Ferri. Antinociceptive activity of salmon calcitonin injected intrathecally in the rat. Neurosci Lett, 1984, 45, 135.

Spampinato S, S Candeletti. Characterization of dynorphin a - induced antinociception at spinal level. Eur J Pharm, 1985, 110, 21.

Spence AA. Relieving acute pain. Brit J Anaesth, 1980, 52, 245.

Sprotte G. Falldarstellung: Therapie am Sympathikus, Anwendung von Opiaten. In: J Schara (Ed.): Anaesthesiologie und Intensivmedizin, Deutscher Anaesthesiekongress 1982, Springer Verlag, Berlin, 1986, 174, 106.

Srinivasan T. Intrathecal morphine for obstetric analgesia. Anesthesiology, 1981, 55, A298.

Srivastava S. Epidural buprenorphine for postoperative pain relief (letter). Anaesthesia, 1982, 37, 699.

Stanley TH, GD Lathrop. Urinary excretion of morphine during and after valvular and coronary artery surgery. Anesthesiology, 1977, 46, 166.

Stanley TH. Intrathecal opiates, a potent tool to be used with caution. Anesthesiology, 1980, 53, 523.

Stanski DR. Alfentanil, a kinetically analgesia predictable narcotic. Anesthesiology, 1982, 57, 935.

Stanski DR. Narcotic pharmacokinetics and dynamics: the basis of infusion applications. Anaesth Intens Care, 1987, 15, 21.

Stanton-Hicks M. Subarachnoid and extradural analgesic techniques. In: G Smith, BG Covino (Eds.): Acute Pain, Butterworth 1985, 237.

Stanton-Hicks M, M Gielen, M Hasenbos, C Matthyssen. High thoracic epidural sufentanil for post-thoracotomy pain. ESRA 6th Congress Eur Soc Reg Anaesth, Publ. MAPAR Paris 1987, Report 89.

Stanton-Hicks M, M Gielen, M Hasenbos, C Matthijssen, JA van Heteren, J Crul. High Thoracis epidural with sufentanil for post-thoracotomy pain. Regional Anesthesia, 1988, 23, 62.

Starkman M, A Abergel, JL Sebbah, T Marsepoil. Morphine intrathécale et dépression respiratoire. Ann Fr Anesth Réanim, 1984, 3, 237.

Stehr CH, Stehr DL. Epidural morphine in the clinical setting. Anesthesiology Rev, 1985, 12, 21.

Steidl L J, G A Fromme, D R Danielson. Lumbar versus thoracic epidural morphine for post-thoracotomy pain. Anesth Analg, 1984, 63, 277.

Steiner G, W Seeling, V Schusdziarra. Wirkungen und Nebenwirkungen von Somatostatin. Anaesthesist, 1987, 36, 669.

Stenkamp SJ, TR Easterling, HS Chadwick. Effect of epidural and intrathecal morphine on the length of hospital stay after cesarean section. Anesth Analg, 1989, 68, 66.

Stenseth R, O Sellevold, H Breivik. Epidural morphine for postoperative pain: experience with 1085 patients. Acta Anaesth Scand, 1985, 29, 148. (a)

Stenseth R, O Sellevold, H Breivik, SE Gisvold. Epidural morphine for postoperative pain relief. Acta Anaesth Scand (Suppl.), 1985, 29, 81. (b)

Steppe J, F Camu. Epidural morphine for postoperative analgesia following abdominal surgery in elderly patients. Acta Anaesth Belgica, 1982, 33, 43.

Steppe J, JP Alexander, J Heykants, F Camu. Continuous peridural fentanyl for pain after abdominal surgery. Acta Anaesth Belgica (Suppl.), 1983, 34, 86.

Stevens RA, M D'Arcy Stanton-Hicks. Subdural injection of local anesthetic: a complication of epidural anesthesia. Anesthesiology, 1985, 63, 323.

Stillman MJ, DE Moulin, KM Foley. Paradoxical pain following high-dose spinal morphine. Pain, 1987, S4, S389.

St Marie B, K Henrickson. Intraspinal narcotic infusions for terminal cancer pain. JIN, 1988, 11, 161.

Stoelting RK. Current views on the role of opioid receptors and endorpins in anesthesiology. Int Anesth Clin, 1986, 24, 17.

Stoelting RK. Intrathecal morphine - an underused combination for postoperative pain management. Anesth Analg, 1989, 68, 707.

Stoffregen J, Codic. Die Mikroprozessor programmierte Intelligenz für Infusionsmaschinen. Anaesthesist (Suppl.), 1983, 32, 161.

Stoner HB, GM Hall. The relationships between plasma substrates and hormones and the severity of injury in 277 recetly injuried patients. Clin Sci, 1979, 56, 563.

Stonham J, BW Perriss, SM Wood. Comparison of epidural and intramuscular pethidine for analgesia in labour (letter). Brit J Obstet Gynaecol, 1981, 88, 1166.

Stoyanov M, H Müller, G Hempelmann. Traitement des douleurs chroniques. Utilisation des morphiniques par la voie péridurale. Anesth Analg Réanim, 1981, 38, 375. (a)

Stoyanov M, H Müller, U Börner, G Hempelmann. L'intérét des dérivés morphiniques par voie péridurale. Ann Anesth Franc, 1981, 4, 311. (b)

Stoyanov M, H Müller, G Hempelmann. Traitement des douleurs chroniques d'origine cancéreuse par l'administration morphinique périmédullaire continue au moyen d'une pompe. Eurométecine 1986, Montpellier (France), Report, Editel France,155.

Strube PJ, JW Downing, JG Brock-Utne. CSF pharmakokinetics of extradural morphine (letter). Brit J Anaesth, 1984, 56, 921. (a)

Strube PJ, NG Lavies, J Rubin. Epidural clonidine. Anaesthesia, 1984, 39, 834. (b)

Struppler A, B Burgmayer, GB Ochs, HG Pfeiffer. The effect of epidural application of opioids on spasticity of spinal origin. Life Sci (Suppl.), 1983, 33, 607.

Strutigi P, L Papadimitriou, L Anagnostopoulou. Epidural sufentanil for postoperative analgesia. ESRA 6th Congress Eur Soc Reg Anaesth, Publ. MAPAR, Paris, 1987, Report 90.

Su CF, MY Liu, MT Lin. Intraventricular morphine produces pain relief, hypothermia, hyperglycaemia and increased prolactin and growth hormone levels in patients with cancer pain. J Neurol, 1987, 235, 105.

Suguzini A, S Grsili. Cervical epidural morphine for malignant pain in the neck. Proc of the Joint Meeting Eur IASP, 1983, Abono Terne May.

Sullivan SP, DA Cherry. Pain from an invasive facial tumor relieved by lumbar epidural morphine. Anesth Analg, 1987, 66, 777.

Sun S, D Dolar, E Oezenç. Intrathecal morphine in tetanus. Brit J Anaesth, 1982, 54, 699.

Suzukawa M, M Matsumoto, JG Collins, LM Kitahata, O Yuge. Dose-response suppression of noxiously evoked activity of WDR neurons by spinally administered fentanyl. Anesthesiology, 1983, 58, 510.

Suzuki M, S Hori, M Oda, T Sato. Side effects of epidural morphine with special reference to age and sex. Masui, 1985, 34, 675.

Swerdlow M. Principles of cancer pain treatment. Eur1médecine, 1986 Montpellier, France, Abstract Editel, Paris, 176.

Swerts JP, R Perdrisot, B Malfroy, JC Schwartz. Is "enkephalinase" identical with "angiotensin-converting enzymes"? Eur J Pharm, 1979, 53, 209.

Szulc R, W Jurczyk, E Rozwadowska. Epidural application of buprenorphine and marcaine in treatment of the patients with chronic pain of vascular origin. Eur J Anaesth, Congress Report, 1984.

Taiwo YO, A Fabian, CJ Pazoles, HL Fields. Potentiation of morphine antinociepetion by monoamine reuptake inhibtiors in the rat spinal cord. Pain, 1985, 21, 329.

Takasaki M, M Asano. Intrathecal morphine with hyperbaric tetracaine. Anaesthesia, 1983, 38, 76.

Talafre ML, P Jacquinot, F Legagneux, J Jasson, C Conseiller. Intrathecal administration of meperidine versus tetracaine for elective cesarean section. Anesthesiology, 1987, 67, A620.

Tamsen A, P Hartvig, B Dahlström, A Wahlström, L Terenius. Endorphins and on demand pain relief. Lancet, 1980, 1, 769.

Tamsen A, S Sjöström, P Hartvig, P Persson, J Gabrielsson, L Paalzow. CSF and plasma kinetics of morphine and meperidine after epidural administration. Anesthesiology, 1983, 59, A196.

Tamsen A, T Gordh. Epidural clonidine produces analgesia. Lancet, 1984, 2, 231.

Tan S, PF White, SE Cohen. Sufentanil for post cesarean analgesia: epidural versus intravenous administration. Anesthesiology, 1986, 65, A398. (b)

Tan S, SE Cohen, PF White. Sufentanil for analgesia after cesarean section: intravenous versus epidural administration. Anesth Analg, 1986, 65, S158. (a)

Tan S, V Bresson, D Brockmann, FS Brauer. Safety and efficacy of epiudral butorphanol in post-cesarean patients in regular clinical setting. Anesthesiology, 1987, 67, A623.

Tanelian DL, MJ Cousins. Failure of epidural opioid to control cancer pain in a patient previously treated with massive doses of intravenous opioid. Pain, 1989, 36, 359.

Tashiro C, M Iwasaki, K Nakahara, I Yoshiya. Postoperative paraplegia associated with epidural narcotic administration. Can J Anaesth, 1987, 34, 190.

Tasker RR, T Tsuda. Clinical neurophysiological investigation of deafferentation pain. In: JJ Bonica (Ed.): Advances in Pain Research and Therapy, Raven Press, New York, 1982, 5, 713.

Tauzin-Fin P, P Ragot, Ph Crozat, B Rossignol, Ph Ballanger, MM Sabathié. Intérets de l'anesthésie loco-régionale (péthidine sous arachnoidienne) associée à l'anesthésie générale en chirurgie urologique lourde. Forum Club, AFAR, 1984, Paris.

Tauzin-Fin P, Crozat, H Albin, A Brachet-Liermain, M Sabathié. Pharmacocinétique de la péthidine apres rachianesthésie, implications cliniques. Ann Fr Anesth Réanim, 1987, 6, 33. (a)

Tauzin-Fin P, MC Houdek, MC Saux, D Hecquet, et al. Etude pharmacocinétique de la péthidine apres rachianesthésie par association péthidine prilocaine. Ann Fr Anesth Reanim, 1987, 30° Congrès SFAR, R 86. (b)

Taveras JM, EH Wood. Diagnostic neuroradiology. 2nd ED, Williams and Wilkins, Baltimore, 1976, p 1130.

Taverne RHT, TI Ionescu. Changes of some renal clearances during epidural bupivacaine and morphine anesthesia for abdominal aortic surgery. VII Eur Congress of Anaesth, 1986, Vienna (Austria), Report, Abst 372.

Teddy PJ, CBT Adams, M Briggs, MA Jamous, JH Kerr. Extradural diamorphine in control of pain following lumbar laminectomy. J Neurol Psych, 1981, 44, 1074.

Terenius L, A Wahlström. Search for an endogenous ligand for the opiate receptor. Acta Physiol Scand, 1975, 94, 74.

Terenius L. Somatostatin and ACTH are peptides with antagonist like selectivity for opiate receptors. Eur J Pharm, 1976, 38, 211.

Teschemacher HJ. Permeationsverhalten morphinartiger Substanzen nach intraventrikulärer und intracerebraler Injektion. Naunyn Schmiedebergs Archiv für Pharmakologie, 1970, 266, 466.

Tessler MJ, DR Biehl, MA Naughler. Caesarean section with epidural carbonated lidocaine and fentanyl. Can J Anaesth, 1988, Abstract S110.

Tewes PA, LM Vella, S Thomas, HH Goll. Epidural fentanyl and bupivacaine combinations in patients undergoing pelvic surgery. Anesthesiology, 1988, 69 (3A), A406.

Thangathurai D, HF Bowles, HW Allen, M Mikhail. The incidence of pruritus after epidural morphine. Anaesthesia, 1988, 43, 1055.

Thangathurai D, HF Bowles, HW Allen, MS Mikhail. Epidural morphine and headache secondary to dural puncture. Anaesthesia, 1988, 43, 519.

Thiebaut JB, S Blond, JM Farcot, C Thurel, G Matge, G Schach, J Meynadier, F Buchheit. La morphine par voie intra-ventriculaire dans le traitement des douleurs néoplasiques. Méd et Hyg, 1985, 43, 636.

Thind GS, JCD Wells, RG Wilkes. The effects of continuous intravenous naloxone on epidural morphine analgesia. Anaesthesia, 1986, 41, 582.

Thompson WR, PT Smith, M Hirst, GP Varkey, RL Knill. Regional analgesic effect of epidural morphine in volunteers. Can Anaesth Soc J, 1981, 28, 530.

Thorén T, M Wattwil. Effects on gastric emptying of thoracic epidural analgesia with morphine or bupivacaine. Anesth Analg, 1988, 67, 687.

Thorén T, H Tanghöj, M Wattwil, G Järnerot. Epidural morphine delays gastric emptying and small intestinal transit in volunteers. Acta Anaesthesiol Scand, 1989, 33, 174.

Thorén T, A Sundberg, M Wattwil, JE Garvill, U Jürgensen. Effects of epidural bupivacaine and epidural morphine on bowel function and pain after hysterectomy. Acta Anaesthesiol Scand, 1989, 33, 181.

Thurston CL, ES Culhane, E Carstens, LR Watkins. Intrathecal vasopressin induced tail flick suppression. Pain (Suppl.), 1987, 4, S37.

Tiengo M, C Ambrosoni, C Nobili, L Piva, M Buscaglia, E Zuliani. Assessment of epidural morphine analgesia in second- trimester induced abortion. Eur J of Anaesth, Congress Report. 1984.

Tolksdorf W, M Hartung, H Usadel, E Wetzel. Four severe withdrawal reactions in two patients receiving epidural morphine for the treatment of cancer pain. Pain, 1987, S4, S69.

Torda TA. Epidural analgesia with morphine a preliminary communication. Anaesth Intens Care, 1979, 7, 367.

Torda TA. Epidural morphine (letter). Anaesth Intens Care, 1980, 8, 217. (a)

Torda TA, DA Pybus, H Liberman, M Clark, M Crawford. Experimental comparison of extradural and i.m. morphine. Brit J Anaesth, 1980, 52, 939. (b)

Torda TA, DA Pybus. Clinical experience with epidural morphine. Anaesth Intens Care, 1981, 9, 129.

Torda TA, DA Pybus. A comparison of four opiates for epidural analgesia. Br J Anaesth, 1982, 54, 291.

Torda TA, DA Pybus. Extradural administration of morphine and bupivacaine. A controlled comparison. Brit J Anaesth, 1984, 56, 141.

Traynor C, GM Hall. Endocrine and metabolic changes during surgery: Anaesthetic implications. Brit J Anaesth, 1981, 53, 153.

Traynor C, J Patterson, ID Ward, M Morgan, GM Hall. Effects of extradural analgesia and vagal blockade on the metabolic and endocrine response to upper abdominal surgery. Brit J Anaesth, 1982, 54, 319.

Treissman DA, JT Bate, PT Randall. Epidural use of morphine in managing the pain of carcineous degeneration of a uterine leiomyoma during pregnancy. Can Med Assoc J, 1982, 126, 505.

Trinh-Duc P, JP Fontes. Intéret de l'association bupivacaine - fentanyl isobare en rachianesthésie. Ann Fr Anesth Réanim, 1987, 6, 142.

Tsai SK, MS Mok, HL Hung, M Lippmann. Analgesic effect of intrathecal ketamine in primates. Anesth Analg, 1988, 67, S234.

Tschirner M, L Zeuner. Die Technik der subkutanen Tunnelung des Epiduralkatheters. Anaesth Reanimat, 1987, 12, 19.

Tseng LF. Tolerance and cross tolerance to morphine after chronic spinal D-Ala2-D-Leu5-Enkephalin infusion. Life Sci, 1982, 31, 987.

Tseng LF. Partial cross tolerance to C-Ala-2-Leu5-Enkephalin after chronic spinal morphine infusion. Life Sci, 1983, 32, 2545.

Tseng LF, JM Fujimoto. Evidence that spinal endorphin mediates intraventricular beta-endorphin-induced tail flick inhibiton and catalepsy. Brain Res, 1984, 302, 231.

Tseng LF, JM Fujimoto. Differential actions of intrathecal naloxone on blocking the tail-flick inhibition induced by intraventricular beta-endorphin and morphine in rats. J Pharm Exp Ther, 1985, 232, 74.

Tsuji H, C Shirasaka, T Asoh, I Uchida. Effects of epidural administration of local anaesthetics or morphine on postoperative nitrogen loss and catobolic hormones. Brit J Surg, 1987, 74, 421.

Tulunay FC, V Ischiro, EE Takemori. The effect of biogenic amine modifiers on morphine analgesia. Eur J Pharm, 1976, 35, 285.

Tung AS, K Maliniak, R Tenicela, PM Winter. Intrathecal morphine for intraoperative and postoperative analgesia. JAMA, 1980, 244, 2637. (a)

Tung AS, R Tenicela, PM Winter. Opiate withdrawal syndrome following intrathecal administration of morphine. Anesthesiology, 1980, 53, 340. (b)

Tung AS, TL Yaksh. Evaluation of epidural opiates in the cat. Anesthesiology, 1981, 55, A155.

Tung AS, TL Yaksh. The antinociceptive effects of epidural opiates in the cats: studies of the pharmacology and the effects of lipophylicity in spinal analgesia. Pain, 1982, 12, 343. (a)

Tung AS, TL Yaksh. In vivo evidence of multiple opiate receptors mediating analgesia in the rat spinal cord. Brain Research, 1982, 247, 75. (b)

Tuohy EB. Continuous spinal anesthesia: Its usefulness and technic involved. Anesthesiology, 1944, 5, 142.

Tuominen M, H Valli, E Kalso, PH Rosenberg. Efficacy of 0.3 mg morphine intrathecally in preventing tourniquet pain during spinal anaesthesia with hyperbaric bupivacaine. Acta Anaesth Scand, 1988, 32, 113.

Tuttle CB. Drug management of pain in cancer patients. Can Med Assn J, 1985, 132, 121.

Twycross RG. Morphine and diamorphine in the terminal ill patient. Acta Anaesth Scand (Suppl), 1982, 74, 128.

Twycross RG, M Zenz. Die Anwendung von oralem Morphin bei inkurablen Schmerzen. Anaesthesist, 1983, 32, 279. (a)

Twycross RG, SA Lack. (Eds.) Symptom control in far advanced cancer: pain relief. Pitman Press, 1983. (b)

Twycross RG. Round Table on pain treatment with spinal opioids. II Int Symposium: Pain Clinic, Lille (France) 1986.

Tyler DC. Respiratory effects of pain in a child after thoracotomy. Anesthesiology, 1989, 70 873.

Ullman DA, RE Wimpy, JB Fortune, TM Kennedy, BB Greenhouse. The treatment of patients with multiple rib fractures using continuous thoracic epidural narcotic infusion. Regional Anesthesia, 1989, 14, 43.

Umans J G, C E Inturrisi. Antinociceptive activity and toxicity of meperidine and normeperidine in mice. J Pharm Ther, 1982, 223, 203.

Usubiaga JE, J Wilinski, R Wilinski, LE Usibiaga, M Pontremoli. Transfer of local anaesthetics to the subarachnoidal space and mechanisms of epidural block Anesthesiology, 1964, 25, 752.

Vaccarino AL, RAR Tasker, R Melzack. Analgesia produced by normal doses of opioid antagonists alone and in combination with morphine. Pain, 1989, 36, 103.

Vainio A, I Tigerstedt. Opioid treatment for radiating cancer pain: oral administration vs epidural techniques. Acta Anaesth Scand, 1988, 32, 179.

Valenti S, et al. Buprenorphine vs morphine both spinally injected in postoperative pain relief. Anaesthesist, 1987, S 73, Poster 190, Hamburg.

Valls JM, MM Mabrok, A Teixidor, B González, JMV Claramunt, JE Banos. Analgesia postoperatoria con morfina por via caudal en cirugia pediátrica: estudio aleatorio y a doble ciego comparado con bupivacaina. Rev Esp Anestesiol Reanim, 1989, 36, 88.

Valverde A, DH Dyson, WN McDonell. Epidural morphine reduces halothane MAC in the dog. Can J Anaesth, 1989, 36, 629.

Van de Woerd A, T Oyama, A Trouwborst, W Erdmann. Intrathecal beta- endorphin treatment in man with intractable cancer pain. In: W Erdmann, T Oyama, MJ Pernak (Eds.): The Pain Clinic I VNU Science Press, Utrecht, 1985, 99.

Van den Hoogen RHWM, FC Colpaert. Long term catheterization of the lumbar epidural space in rats. Pharm Biochem Behav, 1981, 15, 515.

Van den Berg B, E Van den Berg, M Zenz. Peridurale Morphin- Analgesie und Sympathikusblockade. In: M Zenz (Ed.): Peridurale Opiat-Analgesie, Gustav Fischer Verlag, Stuttgart, 1981, 31.

Van den Berg B. Anwendung der periduralen Opiatanalgesie bei Karzinomschmerzen. In: J Brückner (Ed.): Schmerzbehandlung, Springer Verlag, Berlin,1982, 35. (a)

Van den Berg B, E van den Berg, M Zenz. Sympathikusblockade bei Periduralanaesthesie und periduraler Opiatanalgesie. In: JB Brückner (Ed.): Anaesthesiologie und Intensivmedizin, Schmerzbehandlung Epidurale Opiatanalgesie, Springer Verlag, Berlin, Heidelberg, New York, 1982, 153, 65. (b)

Van den Hoogen RHWM. Pharmacology of epidural opiates. II Int Symposium: Pain Clinic, Lille (France) 1986. In: Ph Scherpereel, J Meynadier, S Blond (Eds.): Pain Clinic II, VNU Science Press, Utrecht, 1987, 291. (a)

Van den Hoogen RHWM. In vivo pharmacological effects of ED and SC opiates (sufentanil) in the rat. Proefschrift Rijksuniversiteit, Leiden, 1987, 11, 3. (b)

Van den Hoogen RHWM, FC Colpaert. Epidural and subcutaneous morphine, meperidine, fentanyl and sufentanil in the rat: analgesia and other in vivo pharmacological effects. Anesthesiology, 1987, 66, 186. (c)

Van den Hoogen RHWM, KJW Bervoets, FC Colpaert. Respiratory effects of epidural and subcutaneous morphine, meperidine, fentanyl and sufentanil in the rat. Anesth Analg, 1988, 67, 1071.

Van den Hoogen RHW, K Bervoets, FC Colpaert. Enhancement by pain and stress of analgesia produced by epidural sufentanil in the rat. Anesthesiology, 1988, 69, 24.

Van den Hoogen RHW, KJW Bervoets, FC Colpaert. Respiratory effects of epidural morphine and sufentanil in the absence and presence of chlordiazepoxide. Pain, 1989, 37, 103.

Van der Auwera D, C Verborgh, F Camu. The analgesic effect of 30-50-75 µg sufentanil administered epidurally for postoperative pain in man. Acta Anaesth Belgica, 1985, 76, 6.

Van der Auwera D, C Verborgh, F Camu. Analgesic and cardiorespiratory effects of epidural sufentanil and morphine in man: a double-blind evaluation. VII Eur Congress of Anaesth, 1986, Vienna (Austria), Report, Abst 414.

Van der Auwera D, C Verborgh, F Camu. Analgesic and cardiorespiratory effects of epidural sufentanil and morphine in humans. Anesth Analg, 1987, 66, 999.

Van Diejen D, JJ Driessen, JH Kaanders. Spinal cord compression during chronic epidural morphine administration in a cancer patient. Anaesthesia, 1987, 42, 1201.

Van Droogenbroeck E, D Van der Auwera, C Verborgh, F Camu. The analgesic effect of 30, 50, 75 µg sufentanil administered epidurally for postoperative pain in man. Acta anaesth Belgica, 1985, 76, 6.

Van EE R. Epidural morphine in the terminally ill: How long and how high? The Pain Clinic, 1986, 1, 69.

Van Essen EJ, JG Bovill, EJ Ploeger, H Beerman. Intrathecal morphine and clonidine for control of intractable cancer pain: a case report. Acta Anaesth Belg, 1988, 39, 110.

Van Steenberge A. Epidural lofentanil for pain relief in labor. Anesth Intensiv Med Obstet Anesth Digest, 1983, 3, 365. (c).

Van Steenberge A. The best of two worlds: combination of local anesthetic and narcotic for epidural analgesia during labor. Obst Anesth Digest, 1983, 3, 65. (a)

Van Steenberge A. Choice of local anaesthetic agents for obstetric purposes. Eur J Obst Gyn and Reprod Biology, 1983, 15, 355. (b)

Van Steenberge A, MC Debroux, H Noorduin. Peridural bupivacaine with sufentanil in vaginal deliveries. II Int Symposium: Pain Clinic, Lille (France)1986. In: Ph Scherpereel, J Meynadier, S Blond (Eds.): Pain Clinic II, VNU Science Press, Utrecht, 1987, 303. (a)

Van Steenberge A, HC Debroux, H Noorduin. Extradural bupivacaine with sufentanil for vaginal delivery. Brit J Anaesth, 1987, 59, 1518. (b)

Van Steenberge A. Epidural lofentanil for pain relief in labor. In: HJ Wüst, M Stanton-Hicks (Eds.): Anaesthesiologie und Intensivmedizin, New Aspects in Regional Anesthesia, Springer Verlag, Berlin, Heidelberg, New York, 1986, 176, 145.

Van Wimersma Greidanus TJ, JT ten Haaf. The effects of opiates and opioid peptides on oxytocin release. In: JA Amico, AG Robinson (Eds.): Oxytocin: clinical and laboratory studies, Elsevier Science Publishers B.V., 1985, 145.

Vandalouca A, K Mistakidon, F Antoniou, H Gyftonidon, G Tolis. Comparison of the effects of ketamine HCl, SMS 201995 and fentanyl administered epidurally for postoperative analgesia. Reports 5th Int. Congress Belgiums Society of Anaesthesia and Reanimation, Brussels, 1988.

Vandermeulen E, J Vertommen, H Van Aken, H Noorduin, A Van Steenberge. Epidural bupivacaine with sufentanil in labor. Anesthesiology (Suppl), 1989, 71, 844.

Vanstrum GS, KM Bjornson, R Ilko. Postoperative effects of intrathecal morphine in coronary artery bypass surgery. Anesth Analg, 1988, 67, 261.

Vasko MR, IH Pang, M Vogt. Involvement of 5-hydroxytryptamine-containing neurons in antinocieption produced by injection of morphine into nucleus raphe magnus or onto spinal cord. Brain Res, 1984, 306, 341.

Vatashsky E, Y Haskel, B Beilin, HB Aronson. Common bile duct pressure in dogs after opiate injection-epidural versus intravenous route. Can Anaesth Soc J, 1984, 31, 650.

Vaught JL, RE Chipkin. A characterization of kyotorphin (tyr-arg)-induced antinociception. Eur J Pharm, 1982, 79, 167.

Vaught JL, A Cowan, DE Gmerek. A species difference in the slowing effect of intrathecal morphine on gastrointestinal transit. Eur J Pharm, 1983, 94, 181.

Vedrenne JB, M Esteve. Traitement ambulatoire de la douleur cancéreuse par la morphine en péridural. La nouvelle presse médicale, 1984, 13, 99.

Veillette Y, D Benhamou, T Labaille. Addition of clonidine and / or epinephrine to epidural lidocaine: clinical effects. Anesthesiology (Suppl), 1989, 71, 645.

Vella LM, D Francis, P Houlton, F Reynolds. Comparison of the antiemetics metoclopramide and promethazine in labour. Brit Med J [Clin Res], 1985, 290, 1173. (a)

Vella LM, DG Willatts, HC Kuo, DJ Lintin, DM Justins, F Reynolds. Epidural fentanyl in labour, an evaluation of the systemic contribution to analgesia. Anaesthesia, 1985, 40, 741. (b)

Ventafridda V, M Figliuzzi, M Tamburini, E Gori, D Porolaro, M Sala. Clinical observation on analgesia elecited by intrathecal morphine in cancer patients. In: JJ Bonica (Ed.): Advances in Pain Research and Therapy, Raven Press, New York, 1979, 559.

Ventafridda V. Intraspinal narcotics for cancer pain. Abstracts in Recent advances in intraspinal pain therapy, Vicenza, Sept 1985, 14.

Ventafridda V, F De Conno, M Tamburini, M Pappalettera. Clinical evaluation of chronic infusion of intrathecal morphine in cancer pain. In: KM Foley, CE Inturrisi (Eds.): Advances in Pain Research and Therapy, Raven Press, New York, 1986, 8, 391.

Ventafridda A, E Spoldi, A Caraceni, F De Conno. Intraspinal morphine for cancer pain. Acta Anesth Scand (Suppl.), 1987, 31, 47. (a)

Ventafridda A, M Tamburini, F DeConno. Comprehensive treatment in cancer pain. In: Fields H et al. (Eds.) Advances in pain research and therapy, vol. 9, Raven Press, New York, 1987, 617. (b)

Verborgh C. Epidural sufentanil administration for pain relief after abdominal surgery. II Int Symposium: Pain Clinic, Lille (France) 1986. In: Ph Scherpereel, J Meynadier, S Blond (Eds.): Pain Clinic II, VNU Science Press, Utrecht, 1987, 297. (a)

Verborgh C, D Van der Auwera, F Camu. Meptazinol for postoperative pain relief in man. Comparison of i.t. and i.m. administration. Brit J Anaesth, 1987, 59, 1134. (b)

Verborgh C, D Van der Auwera, E Van Droogenbroeck, F Camu. Epidural sufentanil for postsurgical pain relief. Eur J Anaesth, 1986, 3, 313.

Verborgh C, D Van der Auwera, F Camu. Epidural sufentanil for postsurgical pain relief: Is there a difference between lumbar and thoracic administeration? Reports: 5th Intern. Congress of the Belgiens Society of Anaesthesia and Reanimation, Brussels, 1988.

Verborgh C, D van der Auwera, H Noorduin, F Camu. Epidural sufentanil for postoperative pain relief: effects of adrenaline. Eur J Anaesth, 1988, 5, 183.

Vercauteren M, H Noorduin, G Van den Bussche, G Hanegreefs. Epidural sufentanil in postoperative pain: effect of volume and association with bupivacaine. IV Int. Meeting, Eur Soc Regional Anaesthesia, Roma (Italia) june 1985.

Vercauteren M, G Hanegreefs. Modification of analgesic quality and side effects of epidural sufentanil. II Int Symposium: Pain Clinic, Lille (France), 1986. In: Ph Scherpereel, J Meynadier, S Blond (Eds.): Pain Clinic II, VNU Science Press, Utrecht, 1987, 299.

Vercauteren M, E Boeckx, H Noorduin. Respiratory arrest after sufentanil. Anaesthesia, 1988, 43, 69.

Verdrienne JB, M Esteve. Traitement ambulatoire de la douleur par le morphine en péridural. La Nouvelle Presse Medicale, 1984, 13, 99.

Vertommen J, E Vandermeulen, SM Shnider, H Van Aken. The effect of the addition of epidural sufentanil to bupivacaine 0.5% for elective cesarean section. Anesthesiology (Suppl), 1989, 71, 868.

Vestergaard-Madsen J, L Rybro, BA Schurizek, HC Husegaard, F Joensen, LV Møller, M Wernberg. Respiratory depression following postoperative analgesia with epidural morphine. Acta Anaesth Scand, 1986, 30, 417.

Vickery RG, BC Sheridan, IS Segal, M Maze. Anesthetic and hemodynamic effects of the stereoisomers of medetomidine, an alpha-2-adrenergic agonist, in halothane-anesthetized dogs. Anesth Analg, 1988, 67, 611.

Viel EJ, F D'Athis, JJ Eledjam, JE de la Coussaye. Brachial plexus block with opioids for postoperative pain relief: comparison between buprenorphine and morphine. Regional Anaesthesia, 1989, 14, 274.

Villalonga Morales A, C Lapena Bayo, P Taura Reverter, J Castillo Monsegur, MA Nalda Felipe. Retencion urinaria tras analgesia epidural morfinica postoperatoria. Rev Esp Anest Rean, 1984, 31, 238.

Villalonga A, J Castillo, C Hernandez, MA Nalda. Peridural morphine in opiate addicts. Medicina

Clinica, 1985, 85, 729.

Villoria CM, UDF Miro, CR Hernández. Alteraciones del AMPc tras administración crónica de morfina en el espacio epidural. Rev Espagnola de Anasthesiolgiy Rean, 1987, 34, 5.

Vincenti E, B Tambuscio. Epidural narcotics and control of arterial pressure in a pre-eclamptic patient (letter). Can Anaesth Soc J, 1982, 29, 405. (a)

Vincenti E, B Tambuscio, D Magaldi, L Becagli, M Gambato, D De Salvia, A Ambrosini. Recent trends in the peri-surgical use of continuous epidural anesthesia in elderly patients with vulvar neoplasia. Clin Exp Obst Gyn, 1982, 9, 156. (b)

Vincenti E, M Chiaranda, A Ambrosini, L Becagli, D De Salvia, T Maggino, D Marchesoni. New trends for pain relief in gynaecologic oncology. Eur J Gynaecol Oncol, 1983, 4, 122.

Viscomi CM, JC Eisenach. Patient controlled epidural analgesia (PCEA) for labor. Anesthesiology (Suppl), 1989, 71, 848.

Wakefield RD, M Mesaros. Reversal of pruritis, secondary to epidural morphine, with the narcotic/ antagonist nalbuphine (Nubain). Anesthesiology, 1985, 63, A255.

Wakerlin G, MS Shulman, LY Yamaguchi, JB Brodsky JBD Mark. Experience with lumbar epidural hydromorphone for pain relief after thoracotomy. Anesth Analg (Suppl.), 1986, 65, S163.

Waldman SD, Feldstein GS, Allen ML, G Turnage. Selection of patients for implantable intraspinal narcotic delivery systems. Anesth Analg, 1986, 65, 883.

Waldman SD, GS Feldstein, ML Allen. Troubleshooting intraspinal narcotic delivery systems. Amer J Nursing, 1987, Jan., 63. (a)

Waldman SD, GS Feldstein, ML Allen, M Landers, G Turnage. Cervical epidural implantable narcotic delivery systems in the management of upper body cancer pain. Anaesth Analg, 1987, 66, 780. (b)

Waldman SD, DW Coombs. Selection of implantable narcotic delivery systems. Anesth Analg, 1989, 68, 377.

Waldmann V, C Leveque, JC Levron, G Guerin, MT Cousin. Pharmacokinetics of alfentanil administered epidurally during labor. Anesthesiology (Suppl), 1989, 71, 901.

Waldvogel HH, M Fasano. Extradural administration of lofentanil for balanced postoperative analgesia. Anaesthesist (Suppl.), 1983, 32, 256.

Wallenstein SL. Measurement of pain and analgesia in cancer patients. Cancer (Suppl.), 1984, 53, 2260.

Walmsley PNH, GW Colclough, M Mazloomdoost, FJ McDonnell. Epidural PCA/infusion for post-nephrectomy pain: shorter hospitalization. Anesthesiology (Suppl), 1989, 71, 684.

Walsh TD. Oral morphine in chronic cancer pain. Pain, 1984, 18, 1.

Walts LF, RD Kaufman, JR Moreland, M Weiskopf. Total hip arthroplasty, an investigation of factors related to postoperative urinary retention. Clinical Orthepedics and Related Research, 1985, 194, 280.

Wang BC, JM Hiller, MJ Holland, EJ Simon, DE Hillman, H Turndorf. Distribution of 3H-Morphine following lumbar epidural administration in rabbits. Anesthesiology, 1987, 67, A253. (a)

Wang BC, JM Hiller, MJ Holland, EJ Simon, DE Hillman, H Turndorf. Distribution of 3H Morphine following lumbar subarachnoid administration in rabbits. Regional Anesthesia, 1987, 12, 30. (b)

Wang BC, JM Hiller, EJ Simon, H Turndorf. Epidural methadone does not significantly increase urinary bladder size in unanesthetized rabbits. Anesthesiology, 1988, 69 (3A), A385.

Wang BC, JM Hiller EJ Simon, DE Hillman, C Rosenberg, H Turndorf. Distribution of 3H-morphine following lumbar subarachnoid injection in unanesthetized rabbits. Anesthesiology, 1989, 70, 817.

610

Wang JJ, KH Chan, MS Mok, M Lippmann. Epidural nalbuphine for postoperative pain relief. 8th World Congress of Anesth, Manila 1984, Abstracts 2, A436.

Wang JJ, SP Shuai, TY Lee, M Lippmann, MS Mok. Analgesic effect of epidural nalbuphine: a comparative study. VII Eur Congress of Anaesth, 1986, Vienna (Austria), Report, Abst 413.

Wang JJ, MS Mok, M Lippmann. Comparative analgesic efficacy of epidural nalbuphine, butorphanol, meperidine and morphine. Anesth Analg, 1988, 67, S248.

Wang JJ, MS Mok, M Lippmann. Analgesic effect of epidural morphine and nalbuphine in combined use. Anesthesiology (Suppl), 1989, 71, 703.

Wang JK. Analgesic effect of intrathecally administered morphine. Regional Anesthesia, 1977, 2, 3.

Wang JK, LE Nauss, JE Thomas. Pain relief by intrathecally applied morphine in man. Anesthesiology, 1979, 50, 149.

Wang JK. Intrathecal morphine for intractable pain secondary to cancer of pelvic organs. Pain, 1985, 21, 99.

Wanscher M, L Rishede, B Krogh. Fistula formation following epidural catheter: a case report. Acta Anaesth Scand, 1985, 29, 552.

Warfield CA, LE Dohlman. Intraspinal narcotics for pain control. Hosp Pract [Off], 1984, 19, 148B, 148F, 148H Pasim.

Watkins LR, H Frenk, J Miller, DJ Mayer. Effect of spinal cord lesions on convulsive activity induced by intrathecal morphine. Brain Res, 1984, 310, 337. (a)

Watkins LR, H Frenk, J Miller, DJ Mayer. Cataleptic effects of opiates following intrathecal administration. Brain Res, 1984, 299, 43. (b)

Watkins LR, IB Kinscheck, DJ Mayer. Potentiation opiate analgesia and apparent reversal of morphine tolerance by proglumide. Science, 1984, 224, 395. (c)

Watkins LR, IB Kinscheck, EFS Kaufman, J Miller, H Frenk, DJ Mayer. Cholecystokinin antagonists selectively potentiate analgesia induced by endogenous opiates. Brain Research, 1985, 327, 181.(a)

Watkins LR, IB Kinscheck, DJ Mayer. Potentiation of morphine analgesia by cholecystokinin antagonist proglumide. Brain Research, 1985, 327, 169. (b)

Watson J, A Moore, H McQuay, P Teddy, D Baldwin, M Allen, R Bullingham. Plasma morphine concentration and analgesic effects of lumbar extradural morphine and heroin. Anesth Analg, 1984, 63, 629.

Watson SJ, H Akil, VE Ghazarossian, A Goldstein. Dynorphin immunocytochemical localization in brain and peripheral nervous system. Proc Natl Acad Sci USA, 1981, 78, 1260.

Way L. Studies on the local anesthetic properies os isonipecaine. J. Am. Pharm Assoc, 1946, 35, 44.

Weddel SJ, RR Ritter. Epidural morphine: serum levels and pain relief. Anesthesiology, 1980, 53, S419.

Weddel SJ, RR Ritter. Serum levels following epidural administration of morphine and correlation with relief of postsurgical pain. Anesthesiology, 1981, 54, 210.

Wei TT, MS Mok, YC Cheng, M Lippmann. Evaluation of ketamine as a local anesthetic in humans. Regional Anesthesia, 1987, 12, 100.

Weigel K, J Chrubasik, F Mundinger. Die intraventrikuläre Infusion von Morphin: Eine alternative Methode zur Schmerzbehandlung bei "intractable cancer pain" . Schmerz-Pain-Douleur, 1985, 6, 6. (a)

Weigel K, F Mundiger, JA Chrubasik. Continuous intraventricular morphine infusion for intractable cancer pain. Intern. Symposium Pain Therapy, 1985, abstract, 34. (b)

Weigel K, JA Chrubasik, F Mundiger. Continuous intraventricular morphine infusion for intractable cancer pain. II Int Symposium Pain Clinic, Lille (France), 1986, abstract, III P 8. I

Weiler RL, GC Wardell. Hemodynamic study of epidural clonidine in awake sheep. Anesth Analg, 1988, 67, S252.

Weinger MB, SR Furst The selective alpha-2 agonist dexmedetomidine does not potentiate alfentanil induced respiratory depression in the rat Anesthesiology, (Suppl), 1989, 71, 1094

Weinger MB, IS Segal, M Maze Dexmedetomidine, acting through central alpha-2 adrenoceptors, prevents opiate-induced muscle rigidity in the rat Anesthesiology, 1989, 71, 242

Weintraub SJ, JS Naulty. Acute abstinence syndrome after epidural injection of butorphanol. Anesth Analg, 1985, 64, 452.

Welch DB. Epidural narcotics and dural puncture (letter). Lancet, 1981, 1, 55. (a)

Welch DB, A Hrynaszkiewicz. Postoperative analgesia using epidural methadone administration by lumbar route for thoracic pain relief. Anaesthesia, 1981, 36, 1051. (b)

Welch K, K Salder. Permeability of the chorioid plexus of the rabbit to several solutes. Am J Physiol, 1966, 210, 652.

Welchew EA, JA Thornton. Control of postoperative pain by thoracic fentanyl epidural and its effect upon the stress response. 7th World Congress of Anaesth, Hamburg (W Germany), 1980. Excerpta Medica, Int Congress series 533, p 456.

Welchew EA, JA Thornton. Continuous thoracic epidural fentanyl. A comparison of epidural fentanyl with intramuscular papaveretum for postoperative pain. Anaesthesia, 1982, 37, 309. (a)

Welchew EA, J Hosking. Epidural fentanyl - The optimal concentration, with and without adrenaline. 6th Eur Congress of Anaesth, London, 1982, volume of summaries, p 48. (b)

Welchew EA, D Reid. The metabolic consequences of different forms of postoperative analgesia. 6th Eur Congress of Anaesth, London, 1982, volume of summaries, p 32. (c)

Welchew EA. The optimum concentration for epidural fentanyl. A randomised, double-blind comparison with and without 1:200,000 adrenaline. Anaesthesia, 1983, 38, 1037.

Welchew EA. An open comparison of patient-controlled on-demand fentanyl delivered either extradurally or i.v. Brit J Anaesth, 1985, 57, 346P.

Wells DG, G Davies, D Wagner. Accidental injection of epidural methohexital. Anesthesiology, 1987, 67, 846. (a)

Wells DG, G Davies. Profound central nervous system depression from epidural fentanyl for extracorporeal shock wave lithotripsy. Anesthesiology, 1987, 67, 991. (b)

Wells JCD. The use of spinal opioids in the management of cancer pain. II Int Symposium: The Pain Clinic, 1986, Lille (France): In: Ph Scherpereel, J Meynadier, S Blond (Eds.): Pain Clinic II, VNU Science Press, Utrecht, 1987, 305. (a)

Wells JCD. Routes for opiate administrations. II Int Symposium: The Pain Clinic, 1986, Lille (France). In: Ph Scherpereel, J Meynadier, S Blond (Eds.): Pain Clinic II, VNU Science Press Utrecht, 1987, 309. (b)

Wenningsted-Torgard K, J Heyn, L Willumsen. Spondylitis following epidural morphine. A case report. Acta Anaesth Scand, 1982, 26, 649.

Wermeling DP, TS Foster, KE Record, JE Chalkley. Drug delivery for intractable cancer pain: use of a new disposable parenteral infusion device for continuous outpatient epidural narcotic infusion. Cancer, 1987, 60, 875.

Wheatley RG, ID Somerville, JG Jones. The effect of diamorphine administered epidurally or with a patient-controlled analgesia system on long-term postoperative oxygenation. Eur J Anaesth, 1989, 6, 64.

White PF. Management of postoperative pain. Int Anaesth Res Soc, 61th Congress Report, 1987, 85.

White WD. Fentanyl infusion and epidural bupivacaine in postoperative pain relief after vascular surgery. Brit Med J, 1979, 2, 166.

Whiting WG, AN Sandler, LC Lau, PM Chovaz. Analgesic and respiratory effects of epidural sufentanil in post-thoracotomy patients. Anesthesiology, 1986, 65, A176.

Whiting WC, AN Sandler, LC Lau, PM Chovaz, P Slavchenko, D Daley, G Koren. Analgesic and respiratory effects of epidural sufentanil in patients following thoracotomy. Anesthesiology, 1988, 69, 36.

Whitwam JG, D Niv, L Loh, RD Jack. Effects of subarachnoid midazolam in dogs. Lancet, 1982, 2, 1465.

Whizar-Lugo V, C Cortex Gomez. Epidural ketamine vs epidural morphine in severe cancer pain. Pain (Suppl.), 1987, 4, S142.

Wiesenfeld Z, LL Gustafsson. Continuous intrathecal administration of morphine via an osmotic minipump in the rat. Brain Res, 1982, 247, 195.

Wiesenfeld-Hallin Z. The effects of intrathecal morphine and naltrexone on autotomy in sciatic nerve sectioned rats. Pain, 1984, 18, 267. (a)

Wiesenfeld-Hallin Z, A Persson. Subarachnoid injection of salmon calcitonin does not induce analgesia in rats. Eur J Pharm, 1984, 104, 375. (b)

Wiesenfeld-Hallin Z, P Soedersten. Spinal opiates affect sexual behaviour in rats. Nature, 1984, 309, 257. (c)

Wiesenfeld-Hallin Z. Subarachnoid lidocaine and calcitonin for postoperative analgesia (letter). Anesth Analg, 1988, 67, 298.

Wilde GP, AJ Whitaker, A Moulton. Epidural buprenorphine for pain relief after spinal decompression. J Bone Joint Surg, 1988, 70B, 448.

Wilhite AO, NH Blass. Comparison of analgesic efficacy of alfentanil, fentanyl and sufentanil in continuous epidural infusions of 0.125% bupivacaine for labor and delivery. Anesthesiology (Suppl), 1989, 71, 902.

Willer JC, S Bergeret, M Szatan, JH Gaudy. Peridural morphine analgesia is mediated by a direct spinal effect. New Eng J Med, 1984, 311, 602.

Willer JC, S Bergeret, JH Gaudy. Epidural morphine strongly depress nociceptive flexion reflexes in patients with postoperative pain. Anesthesiology, 1985, 63, 675.

Willer JC, S Bergeret, T De Broucker, JH Gaudy. Low dose epidural morphine does not affect non-nociceptive spinal reflexes in patients with postoperative pain. Pain, 1988, 32, 9.

Williams P, R Warwick. (Eds.) Gray's anatomy. In: Gray's anatomy, 1980, Churchill Livingstone Edinburgh.

Wilson PR, GA Power. Analgetic action of epidural narcotics in animals. Intern Association of the Study of Pain, 1979, 371.

Wilson PR, TL Yaksh. Baclofen is antinociceptive in the spinal intrathecal space of animals. Eur J Pharm, 1978, 51, 323.

Wimpy R, LL Hubbard, M McCormick, JB Fortune. The treatment of patients with multiple rib fractures using continuous thoracic epidural narcotic infusions. Regional Anesthesia, 1987, 12, 48.

Wishart JM. Epidural morphine at home. Can Anaesth Soc J, 1981, 28, 492.

Woerd VD A, T Oyama, A Trouwborst, W Erdmann. Intrathecal beta- endorphin treatment in man with intractable cancer pain. In: W Erdmann, T Oyama, MJ Pernak (Eds.): The Pain Clinic I, VNU, Science Press, Utrecht,1985, 99.

Wolf AR, AJ Hobbs, D Hughes, C Prys-Roberts. Combined bupivacaine/morphine caudals: duration of analgesia and plasma morphine concentration. Anesthesiology (Suppl), 1989, 71, 1015.

Wolfe MJ, ADG Nicholas. Selective epidural analgesia (letter). Lancet, 1979, 2, 150.

Wolfe MJ, GK Davies. Analgesic action of extradural fentanyl (letter). Brit J Anaesth, 1980, 51, 357.

Wolff J, P Carl, ME Crawford. Epidural buprenorphine for postoperative analgesia. A controlled comparison with epidural morphine. Anaesthesia, 1986, 46, 76.

Woods WA, SE Cohen. High-dose epidurale morphine in a terminally ill patient. Anesthesiology, 1982, 56, 311.

Woolf CJ. Intrathecal high dose morphine produces hyperalgesia in the rat. Brain Res, 1981, 209, 491.

Worthley LIG. Thoracic epidural in the management of chest trauma - a study of 161 cases. Intens Care Med, 1985, 11, 312.

Wright JT. Abnormal labour and pain relief. Nursing (Oxford), 1981, 21, 921.

Wright RM, T Goroszeniuk. Epidural fentanyl for pain of multiple fractures (letter). Lancet, 1980, 2, 1033.

Writer WD, FM James, AS Wheeler. Double blind comparison of morphine and bupivacaine for continuous epidural analgesia in labor. Anesthesiology, 1981, 54, 215.

Writer WDR, JB Hurtig, D Evans, RE Needs, CE Hope, JB Forrest. Epidural morphine prophylaxis of postoperative pain: report of a double blind multicentre study. Can Anaesth Soc J, 1985, 32, 330.

Writer WDR, GS Fox, JB Hurtig. Epidural morphine for postoperative analgesia (letter). Can Anaesth Soc J, 1986, 33, 116.

Wüst HJ, KG Moritz, W Sandmann, O Richter. Modifikation der Analgetikawirkung (Buprenorphin, Pentazocine, Pethidine) auf Atmung und Kreislauf durch die Epidural-, Halothan- oder Neuroleptanaesthesie. Anaesthesie Intensivtherapie Notfallmedizin, 1980, 15, 119.

Wust HS, PR Bromage. Delayed respiratory arrest after epidural hydromorphine. Anaesthesia, 1987, 42, 404.

Wyant GM, BJ Miller. Complications with the Holter-Hausner implantable epidural system. Pain Clinic, 1986, 1, 63.

Yablonski-Peretz T, B Klin, Y Beilin, E Warner, S Baron, D Olshwang, R Gatane. Continuous epidural narcotic analgesia for intractable pain due to malignancy. J Surg Oncology, 1985, 29, 8.

Yaksh TL. Analgetic actions of intrathecal opiates in cat and primate. Brain Res, 1978, 153, 205. (b)

Yaksh TL, PR Wilson PR, RF Kaiko, CE Inturissi. Analgesia produced by a spinal action of morphine and effects upon parturition in the rat. Anesthesiology, 1979, 51, 386.

Yaksh TL, TA Rudy. Analgesia mediated by a direct spinal action of narcotics. Science, 1976, 192, 1357.

Yaksh TL, TA Rudy. Narcotic analgetics : CNS sites and mechanisms of action as revealed by intracerebral injection techniques. Pain, 1978, 4, 299. (a)

Yaksh TL, TA Rudy. Studies on the direct spinal action of narcotics in the production of analgesia in the rat. J Pharm and Exper Therapeutics, 1977, 202, 411.

Yaksh TL, SV Reddy. Studies in the primate on the analgesic effects associated with intrathecal actions of opiates, alpha-adrenergic agonists and baclofen. Anesthesiology, 1981, 54, 451.

Yaksh TL, DL Hammond. Peripheral and central substances involved in the rostral transmission of nociceptive information. Pain, 1982, 13, 1. (a)

Yaksh TL, GJ Harty. Effects of thiorphan on the antinociceptive actions of intrathecal (D-Ala2, Met2) Enkephalin. Eur J Pharm, 1982, 79, 293. (b)

Yaksh TL. Spinal opiate analgesia. Characteristics and principles of action. Pain, 1982, 11, 293. (c)

Yaksh TL, H Müller (Eds.) Spinal opiate analgesia. Experimental and clinical studies. Anaesth Intensivmed, 1982, Springer Verlag, Berlin Heidelberg New York. (d)

Yaksh TL, KE Gross, CH Li. Studies on the intrathecal effect of beta-endorphin in primate. Brain Res, 1982, 241, 261. (e)

Yaksh TL. The limiting issue-tolerance. Intraspinal narcotic analgesia for acute and chronic pain. Palm Springs, USA, 1983, Symposium report. (a)

Yaksh TL. Advances in pharmacology of pain control by spinal drug therapy. Intraspinal narcotic analgesia for acute and chronic pain. Palm Springs, USA, 1983, Symposium report. (b)

Yaksh TL. Principles of spinal pain processing. Intraspinal narcotic analgesia for acute and chronic pain. Palm Springs, USA, 1983, Symposium report. (c)

Yaksh TL. Effects of spinally administered agents on spinal cord blood flow: a need for further studies. Anesthesiology, 1983, 59, 173. (d)

Yaksh TL. In vivo studies on spinal opiate receptor systems mediation antinociception. I. mu and delta receptor profiles in the primate. J Pharm Exp Ther, 1983, 226, 303. (e)

Yaksh TL. The principles behind the use of spinal narcotics. Clinics in Anaesthesiology, 1983, 1, 219. (f)

Yaksh TL, R Noueihed, PhA Durant. Preliminary studies on the anti nociceptive effects of intrathecal alfentanil in animal models. In: FG Estefanous (Ed.): Opioids in Anesthesia, Butterworth, Boston, 1984, 161.

Yaksh TL. Pharmacology of spinal adrenergic systems which modulate spinal nociceptive processing. Pharm Biochem Behav, 1985, 22, 845. (a)

Yaksh TL, R Noueihed. The physiology and pharmacology of spinal opiates. Ann Rev Pharmacol Toxicol, 1985, 25, 433. (b)

Yaksh TL, SR Atchison, PhAC Durant. Characteristics of action and pharmacology of intrathecally administered D-Ala-D-Leu-Enkephalin. In: KM Foley, CE Inturrisi (Eds.): Advances in Pain Reseach and Therapy, vol 8, Raven Press, New York, 1986, 303. (a)

Yaksh TL, GJ Harty, BM Onofrio. High doses of spinal morphine produce a nonopiate receptor-mediated hyperesthesia: clinical and theoretical implications. Anesthesiology, 1986, 64, 590. (b)

Yaksh TL, R Noueihed, P Durant, et al. Studies of the pharmacology and pathology of intrathecally administered 4-anilinopiperidine analogues et al. Anesthesiology, 1986, 64, 54. (c)

Yaksh TL. Neurochemical mediaton of analgesia in the spinal cord. Pain, 1987, S4, S224. (a)

Yaksh TL. Spinal opiates: a review of their effect on spinal function with emphasis on pain processing. Acta Anaesth Scand (Suppl.), 1987, 31, 25. (b)

Yaksh TL, BM Onofrio. Retrospective consideration of the doses of morphine given intrathecally by chronic infusion in 163 patients. Pain, 1987, 31, 211. (c)

Yaksh TL, E Mjanger, CW Stevens. Pharmacology of the analgesic effects of opioid and non-opioid receptor selective agents in the spinal cord. Acta 20th Int. Meeting Anaesthesia and Critical care, JEPU Publ. Arnette Paris, 1988. (a)

Yaksh TL, MRF Al-Rodhan, TS Jensen. Sites of action of opiates in production of analgesia. In: HL Fields (Ed.): Progress in brain Res. 1988. (b)

Yaksh TL, CW Stevens. Properties of the modulation of spinal nociceptive transmission by receptor-selective agents. In: R Dudner, GF Gebhart, MR Bond (Eds.): Proceedings of the Vth World Congress on Pain. Elsevier, 1988, 417.

Yaksh TL, JG Collins. Studies in animals should precede human use of spinally administered drugs. Anesthesiology, 1989, 70, 4.

Yamada K, Y Ishihra, S Shimada. Epidural morphine for postoperative pain relief after tonsillectomy. Pain, 1987, S4, S390.

Yamaguchi H, S Watanabe, T Fukuda, H Takahashi, K Motokawa, Y Ishizawa. Minimal effective dose of intrathecal morphine for pain relief following transabdominal hysterectomy. Anesth Analg 1989, 68, 537.

Yamamoto M, S Tachikawa, H Maeno. Effects of porcine calcitonin on behavioral and electrophysiological responses elicited by electrical stimulation of the tooth pulp in rabbits. Pharmacology, 1982, 24, 337.

Yanagida H, T Nonoyama, Yamamura H. Electroencephalographic study of the direct injection of anesthetics into the pontine reticular formation. Jap J Anesth, 1971, 20, 290. (a)

Yanagida H, H Yamamura. The site of action of Innovar in the brain. Can Anaesth Soc J, 1971, 18, 552. (b)

Yasuda S, Y Takino, J Takahashi. Effect of epidural morphine on urinary catecholamine excretion during postoperative period. Keio J Med, 1985, 34, 25.

Yasuoka S, TL Yaksh. Effects on nociceptive threshold and blood pressure of intrathecally administered morphine and alpha-adrenergic agonists. Neuropharmacology, 1983, 22, 309.

Yate PM, D Thomas, SM Short, PS Sebel, J Morton. Comparison of infusions of alfentanil or pethidine for sedation of ventilated patients on the ITU. Brit J Anaesth, 1986, 58, 1091.

Yeager MP, DD Glass, RK Neff, T Brink-Johnsen. Epidural anaesthesia and analgesia in high risk surgical patients. Anesthesiology, 1987, 66, 729.

Youngstrom PC, RI Cowan, C Sutheimer, JDW Eastwood, JC Yu. Pain relief and plasma concentrations from epidural and intramuscular morphine in post-cesarean patients. Anesthesiology, 1982, 57, 404.

Youngstrom PC, D Eastwood, H Patel, R Bhatia, R Cowan, C Sutheimer. Epidural fentanyl and bupivacaine in labor: double-blind study. Anesthesiology, 1984, 61, A414.

Youngstrom P, M Sedensky, D Frankmann, S Spagnuolo. Continuous epidural infusion of low-dose bupivacaine-fentanyl for labor analgesia. Anesthesiology, 1988, 69 (3A), A686.

Younker D, R Clark, J Tessem, TH Joyce, M Kubicek. Bupivacaine-fentanyl epidural analgesia for a parturient in status asthmaticus. Can J Anaesth, 1987, 34, 609.

Youssef MS, PA Wilkinson. Epidural fentanyl and monoamine oxidase inhibitors. Anaesthesia, 1988, 43, 210.

Youssef MS. Extradural fentanyl and dystrophia myotonica. Anaesthesia, 1989, 44, 360.

Yu CM, PC Youngstrom, RI Cowan, SET Spagnuolo, C Sutheimer, DW Eastwood. Post cesarean epidural morphine: double blind study. Anesthesiology, 1980, 53, S216.

Yu PYH, DR Gamling, GH McMorland. A comparative study of patient controlled epidural fentanyl and single dose epidural morphine for post-caesarean section analgesia. Can J Anaesth, 1989, 36, S55.

Yuge O, M Matsumoto, LM Kitahata, JG Collins, M Senami. Direct opioid application to peripheral nerves does not alter compound action potentials. Anesth Analg, 1985, 64, 667.

Zakowski M, S Ramanathan, H Turndorf. Experience with two epidural morphine doses in post-cesarean section analgesia. Anesthesiology (Suppl), 1989, 71, 833.

Zakowski M, S Ramanathan, H Turndorf. Intrathecal morphine for post-cesarean section analgesia. Anesthesiology (Suppl), 1989, 71, 870.

Zenz M, S Piepenbrock, B Otten, G Otten. Epidurale Morphin-Injektion zur postoperativen Schmerzbekämpfung. Fortschr Med, 1980, 98, 306.

Zenz M, S Piepenbrock, M Hüsch, B Otten, G Otten. Peridurale Morphin-Analgesie (epidural morphine analgesia) Anaesthesist, 1981, 30, 28. (a)

Zenz M, S Piepenbrock, M Hüsch, B Otten, G Otten, R Neuhaus. Peridurale Morphin-Analgesie, I. Postoperative Phase. Anaesthesist, 1981, 30, 77. (b)

Zenz M. Peridurale Morphin-Analgesie zur Schmerztherapie bei Karzinompatienten. In: M Zenz (Ed.): Peridurale Opiat-Analgesie, Gustav Fischer Verlag, Stuttgart, 1981, 83. (c)

Zenz M, S Piepenbrock, B Hübner, M Glocke. Peridurale Analgesie mit Buprenorphin und Morphin bei postoperativen Schmerzen. Anaesth Intensivther Notfallmed, 1981, 16, 333. (d)

Zenz M, S Piepenbrock, B Schappler-Scheele, M Hüsch. Epidural morphine analgesia (PMA). III. Cancer pain. Anaesthesist, 1981, 30, 508. (e)

Zenz M, B Schappler-Scheele, R Neuhans, S Piepenbrock, J Hilfrich. Long term peridural morphine

616

analgesia in cancer pain. Lancet, 1981, 1, 91. (f)

Zenz M, B van den Berg, E van den Berg. Plethysmographic study on sympathetic block in peridural anaesthesia and peridural morphine analgesia. Regional Anaesthesie, 1981 4, 70. (g)

Zenz M. Peridurale Opiat-Analgesie. Deut Med Wochenschr, 1981, 106, 483. (h)

Zenz M. Peridurale versus intrathekale Opiat-Analgesie. Zentraleuropäischer Anaesthesiekongress, 1981, Berlin. (i)

Zenz M, S Piepenbrock, M Hüsch, B Schappler-Scheele, R Neuhaus. Erfahrungen mit längerliegenden Periduralkathetern. Peridurale Morphin-Analgesie bei Karzinompatienten. Regional Anaesthesie, 1981, 5, 26. (j)

Zenz M, J Hilfrich, S Burkert, S Dammenheim. Schmerztherapie durch peridurale Morphin-Applikation bei Patienten mit terminaler gynaekologischer Karzinomerkrankung. Arch Gynecol, 1981, 232, 310. (k)

Zenz M, S Piepenbrock, G Otten, M Hüsch. Postoperative pain therapy by epidural morphine. In: TL Yaksh, H Müller (Eds.): Anaesthesiologie und Intensivmedizin, Spinal Opiate Analgesia, Experimental and clinical studies. Springer Verlag, Berlin, Heidelberg, New York, 1982, 144, 109. (a)

Zenz M, S Piepenbrock, J Hilfrich, M Hüsch. Pain Therapy by epidural morphine in patients with terminal cancer. In: TL Yaksh, H Müller (Eds.): Anaesthesie und Intensivmedizin, Spinal Opiate Analgesia, Experimental and clinical studies, Springer Verlag, Berlin, Heidelberg, New York, 1982, 144, 141. (b)

Zenz M, S Piepenbrock. Extradural buprenorphine. Brit J Anaesth, 1982, 54, 1146. (c)

Zenz M, S Piepenbrock, B Huebner, M Glocke. Buprenorphin und Morphin zur periduralen Analgesie bei postoperativen Schmerzen. In: JB Brueckner (Ed.): Anaesthesiologie und Intensivmedizin, Schmerzbehandlung Epidurale Opiatanalgesie, Springer Verlag, Berlin, Heidelberg, New York, 1982, 153, 78. (d)

Zenz M, S Piepenbrock, H Brämswig, M Hüsch, G Otten. Postoperative Komplikationen bei zwei Analgesiemethoden: 2-Jahres-Studie. In: JB Brueckner (Ed.): Anaesthesiologie und Intensivmedizin, Schmerzbehandlung Epidurale Opiatanalgesie, Springer Verlag, Berlin, Heidelberg, New York, 1982, 153, 116. (e)

Zenz M. Peridurale versus intrathekale Opiat-Analgesie. In: JB Brückner (Ed.): Anaesthesiologie und Intensivmedizin, Schmerzbehandlung Epidurale Opiatanalgesie, Springer Verlag, 1982, 153, 4. (f)

Zenz M, S Piepenbrock. Erwiderung zu den vorstehenden Bemerkungen von KU Josten. Regional Anaesthesie, 1982, 5, 48. (g)

Zenz M, S Piepenbrock, M Tryba, H Brämswig. Peridurale Opiat- Analgesie. Klinische Ergebnisse einer 2-Jahres-Studie. Anaesthesist, 1983, 32, 289. (a)

Zenz M, S Piepenbrock. Utilisation de morphiniques par voie péridurale pour le traitement des douleurs cancéreuses. Résultats d'un traitement prolongé chez 104 patients. In: Ars Medici, Bruxelles, Congress Series 3, II, 1983, 3, 441. (b)

Zenz M. Der Periduralkatheter in der Langzeittherapie. In: J Meyer, H Nolte (Eds.): Die kontinuierliche Periduralanaesthesie, G Thieme Verlag, Stuttgart, New York, 1983, 79. (c)

Zenz M. Medikamentöse Schmerztherapie. In: M Zimmerman, HO Handwerker (Eds.): Schmerz, Springer Verlag, 1984, 189. (a)

Zenz M. Epidural opiates in cancer pain. In: M Zimmermann, P Drings, HU Gerbershagen, G Wagner (Eds.): Recent Results in Cancer Research. Springer Verlag, Heidelberg, 1984, 89, 107. (b)

Zenz M. Therapiemöglichkeiten bei Krebsschmerzen. Münch Med Wochenschr, 1984, 126, 929. (c)

Zenz M. Spinale Opioid-Therapie: Derzeitiger Stand. In: K Steinbereithner, H Bergmann (Eds.): Beiträge zur Anaesthesiologie und Intensivmedizin, Verlag Maudrich, Wien, 1984, 122. (d)

Zenz M. Spinale Opiat-Analgesie. Arzneim Forsch/Drug Res, 1984, 34, 1089. (e)

Zenz M, S Piepenbrock, M Glocke. A double blind comparison of epidural buprenorphine and epidural morphine in post-operative pain. In: P Bevan, M Firth (Eds.): Buprenorphine and anaesthesiology, Royal Society of Medicine, Oxford University Press, 1984, 65, 115. (f)

Zenz M, S Piepenbrock, M Tryba. Epidural opiates: long-term experiences in cancer pain. Klin Wochenschr, 1985, 63, 225. (a)

Zenz M. Ambulante Schmerztherapie mit Opiaten. Diagnostik, 1985, 18, 24. (b)

Zenz M, C Panhans, HC Niesel, H Kreuscher (Eds.). Regional-Anaesthesie: Operativer Bereich - Geburtshilfe.- Schmerztherapie. (2. Auflage), Gustav Fischer Verlag, Stuttgart, 1985. (c)

Zenz M. Rückenmarksnahe Opiattherapie beim Tumorpatienten. In: J Schara (Ed.): Anesthesiologie und Intensivmedizin, Deutscher Anaesthesiekongress 1982, Springer Verlag, Berlin, Heidelberg, New York, 1986, 174, 85. (a)

Zenz M. Rückenmarksnahe Opioidtherapie. In: Schmerztherapie - eine interdisziplinäre Aufgabe. Reihe Klinische Anaesthesiologie und Intensivtherapie. Springer Verlag, 1986, 111. (b)

Zenz M. Postoperative Analgesie: Plädoyer für epidurale Opiate. In: G Hossli, P Frey, G Kreienbühl (Eds.): Anaesthesiologie und Intesivemedizin, ZAK, Zürich II, Springer Verlag, 1986, 188, 332. (c)

Zenz M. Epidural opioid in cancer pain. Personal communication, 1988.

Zieglgänsberger W, M Gessler, M Rust, A Struppler. Neurophysiologische Grundlagen der spinalen Opiatanalgesie. Anaesthesist, 1981, 30, 343.

Zieglgänsberger W, B Butor. Opioidergic interneurons in the dorsal horn of the spinal cord as basis for the epidural opioid analgesia. Schmerz-Pain-Douleur, 1985, 6, 110.

Zimman Mansfeld HM, A Gonzalez Navarro, MJ Gonzalez Hernandez, T Molinero Aparicio. Epidural morphine for pain (letter). Neurosurgery, 1984,14, 383.

Zimmermann M. Physiologie von Nozizeption und Schmerz. In: M Zimmermann, HO Handwerker (Eds.): Schmerz, Spinger-Verlag, 1984, 1.

Zinck B, KW Fritz. Atemdepression nach epiduraler Opiate-Analgesie mit Buprenorphin-Hydrochloride? Anaesth Intensivther Notfallmed, 1982, 17, 345. (a)

Zinck B, KW Fritz, E Luellwitz. Epidurale Opiat-Analgesie mit Buprenorphine-Hydrochlorid. Erfahrungen mit thorakaler Applikationsweise nach Oberbaucheingriffen. Referat: Deutscher Anaesthesiekongress Anaesthesist, 1982, 31. (b)

Zinck B, KW Fritz. Allgemeinanaesthesie versus Regionalanaesthesie. Konkurrierende Verfahren oder sinnvolle Ergänzungen? Referat: 3. Internationales Symposium über Anaesthesia - Reanimations - und Intensiv-Behandlungsprobleme, in Zürs/Arlberg, 06.02-13.02.1982. (c)

Zinck B. Epidurale Opiat-Analgesie mit Buprenorphin - Untersuchungen mit thorakaler Applikation nach Oberbauchlaparotomien. Internat. Sertürner Symposium: Schmerz. Schmerzforschung und Therapie, Göttingen, 15.-18.06.1983.

Zinck B. Blutgasanalytische Untersuchungen nach thorakaler Epiduraler Opiat-Analgesie. VII Eur Congress of Anaesth, 1986, Vienna (Austria) Report, Abst 424.

Zindler M, E Hartung. Alfentanil ein neues ultrakurzwirkendes Opioid. Publ. Urban u Schwarzenberg, München 1985.

Zornow MH, JE Fleischer, MS Scheller, K Nakakimura, JC Drummond. Cerebral effects of the alpha-2 agonist, dexmedetomidine. Anesthesiology (Suppl), 1989, 71, 612.

Zucker-Pinchoff B, S Ramanathan. Anaphylactic reaction to epidural fentanyl. Anesthesiology, 1989, 71, 599.

Zukin RS, SR Zukin. Multiple opiate receptors and emerging concepts. Life Sci, 1981, 29, 2681.

Addendum to the Bibliography and references

Abboud TK, A Afrasiabi, J Davidson, J Zhu, A Reyes, N Khoo, Z Steffens. Prophylactic oral naltrexone with epidural morphine: effect on adverse reactions and ventilatory responses to carbon dioxide. Anesthesiology, 1990, 72, 233.

Abouleish E, N Rawal, J Shaw, MN Rashad, T Lorenz. Subarachnoid morphine prolongs labor compared to epidural bupivacaine. Anesth Analg (Suppl.), 1990, 70, S4.

Ang ET, S Khon, G Goldfarb, B Debaene, C Galet, P Jolis. Duree de l'analgesie apres bloc du nerf crural: effet de l'addition de clonidine à la xylocaine. Ann Fr Anesth Réanim, 1989, 8, R213.

Bastide R, Y Lazorthes, B Caute-Sallerin, JCl Verdie. Intrathecal spinal versus intra-cerebroventricular opioids for cancer pain control. Pain (Suppl.), 1990, 5, S114.

Berde CB, NF Sethna, JM De Jesus, TA Yemen, J Mandell. Continuous epidural bupivacaine-fentanyl infusions in children undergoing urologic surgery. Anesth Analg (Suppl.), 1990, 70, S22.

Bisgaard C, P Mouridsen, JB Dahl. Continuous epidural bupivacaine plus morphine versus epidural morphine after colonic surgery. Acta Anaesth Scand (Suppl.), 1989, 71, 77.

Bisgaard C, P Mouridsen, JB Dahl.Continuous lumbar epidural bupivacaine plus morphine versus epidural morphine after major abdominal surgery. Eur J Anaesth, 1990, 7, 219.

Boersma FP, H Noorduin, V vanden Bussche. Epidural sufentanil for cancer pain control in outpatients. Regional Anesthesia, 1989, 14, 293.

Boico O, F Bonnet, JX Mazoit, PL Darmon, P Catoire, B Rey. Effets de l'adjonction d'adrenaline et de clonidine sur la cinetique de la bupivacaine par voie spinale. Ann Fr Anesth Réanim, 1989, 8, R210.

Bonnet F, A Diallo, P Catoire, M Belon, M Saada, M Guilbaud. Incidence des douleurs au garrot sous rachianesthesie associant bupivacaine et clonidine. Ann Fr Anesth Réanim, 1989, 8, R208.

Bonnet F, VB Buisson, Y Francois, P Catoire, M Saada, K Abhay. La prolongation de l'anesthesie spinale par la clonidine depend du mode d'administration. Ann Fr Anesth Réanim, 1989, 8, R209.

Bonnet F, O Boico, S Rostaing, JF Loriferne, M Saada. Clonidine- induced analgesia in postoperative patients: epidural versus intramuscular administration. Anesthesiology, 1990, 72, 423.

Brockway MS, DW Noble, GH Sharwood-Smith, JH McClure. Profound respiratory depression after extradural fentanyl. Brit J Anaesth, 1990, 64, 243.

Buisson VB, F Bonnet, P Catoire, M Saada, S Rostaing, O Boico. Anesthesie spinale associant tetracaine hyperbare et clonidine: effet-dose. Ann Fr Anesth Réanim, 1989, 8, R207.

Capogna G, D Celleno, M Tomassetti. Maternal analgesia and neonatal effects of epidural sufentanil for cesarean section. Regional Anesthesia, 1989, 14, 282.

Celleno D, G Capogna, M Emanuelli, M Sebastiani, P Costantino, G Cipriani, M Tomasetti. Ventilatory effects of subarachnoid fentanyl in the elderly. Anesth Analg (Suppl.), 1990, 70, S53.

Cheng DCH, F Chung, KR Chapman, J Romanelli. Low-dose sufentanil and lidocaine supplementation of general anaesthesia. Can J Anaesth, 1990, 37, 521.

Cherry DA, JL Plummer, MM Wood, GK Gourlay, MM Onley, MJ Cousins. Comparison of intermittent bolus with continuous infusion of epidural morphine in the treatment of cancer pain. Pain (Suppl.), 1990, 5, S115.

Chestnut DH, LJ Laszewski, KL Pollack, JN Bates, NK Manago, WW Choi. Continuous epidural infusion of 0.0625% bupivacaine -0.002% fentanyl during the second stage of labor. Anesthesiology, 1990, 72, 613.

Chrubasik J. Spinal somatostatin studies in animals. Anesth Analg, 1990, 70, 222.

Chrubasik J, F Magora. Relative epidural analgesic potencies of opiates in treatment of postoperative pain. Anesth Analg (Suppl.), 1990, 70, S60.

Connelly M, J Shagrin, C Warfield. Epidural opioids for the management of pain in a patient with the Guillain-Barré syndrome. Anesthesiology, 1990, 72, 381.

Coombs DW. Effect of spinal adrenergic analgesia on opioid resistant pain. Acta Anaesth Scand (Suppl.), 1989, 91, 37.

Crul BJP, EM Delhaas. Long-term spinal morphine infusion. Experience from 140 cases yields preference for the intrathecal route. Acta Anaesthesiol Scand (Suppl.), 1989, 91, 105.

Dahl JB, JB Jacobsen. Accidental epidural narcotic overdose. Anesth Analg, 1990, 70, 321.

De Sousa H, E Klein. Intrathecal and epidural oxymorphone. Anesthesiology (Suppl.), 1989, 71, A699.

Eisenach JC, RL Rauck, C Buzzanell, SZ Lysak. Epidural clonidine analgesia for intractable cancer pain: phase I. Anesthesiology, 1989, 71, 647.

Eisenach JC, SZ Lysak, CM Viscomi. Epidural clonidine analgesia following surgery: phase I. Anesthesiology, 1989, 71, 640.

Eisenach JC, DM Dewan. Intrathecal clonidine in obstetrics: sheep studies. Anesthesiology, 1990, 72, 663.

Elliott RD, M Stockwell. Continuous infusion epidural anaesthesia for obstetrics: bupivacaine vs bupivacaine-fentanyl. Can J Anaesth (Suppl.), 1990, 37, S6.

Ellis DJ, WL Millar, LS Reiner. A randomized double-blind comparison of epidural versus intravenous fentanyl infusion for analgesia after cesarean section. Anesthesiology, 1990, 72, 981.

Fenollosa P, J Pallarces, MJ Pallares, T Santonja, R Montero, A Camba. Spinal morphine in malignant facial pain. Pain (Suppl.), 1990, 5, S121.

Ferrer-Brechner T, Z Hoh, G Abraham. Intrathecal narcotic analgesia (ITA) vs patient controlled analgesia (PCA) for postoperative pain control after major abdominal surgery. Pain (Suppl.), 1990, 5, S142.

Girota S, S Kumar, KM Rajendran. Postoperative analgesia in children who have genito-urinary surgery. A comparison between caudal buprenorphine and bupivacaine. Anaesthesia, 1990, 45, 406.

Glaze GM, RB Salsitz, LT Baker, WF Spillane. Continuous epidural analgesia with an elastomeric infusion device: simple, safe, effective. Pain (Suppl.), 1990, 5, S143.

Goodchild CS. The mechanisms by which benzodiazepines produce spinally mediated analgesia. Eur J Anaesth, 1990, 7, 254.

Gordh T. Cholinergic mechanisms for analgesia. Acta Anaesth Scand (Suppl.), 1989, 91, 75.

Gourlay GK. Spinal versus systemic application of opioids. Eur J Pain, 1990, 1, 38.

Grant GJ, M Zakowski, S Ramanathan, H Turndorf. Lumbar versus thoracic administration of epidural morphine for post-thoracotomy analgesia. Anesth Analg (Suppl.), 1990, 70, S134.

Grant RP, JF Dolman, JA Harper, SA White, DG Parsons, KG Evans, P Merrick. Patient controlled lumbar epidural fentanyl for post-thoracotomy pain. Can J Anaesth (Suppl.), 1990, 37, S45.

Grice SC, JC Eisenach, DM Dewan. Labor analgesia with epidural bupivacaine plus fentanyl: enhancement with epinephrine and inhibition. Anesthesiology, 1990, 72, 623.

Gwirtz KH. Intrathecal combination of bupivacaine-fentanyl-morphine. Anesth Analg, 1990, 71, 106.

Herman NL, FL Hussain, KG Knape, JW Downing. Extradural opioids in labour. Brit J Anaesth, 1990, 64, 528.

Ilsley AH, H Owen, J Currie, RRL Fronsko. A laboratory evaluation of a new generation programmable infusion device. Pain (Suppl.), 1990, 5, S183.

Immelman L, S Roth, MA Sabourin, L Strunin. Analgesia and serum concentrations of extradural, subdural and intraperitoneal fentanyl in a rat model. Can J Anaesth, 1990, 37, 63.

Jacobson L, C Chabal. Antinociceptive opioid activity ratio. Reply. Anesthesiology, 1990, 72, 1097.

Jain S, A Kestenhaus, Y Khan, N Shah. Does epidural morphine predispose to herpes simplex in cancer patients? A comparison with epidural lidocaine. Anesth Analg (Suppl.), 1989, 70, S174.

James CF, TCE Banner. High-volume fentanyl compared with other narcotics after cesarean section: analgesia and respiratory status. Anesth Analg (Suppl.), 1990, 70, S178.

Johnson C, N Oriol. Comparison of onset time between bupivacaine 0.5% and 2-chloroprocaine 3% with and without fentanyl 75 mcg. Anesth Analg (Suppl.), 1990, 70, S179.

Jorrot JC, JD Lirzin, Ph Dailland, P Jacquinot, Ch Conseiller. Interet de l'association du sufentanil à la bupivacaine 0.25% par voie peridurale pour l'analgesie obstetricale? Ann Fr Anesth Réanim, 1989, 8, R64.

King MJ, MI Bowden, GM Cooper. Epidural fentanyl and 0.5% bupivacaine for elective caesarean section. Anaesthesia, 1990, 45, 285.

Kirson L, JM Goldman, RB Slover. Postoperative care following intrathecal or epidural opioids. II. Reply Anesthesiology, 1990, 72, 213.

Kreitzer JM, LP Kirschenbaum, JB Eisenkraft. Epidural fentanyl by continuous infusion for relief of postoperative pain. Clin J Pain, 1989, 5, 283.

Lamb SA, Y Hosobuchi. Intrathecal morphine sulfate for chronic benign pain, delivered by implanted pump delivery systems. Pain (Suppl.), 1990, 5, S120.

Langeman L, E Golomb, S Benita, M Tverskoy. Intrathecal opiates: a new way for prolongation of pharmacological effect. Anesthesiology, 1989, 71, A697.

Lazorthes Y. Morphinothérapie intrathécale chez l'homme. Rec Méd Vét, 1985, 162, 1409.

Lazorthes Y, JC Verdie, B Caute, R Maranhao, M Tafani. Intracerebroventricular morphinotherapy for control of chronic cancer pain. In: HI Fields, JM Besson (Eds.): Progress in brain research. Elsevier Science Publishers B.V., 1988, 395.

Leicht CH, AJ Kelleher, DE Robinson, SE Dickerson. Prolongation of postoperative epidural sufentanil analgesia with epinephrine. Anesth Analg, 1990, 70, 323.

Leigh J, SJ Fearnley, KG Lupprian. Intrathecal diamorphine during laparatomy in a patient with advanced multiple sclerosis. Anaesthesia, 1190, 43, 640.

Loper KA, LB Ready, MN Nessly, BS Lorie Wild. Epidural morphine provides safe and effective analgesia on hospital wards. Anesth Analg (Suppl.), 1990, 70, S248.

Lubenow TR, RJ McCarthy, S Grande, AD Ivankovich. Comparison of continuous epidural narcotic bupivacaine mixtures to patient-controlled analgesia after major orthopedic surgery. Anesth Analg (Suppl.), 1989, 70, S250.

Lund C, S Qvitzau, A Greulich, NC Hjortsø, H Kehlet. The effect of epidural clonidine and morphine on postoperative pain, stress response, blood pressure and pulmonary function. Act Anaesth Scand (Suppl.), 1989, 91, 103.

Lysak SZ, JC Eisenach, CE Dobson. Patient-controlled epidural analgesia during labor: a comparison of three solutions with a continuous infusion control. Anesthesiology, 1990, 72, 44.

Magora F. Antinociceptive opioid activity ratio. Anesthesiology, 1990, 72, 1097.

Mahesh KT, JE Heavner. Post cesarean section analgesia requests are independent of when epidural fentanyl is given. Anesth Analg (Suppl.), 1990, 70, S255.

Martin CS, EM McGrady, A Colquhoun, J Thorburn. Extradural methadone and bupivacaine in labour. Brit J Anaesth, 1990, 65, 330.

McClure JH. Comparison of bupivacaine and bupivacaine with fentanyl in continuous extradural analgesia during labour. Brit J Anaesth, 1989, 63, 637.

McDonald JS, AK Rattan, GA Tejwani. Effect of intrathecal bupivacaine on morphine analgesia. Anesthesiology (Suppl.), 1989, 71, A680.

McMorland GH, MJ Douglas, JHK Kim, AA Kamani, JE Swenerton, J Berkowitz, PLE Ross, L Palmer. Epidural sufentanil for post-caesarean section analgesia: lack of benefit of epinephrine. Can J Anaesth, 1990, 37, 432.

Meert TF, H Noorduin, H van Craenendonck, P Vermote, FP Boersma, PAJ Janssen. Effects of adrenaline, an alpha2-adrenoceptor agonist, the volume of injection, and the global pain state of the animal on the activity of epidural sufentanil. Acta Anaesth Belg, 1989, 40, 247.

Moine P, C Ecoffey. Analgesie et effets respiratoires de l'anesthesie caudale avec une association bupivacaine-fentanyl chez l'enfant. Ann Fr Anesth Réanim, 1989, 8, R71.

Mok MS, JJ Wang, M Lippmann. Epidural nalbuphine attenuates the adverse effect of epidural morphine. Pain (Suppl.), 1990, 5, S137.

Moore AK, S Vilderman, W Lubenskyi, J McCans, GS Fox. Differences in epidural morphine requirements between elderly and young patients after abdominal surgery. Anesth Analg, 1990, 70, 316.

Morisot P, JF Dessangers, J Regnard, A Lockhart. Effet depresseur respiratoire du fentanyl a faible dose (50 μg) par voie peridurale. Ann Fr Anesth Réanim, 1989, 8, R175.

Naji P, M Farschtschian, OH Wilder-Smith, CH Wilder-Smith. Epidural droperidol and morphine for postoperative pain. Anesth Analg, 1990, 70, 583.

Nielsen TH, HK Nielsen, SE Husted, SL Hansen, KH Olsen, N Fjeldborg. Stress response and platelet function in minor surgery during epidural bupivacaine and general anaesthesia: effect of epidural morphine addition. Eur J Anaesth, 1989, 6, 409.

Noorduin H, L Tritsmans, TF Meert. Clinical experience with epidural sufentanil. Pain (Suppl.), 1990, 5, S115.

Pallares MJ, J Pallares, P Fenollosa, T Santonja, F Pelegrin, R Montero, A Camba. Intrathecal morphine in spinal cord injuried patients. Pain (Suppl.), 1990, 5, S120.

Panos L, AN Sandler, DG Stringer, N Badner, S Lawson, G Koren. Continuous infusions of lumbar epidural fentanyl and intravenous fentanyl for post-thoracotomy pain relief. I: Analgesic and pharmacokinetic effects. Can J Anaesth (Suppl.), 1990, 37, S66.

Parker RK, M Baron, DL Helfer, N Berberich, PF White. Use of epidural PCA for post-operative pain management: effect of local anesthetic on the opioid requirement. Anesth Analg (Suppl.), 1990, 70, S297.

Parker RK, M Baron, DL Helfer, N Berberich, PF White. Epidural PCA: effect of a continuous (basal) infusion on the postoperative opioid requirement. Anesth Analg (Suppl.), 1990, 70, S296.

Patel D, Y Janardhan, B Marai. Comparison of intrathecal meperidine and lidocaine in endoscopic urological procedures. Can J Anaesth, 1990, 37, 567.

Perreault C, JF Albert, P Couture, R Meloche. Epidural alfentanil during labor, in association with a continuous infusion of bupivacaine. Can J Anaesth (Suppl.) 1990, 37, S5.

Perriss BW, BV Latham, IH Wilson. Analgesia following extradural and i.m. pethidine in post-caesarean section patients. Brit J Anaesth, 1990, 64, 355.

Power KJ, AF Avery. Extradural analgesia in the intrapartum management of a patient with pulmonary hypertension. Brit J Anaesth, 1989, 63, 116.

Racle JP Utilisation des alpha-stimulants par voies intrathécale et péridurale. Ann Fr Anesth Réanim, 1990, 9, 338.

Rattan AK, KP Gudehithlu, JS McDonald, GA Tejwani. Differential effect of intrathecal midazolam on morphine analgesia. Anesthesiology (Suppl.), 1989, 71, A681.

Rawal N, L Nuutinen, P Raj, L Lovering, E Abouleish. Histopathological effects of intrathecal sufentanil. Pain (Suppl.), 1990, 5, S130.

Reimer EJ, NH Badner, CA Moote, WE Komar. Bupivacaine added to epidural fentanyl does not improve postoperative analgesia. Can J Anaesth (Suppl.), 1990, 37, S54.

Rosen MA, SC Hughes, SM Shnider, GR Curry, GM Glaze, AV Thirion, JD Vertommen. Continuous infusion epidural sufentanil for postoperative analgesia. Anesth Analg (Suppl.), 1990, 70, S331.

Ross NL. Postoperative care following intrathecal or epidural opioids. Anesthesiology, 1990, 72, 212.

Sandler AN. Epidural opiate analgesia for acute pain relief. Can J Anaesth (Suppl.), 1990, 37, Sxxxiii. Spangsberg N, E Anker-Møller, S Dyring, P Carlsson. Pain relief with epidural catheters - experiences from routine use. Acta Anaesth Scand (Suppl.), 1989, 91, 104.

Steinstra R, F van Poorten. Immediate respiratory arrest after caudal epidural sufentanil. Anesthesiology, 1989, 71, 993.

Stringer DG, AN Sandler, L Panos, S Lawson, TR Einarson, N Badner. Continuous infusions of lumbar epidural fentanyl and intravenous fentanyl for post-thoracotomy pain relief. II: Respiratory effects. Can J Anaesth (Suppl.), 1990, 37, S16.

Tauzin-Fin P, P Maurette, G Vincon, A Brachet-Liermain, T Rian. Association pethidine prilocaine en rachianesthesie. Aspects cliniques et pharmacocinetiques. Ann Fr Anesth Réanim, 1989, 8, R148.

Tsai SK, MS Mok, LF Hung, M Lippmann. Sacral epidural morphine vs. bupivacaine for the relief of postoperative pain in children. Anesth Analg (Suppl.), 1990, 70, S411.

Tuman KJ, RJ McCarthy, BD Spiess, AD Ivankovich Epidural anesthesia and analgesia decreases postoperative hypercoagulability in high-risk vascular patients. Anesth Analg (Suppl.), 1990, 70, S414.

Vaidya D, B Merai, J Robalino, K Shevde. Intrathecal hypobaric fentanyl with lidocaine for hip surgery. Can J Anaesth (Suppl.), 1990, 37, S60.

Van Essen EJ, JG Bovill, EJ Ploeger, BC Schout. A comparison of epidural clonidine and morphine for post-operative analgesia. Eur J Anaesth, 1990, 7, 211.

Veillette Y, D Benhamou, T Labille. Effects cliniques de l'addition de clonidine avec ou sans adrenaline lors de l'administration de lidocaine en peridurale. Ann Fr Anesth Réanim, 1989, 8, R206.

Vercauteren M; G Meese, E Lauwers, K Hendrickx, H Adriaensen. Addition of clonidine potentiates postoperative analgesia of epidural sufentanil. Anesth Analg (Suppl.), 1990, 70, S416.

Volk B, E Rosenmann. Somatostatin neurotoxicity in animals. Anesth Analg, 1990, 70, 669.

Ward NG. Akathisia associated with droperidol during epidural anesthesia. Anesthesiology, 1989, 71, 786.

Wasnick J, W Hurford, C Gelb, B Chernow. Epidural opioid analgesia does not alter the neuro-endocrine response to thoracotomy. Anesth Analg (Suppl.), 1990, 70, S422.

Wheatley RG, ID Somerville, DJ Sapsford, JG Jones. Postoperative hypoxaemia: comparison of extradural, i.m. and patient-controlled opioid analgesia. Brit J Anaesth, 1990, 64, 267.

Wilder-Smith CH, P Naji, M Farschtschian, O Wilder-Smith. Reduction of side-effects of epidural morphine with epidural droperidol. Pain (Suppl.), 1990, 5, S151.

Yaksh TL. The role of multiple spinal receptor systems in the modulation of different types of pain. Acta Anaesth Scand (Suppl.), 1989, 91, 36.

Yaksh TL. Extradural somatostatin. Brit J Anaesth, 1990, 65, 152. Yamaguchi H, S Watanabe, K Motokawa, Y Ishizawa. Intrathecal morphine dose-response data for pain relief after cholecystectomy. Anesth Analg, 1990, 70, 168.

Zakowski M, S Ramanathan, P Khoo, H Turndorf. Plasma histamine with intraspinal morphine in cesarean section. Anesth Analg (Suppl), 1990, 70, S448.

Index of subjects

In Memoriam Joris de Castro

9.11.1918	Born in Hamme, Belgium
1938–1945	Medical studies in Ghent, Belgium
1945	Medical doctor
1945	Doctor in tropical medicine
1946–1954	General practitioner in Belgium
1946–1983	Founder and editor of *Ars medici*
1954–1956	Postgraduate in Anaesthesiology
1956	Established as specialist in Anaesthesiology, Hôpital St. Pierre, Université Libre de Bruxelles
1956–1970	Université Libre de Bruxelles
1972	Medical thesis, Agrégé de l'enseignement superieur in Anaesthesiology, Université Libre de Bruxelles
1970–1983	Chairman of the Department of Anaesthesiology and Intensive Care, University Hospital Tivoli, La Louvière, Université Libre de Bruxelles
8.10.1990	Died in Moscow, USSR

A great man from the field of international anaesthesiology is dead. Shortly before this book was printed, on October 8, 1990, Prof. Joris de Castro died while attending a congress on anaesthesiology in Moscow. I feel extremely sad that he never had the chance to see this book in print after having worked so hard on it for the last 5 years.

He had the idea of collecting all the results on spinal opioids when this method was at the height of its appeal. As time passed, more and more information had to be included, and the book's content was changed 13 times. Each version was typed by Joris de Castro and his wonderful wife, Dr. Suzanne Andrieu, who is also an anaesthesiologist and was co-author of many of her husband's papers. They worked together for more than 20 years and travelled throughout the world to give lectures and attend conferences. Only once in all those years did I meet Joris without the company of his wife Suzanne.

International anaesthesiology has lost in Joris de Castro one of the most important researchers and clinicians. He was a true "workaholic" in his lifetime, even after his retirement 7 years ago. Joris de Castro introduced neuroleptanalgesia to clinical practice in 1959 together with Mundeleer. The first report on this was given at the 10th French Congress of Anaesthesiology in Lyon in

1959, and the first paper on this new method was published in the same year: 'Anesthésie sans barbituriques: la neuroleptanalgésie (R. 1406, R. 1625, Hydergine, Procaine)' by J. de Castro and P. Mundeleer, in *Anesthésie Analgésie Réanimation*, XVI, No. 5, pp. 1022–1056, Nov-Dec 1959.

De Castro made an enormous contribution to the development of modern anaesthesia as a result of this report. Many fields of operative medicine are nowadays closely bound to the possibilities of intravenous anaesthesia; neuroanaesthesia, cardioanaesthesia, and anaesthesia in uncommon diseases is usually performed under neuroleptanalgesia or its modifications. So, too in these newer modifications it was de Castro who took the first steps and introduced them into clinical practice. He was the first to present anaesthesiological experiences with haloperidol (1959), dextromoramide (1959), phenoperidine (1959), droperidol (1962), fentanyl (1962), flunitrazepam (1972), sufentanil (1975), alfentanil (1976), and ketanserine (1982). Due to this pioneering work he had a huge influence on the development and progress of anaesthesia. As recognition for his valuable work he received honorary professorships and honorary memberships of universities and societies from all over the world. However, he always remained modest and obliging and never stopped working towards further advancement, always allowing colleagues to share in his experiences.

Joris de Castro wrote more than 200 papers and over 20 monographs. He gave more than 1000 lectures, never refusing offers if feasible. We all thank him for his enormous efforts in modern anaesthesia, for his kindness and for his imagination which influenced our daily work in anaesthesia without any comparison over the last 30 years. Some of us have the honour of thanking him for his friendship and for the many happy hours we were able to spend together with him and his wife Suzanne. At these times we realised that anaesthesia was by no means the only interest in his life, but that modern art, theatre, literature, good food and French wine were also matters on which Joris de Castro was an authority. He will continue to live on in our hearts and in our minds as an important anaesthesia researcher, a wonderful friend and a very modest and wise man who was an inspiration to many, not just in the field of anaesthesiology.

Bochum, November 1990   Michael W. Zenz

DEVELOPMENTS IN
CRITICAL CARE MEDICINE AND ANESTHESIOLOGY

KLUWER ACADEMIC PUBLISHERS – DORDRECHT / BOSTON / LONDON

CPSIA information can be obtained
at www.ICGtesting.com
Printed in the USA
LVHW081404200619
621858LV00009B/272/P

9 789401 075435